JON AYRES

January 2002

PARTICLE–LUNG INTERACTIONS

LUNG BIOLOGY IN HEALTH AND DISEASE

Executive Editor

Claude Lenfant
Director, National Heart, Lung and Blood Institute
National Institutes of Health
Bethesda, Maryland

1. Immunologic and Infectious Reactions in the Lung, *edited by C. H. Kirkpatrick and H. Y. Reynolds*
2. The Biochemical Basis of Pulmonary Function, *edited by R. G. Crystal*
3. Bioengineering Aspects of the Lung, *edited by J. B. West*
4. Metabolic Functions of the Lung, *edited by Y. S. Bakhle and J. R. Vane*
5. Respiratory Defense Mechanisms (in two parts), *edited by J. D. Brain, D. F. Proctor, and L. M. Reid*
6. Development of the Lung, *edited by W. A. Hodson*
7. Lung Water and Solute Exchange, *edited by N. C. Staub*
8. Extrapulmonary Manifestations of Respiratory Disease, *edited by E. D. Robin*
9. Chronic Obstructive Pulmonary Disease, *edited by T. L. Petty*
10. Pathogenesis and Therapy of Lung Cancer, *edited by C. C. Harris*
11. Genetic Determinants of Pulmonary Disease, *edited by S. D. Litwin*
12. The Lung in the Transition Between Health and Disease, *edited by P. T. Macklem and S. Permutt*
13. Evolution of Respiratory Processes: A Comparative Approach, *edited by S. C. Wood and C. Lenfant*
14. Pulmonary Vascular Diseases, *edited by K. M. Moser*
15. Physiology and Pharmacology of the Airways, *edited by J. A. Nadel*
16. Diagnostic Techniques in Pulmonary Disease (in two parts), *edited by M. A. Sackner*
17. Regulation of Breathing (in two parts), *edited by T. F. Hornbein*
18. Occupational Lung Diseases: Research Approaches and Methods, *edited by H. Weill and M. Turner-Warwick*
19. Immunopharmacology of the Lung, *edited by H. H. Newball*
20. Sarcoidosis and Other Granulomatous Diseases of the Lung, *edited by B. L. Fanburg*
21. Sleep and Breathing, *edited by N. A. Saunders and C. E. Sullivan*
22. *Pneumocystis carinii* Pneumonia: Pathogenesis, Diagnosis, and Treatment, *edited by L. S. Young*
23. Pulmonary Nuclear Medicine: Techniques in Diagnosis of Lung Disease, *edited by H. L. Atkins*
24. Acute Respiratory Failure, *edited by W. M. Zapol and K. J. Falke*
25. Gas Mixing and Distribution in the Lung, *edited by L. A. Engel and M. Paiva*

26. High-Frequency Ventilation in Intensive Care and During Surgery, *edited by G. Carlon and W. S. Howland*
27. Pulmonary Development: Transition from Intrauterine to Extrauterine Life, *edited by G. H. Nelson*
28. Chronic Obstructive Pulmonary Disease: Second Edition, *edited by T. L. Petty*
29. The Thorax (in two parts), *edited by C. Roussos and P. T. Macklem*
30. The Pleura in Health and Disease, *edited by J. Chrétien, J. Bignon, and A. Hirsch*
31. Drug Therapy for Asthma: Research and Clinical Practice, *edited by J. W. Jenne and S. Murphy*
32. Pulmonary Endothelium in Health and Disease, *edited by U. S. Ryan*
33. The Airways: Neural Control in Health and Disease, *edited by M. A. Kaliner and P. J. Barnes*
34. Pathophysiology and Treatment of Inhalation Injuries, *edited by J. Loke*
35. Respiratory Function of the Upper Airway, *edited by O. P. Mathew and G. Sant'Ambrogio*
36. Chronic Obstructive Pulmonary Disease: A Behavioral Perspective, *edited by A. J. McSweeny and I. Grant*
37. Biology of Lung Cancer: Diagnosis and Treatment, *edited by S. T. Rosen, J. L. Mulshine, F. Cuttitta, and P. G. Abrams*
38. Pulmonary Vascular Physiology and Pathophysiology, *edited by E. K. Weir and J. T. Reeves*
39. Comparative Pulmonary Physiology: Current Concepts, *edited by S. C. Wood*
40. Respiratory Physiology: An Analytical Approach, *edited by H. K. Chang and M. Paiva*
41. Lung Cell Biology, *edited by D. Massaro*
42. Heart–Lung Interactions in Health and Disease, *edited by S. M. Scharf and S. S. Cassidy*
43. Clinical Epidemiology of Chronic Obstructive Pulmonary Disease, *edited by M. J. Hensley and N. A. Saunders*
44. Surgical Pathology of Lung Neoplasms, *edited by A. M. Marchevsky*
45. The Lung in Rheumatic Diseases, *edited by G. W. Cannon and G. A. Zimmerman*
46. Diagnostic Imaging of the Lung, *edited by C. E. Putman*
47. Models of Lung Disease: Microscopy and Structural Methods, *edited by J. Gil*
48. Electron Microscopy of the Lung, *edited by D. E. Schraufnagel*
49. Asthma: Its Pathology and Treatment, *edited by M. A. Kaliner, P. J. Barnes, and C. G. A. Persson*
50. Acute Respiratory Failure: Second Edition, *edited by W. M. Zapol and F. Lemaire*
51. Lung Disease in the Tropics, *edited by O. P. Sharma*
52. Exercise: Pulmonary Physiology and Pathophysiology, *edited by B. J. Whipp and K. Wasserman*
53. Developmental Neurobiology of Breathing, *edited by G. G. Haddad and J. P. Farber*
54. Mediators of Pulmonary Inflammation, *edited by M. A. Bray and W. H. Anderson*
55. The Airway Epithelium, *edited by S. G. Farmer and D. Hay*

56. Physiological Adaptations in Vertebrates: Respiration, Circulation, and Metabolism, *edited by S. C. Wood, R. E. Weber, A. R. Hargens, and R. W. Millard*
57. The Bronchial Circulation, *edited by J. Butler*
58. Lung Cancer Differentiation: Implications for Diagnosis and Treatment, *edited by S. D. Bernal and P. J. Hesketh*
59. Pulmonary Complications of Systemic Disease, *edited by J. F. Murray*
60. Lung Vascular Injury: Molecular and Cellular Response, *edited by A. Johnson and T. J. Ferro*
61. Cytokines of the Lung, *edited by J. Kelley*
62. The Mast Cell in Health and Disease, *edited by M. A. Kaliner and D. D. Metcalfe*
63. Pulmonary Disease in the Elderly Patient, *edited by D. A. Mahler*
64. Cystic Fibrosis, *edited by P. B. Davis*
65. Signal Transduction in Lung Cells, *edited by J. S. Brody, D. M. Center, and V. A. Tkachuk*
66. Tuberculosis: A Comprehensive International Approach, *edited by L. B. Reichman and E. S. Hershfield*
67. Pharmacology of the Respiratory Tract: Experimental and Clinical Research, *edited by K. F. Chung and P. J. Barnes*
68. Prevention of Respiratory Diseases, *edited by A. Hirsch, M. Goldberg, J.-P. Martin, and R. Masse*
69. *Pneumocystis carinii* Pneumonia: Second Edition, *edited by P. D. Walzer*
70. Fluid and Solute Transport in the Airspaces of the Lungs, *edited by R. M. Effros and H. K. Chang*
71. Sleep and Breathing: Second Edition, *edited by N. A. Saunders and C. E. Sullivan*
72. Airway Secretion: Physiological Bases for the Control of Mucous Hypersecretion, *edited by T. Takishima and S. Shimura*
73. Sarcoidosis and Other Granulomatous Disorders, *edited by D. G. James*
74. Epidemiology of Lung Cancer, *edited by J. M. Samet*
75. Pulmonary Embolism, *edited by M. Morpurgo*
76. Sports and Exercise Medicine, *edited by S. C. Wood and R. C. Roach*
77. Endotoxin and the Lungs, *edited by K. L. Brigham*
78. The Mesothelial Cell and Mesothelioma, *edited by M.-C. Jaurand and J. Bignon*
79. Regulation of Breathing: Second Edition, *edited by J. A. Dempsey and A. I. Pack*
80. Pulmonary Fibrosis, *edited by S. Hin. Phan and R. S. Thrall*
81. Long-Term Oxygen Therapy: Scientific Basis and Clinical Application, *edited by W. J. O'Donohue, Jr.*
82. Ventral Brainstem Mechanisms and Control of Respiration and Blood Pressure, *edited by C. O. Trouth, R. M. Millis, H. F. Kiwull-Schöne, and M. E. Schläfke*
83. A History of Breathing Physiology, *edited by D. F. Proctor*
84. Surfactant Therapy for Lung Disease, *edited by B. Robertson and H. W. Taeusch*
85. The Thorax: Second Edition, Revised and Expanded (in three parts), *edited by C. Roussos*

86. Severe Asthma: Pathogenesis and Clinical Management, *edited by S. J. Szefler and D. Y. M. Leung*
87. *Mycobacterium avium*–Complex Infection: Progress in Research and Treatment, *edited by J. A. Korvick and C. A. Benson*
88. Alpha 1–Antitrypsin Deficiency: Biology • Pathogenesis • Clinical Manifestations • Therapy, *edited by R. G. Crystal*
89. Adhesion Molecules and the Lung, *edited by P. A. Ward and J. C. Fantone*
90. Respiratory Sensation, *edited by L. Adams and A. Guz*
91. Pulmonary Rehabilitation, *edited by A. P. Fishman*
92. Acute Respiratory Failure in Chronic Obstructive Pulmonary Disease, *edited by J.-P. Derenne, W. A. Whitelaw, and T. Similowski*
93. Environmental Impact on the Airways: From Injury to Repair, *edited by J. Chrétien and D. Dusser*
94. Inhalation Aerosols: Physical and Biological Basis for Therapy, *edited by A. J. Hickey*
95. Tissue Oxygen Deprivation: From Molecular to Integrated Function, *edited by G. G. Haddad and G. Lister*
96. The Genetics of Asthma, *edited by S. B. Liggett and D. A. Meyers*
97. Inhaled Glucocorticoids in Asthma: Mechanisms and Clinical Actions, *edited by R. P. Schleimer, W. W. Busse, and P. M. O'Byrne*
98. Nitric Oxide and the Lung, *edited by W. M. Zapol and K. D. Bloch*
99. Primary Pulmonary Hypertension, *edited by L. J. Rubin and S. Rich*
100. Lung Growth and Development, *edited by J. A. McDonald*
101. Parasitic Lung Diseases, *edited by A. A. F. Mahmoud*
102. Lung Macrophages and Dendritic Cells in Health and Disease, *edited by M. F. Lipscomb and S. W. Russell*
103. Pulmonary and Cardiac Imaging, *edited by C. Chiles and C. E. Putman*
104. Gene Therapy for Diseases of the Lung, *edited by K. L. Brigham*
105. Oxygen, Gene Expression, and Cellular Function, *edited by L. Biadasz Clerch and D. J. Massaro*
106. Beta$_2$-Agonists in Asthma Treatment, *edited by R. Pauwels and P. M. O'Byrne*
107. Inhalation Delivery of Therapeutic Peptides and Proteins, *edited by A. L. Adjei and P. K. Gupta*
108. Asthma in the Elderly, *edited by R. A. Barbee and J. W. Bloom*
109. Treatment of the Hospitalized Cystic Fibrosis Patient, *edited by D. M. Orenstein and R. C. Stern*
110. Asthma and Immunological Diseases in Pregnancy and Early Infancy, *edited by M. Schatz, R. S. Zeiger, and H. N. Claman*
111. Dyspnea, *edited by D. A. Mahler*
112. Proinflammatory and Antiinflammatory Peptides, *edited by S. I. Said*
113. Self-Management of Asthma, *edited by H. Kotses and A. Harver*
114. Eicosanoids, Aspirin, and Asthma, *edited by A. Szczeklik, R. J. Gryglewski, and J. R. Vane*
115. Fatal Asthma, *edited by A. L. Sheffer*
116. Pulmonary Edema, *edited by M. A. Matthay and D. H. Ingbar*
117. Inflammatory Mechanisms in Asthma, *edited by S. T. Holgate and W. W. Busse*
118. Physiological Basis of Ventilatory Support, *edited by J. J. Marini and A. S. Slutsky*

119. Human Immunodeficiency Virus and the Lung, *edited by M. J. Rosen and J. M. Beck*
120. Five-Lipoxygenase Products in Asthma, *edited by J. M. Drazen, S.-E. Dahlén, and T. H. Lee*
121. Complexity in Structure and Function of the Lung, *edited by M. P. Hlastala and H. T. Robertson*
122. Biology of Lung Cancer, *edited by M. A. Kane and P. A. Bunn, Jr.*
123. Rhinitis: Mechanisms and Management, *edited by R. M. Naclerio, S. R. Durham, and N. Mygind*
124. Lung Tumors: Fundamental Biology and Clinical Management, *edited by C. Brambilla and E. Brambilla*
125. Interleukin-5: From Molecule to Drug Target for Asthma, *edited by C. J. Sanderson*
126. Pediatric Asthma, *edited by S. Murphy and H. W. Kelly*
127. Viral Infections of the Respiratory Tract, *edited by R. Dolin and P. F. Wright*
128. Air Pollutants and the Respiratory Tract, *edited by D. L. Swift and W. M. Foster*
129. Gastroesophageal Reflux Disease and Airway Disease, *edited by M. R. Stein*
130. Exercise-Induced Asthma, *edited by E. R. McFadden, Jr.*
131. LAM and Other Diseases Characterized by Smooth Muscle Proliferation, *edited by J. Moss*
132. The Lung at Depth, *edited by C. E. G. Lundgren and J. N. Miller*
133. Regulation of Sleep and Circadian Rhythms, *edited by F. W. Turek and P. C. Zee*
134. Anticholinergic Agents in the Upper and Lower Airways, *edited by S. L. Spector*
135. Control of Breathing in Health and Disease, *edited by M. D. Altose and Y. Kawakami*
136. Immunotherapy in Asthma, *edited by J. Bousquet and H. Yssel*
137. Chronic Lung Disease in Early Infancy, *edited by R. D. Bland and J. J. Coalson*
138. Asthma's Impact on Society: The Social and Economic Burden, *edited by K. B. Weiss, A. S. Buist, and S. D. Sullivan*
139. New and Exploratory Therapeutic Agents for Asthma, *edited by M. Yeadon and Z. Diamant*
140. Multimodality Treatment of Lung Cancer, *edited by A. T. Skarin*
141. Cytokines in Pulmonary Disease: Infection and Inflammation, *edited by S. Nelson and T. R. Martin*
142. Diagnostic Pulmonary Pathology, *edited by P. T. Cagle*
143. Particle–Lung Interactions, *edited by P. Gehr and J. Heyder*

ADDITIONAL VOLUMES IN PREPARATION

Tuberculosis: A Comprehensive International Approach, Second Edition, Revised and Expanded, *edited by L. B. Reichman and E. S. Hershfield*

Asthma and Respiratory Infections, *edited by D. P. Skoner*

Pulmonary and Peripheral Gas Exchange in Health and Disease, *edited by J. Roca, R. Rodriguez-Roisen, and P. Wagner*

Environmental Asthma, *edited by R. K. Bush*

Sleep and Breathing in Children: A Developmental Approach, *edited by G. M. Loughlin, J. L. Carroll, and C. L. Marcus*

Combination Therapy for Asthma and Chronic Obstructive Pulmonary Disease, *edited by R. J. Martin and M. Kraft*

Sleep Apnea: Implications in Cardiovascular and Cerebrovascular Disease, *edited by T. D. Bradley and J. S. Floras*

Nosocomial Pneumonia, *edited by W. R. Jarvis and O. Tablan*

Fetal Origins of Cardiovascular and Lung Disease, *edited by D. J. P. Barker*

Lung Surfactants: Basic and Clinical Applications, *edited by R. H. Notter*

The opinions expressed in these volumes do not necessarily represent the views of the National Institutes of Health.

PARTICLE–LUNG INTERACTIONS

Edited by

Peter Gehr
University of Bern
Bern, Switzerland

Joachim Heyder
GSF–Research Center for Environment and Health
Neuherberg/Munich, Germany

MARCEL DEKKER

MARCEL DEKKER, INC. NEW YORK • BASEL

ISBN: 0-8247-9891-0

This book is printed on acid-free paper.

Headquarters
Marcel Dekker, Inc.
270 Madison Avenue, New York, NY 10016
tel: 212-696-9000; fax: 212-685-4540

Eastern Hemisphere Distribution
Marcel Dekker AG
Hutgasse 4, Postfach 812, CH-4001 Basel, Switzerland
tel: 41-61-261-8482; fax: 41-61-261-8896

World Wide Web
http://www.dekker.com

The publisher offers discounts on this book when ordered in bulk quantities. For more information, write to Special Sales/Professional Marketing at the headquarters address above.

Current printing (last digit):
10 9 8 7 6 5 4 3 2 1

PRINTED IN THE UNITED STATES OF AMERICA

INTRODUCTION

In *Verse and Universe: Poems About Science and Mathematics* edited by Kurt Brown (1), one can find the following interesting verses describing the absorption of oxygen in the body:

The Lungs

In the tidal flux, the lobed pair avidly
grasp the invisible.

. . .

Braids of vessels and cartilage descend
in vanishing smallness,

to grape cluster of alveoli, the sheerest
of membranes, where oxygen

crosses the infinite cellular web, where air turns
to blood, spirit to flesh,

in a molecular transubstantiation, to bring rich
food to that red engine,

the heart, which like an equitable mother, pumps
to each organ and appendage

according to need, so even the cells in the darkest
corners can breathe.

For this to occur, the food (oxygen) must be clean, that is, free of particles. Of course, all particles are not the same. Some are deleterious, whereas others are medicinal. Nonetheless, all trigger responses in the lung, albeit varied ones.

Environmental sources of particles, inhalation of drugs, and the reaction of the lungs to pollutants have individually been the subject of several volumes in the Lung Biology in Health and Disease series, but this volume is novel in the sense that it covers all of these aspects. The particle–lung interactions are reviewed from the level of the molecule to that of the organ and even to the body as a whole. Any researcher or medical doctor interested in this area of biology will benefit from reading this text.

In addition to the editors, Peter Gehr and Joachim Heyder, this volume brings together a roster of contributors internationally recognized for their pioneering investigations. As executive editor of this series, I greatly appreciate the opportunity to present this important addition.

Claude Lenfant, M.D.
Bethesda, Maryland

Reference

1. Jones A. In: Brown K, ed. Verse and Universe: Poems About Science and Mathematics. Minneapolis: Milkweed Editions, 1998.

PREFACE

The atmospheric environment is composed of a number of gases in which particles are suspended. As a consequence, millions of particles are inhaled with every breath. A surface area the size of a tennis court is available in the lungs for the deposition of these particles. This huge surface area is in direct contact with the atmospheric environment, and is thus the primary target for inhaled particles. Usually particles in the diameter range of 0.01–10 µm are deposited in the lungs and are therefore available for interactions with pulmonary surfaces. Unfortunately, however, different definitions of particle size ranges are in use so that data are often not comparable. We were not able to cope with this problem, but we hope that Table 1 will help in the interpretation of the presented data.

The deeper a particle is deposited in the lungs the thinner is the barrier

Table 1 Classification of Aerosol Particles

Particle modes	Particle classification	PM particle classification
Nucleation mode: particles smaller than 0.02 µm in diameter	Ultrafine particles: particles smaller than 0.1 µm in diameter (lower limit: 0.001 µm)	
Aitken mode: particles of diameters 0.02–0.1 µm		
Accumulation mode: particles of diameters 0.1–1 µm	Fine particles: particles of diameters 0.1–1 µm	
Coarse mode: particles larger than 1 µm in diameter	Coarse particles: particles larger than 1 µm in diameter (no upper limit defined)	PM_x = particles smaller than x µm in aerodynamic diameter

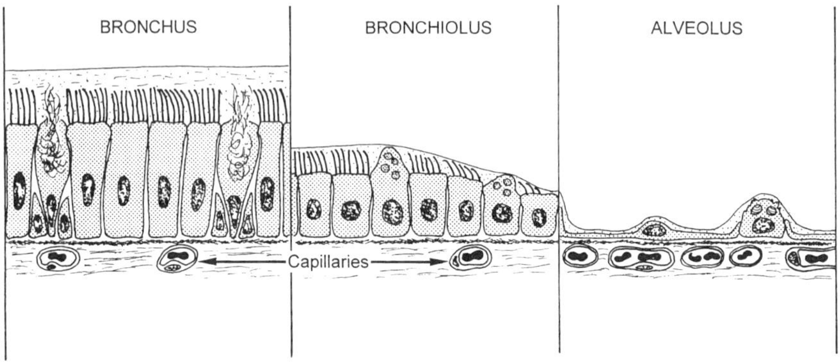

Figure 1 Comparative depths of lumen barriers within areas of the lungs. (Modified from Ref. 1.)

separating the lumen from blood vessels. In airways, it can be as thick as 20 μm; in peripheral airspaces, as thin as 0.5 μm, as illustrated in Figure 1. It is, therefore, most likely that the vulnerability of the epithelium to deposited particles depends on its location within the lungs.

The residence time of the particles on the epithelial surface is rather short. The particles may 1) be readily soluble in the fluid covering the epithelium; 2) be cleared by the mucociliary escalator; 3) be taken up by macrophages or epithelial or dendritic cells; or 4) penetrate into the interstitium. Depending on their disposition, they can activate cells, alter cell function, and interfere with cell-to-cell communication. These responses, on the cellular and molecular level, to deposited particles can often be compensated for by the physiological defense capacity of the lungs, such that respiratory and nonrespiratory lung functions are not affected. However, they can also stimulate processes with which the lungs are unable to cope and thereby initiate cascades of pathophysiological events that can result in altered respiratory and nonrespiratory lung functions.

This all depends on the number of particles deposited in the lungs and on the mass of chemicals they carry into the lungs. Because the concentration and composition of particles in the indoor and outdoor environments vary considerably in space and time, the lungs are exposed to an ever-changing level and mixture of particles. Current research focuses on the question of which levels and mixtures should be considered a health risk. Many epidemiological studies, clinical studies with human volunteers and experimental animals, and studies on cell and tissue cultures are being carried out worldwide in attempts to answer this question.

On the other hand, particles can be used to carry drugs into the lungs for topical or systemic therapy. This field still has many controversial aspects: technical aspects regarding drug formulation and particle generation and the question of how drugs might interfere with pathogenic processes of pulmonary or systemic diseases.

Every human being experiences lifelong exposure to environmental particles, some also experience exposure to particles generated by occupational activities, and others are purposely exposed to therapeutic particles. Therefore, the characteristics of environmental, occupational, and medicinal particles are discussed at the beginning of the book. Their deposition and disposition in the respiratory tract are considered in the next chapter, before the discussion turns toward biological responses initiated by deposited particles. These responses are often physiological responses, without pathophysiological consequences. However, some of them are considered adverse responses. Therefore, health consequences associated with the inhalation of particles are discussed in the last chapter.

Since this monograph first took shape, the field of particle–lung interactions has expanded considerably. The ''bad'' particles are currently ultrafine particles released into the environment from combustion processes. The ''good'' particles are those carrying insulin into the lungs. The treatment of diabetes via the inhalation route will most likely become the first approved aerosol treatment for a systemic disease. Nevertheless, we both hope that established knowledge and controversial issues are sufficiently reflected in this volume on particle–lung interactions.

We are honored to have been asked to edit this monograph and grateful for the support of all the colleagues who contributed to the book. Now that the work is done, we must confess that—once in a while—we went through times of irritation, but the overwhelming sensation remaining is the enjoyment of the stimulating interactions with the executive editor, Claude Lenfant, all the authors, and the publisher while this book was formed. We are very pleased and grateful that this book is now available to the scientific and professional community. We certainly hope that it will serve its purpose and will take its place among the well-received monographs in the Lung Biology in Health and Disease series.

Peter Gehr
Joachim Heyder

Reference

1. Burri P, Weibel ER. Funktionelle aspekte der lungenmorphologie. In: Fuchs WA, Vögeli V, eds. Röntgendiagnostik. Aktuelle Probleme der Röntgendiagnostik, 2nd ed. Bern: Huber, 1973:1–17.

CONTRIBUTORS

Edward G. Barrett, Ph.D. Research Fellow, Department of Environmental Medicine, University of Rochester School of Medicine and Dentistry, Rochester, New York

Peter Brand, Ph.D. Senior Scientist, Institute for Inhalation Biology, GSF–Research Center for Environment and Health, Neuherberg/Munich, Germany

Yung Sung Cheng, Ph.D. Senior Scientist, Inhalation Toxicology Laboratory, Department of Aerosol Science, Lovelace Respiratory Research Institute, Albuquerque, New Mexico

Andrew Churg, M.D. Professor, Department of Pathology, University of British Columbia, Vancouver, British Columbia, Canada

Robert W. Clarke, Ph.D. Research Fellow, Department of Environmental Health, Harvard School of Public Health, and Brigham and Women's Hospital, Boston, Massachusetts

Daniel L. Costa, Sc.D. Chief, Pulmonary Toxicology Branch, National Health and Environmental Research Laboratory, U.S. Environmental Protection Agency, Research Triangle Park, North Carolina

Robert B. Devlin, Ph.D. Chief, Clinical Research Branch, National Health and Environmental Effects Research Laboratory, U.S. Environmental Protection Agency, Research Triangle Park, North Carolina

Douglas W. Dockery, Sc.D. Professor, Department of Environmental Epidemiology, Harvard School of Public Health, Boston, Massachusetts

Jacob N. Finkelstein, Ph.D. Professor, Department of Pediatrics, University of Rochester School of Medicine and Dentistry, Rochester, New York

Mark W. Frampton, M.D. Associate Professor, Pulmonary and Critical Care Unit, University of Rochester Medical Center, University of Rochester School of Medicine and Dentistry, Rochester, New York

Peter Gehr, Ph.D. Professor and Head, Division of Histology, Institute of Anatomy, University of Bern, Bern, Switzerland

Marianne Geiser, Ph.D. Division of Histology, Institute of Anatomy, University of Bern, Bern, Switzerland

Andrew J. Ghio, M.D. Research Medical Officer, Human Studies Division, U.S. Environmental Protection Agency, Research Triangle Park, North Carolina

M. Ian Gilmour, Ph.D. Research Biologist, Experimental Toxicology Division, Immunotoxicology Branch, U.S. Environmental Protection Agency, Research Triangle Park, North Carolina

John J. Godleski, M.D. Associate Professor, Department of Environmental Health, Harvard School of Public Health, and Brigham and Women's Hospital, Boston, Massachusetts

Francis H. Y. Green, M.D., Ch.B., M.B. Professor, Department of Pathology and Laboratory Medicine, University of Calgary, Calgary, Alberta, Canada

Joachim Heyder, Ph.D. Professor and Director, Institute for Inhalation Biology, GSF–Research Center for Environment and Health, Neuherberg/Munich, Germany

Vinzenz Im Hof, M.D. Professor, Department of Medicine, and Director, Institute of Pathophysiology, University of Bern, Bern, Switzerland

Patrick G. Holt, Ph.D., F.R.C.Path., F.R.C.P.I., D.Sc., M.D.(Hon.) Professor, Division of Cell Biology, TVW Telethon Institute for Child Health Research, West Perth, Western Australia, Australia

Mark D. Hoover, Ph.D., C.H.P., C.I.H. Aerosol Scientist, Inhalation Toxicology Laboratory, Department of Aerosol Science, Lovelace Respiratory Research Institute, Albuquerque, New Mexico

Neil F. Johnson, Ph.D., F.R.C.Path. Leader, In Vivo Toxicology Section, Department of Nonclinical Drug Safety, Boehringer Ingelheim Pharma KG, Biberach am Riss, Germany

Cecile M. King, Ph.D. Research Associate, Department of Immunology, The Scripps Research Institute, La Jolla, California

Malcolm King, Ph.D., F.C.C.P. Professor, Pulmonary Research Group, Department of Medicine, University of Alberta, Edmonton, Alberta, Canada

Hillel S. Koren, Ph.D. Director, Human Studies Division, National Health and Environmental Effects Research Laboratory, U.S. Environmental Protection Agency, Research Triangle Park, North Carolina

Wolfgang G. Kreyling, Ph.D. Senior Scientist, Institute for Inhalation Biology, GSF–Research Center for Environment and Health, Neuherberg/Munich, Germany

Martin M. Lee, Ph.D. Canadian Lung Association/Bayer Postdoctoral Fellow, Channing Laboratory, Department of Medicine, Harvard Medical School, and Brigham and Women's Hospital, Boston, Massachusetts

Joe L. Mauderly, D.V.M. Senior Scientist and Director of External Affairs, Lovelace Respiratory Research Institute, Albuquerque, New Mexico

Roger O. McClellan, D.V.M., A.B.T., A.B.V.T. Adjunct Professor, Duke University, Durham, North Carolina State University, Raleigh, and University of North Carolina, Chapel Hill, and President, Chemical Industry Institute of Toxicology, Research Triangle Park, North Carolina

Andrew S. McWilliam, Ph.D. Senior Research Fellow, *H. pylori* Research Laboratory, Department of Medicine, University of Western Australia, Nedlands, Western Australia, Australia

C. Arden Pope III, Ph.D. Professor, Department of Economics, Brigham Young University, Provo, Utah

Clive Robinson, Ph.D. Senior Lecturer, Department of Pharmacology and Clinical Pharmacology, St. George's Hospital Medical School, London, England

Jonathan M. Samet, M.D., M.S. Professor and Chairman, Department of Epidemiology, School of Hygiene and Public Health, Johns Hopkins University, Baltimore, Maryland

Gerhard Scheuch, Ph.D. Senior Scientist, Institute for Inhalation Biology, GSF–Research Center for Environment and Health, Gauting/Munich, and General Manager, Institute for Aerosol Medicine InAMed GmbH, Gemuenden, Germany

Holger Schulz, M.D. Senior Scientist, Institute for Inhalation Biology, GSF–Research Center for Environment and Health, Neuherberg/Munich, Germany

Samuel Schürch, Ph.D. Professor, Department of Physiology and Biophysics, Health Sciences Center, University of Calgary, Calgary, Alberta, Canada

Frank E. Speizer, M.D. E. H. Kass Professor, Department of Medicine, Channing Laboratory, Harvard Medical School, and Brigham and Women's Hospital, Boston, Massachusetts

Geoffrey A. Stewart, Ph.D. Department of Microbiology, University of Western Australia, Nedlands, Western Australia, Australia

Frank Stratmann, Ph.D. Institute for Tropospheric Research, Leipzig, Germany

Katharina Svartengren, M.D., Ph.D. Division of Respiratory and Allergic Diseases, Department of Medicine, Karolinska Institute, Huddinge University Hospital, Stockholm, Sweden

Magnus Svartengren, M.D., Ph.D. Professor, Division of Occupational Medicine, Department of Public Health Sciences, Karolinska Institute, Stockholm, Sweden

Ina Tegen, Ph.D. Department of Applied Physics, Columbia University, New York, New York

Philip J. Thompson, M.B.B.S., F.R.A.C.P., F.C.C.P., M.R.A.C.M.A. Associate Professor, Department of Medicine, University of Western Australia, Nedlands, Western Australia, Australia

Mark J. Utell, M.D. Professor, Department of Medicine and Environmental Medicine, and Director, Divisions of Pulmonary/Critical Care and Occupational Medicine, University of Rochester Medical Center, University of Rochester School of Medicine and Dentistry, Rochester, New York

Alfred Wiedensohler, Ph.D. Institute for Tropospheric Research, Leipzig, Germany

Donovan B. Yeates, Ph.D. Research Professor, Department of Medicine, University of Illinois at Chicago, and Veterans Affairs Chicago Health Care System, Chicago, Illinois

Hsu-Chi Yeh, Ph.D. Scientist Emeritus, Lovelace Respiratory Research Institute, Albuquerque, New Mexico

CONTENTS

Part One

OVERVIEW

1

Particle Interactions with the Respiratory Tract

ROGER O. McCLELLAN

Duke University, Durham
North Carolina State University, Raleigh
University of North Carolina, Chapel Hill
and Chemical Industry Institute of Toxicology
Research Triangle Park, North Carolina

I. Introduction

The purpose of this chapter is to provide an overview of the science related to interactions of particles with the respiratory tract, thereby providing an introduction to the chapters that follow. I have purposefully used the term *respiratory tract*, rather than *lung* to describe the scope of this chapter. The respiratory tract includes the structures from the nares, or nose, to the respiratory bronchioles and alveoli, in which gas exchange occurs. The term *lungs* is used both in a more restricted sense to include only the bronchioles and alveoli and, broadly, to include all of the respiratory tract. The study of interactions between particles and the respiratory tract is extraordinarily rich from a scientific viewpoint and also of immense importance because it relates directly to major societal issues.

The scientific dimensions are rich in part because two broad fields that have very different disciplinary roots must be joined to understand interactions between particles and the respiratory tract. On the one hand, we are concerned with characteristics of airborne particles that draw heavily on the disciplines of chemistry, physics, and engineering. On the other hand, we are concerned with the respiratory tract, for which an understanding of normal biology and of disease is rooted in all the disciplines in biomedical science. Each of these areas, particle science and the biology and pathobiology of the respiratory system, is fascinating in its own right. To join the two areas and understand their interactions adds additional challenges and opportunities.

The science of particle–respiratory interactions relates to very important societal issues. This starts with broad concern for the health of humankind and extends to how exposure to particles may affect human health and the quality of life. To state the obvious, the proper functioning of the respiratory system is essential to survival. Alterations in the functioning of the respiratory system are readily reflected in signs and symptoms that immediately arouse concern and, if left unchecked, are manifest as serious disease and death. Moreover, the respiratory tract is one of the major sites of cancer. Many of the diseases of the respiratory tract are directly linked to inhaled material, as exemplified by cigarette smoking and to a substantially lesser extent, by occupational or environmental exposures to various agents. The control of occupational and environmental exposures to air pollution is a high priority in most countries, as reflected by substantial legislation and related expenditures to maintain or improve air quality. Thus our concern for interactions between particles and the respiratory tract is driven, not just by scientific curiosity, but also by a desire to provide the scientific basis needed to improve air quality in a cost-effective manner and, thereby, improve respiratory health.

In this chapter, I will first provide some historical perspective for research on particle–respiratory tract interactions. Next, I will discuss the respiratory tract as a target organ for inhaled particles, and then proceed to discuss the characteristics of particles that influence their toxicity. This will be followed by a section on basic concepts governing the disposition of inhaled particles and a brief review of the primary health responses of the respiratory tract. The chapter closes with a discussion of regulatory approaches taken to minimize the occupational and environmental effects of airborne materials. The reader who is interested in broad coverage of inhalation toxicology is referred to reference texts by McClellan and Henderson (1) and by Gardner et al. (2) and earlier volumes in the Lung Biology in Health and Disease series.

II. A Source-Exposure–Dose-Response Framework

There are multiple drivers of our quest to obtain an improved understanding of particle–respiratory tract interactions. One of these is the need to devise control strategies that will limit the potential for human disease from airborne materials. Another motivation is the desire to simply expand the boundaries of what is known about particles and the respiratory tract, a motivation grounded in scientific curiosity or our desire to explore the unknown.

In both these cases, placing our quest for new knowledge within an overall framework will help identify gaps in our present knowledge and integrate new information as it is acquired. Such a framework is depicted schematically in Figure 1. The use of this framework is intended to provide guidance for our research and integrative activities, not to impose constraints. The framework is an attempt to link particles, a toxicant, with the target, the respiratory tract. This critical linkage must be understood at all stages, from concern for sources of particles to the focus on the health effects that may be produced. Let me illustrate with several examples.

Frequently, a need develops for devising a sampling strategy for a workplace in which a new material is to be used. Recognition of the multiple factors that influence the disposition and toxicity of particles (to be discussed in detail later) causes us to obtain data on particle size and composition. Because we know the importance of particle size in influencing disposition of airborne particles, primary attention is given to sampling and characterizing particles smaller than 10 µm in aerodynamic size. The use of a high-volume sampler that collects particles of all sizes for chemical characterization, including much mass associated with particles larger than 10 µm in size, would be easy. As is well recognized, however, detailed chemical characterization of a sample dominated by large particles does not yield information relevant to the smaller particles most likely to be inhaled and deposited. This is true even if the large particles predominate in the raw material delivered to the factory. Thus, concern for the source–exposure atmosphere linkage helps guide our research.

Let us continue with this same example and assume that occupational health and regulatory authorities are eager to know the inherent toxicity of this new material, even if large particles predominate at all stages of the manufacturing process. They argue that some small respirable particles are present and could

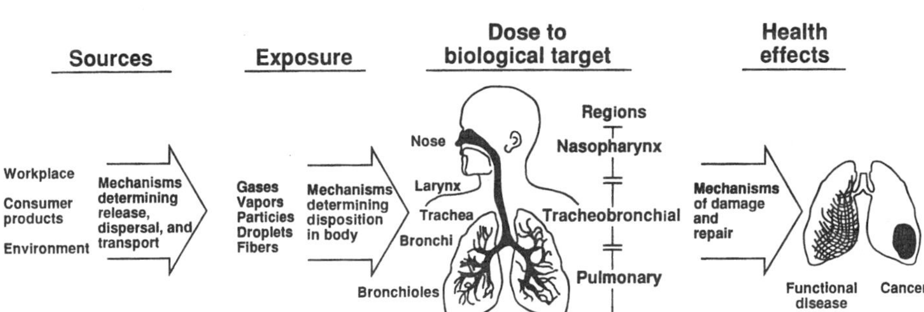

Figure 1 Schematic representation of a framework linking sources, exposure, dose, and health effects to provide an understanding of how particles interact with the respiratory system.

pose a hazard. To get around the fact that most of the particles of the new material cannot even be inhaled, some investigators suggest that the larger particles be instilled in the trachea or implanted in the pleural cavity. I would strongly advise against administering particles by either of these nonphysiological modes of administration. I question the usefulness of data acquired using nonphysiological modes of administration of the toxicants for assessing human risks. Alternatively, a decision could be made to evaluate the inherent toxicity of the material by mechanically grinding the large particles in bulk to produce an abundance of small particles, separate the small from the large particles, and then use the smaller particles for inhalation studies. If this is done and some evidence of toxicity is found when rats are chronically exposed to the ground particles in the range of several hundred micrograms per cubic meter, then the findings must be put into perspective when they are used to assess the potential workplace hazard. This includes recognition that particles of the size studied are present at concentrations of only a few micrograms per cubic meter or less in the workplace environment. Thus, extrapolation from high- to low-exposure concentrations is necessary. Moreover, differences in the deposition and retention of particles of various sizes in rats and humans, as well as possible interspecies differences in sensitivity, must be considered in evaluating the rat data for their relevance for assessing human risks.

The point to be made is that both the sampling strategies at the source and the interpretation of the toxicity data must be linked to likely real-world exposures. Neither information on particle characteristics nor on particle toxicity should be obtained in isolation from how the data will be used. In both situations, consideration of fundamental properties of both particles and the respiratory tract is crucial in planning and interpreting research.

III. Historical Perspective

Concern has existed for centuries about air quality and its effect on human health. There is no doubt that this concern arose soon after humans began using fire for cooking and heating, and it was certainly further exacerbated when utilization of new fuels intensified with the industrial revolution.

In the Western world, concern for air pollution intensified following the return of Marco Polo from the East and the introduction of coal as an energy source. As early as the 13th century, there was concern over coal smoke and odor in London. Reportedly, the Queen of England moved from London to Nottingham because of the smoke in London. A classic publication, *Fumifugium: Or the Inconvenience of the Air and Smoke of London Dissipated*, written by John Evelyn in 1661, called attention to the issue of air pollution. This concern was viewed as an inconvenience and not necessarily as a matter of essential health concern.

During the early years of the industrial revolution, wood served as the primary fuel, and industry was located near forests. This served to restrict the development of industry. With the introduction of coal and the development of the steam engine, the scene changed. The pace of industrialization increased, and factories were located near sources of coal and along waterways that served as efficient arteries for transport of coal, raw materials, and finished products. Very soon concern developed for the smoke and ash from coal-fired boilers in factories, power plants, and locomotives. These early concerns focused on the impaired visibility and soiling caused by air pollution, rather than on concern for health. In addition, damage to vegetation from emissions produced in the smelting of sulfide ores raised concern that pollution that could harm plants might harm people. This kind of concern in the Rhine Valley of Germany led to the design of air ducts leading from smelters in villages in the valley floor to chimneys placed at the top of nearby hills. Clearly, the use of dilution and dispersion to minimize air pollution did not originate with the later development of heavy industry and use of tall stacks in areas such as the Ruhr Valley of Germany and the Ohio River Valley in the United States.

Although air pollution was recognized in many industrial countries and especially in major cities, it was probably nowhere as apparent as in London. The high levels of pollution combined with London's notorious fog created a serious problem. (The term *smog* is reputed to be a contraction of the words smoke and fog.) In the twentieth century, concern for air pollution was heightened by several events. In December 1930, air pollution caused over 60 deaths and hundreds of illnesses in the Meuse Valley of Belgium during a period of stagnant weather conditions. In December 1952, smog in London is reported to have caused 4000 deaths, primarily among the infirm, the old, and those with respiratory disease (Fig. 2). An increase in the daily death rate followed an increase in the level of pollution within hours. As the air pollution subsided, so did the death rate. Indeed, the death rate dropped below normal levels for a time, suggesting that a harvesting of individuals who were on the verge of death had occurred.

Acute respiratory effects were also observed in cattle at the famous Smithfield Club Livestock Show in London. The death rate was highest for the prize cattle, which were well cared for and had their litter promptly removed. The death rate was lower in the cattle that were not so well cared for. Presumably, ammonia produced by microbes acting on the excreta had a beneficial effect in neutralizing sulfur oxides and sulfuric acid in the polluted air. Other pollution episodes were observed in London and served as a major stimulus to institution of control measures. Air pollution episodes with serious effects were not restricted to Europe. In October 1948, a period of particularly calm and stable meteorology,

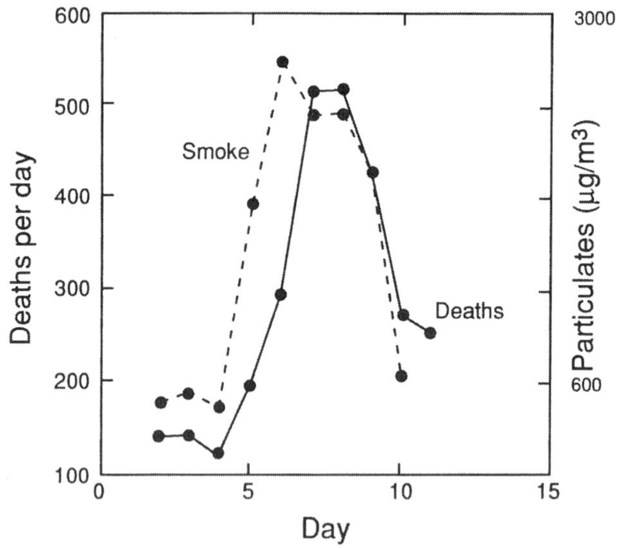

Figure 2 Relation between particulate air pollution and daily mortality in London, December 1952. (From Ref. 104.)

in Donoro, Pennsylvania, resulted in a marked increase in the levels of oxides and inorganic sulfates and an associated increase in morbidity and mortality from respiratory effects. The level of pollution was so high that footprints and tire prints could be observed on the streets much as with a light snowfall.

Despite the early concern for air pollution, remarkably little research was conducted before World War I to improve our knowledge of how air pollution affects health. The unfortunate use of poisonous gas in World War I provided a clear stimulus for developing a better understanding of how these specific agents produced disease. Unfortunately, literature from this era is meager. However, the lack of activity in the field of respiratory health is probably reflective of the general lack of biomedical research in the first third of the 20th century, rather than a lack of interest in respiratory health per se. The strong preventive medicine orientation that exists today for diseases of both occupational and environmental origin was still in its infancy.

However, some of the major roots of the science of particles and the respiratory tract are traceable to the 1920s and 1930s. Especially notable in the United States was the pioneering research in industrial hygiene and inhalation toxicology of T. F. Hatch at the University of Pittsburgh and C. K. and P. Drinker at Harvard University. Their work focused on airborne materials that caused occupational diseases. Two classic texts stand as lasting testimonials to the efforts of these pioneers. They are *Industrial Dust: Hygienic Significance, Measurement and Control* by Drinker and Hatch (3) and *Pulmonary Deposition and Retention of Inhaled Aerosols* by Hatch and Gross (4). Strong research programs on the health effects of air pollutants continue at Harvard today. These programs include basic pulmonary biology research by J. Brain and colleagues and epidemiological and exposure assessment studies by F. Speizer, D. Dockery, J. Schwartz, J. Spengler, and others.

In Germany, the occurrence of pneumoconiosis in miners in the Ruhr Valley served as a research stimulus. This research focused on the role of quartz dust in the mines as the causative factor in coal miners' silicosis. W. Stöber, who contributed much to the development of aerosol science and inhalation toxicology both in Germany and the United States, spent the early portion of his career conducting research on silicosis.

World War II served as a major stimulus for the conduct of research on three markedly different types of airborne materials: chemical and biological agents, radioactive materials, and automotive exhaust emissions. The sad experience of World War I with chemical agents gave rise to a strong sentiment during World War II that the use of such agents should not be repeated. Furthermore, the United States and its allies were committed to being able to defend against their use. This gave impetus to military-sponsored research that would show how airborne materials of either a chemical or a biological nature cause disease. A contributor to the United Kingdom effort in this area was C. N. Davies, who later authored the classic book, *Dust Is Dangerous* (5).

The advent of the Manhattan project, established by the United States to develop an atomic bomb, gave rise to concern for the potential health effects of radioactive materials. Very early, an awareness developed of the potential for occupational exposure to some of the key materials used in the project. This included uranium, which was a starting material for both controlled nuclear fission and the manufacture of atomic bombs. An extensive research program on the toxicity of uranium with special emphasis on the inhalation route of entry was initiated at the University of Rochester under the leadership of Dr. Harold Hodge, pioneer toxicologist who was at that time in the Department of Pharmacology. He and scientists who subsequently provided leadership for the program recognized the need for multidisciplinary input extending from aerosol science to the biomedical sciences and recruited and trained accordingly. Over the years this program and successive efforts involved many scientists, some beginning as graduate students, who made major contributions to the fields of aerosol science and inhalation toxicology. Prominent scientists involved in the University of Rochester program include P. Morrow, W. Stöber, T. Mercer, R. Thomas, B. Boecker, J. N. Stannard, L. Casarett, S. Laskin, W. Bair, H. Stokinger, J. Vostal, B. Dahneke, S. Soderholm, R. Phalen, D. Craig, D. Raabe, R. Cuddihy, O. Moss, B. Chen, B. Stuart, B. Greenspan, J. Ferin, M. Utell, J. Finkelstein, and G. Oberdörster. A brief account of the early years of the University of Rochester program is contained in a Foreword by P. Morrow to the 2nd edition of *Concepts in Inhalation Toxicology* (1) and in *Radioactivity and Health: A History* (6).

Also of early concern was the man-made element plutonium, which resulted from neutron capture by uranium, and the fission product radionuclides, which were produced by controlled nuclear fission in a reactor or by the detonation of a nuclear weapon. Plutonium, an alpha-emitting radionuclide, was used in the manufacture of nuclear weapons. Because plutonium was believed to concentrate in the skeleton, there was concern that various nuclides of plutonium could cause bone cancer, as was observed in the luminous dial painters who had ingested alpha-emitting radium in the early 1900s. Inhalation was recognized as a major potential route of entry into the body for plutonium. During and after World War II, this recognition served as a stimulus for research programs in several laboratories in addition to the University of Rochester. One of the most significant of these was the program at the Hanford Laboratories in Richland, Washington. Under the leadership of W. J. Bair, this group made major contributions to aerosol science and inhalation toxicology on a continuing basis. This program continues today, with a focus on chemical toxicants as a part of the inhalation toxicology unit at Battelle's Pacific Northwest Laboratories.

During the post-World War II years, commercial nuclear power in many countries was rapidly expanded. This gave rise to heightened concern for accidents involving the release of radioactive materials from reactors (as did occur at Chernobyl in the Ukraine), fuel reprocessing plants, or handling of wastes. This concern was the basis for C. S. White's initiation of the Fission Product Inhalation Program at the Lovelace Foundation in Albuquerque, New Mexico, in 1960, a program for which I was responsible from 1966 through 1988 (7). The early focus of the research was on fission product radionuclides, such as radionuclides of strontium, yttrium, cesium, cerium, and iodine. The program later expanded to include plutonium and other actimide elements and, in the late 1970s, motor vehicle exhaust and chemical toxicants. The program continues today under the leadership of J. L. Mauderly and C. H. Hobbs.

Similar efforts focusing on the potential effects of inhaled radioactive materials were carried out in many other countries, with perhaps the largest programs in the former U.S.S.R., France, Germany, Japan, and the United Kingdom. During the post-World War II years, there were also major advances in our understanding of the basic properties of aerosols. Of special note is the work of N. A. Fuchs at the Karpor Institute of Physical Chemistry in Moscow, which is summarized in his classic text, *The Mechanics of Aerosols* (8). The English translation was edited by C. N. Davies, who himself did so much to advance the field of aerosol science. During this period, significant advances were made in our understanding of the basic biology and pathobiology of the respiratory tract. This is illustrated by the now-classic reference, *Morphometry of the Human Lung*, by E. R. Weibel (9).

The substantial research efforts on radioactive materials provided the information needed to establish stringent standards and control procedures that were effective in minimizing disease from occupational and environmental exposures to radioactive materials. Unfortunately, the catastrophic accident that occurred at the Chernobyl nuclear power station in 1986 has left an unfortunate legacy of radioactive contamination of the environment and associated increased potential for radiation-induced disease. The exact influence of this accident and of the radioactive contamination near Russian facilities associated with the nuclear weapons program of the U.S.S.R. will not be known for many decades.

In contrast to the concern and proactive approach taken with plutonium and the fission products, there was a failure to fully appreciate the role of radon, a radioactive gas, and its radioactive progeny in causing lung cancer. This was surprising because we know in retrospect that a high incidence of lung cancer occurred in miners in central Europe over many decades. Some of these mines were used to produce pitchblende for the Curies. The failure to adequately recognize the linkage between exposure to radon and lung cancer resulted in a repeat of history, with an excess of lung cancer observed in uranium miners from these same mines in the 1950s and later in the United States and other countries (10,11). Concern for radon-induced lung cancer is still with us, but the focus has shifted to the potential danger of much lower levels of radon found in homes. At low levels of radon exposure, excess lung cancer risk cannot be measured. Nonetheless, the use of exposure–response models that assume a linear relation between lung cancer and radon exposure down to zero result in calculated population risks of tens of thousands of lung cancers in the United States when calculations are made for populations of millions of individuals (12). Unfortunately, such estimates rarely convey the uncertainties associated with risk estimates or clearly define the populations at greatest risk. Many of the excess cancers are calculated for exposures below the median exposure for the population at large. Because relative risk models are typically used, most of the excess risk is presumably borne by smokers who already have an excess risk of lung cancer on the order of ten times greater than nonsmokers.

Beyond the institutional effects noted in the foregoing, the atomic era that began in earnest with World War II had a major influence in a general way through its emphasis on the physical sciences and quantitation. The major disciplinary roots of the atomic era were physics and chemistry, both highly quantitative sciences. With the use of radioactive materials and increasingly precise measurement methods, quantitating the amount of a radioactive material in the air and the fraction deposited and retained in the body as a function of time also became possible. Moreover, relating the observed health effects to various quantitative measures of dose, rather than simply to exposure metrics, also became possible. Elements such as plutonium 239 and strontium 90 were specifically of concern because they had radioisotopes. For these radionuclides, the use of radiation dose terms for lung, liver, and skeleton imposed between exposure and response was quite natural (see Fig. 1). This was certainly in keeping with dosimetric developments in the interrelated fields of radiology, radiation biology, and radiation protection. The same approach was extended to radioactively labeled organic compounds using radioisotopes such as ^{3}H, ^{14}C, and ^{32}P. Readers who have an interest in the history of developments in the radiation field, including aspects of inhalation toxicology, are referred to a substantial volume, *Radioactivity and Health: A History*, by J. N. Stannard (6). Stannard was one of the early pioneering toxicologists at the University of Rochester who mentored many in the field of inhalation toxicology. A second classic reference worthy of special note that is traceable to the University of Rochester is *Aerosol Technology in Hazard Evaluation*, by T. T. Mercer (13). The quantitative traditions of inhalation toxicology and aerosol science are reflected in many of the chapters in this volume. Mercer did graduate work at the University of Rochester and returned to the faculty there after having spent 1960 to 1966 with the Lovelace Foundation in Albuquerque, New Mexico, where he laid the groundwork for that organization's strong aerosol science tradition.

World War II provided a springboard for concern about another kind of air pollution: emissions from motor vehicles. Immediately post-World War II, the number of both automobiles and trucks began to increase dramatically, an increase that is continuing even today around the world. Perhaps nowhere was the influence of motor vehicles more apparent than in Los Angeles, California, where industry and population increased along with motor vehicles. The setting—a large basin rimmed by mountains with onshore winds prevailing, was made to order for an air pollution problem. This no doubt was the basis for the explorer Juan Rodriques Cabrillo, in 1542, coining the name ''Bay of Smokers'' for San Pedro Bay on the California coast. The name took on a contemporary tone in the 1950s when high levels of smog became an everyday occurrence in the Los Angeles basin. In the early 1950s, A. J. Haagen-Smit of the California Institute of Technology, who had a strong chemistry background, discovered the critical interactions among the oxides of nitrogen and hydrocarbons from vehicle exhaust and sunlight in producing ozone and other photochemical oxidants as components of Los Angeles smog. Hydrocarbons from other sources, including vegetation, are now known to contribute to these complex interactions, as do oxides of nitrogen from power plants and other sources. The tradition of excellence in aerosol science at the California Institute of Technology was continued by S. Friedlander (who has since relocated to the University of California–Los Angeles), J. Seinfeld, and R. Flagan. A related center of excellence in aerosol science with a strong emphasis on engineering concepts and particle measurement is the program at the University of Minnesota, which was originally led by K. Whitby and is now led by B. Liu. A program with a stronger industrial hygiene orientation developed at the New York University with major input from N. Nelson, R. Albert, S. Laskin, and M. Lippmann. Similar developments occurred in Europe, with one of the most successful programs being that of W. Stahlhofen in Frankfurt, Germany. This program continues today under the leadership of J. Heyder at the GSF Institute for Inhalation Biology, Neuherberg, Germany. An additional laboratory of note is the Fraunhofer Institute of Toxicology and Aerosol Research located in Hannover, Germany, which developed under the leadership of W. Stöber, later U. Mohr, and now U. Heinrich.

The foregoing references to specific laboratories are not intended to be comprehensive, but rather, illustrative of a key point. A careful review of the work of these pioneers is a reminder that advances in understanding what is in the air and how it affects health inevitably involves a joining of the physical and chemical sciences, engineering, and the biomedical sciences.

Another important dimension of this field that is worthy of note from a historical standpoint is its relation to the diagnosis and treatment of disease. Soon after World War II, physicians and allied health personnel recognized the potential value of using radioactive materials to evaluate respiratory tract function. This soon led to the development of instrumentation for measuring radioactivity and techniques for evaluating pulmonary ventilation, diffusion, and perfusion, and the deposition and clearance of inhaled particles. More recently, there has been great interest in using our fundamental understanding of particles and how they interact with the respiratory tract to aid in designing pharmaceutical agents and delivery methods that target specific portions of the respiratory tract. These efforts have been directed both toward agents that affect the respiratory tract directly, such as those used for treating asthma, and toward agents that may be absorbed and influence other body systems.

As we work to continually advance the science that undergirds our understanding of particle–respiratory tract interactions, we must not cast aside our historical roots. We need to periodically review, in some detail, our past findings so that we can use what we already know to the greatest possible advantage, avoid periodic rediscovery of the wheel, and at the same time, make maximum use of new technology, even when it involves using the newest approaches to address old issues. The saying "The past is prologue" is always deserving of careful attention.

IV. The Respiratory Tract as a Target Organ for Inhaled Particles

The respiratory tract serves both as a portal of entry for inhaled materials and as a target organ for effects produced both by the inhaled material and by toxicants transported to the respiratory tract by the bloodstream. There are numerous examples of the respiratory tract as a portal of entry for materials that directly affect it. Examples are inhaled particles and irritant gases, such as ozone and oxides of nitrogen. There are also many materials that enter through the respiratory tract and are transported by the bloodstream to remote sites in the body where effects are produced. Examples are benzene, which is primarily metabolized in both the liver and bone marrow and produces toxic effects in the hematopoietic tissue, and stable lead, which produces damage in both the central nervous system and hematopoietic tissue. Some material such as paraquat may be absorbed from the gastrointestinal tract and transported to the lungs, which become the target organ for effects.

As illustrated in Figure 1, the respiratory tract is a complex and diverse system extending from the nares, or nose, down to the alveoli. Inhaled particles can be deposited in all the regions of the respiratory tract and produce adverse effects. Understanding the unique characteristics of each of these regions is important when evaluating interactions between particles and the respiratory tract. Moreover, both the similarities and differences between the respiratory tracts of laboratory animal species and humans must be recognized. Fortunately, they share many common features in the main, although there are important differences between the respiratory tracts of laboratory animals and humans. This is an important underpinning of our use of laboratory animal species as surrogates for humans in conducting toxicological evaluations for the purpose of assessing potential human risks and the acquisition of fundamental knowledge that can ultimately be used to understand human biology and pathobiology.

A. Structure and Function of the Respiratory Tract

The primary function of the respiratory tract is gas exchange: delivering life-sustaining oxygen to red blood cells circulating through the lungs for transport to the tissues of the body and, in turn, removing released waste carbon dioxide from the body. The respiratory tract has other vital functions, including olfaction; control of acid–base balance of the blood and body as a whole; serving as a blood reservoir and, thereby, aiding in the regulation of blood volume; functioning as part of the body's immune system; contributing to thermal regulation of the body; metabolism of a wide range of compounds; and expiration of certain compounds. In this section, a broad overview will be provided of the structure and function of the respiratory tract. Readers interested in greater detail are referred to more substantial texts (1,2,14).

The structure of the respiratory tract is optimized for gas exchange. Over a lifetime, the average individual will inhale about 400 million L of air. On a volumetric basis, this is about 5000 times more than the volumes of food or water taken into the body. For convenience in describing the respiratory tract structure and function, it can be subdivided into three major compartments, as depicted in Figure 1. This approach, largely based on the pioneering morphometric work of Weibel (9), has contributed greatly to the modeling of respiratory tract function and its handling of toxic materials.

The nasopharyngeal compartment begins at the nares and mouth, where air enters the body, and extends to the larynx. In this compartment, the temperature of the air is equilibrated to approximate that of the body, and the air is humidified. Here olfaction occurs by olfactory sensory cells that are in contact with air and connected to the nervous system. Inspired airborne particles are also removed in the nasopharynx, the largest particles depositing by inertial forces and the smallest particles by diffusion.

The tracheobronchial compartment extends from the larynx to the terminal bronchioles. This set of conducting airways of increasing cross-sectional diameter delivers gases to and collects them from the pulmonary region. The tracheobronchial airways are lined by ciliated cells, with an overlying blanket of mucus that serves an important role in transported macrophages and particulate material from the pulmonary region to the nasopharyngeal compartment.

The pulmonary region consists of the respiratory bronchioles, alveolar ducts, alveolar sacs, and alveoli. The relatively small diameter of the alveoli maximizes the surface area of the pulmonary region, thereby optimizing the exchange of gases between the alveolar air sacs and the blood circulating through the large network of capillaries lying between the alveoli. The alveoli are lined by a thin layer of surfactant material that is essential for maintaining alveolar structure as the gas volume changes in a cyclic manner.

From a cellular viewpoint, the respiratory tract is extraordinarily complex, consisting of more than 40 different individual cell types. The airways of the nasopharyngeal and tracheobronchial compartments are lined by epithelial cells. The most anterior portion is lined by stratified squamous epithelium that in a short distance transitions to respiratory epithelium, with numerous ciliated cells and occasional goblet cells that serve as a source of mucus.

The ciliated epithelial cells extend down the respiratory tract to the respiratory bronchioles. The cilia provide locomotion for the overlying mucous blanket, propelling mucus and associated debris forward in the most anterior portion of the nares or propelling it to the oral cavity in the most posterior portion of the nasopharyngeal compartment. In the tracheobronchial compartment, mucus and associated material are moved upward to the oral cavity.

In the human, the alveoli are about 200–300 μm in diameter and are lined by very thin alveolar epithelial cells. The most prominent of these cells are the type I (also called type A) alveolar epithelial cells, which are only about 0.1 μm in thickness and cover a wide area. The second most prominent of these cells are the type II cells, which are roughly cuboidal. The type II cells, which are capable of division, are thought to serve as precursors of type I cells during lung growth or repair. The type II cells also produce surfactant, a surface tension–lowering material that lines the alveoli and reduces the tendency of the very thin-walled alveoli to collapse. A vast network of small capillaries lined by very thin endothelial cells underlie the alveolar epithelial cells.

Beyond the cell types already mentioned, the respiratory tract contains numerous other cell types, including nerve cells, fibroblasts, lymphoid cells, and macrophages. The macrophages play an important role in removing microbial organisms, cellular debris, and particulate material. The interactions between inhaled particles and macrophages will be a topic of recurring discussion in this book.

The lymphoid tissue of the lungs is concentrated in the human in four major groups of lymph nodes: (1) bronchopulmonary lymph nodes around the divisions of the lobar bronchi, (2) hilar nodes around the upper and lower bronchi, (3) paratracheal nodes, and (4) the azygous node at the junction of the right upper lobar bronchus and the right main bronchus. A network of lymphatic vessels drains from both superficial and deep portions of the lungs into the lymph nodes. Lymph flows from the nodes into thoracic duct, which, in turn, drains into the systemic venous circulation. The lymphatic vessels of the respiratory tract also communicate with other lymphatic vessels, including drainage to deep cervical nodes and to abdominal nodes. The lymphatic vessels can serve as a vehicle for translocation of inhaled particles, not only to lymph nodes associated with the respiratory tract, but also to lymph nodes associated with adjacent organs.

Among the various species, from mice to humans, the respiratory tracts vary greatly in their size, especially in the dimensions of airways that serve to conduct gas and particles between the nares and the alveoli. As will be discussed later, these differences do have a profound influence on the fractional regional deposition of inhaled particles of varied size. These biological differences in respiratory tract dimension may also be a factor in the marked species differences in the long-term pulmonary retention of particles observed among mice, rats, dogs, and humans.

B. Pathology of the Respiratory Tract

The respiratory tract can develop a wide range of diseases partly owing to the numerous cell types it contains. In this section, a brief description is provided of the major mechanisms by which the respiratory tract responds to injury. This summary is intended primarily for nonbiologists. More detailed coverage is provided in Chapters 8–19.

Perhaps the most profound response of cells is death. Indeed, numerous toxic agents, including some reaching the respiratory tract as particles, can kill various lung cells. If the dying cells are not replaced, atrophy occurs. Atrophy plays a significant role in pulmonary emphysema, a disease characterized by a loss of alveolar walls. Adjacent alveoli then coalesce, resulting in larger alveoli, a loss of alveolar surface area, and reduced opportunity for gas exchange.

In addition to induced injury giving rise to cell death, cells also undergo programmed cell death, or apoptosis, as a part of the normal cell cycle. These cells must then be replaced, giving rise to cell proliferation. Compared with some other systems (e.g., the lining cells of the gastrointestinal tract), cells in the respiratory tract turn over at a relatively slow rate in the absence of injury. In response to some types of injury, individual cells may simply increase in size, a process called hypertrophy. In other situations, the number of cells may actually increase, a process called hyperplasia. Both hypertrophy and hyperplasia are observed in response to many different kinds of toxic insults to the respiratory tract.

Deposition of some kinds of microbial agents or particulate materials may give rise to inflammation, in which the response is characterized not only by changes in the cell types already present in the region, but also by recruitment of other inflammatory cells. This includes macrophages and a wide range of hematopoietic cells, especially neutrophils and peripheral monocytes. Inflammatory processes can occur throughout the respiratory tract. The inflammation is called rhinitis if it occurs in the nose, bronchitis if it occurs in the bronchi, and pneumonitis if it involves the lung parenchyma.

The inflammatory process involves complex signaling between cells. The cytokines, which make up one set of signals, are small, typically glycosylated proteins that play a crucial role in regulating cell proliferation, differentiation, and activation. The role of cytokines in pulmonary inflammation and fibrosis is described in an excellent review (15).

Persistent injury can give rise to transdifferentiation or metaplasia in addition to hyperplasia, hypertrophy, and inflammation. With inhaled toxicants, both secretory metaplasia and squamous metaplasia are the most obvious forms of epithelial cell adaptation to injury. Squamous metaplasia tends to be associated with more severe and persistent injury.

Frequently, a late sequelae to chronic inflammation is the development of fibrosis, which is characterized by increased quantities of connective tissue laid down by fibroblasts. Some toxic agents, such as silica, have a special capacity for triggering pulmonary injury and the development of severe fibrosis; when the etiologic agent is silica, the condition is called silicosis. A similar condition seen in coal miners with chronic exposure to coal dust is called coal miners' pneumoconiosis.

One of the disease states of greatest concern for all organ systems, including the respiratory tract, is the development of cancer, which is shorthand for the development of neoplasia, or new growth. In contrast with the disease conditions discussed earlier, neoplasia is manifest after there is a permanent change or, perhaps more accurately, a series of permanent changes in the genetic material of the somatic cells. These permanent changes are called mutations. In reality, cancer is a family of diseases. The specific neoplasms are defined by their histological and cytological characteristics. In general, neoplasms are divided into benign or malignant neoplasia depending on their growth characteristics. Two of the most common respiratory tract neoplasms in humans are bronchial carcinomas, which arise from the bronchial epithelium, and mesothelioma, which arises from the mesothelium lining the pleural cavity.

In evaluating the potential human effects of various kinds of inhaled particles, it is important to recognize that responses of the respiratory tract are rarely unique to a specific toxicant. The respiratory tract has a repertoire of responses that are common to multiple toxicants. Even the few conditions that are described by a term incorporating the agent (e.g., silicosis) share many similarities with diseases caused by other agents, such as coal dust. There are frequently subtle differences in the nature of the diseases; and, most importantly, there may be dramatic differences in the potency of the agents (i.e., the quantity of the agent inhaled to produce the disease). The similarity in the end disease produced by exposure to different agents (e.g., bronchial carcinomas produced by both radon and cigarette smoke) is one of the reasons why conducting epidemiological investigations and detecting low incidences of disease attributable to single toxicants is so difficult. Without question, the overriding influence of cigarette smoking as an etiologic risk factor for most cancers makes the identification of other potential lung carcinogens from epidemiological studies more difficult. Thus, information must be obtained and integrated for human risk assessment purposes from multiple studies using epidemiological approaches, in vitro methods with cells and tissues, and in vivo investigations in both laboratory animals and in human subjects when ethically feasible.

V. Particle Characteristics That Influence Respiratory Tract Toxicity

The physical and chemical characteristics of inhaled particles can have a profound effect on the nature of the toxic effects produced in both laboratory animals and humans. Clearly, not all particles are equivalent from a biological standpoint. A major determinant of how a particle is deposited, retained in the body, and produces effects depends on particle size, as will become apparent in the discussion that follows.

As an aid to the reader, some of the common nomenclature and basic concepts of the field are reviewed. The reader desiring more in-depth coverage is referred to other reviews and authoritative texts (16–18). Systems for conducting inhalation exposures have also been described (19).

A starting point for considering nomenclature is the generic term *aerosol*, which is defined as a relatively stable suspension of solid particles or liquid droplets in a gaseous medium. *Fibers* are a special class of particles, defined as elongated objects for which the aspect ratio—the ratio of the length of the object to its diameter—is greater than 3. The toxicity of fibers is a highly specialized area and will not be dealt with in this chapter. The reader interested in fibers is referred to recent reviews (20,21). The relation between gases and particles and droplets is dynamic (Fig. 3). This figure also shows the terms applied to each of the three modes, as well as related terms used to describe aerosols.

Within the trimodal distribution (see Fig. 3), the largest aerosol particles contained in the largest mode are typically considered to be *dust*, which is classically defined as fine particles of matter (i.e., earth). In common usage, however, the term has been used to describe a wide range of airborne materials originating in the broadest sense from the earth. In the interest of completeness, some related terms are defined. *Fumes* are formed by combustion, sublimation, or condensation, usually with a change in chemical form; metal oxide fumes are a good example. They typically start as very small particles of angstrom size and coagulate or flocculate to form larger particles. *Smokes* are formed by combustion of organic materials, and their particles are usually smaller than 0.5 μm in diameter.

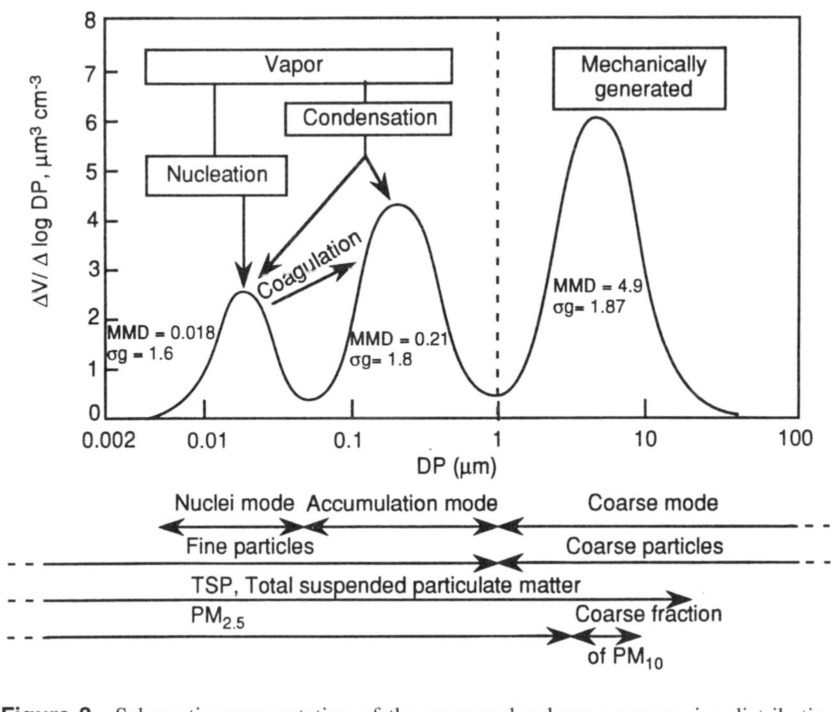

Figure 3 Schematic representation of the measured volume or mass size distribution of airborne particles illustrating the dynamic relation between the suspending medium and particles of varied size. (From Ref. 105.)

Mists and *fogs* are liquid aerosols formed either by condensation of a liquid on particulate nuclei in air, or by uptake of liquid by hygroscopic particles. The term *smog*, a contraction of smoke and fog, has usually been applied to a complex mixture of particles and gases in an atmosphere originating from combustion. Although the term smog dates to episodes of pollution in London at the beginning of the industrial revolution, more recently, it has been used to describe polluted atmospheres arising from solar irradiation of vehicle emissions and other combustion products.

In the United States, *particulate matter* is a term that has found wide usage as a result of legislated requirements under the Clean Air Act (CAA; 22). The CAA requires the US Environmental Protection Agency (EPA) to list pollutants that may reasonably be anticipated to endanger public health or welfare and to issue air quality criteria for them; hence, the term *criteria pollutants*. Particulate matter is identified as a criteria pollutant for which the EPA will develop criteria and establish National Ambient Air Quality Standards (NAAQS), as will be discussed in detail later.

The first NAAQS for particulate matter was set in 1971 and was based on *total suspended material* (TSP; Fig. 4). Basically, compliance with this standard involved collection of particulate matter on a filter that sampled all the air that could be drawn through a high-volume sampler. Only the wide-range aerosol collector (WRAC) samples a wider range of particle sizes than does the TSP sampler. Many of the large particles collected by a TSP or WRAC have a very low probability of being inhaled, and an even smaller fraction have potential for being deposited in the pulmonary region. In 1987, the TSP standard was replaced with a standard based on collection of particles using an aerodynamic-sampling system with 50% efficiency for particles with a 10-μm–aerodynamic diameter. Hence, the term *particulate material, 10 μm* (PM_{10}). The corresponding term for a sample with 50% efficiency at 2.5 μm is $PM_{2.5}$. The term *fine particle fraction* has been used for particles smaller than 2.5 μm in diameter, and the term *coarse particle fraction* for particles in the range of 2.5- to 10-μm–aerodynamic diameter. The EPA is giving consideration in 1996 to adding a $PM_{2.5}$ standard as a NAAQS for PM.

Particles can be characterized in several ways to aid in evaluating their potential health consequences. Three interrelated size parameters are of interest: volume, surface, and number (Fig. 5). Toxicologists have traditionally given greatest emphasis to characterizing the volume or mass characteristics of airborne particles being studied. Only in recent years has appropriate consideration been given to characterizing aerosols based on the distribution of the aerosol being studied. The importance of characterizing aerosols by their size distribution for biological studies first gained prominence in work with radioactive aerosols and has only recently been extended to work with chemical toxicants. Very recently

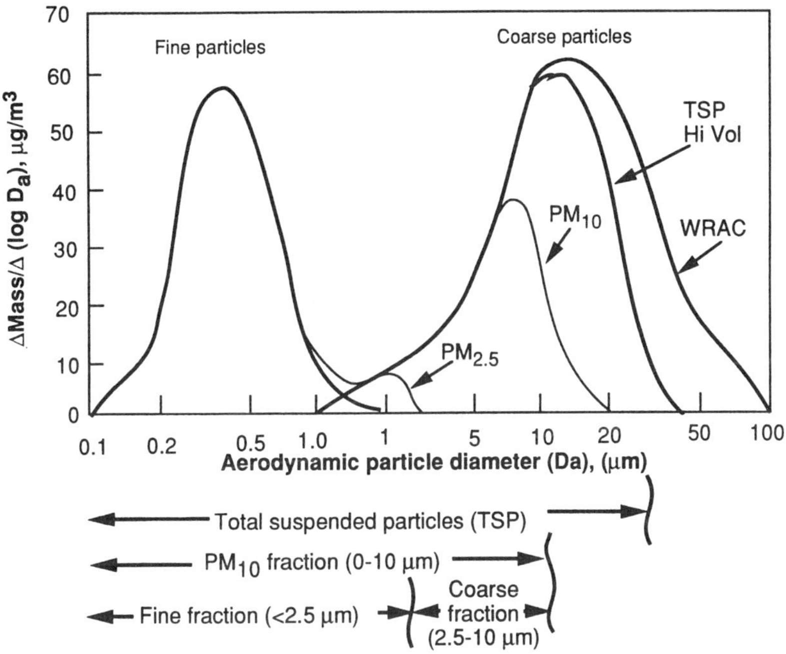

Figure 4 Schematic representation of the relation between different parameters used to describe the size distribution of airborne particles. (From Ref. 106.)

concern has developed for the potential toxicity of ultrafine particles for which particle number may be a more appropriate ''dose metric'' than particle mass.

Deposition in the human respiratory tract of airborne particles is now well known to be governed largely by the aerodynamic and diffusion size characteristics of the particles. For particles smaller than about 0.5 μm, the relevant parameter is the *diameter* of the particles. Diffusion diameter is measured using a sampling device such as one that uses multiple fine screens to measure diffusional characteristics of the particles. For particles larger than a few tenths of a micron, the inertial characteristics (determined by aerodynamic drag) of the particles dominate the deposition process. These characteristics are taken into account when an aerosol sampling device, such as a cascade impactor, is used that characterizes the aerosol particles' aerodynamic diameter and its geometric standard deviation. The parameter measured, *aerodynamic diameter*, represents the diameter of a unit density sphere having the same terminal setting velocity as the particle sampled, whatever its size, shape, and density. It is important to characterize

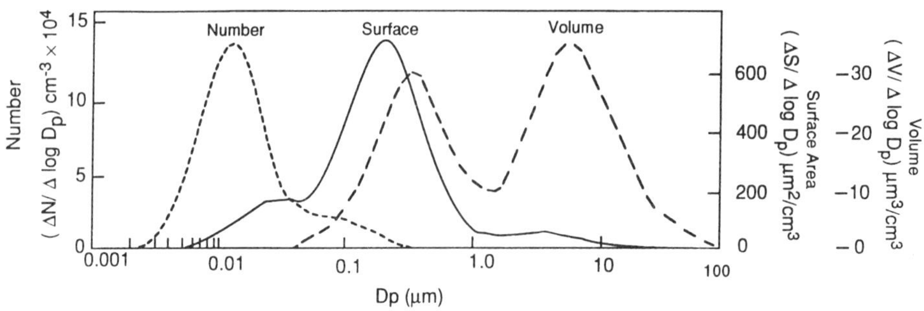

Mode

number	Nucleation or ultrafine	Accumulation or fine	Coarse
DGN	7.7×10^4	1.3×10^4	–
δg	0.013	0.069	–
Surface ($\mu m^2/cm^3$)	1.7	2.03	–
DGS	74	535	41
δg	0.023	0.19	3.1
Volume ($\mu m^3/cm^3$)	–	–	2.15
DGV	0.33	22	29
	0.031	0.31	5.7

DGN = geometric mean diameter by number

DGS = geometric mean diameter by surface area

DGV = geometric mean diameter by volume

Figure 5 Distribution of coarse, accumulation, or fine, and nucleation or ultrafine mode particles by three characteristics: DGV, geometric mean diameter by volume; DGS, geometric mean diameter by surface area; DGN, geometric mean diameter by number. (From Ref. 107.)

the median particle size, the *mass median aerodynamic diameter*, and the degree of dispersity, expressed as the geometric standard deviation, assuming that the particle sizes are normally distributed. If radioactivity is measured, rather than mass, the appropriate term is *activity median* aerodynamic diameter. The *aerodynamic size distribution* of the aerosol is important because aerodynamic size governs particle deposition by factors that involve inertia, such as impaction and sedimentation.

The potential toxicological importance of particle number has only recently been recognized. Unfortunately, sufficient experimentation has not been performed under rigorously controlled conditions to determine if particle number, rather than particle mass, is more important for producing toxic effects for some particles. From Figure 5, one can recognize that particle number might be of special importance when there are many particles smaller than 0.1 μm in diffusion diameter. In that size range, distinguishing between the closely related parameters of particle number and surface area is also a challenge (i.e., surface area per unit mass of particle increases with decreased particle size and increasing particle number). From a practical standpoint, recognizing that such small particles quickly aggregate in the atmosphere to become larger particles is necessary (see Fig. 3).

Before concluding this discussion of the characterization of airborne particulate material, three concepts should be emphasized: (1) Aerosols are typically heterogeneous in size; rarely is an aerosol encountered in which particles are all of the same size (i.e., a monodisperse aerosol). Typically, a given atmosphere contains a distribution of particle sizes. This is usually true in laboratory settings and is almost always true in occupational and environmental settings. (2) The chemical composition of atmospheres encountered in the real world is almost always heterogeneous. Usually, chemically homogenous experimental atmospheres are created only in the laboratory. (3) The atmosphere is a dynamic system. Both chemical reactions, such as those that occur with formation of photochemical oxidants, and physical forces produce continuous change. Diffusion, or brownian motion, serves to bring particles together and into contact with surfaces. Diffusion is especially dominant for very small particles. For larger particles,

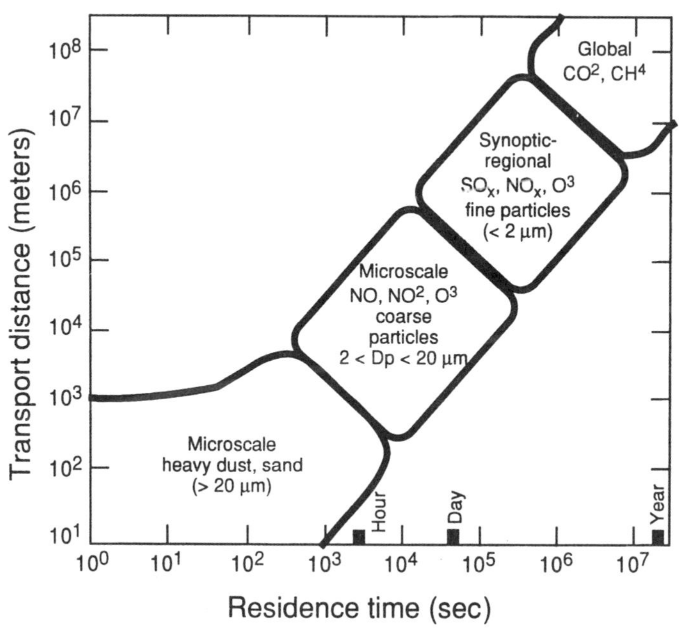

Figure 6 Relation of spatial and temporal scales for coarse and fine particles in the atmosphere.

gravitational settling is most important and serves to cleanse the air. Rainout and washout are important for particles of intermediate size. The relations of the spatial and temporal scales to particle size characteristics are shown in Figure 6. Larger particles, including those characterized as nuisance dusts, are of greatest concern in the micro- and mesoscale dimensions and in close proximity to the sources. Conversely, longer time scales and larger spatial distributions are dominated by smaller particles. However, one should remain alert to mesoscale events in pollution episodes, which involve short-lived chemical species associated with small particles.

VI. Sources of Particulate Material

Particulate material is ubiquitously distributed, partly because there are many sources. The concentration, particle size, and chemical characteristics of particulate material vary widely in both space and time. Distinctions are commonly drawn between occupational and environmental (or perhaps, more appropriately, nonoccupational) settings, with the latter subdivided into the outdoor (or ambient) versus indoor environment. For the ambient environment, a distinction is customarily made between stationary point sources (e.g., a factory or refinery) and mobile sources (e.g., automobiles and trucks). Roadways are line sources. The occupational environment also has subdivisions that can vary markedly in their particulate matter content, depending on the particular processes being carried out in different work areas. The document *Air Quality Criteria for Particulate Material* (23) is an excellent summary of information on sources and characteristics of particulate matter, with special reference to the United States.

The exposure of any individual depends upon the amount of time spent in various microenvironments and the particulate matter content of each area. The range of microenvironments encountered by individuals is quite varied, with the indoor residential environment predominating. On the average, individuals spend nearly 70% of their time indoors, either at home or at work.

Concern for relations between exposure to particulate matter and health centers primarily on two microenvironments, the workplace and the ambient outdoor environment, which is perhaps surprising, considering the distributions of time individuals spend in the various environments. Attention has focused on the workplace because workplace exposures to particulate matter have clearly yielded health effects in the past. As a result, responsible employers have voluntarily taken steps to limit occupational exposures. In addition, various national and international agencies have developed guidelines and standards to limit workplace exposures.

A consideration of the myriad of occupational situations and the wide range of particulate matter environments is beyond the scope of this chapter. A key point to bear in mind is that a spectrum of conditions exists in the range of current occupational standards from very dusty environments, to very well controlled environments, such as clean rooms in the microelectronics industry that are virtually free of particles. If an attempt is to be made—and it should be—to use particles for experimental toxicological studies, industrial hygiene measurements to characterize the particles in the specific occupational setting that is of interest should be obtained. The particulate matter in a facility producing or using carbon black is very different from that in a facility in which plastics are being machined versus a metalworking shop.

The ambient environment also varies widely in particle content. Although such information is country-specific, information for the United States will be briefly reviewed to illustrate the general characteristics of such data.

Significant geographic differences in particulate matter exist in the United States. In the western United States, annual PM_{10} concentrations were about 50 $\mu g/m^3$ in 1985 and decreased by about one-half by 1993. In the eastern United States, the annual PM_{10} average was about 35 $\mu g/m^3$ in 1985 and decreased by one-third by 1993. The second highest maximum 24-hr concentration of PM_{10} for most areas ranged from 35 up to about 90 $\mu g/m^3$. However, some metropolitan areas had second highest maximum daily PM_{10} measurements in the 100- to 200-$\mu g/m^3$ range. In general, PM_{10} measurements are usually somewhat higher in the

Table 1 Concentration Ranges of Various Elements Associated with Particulate Matter in the U.S. Atmosphere

	Concentration range (ng/m^3)		
Element	Remote	Rural	Urban
As	0.007–1.9	1.0–28	2–2320
Cd	0.003–1.1	0.4–1000	0.2–7000
Ni	0.01–60	0.6–78	1–328
Pb	0.007–64	2–1700	30–96,270
V	0.001–14	2.7–97	0.4–1460
Zn	0.03–460	11–403	15–8328
Co	0.001–0.9	0.08–10.1	0.2–83
Cr	0.005–11.2	1.1–44	2.2–124
Cu	0.029–12	3–280	3–5140
Fe	0.62–4160	55–14,530	130–13,800
Hg	0.005–1.3	0.05–160	0.58–458
Mn	0.01–16.7	3.7–99	4–488
Se	0.0056–0.19	0.01–3.0	0.2–30
Sb	0.0008–1.19	0.6–7	0.5–171

Source: Ref. 102.

western than in the eastern United States. In addition, peak concentrations of PM_{10}, and especially of $PM_{2.5}$, occur in winter in the West, whereas they peak in the summer in the East. Significant regional differences also exist in the chemical composition of particulate matter. Minerals of crustal origin are high in the West: 70% of the coarse fraction and 15% of the $PM_{2.5}$ fraction, versus only 52 and 4% of the same fractions in the East. Carbon of organic origin is a higher proportion (39%) in the West compared with the East (21%). Likewise, elemental carbon is higher in the West (15%) than in the East (4%). Conversely, ammonium sulfate represents a much higher proportion of particulate matter in the East (47%) than in the West (15%).

Concentration ranges for various elements associated with particulate material are given in Table 1. There is a broad range of concentrations for a given element in samples collected in urban, rural, or remote sites and within a given site classification. There is a difference of nearly three orders of magnitude in measured concentration from the least abundant element, selenium, to the most abundant element, lead. The higher concentrations of lead are partly related to its previous wide use in commerce, particularly as a gasoline additive, and in paint.

VII. Disposition of Inhaled Particles

The dose to the respiratory tract has a central role in linking what is in the air to the health responses the particles may cause (see Fig. 1). This requires an understanding of the disposition of particles in the body; their deposition in the respiratory tract, and subsequent retention (and conversely, clearance) in the respiratory tract and translocation to other organs. These topics are covered in detail in Chapters 5–7. Schlesinger (24) has also provided a useful review, and this chapter provides a broad overview of these topics.

A. Deposition of Inhaled Particles

The site and magnitude of deposition of particles in the respiratory tract is determined by physical mechanisms and the biology of the subject inhaling the particles. The five most significant mechanisms of deposition are sedimentation, impaction, diffusion, interception, and electrostatic precipitation (Fig. 7).

Deposition by sedimentation and impaction is a function of the inertial aerodynamic size characteristics of the aerosol particles. Deposition by diffusion is a function of the diffusional properties of the aerosol. Deposition by interception occurs when one of the edges of a particle touches the surface of the respiratory tract. Interception is an especially important determinant of deposition of fibers. Deposition of particles in the respiratory tract by electrostatic precipitation

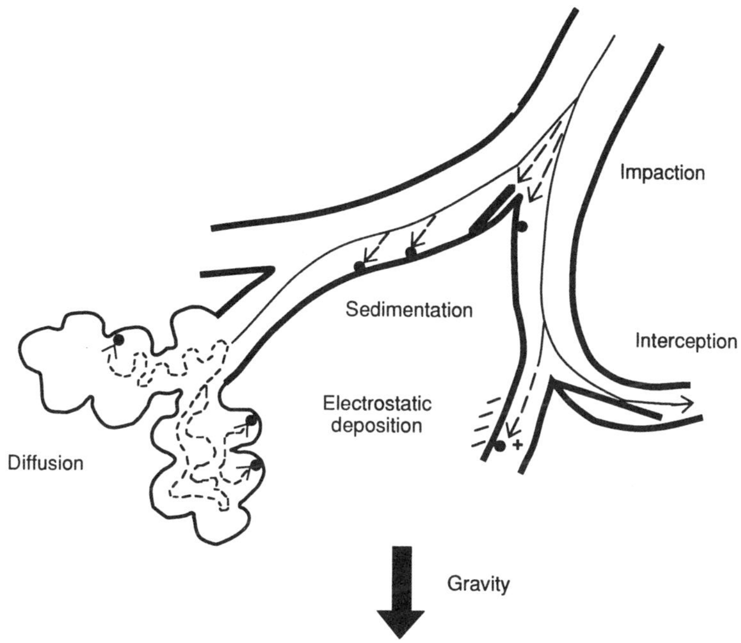

Figure 7 Primary mechanisms of deposition of inhaled particles in the respiratory tract.

is usually negligible because suspended particles in air are at equilibrium charge distribution.

The biological characteristics of the individual inhaling the particles also influences deposition. The two major determinants are the volumes of air inhaled, as determined by respiratory rate and tidal volume, and the dimensional characteristics of the respiratory tract. Dimension is especially critical in scaling between species and as influenced by age (and growth) within a species. Miller et al. (25) raised the possibility of altered patterns of deposition of particles within the lungs of individuals with respiratory disease.

In evaluating potential health consequences of airborne particles, it is important to consider fractional deposition within the three major subdivisions of the respiratory tract (Fig. 8), the airways of the nasopharyngeal (head), tracheobronchial, and pulmonary regions, as well as a summation representing total deposition. Fractional deposition in various regions is related to particle size. For sizes larger than about 0.5 μm in diameter, the metric most relevant for determining deposition is the aerodynamic diameter of the particles. For the smallest particles, the appropriate particle characterization metric related to deposition is the diffusion equivalent diameter. When considering the potential deposition and

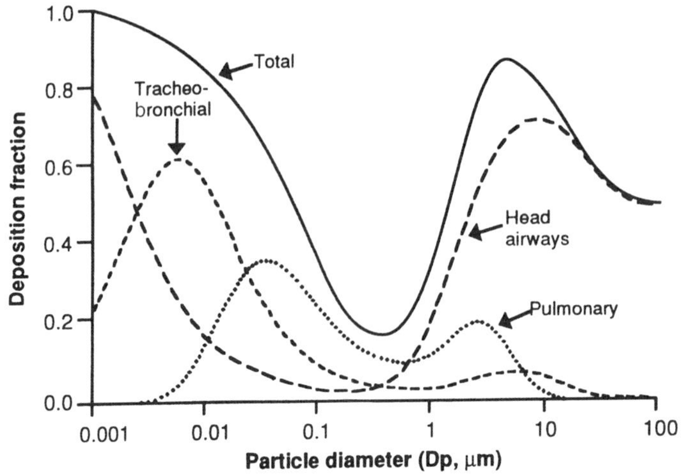

Figure 8 Deposition of particles in the major regions of the human respiratory tract related to particle size. (From Ref. 108.)

subsequent clearance of particles, both the median size and the dispersity of the aerosol must be considered. For example, even an aerosol with a mass median aerodynamic diameter of 5.0 μm could have a large number of particles in the aerodynamic size range of 2.0–3.0 μm if the aerosol is sufficiently polydisperse in size distribution.

Evaluation of the toxicity of airborne particulate matter frequently requires that studies be conducted in laboratory animals to complement and extend the limited data usually available from direct observation of humans. In developing and evaluating data obtained in laboratory animal species, a recognition of the marked differences observed between species in the fractional and spatial deposition of inhaled particles is critically important (24,26).

These species differences are of profound importance when making extrapolations from laboratory animals to humans. For example, particles larger than 3.0-μm–median aerodynamic diameter have a low probability of being inhaled and deposited in the alveolar region of rats, whereas particles 3.0–5.0 μm in median aerodynamic diameter still have a relatively high probability of being deposited in the alveolar region of humans. Because of these species differences, the use of rats to evaluate a particulate test material with a mass median aerodynamic diameter larger than about 3.0 μm may not be appropriate. Certainly, if such particulate matter were studied using rats, species differences must be considered in making the extrapolation to humans. Such an extrapolation would be greatly facilitated by having measured the lung burden of the test material at various times during the study. An example is the classic study of the disposition of inhaled exhaust particles by Wolff et al. (27). Extrapolations based on the measured lung burdens in rats and the projected lung burdens for humans exposed to particulate matter of that size have far greater validity than extrapolations made solely on measurements of particulate matter in air. We must move beyond measurements of exposure and measure or assess the delivered dose to individuals.

To overcome the difficulties associated with studying materials consisting of large particles, some investigators have either physically reduced the size of the particles by grinding or have size-separated the material and only used fractions of the smallest size. If either of these approaches is used, the use of size-selected particulate material must be taken into account when the data are extrapolated back to human exposure situations. For example, a material that normally consists primarily of particles 100 μm or larger, as it is delivered for use in an industrial process, could be reduced to particles a few micrometers in aerodynamic diameter and studied in rats. The studies of Bellmann et al. (28) and Muhle et al. (29) with toner are examples of using such an approach. If the particles studied represent only a very small fraction of the mass of particulate material found in workplace samples, that some large quantity of the particles of reduced size produce mild or moderate toxic effects in rats may still translate to limited significance for humans.

The foregoing discussion has focused on the lung, or pulmonary, burden of particulate matter. Marked differences in both upper respiratory and tracheobronchial fractional deposition also exist between rats and humans over the size range of 0.1–3.0 μm. For particles in the size range of 0.1–0.3 μm, fractional deposition is high in the upper respiratory tract of rats, whereas it is very low in humans. Thus particles of 0.1–0.3 μm might produce toxicity in the noses of rats, but have limited relevance for humans. Likewise, for particles 2.0–4.0 μm in aerodynamic diameter, the low fractional deposition in the tracheobronchial region of rats may result in an underestimation of the likely human toxicity of the material, recognizing that a human might deposit some 10–20% of material of this size in the tracheobronchial region.

Most of the fractional deposition data that are available have been obtained with particles larger than 0.5 μm in aerodynamic size using mass as the particle metric or radioactivity as a surrogate for mass. Relatively little quantitative data are available for particles smaller than 1.0 μm aerodynamic diameter or in the range of 0.5 μm, either aerodynamic diameter or diffusion-equivalent diameter, a size for which both aerodynamic and diffusion characteristics are important influences on deposition. A related consideration is the extent to which both the particle number and particle surface area per unit mass increase markedly as particle size decreases. These factors need to be taken into account when attempting to use laboratory animals to obtain data relevant to assessing human risks of fine particles.

When conducting studies using the inhalation route of entry, interindividual differences will be observed in the amount of material deposited, much more so than with parenteral administration of a toxicant. This is illustrated in Figure 9, with data on the lung burdens of dogs exposed once to relatively insoluble particles labeled with a radioactive tracer to aid in quantitating the amount of material inhaled and deposited (30). For comparison, data are shown for lung burdens of titanium measured in humans. The variability shown for the dogs reflects both the true interindividual variability as well as intraindividual variability for multiple studies of deposition conducted on the same animal. When groups of animals are exposed repeatedly, the range of lung burdens is reduced substantially.

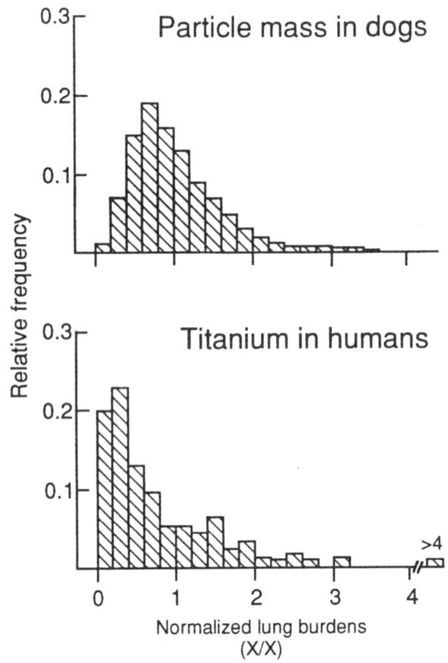

Figure 9 Lung burdens in dogs following single brief exposures to relatively insoluble particles labeled with radioactive tracers and measured human lung burdens of titanium. (From Ref. 30.)

B. Particle Clearance and Retention

The clearance of particles from the respiratory tract may be viewed as the first line of defense of the respiratory tract to protect the body from toxic effects of the deposited particles. The responses of the respiratory tract will also vary depending on where the particles are deposited, extending from the nares to the alveolar spaces (see Fig. 8). Although the clearance of particles and related activities are initiated as physiologically adaptive responses, they can progress and become pathological responses, as will be discussed later.

Let us first consider particle clearance from the respiratory tract when exposure concentrations are lower than those that elicit pathological alterations. Clearance at low-exposure concentrations involves interplay between mechanical and biological mechanisms. In all regions of the respiratory tract, macrophages are present that begin engulfing particles as soon as they are deposited. Both the free particles and those that are engulfed are available for mechanical removal.

Particulate matter deposited in the nasopharyngeal portions of the respiratory tract can trigger serous or mucous secretion and flow. The serous fluid or mucus moves either anteriorly to the nares, where it is removed by blowing or dripping, or posteriorly into the pharynx, where it may be swallowed. Sensory elements may also be triggered that evoke sneezing to drive out the fluid or mucus. (Chapters 13 and 14 reviews the biology and pathobiology of respiratory tract mucus.)

Particulate matter deposited in the trachea and conducting airways encounters a blanket of mucus moving on top of beating cilia in normal persons (Fig. 10). The particles entrapped within macrophages or directly within the mucus are carried up the mucociliary escalator to the pharynx, where the material is swallowed. Because of the clearance of particulate matter to the pharynx from either the nasopharynx or the trachea, with subsequent ingestion, essentially all inhalation exposures also involve ingestion of particulate matter. The time period for tracheobronchial clearance for most of the particulate matter is on the order of hours. A small fraction may be cleared more slowly, and there is evidence that a very small fraction may actually be carried into the epithelial cells and the underlying tissue. In some individuals, neurogenic receptors may be stimulated, triggering coughing and also causing constriction of airways and altered resistance to airflow.

Particulate matter that reaches the alveolar spaces has a high probability of being ingested by macrophages. If the particles are nontoxic, they reside in individual macrophages until they die, and then the particulate matter and debris are engulfed by other macrophages. Over time, some portion of the particles, presumably largely within macrophages, reaches the terminal bronchioles, gains access to the mucociliary escalator, and is removed from the body. Other particles

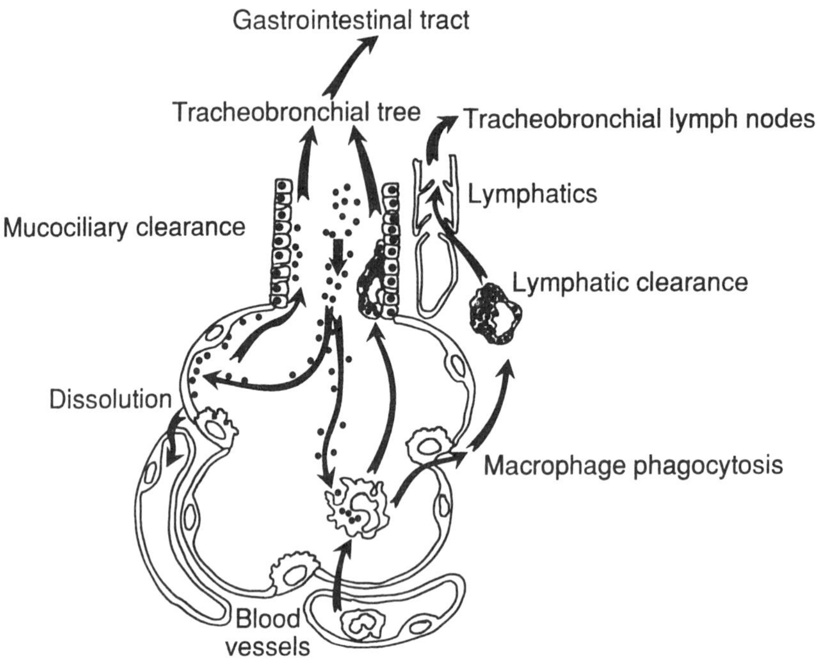

Figure 10 Schematic rendering of the mechanisms of clearance of inhaled particles deposited in the respiratory tract. (Courtesy of Dr. Patrick J. Haley, Nycomed R&D, Inc., Collegeville, PA.)

may be carried to the interstitial spaces by macrophages or other inflammatory cells or by direct penetration. Some particulate matter is transported to the regional lymph nodes through the lymphatics, and some particulate matter may gain access directly to the bloodstream. The chemical form of the particles and their real size (i.e., their surface area) determines their rate of dissolution and, therefore, their clearance, as contrasted with the aerodynamic and diffusion properties that govern deposition. The solutes from the particulate matter form complexes with macromolecules and are retained in the immediate area or transported away (31). The smaller the particles, the greater the ratio of surface area to particle mass and the more rapid the rate of dissolution. The rate of dissolution of particulate matter also depends on its chemical composition.

Significant differences exist among species in the rate of removal of inhaled particulate matter. These differences are perhaps most evident for long-term clearance of PM from the pulmonary region (Fig. 11a) and translocation to lung-associated lymph nodes (see Fig. 11b). The basis for the marked difference in

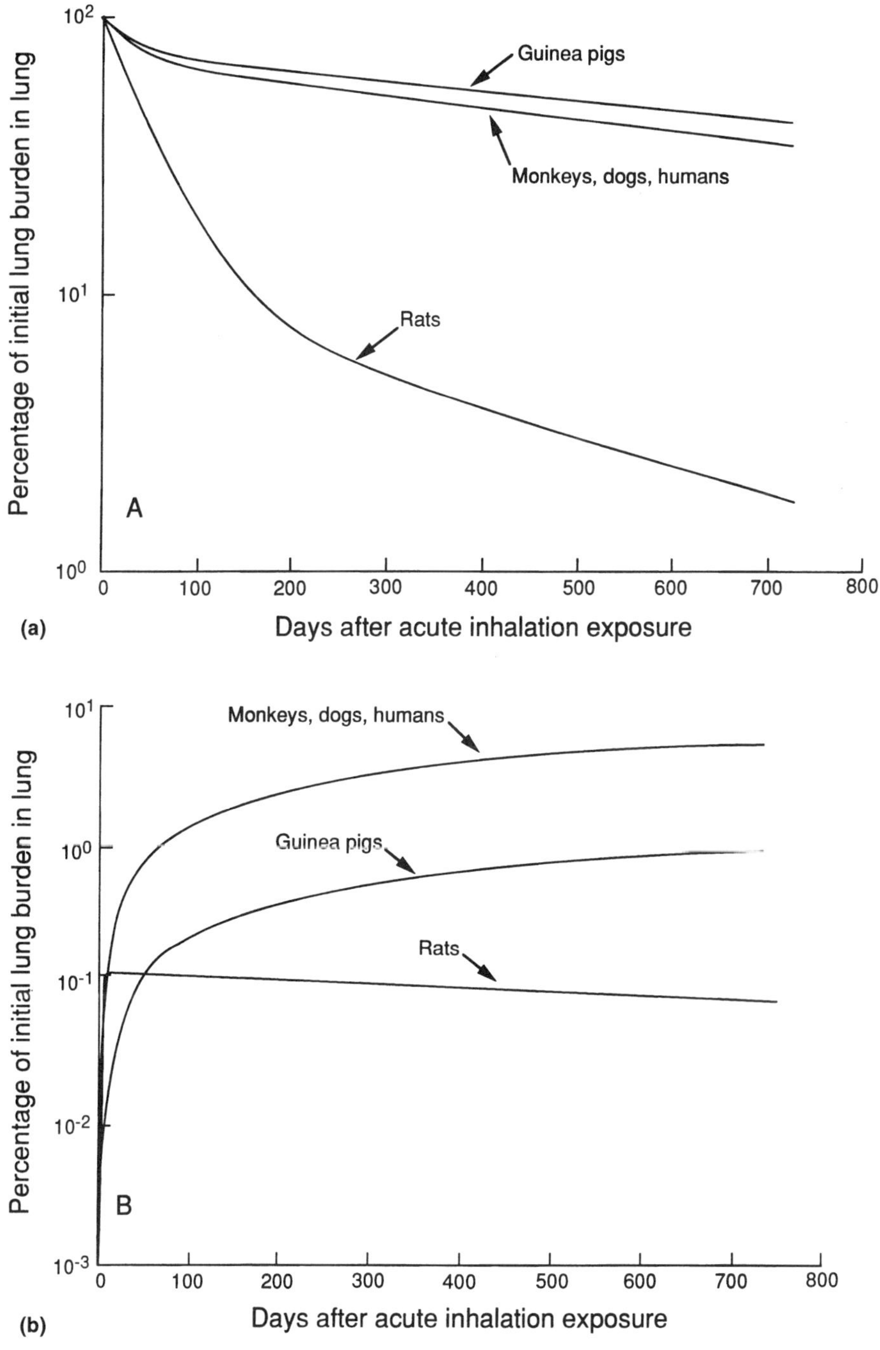

Figure 11 Schematic rendering of the clearance of relatively insoluble particles from (a) pulmonary region and (b) accumulation in lung-associated lymph nodes in several species following a single brief inhalation exposure. (From Ref. 32.)

clearance among mice, rats, dogs, and humans is not well understood. This is an intriguing basic biology issue with influence on toxicology and risk assessment that deserves additional attention. Quite possibly differences in macrophage trafficking in the several species could play a role. The existence of these interspecies' differences must be kept in mind when extrapolating data on the toxicity of inhaled particles from laboratory animals to humans. When considering clearance, the real concern is not for what has been cleared, but rather, the converse, what is retained and its potential for causing toxic effects.

This is illustrated in Figure 12 with the results of simulation modeling of the deposition and retention in the lungs of inhaled relatively insoluble particles. Both the shape of the build-up curves and the differences among species should be noted. The lung burdens always slowly increase over a period of months to ultimately reach lung burdens that are at equilibrium with the concentration of particles in the air. This equilibrium relation varies among the several species commonly used for inhalation toxicity studies and humans.

Occasionally, the equilibrium relation between air concentration and lung

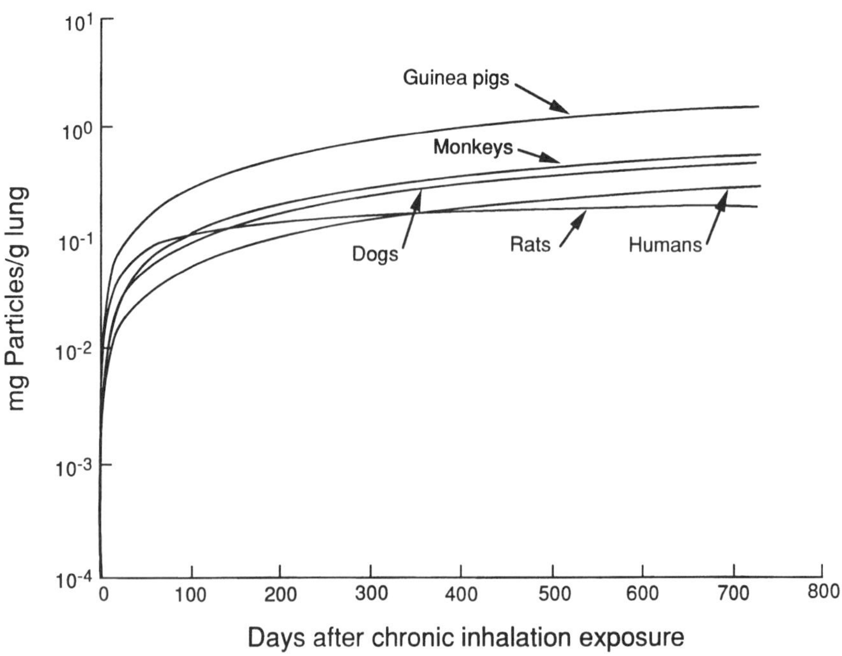

Figure 12 Simulation model results of the accumulation of particles in the lungs of several species after chronic exposure to an atmosphere containing 0.5 mg/m^3 of particulate matter. (From Ref. 32.)

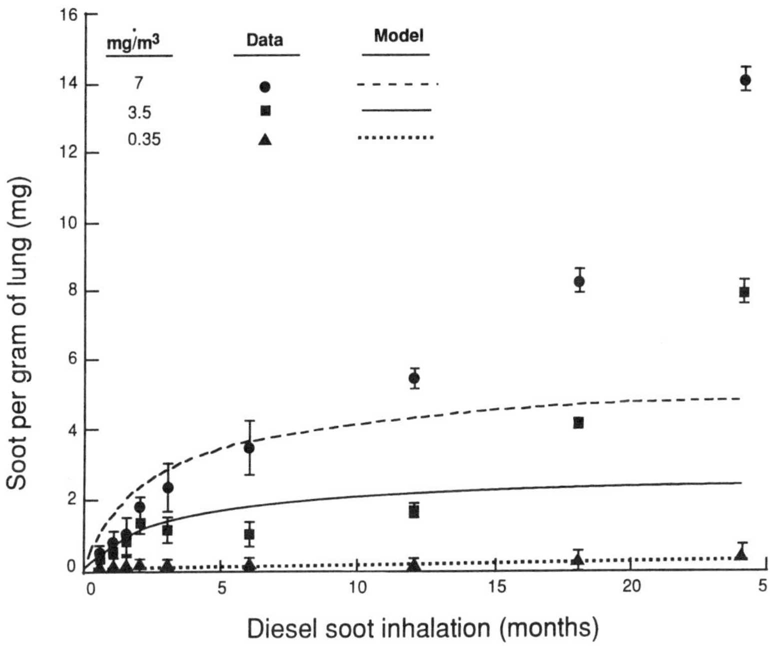

Figure 13 Lung burdens of diesel soot particles in rats chronically exposed to diesel exhaust: The means and standard errors are plotted for data from animals killed at various times after exposures were initiated and compared with simulation model results, assuming no effect of exposure concentration on deposition or clearance of particles.

burden may be perturbed by pathological changes associated with the rate of particle deposition, the accumulated lung burden of particles, or both. This is illustrated in Figure 13 with data from a study with rats exposed to various air concentrations of diesel soot (27,32). As will be discussed in greater detail later, exposure concentration–related pathology developed. Lung burdens at the two highest exposure concentrations (3.5 and 7.0 mg/m^3) were much greater than predicted based on the kinetics observed at the lowest exposure concentration (0.35 mg/m^3). This is the so-called overload phenomenon described by McClellan (33) and Morrow (34). These and related data from other studies with diesel soot and other insoluble particulate materials have been modeled (35–38).

VIII. Responses of the Respiratory Tract

The respiratory tract has a limited number of ways it can respond to inhaled particles. The initial responses are intended to clear the particles from the respiratory tract and, indeed, from the body. However, responses that begin as physiologically adaptive can also progress and become pathological.

A. Noncarcinogenic Responses

Chapters 8 to 19 review the noncarcinogenic responses to particulate material. The initial responses of coughing and sneezing triggered by stimulation of neurogenic receptors are generally viewed as being physiological, but even they can continue to the extent that the afflicted person may begin to wonder if they are more than a nuisance. Production of serous fluid and mucus is initially increased by discharging of intracellular stores and may then progress to hypertrophy of the existing cells and, at the extreme, hyperplasia of these cells.

The continuous insult of cells lining the nasal cavity and trachea, bronchi, and lower airways can be sufficient to result in metaplastic transformations. Sometimes, this may progress to sheets of squamous cells lining portions of the conducting airways.

With prolonged exposure to particulate matter at sufficiently high concentrations, the particulate matter continuously deposited in the alveolar spaces can trigger a sustained inflammatory reaction. The inflammation can alter particle clearance, initially increase the rate of clearance, and then later cause inhibition of clearance. This, in turn, intensifies the inflammatory reaction, which further impairs clearance and enhances the rate of particle accumulation in the alveolar region. Some of these particles are found in the interstitial areas and others in the alveolar spaces, where aggregates of macrophages, particles, and proteinaceous material may be observed. Adjacent epithelial cells become hypertrophic, hyperplastic, and occasionally, metaplastic. Frequently, bronchiolar epithelium may appear to be extending down into the alveoli. This pattern of particle-induced overload disease has been described in detail in rats chronically exposed to diesel exhaust or carbon black particles (39,40). The extent to which similar lesions are produced in humans exposed to similar levels of diesel soot or carbon black is not well understood.

Traditionally, many kinds of particulate matter have not been considered to produce significant structural changes in the respiratory tract and, hence, were traditionally called *nuisance dusts*. The relative lack of response to particulate matter was viewed as contrasting with the responses to materials that produced a clear adverse effect in the form of granulomas or fibrosis. The pulmonary reaction to these dusts has occasionally been termed a benign pneumoconiosis to distinguish a mild reaction from the very severe pulmonary reaction to a fibrogenic material, such as silica.

Recent studies with rats exposed for 2 years or longer to high concentrations of particulate material, which formerly might have been classified as a nuisance or inert dust, have demonstrated that even these materials are not inert when the exposure rate, exposure time, and total exposure are substantial. One view of the results is that they, again, demonstrate, the universality of the axiom, ''The dose makes the poison.'' An alternative view is that the studies provide a signal for possible human responses to these materials and in doing so suggest the need for caution and the use of appropriate protective procedures (limiting workplace exposure concentrations, respiratory protection, or both) when working with any kind of particulate matter to minimize the potential for human disease (41,42).

One way to consider the possible health effects of inhaled particles is to consider the statistics on both acute and chronic respiratory diseases in humans, with the assumption that some portion of these diseases may be attributed to particles. Such statistics for the United States are shown in Tables 2 and 3. In considering these data, it is important to recall the overwhelming influence of cigarette smoking on respiratory disease. This influence is so great that it complicates attempts to establish the role of occupational or environmental factors, including particulate matter, in causing respiratory disease. Nonetheless, as reviewed in the Criteria Document for particulate matter (23) and in Chapters 18 and 19, some portion of these conditions can be attributed to particulate matter other than cigarette smoke.

The magnitude of morbidity for respiratory tract conditions is such that mortality also results. As reviewed in Chapter 19, several studies have demonstrated excess mortality associated with elevated levels of PM exposure. The results of one such study are shown in Figure 14. In this study, excess deaths were apparent in those individuals older than 65 years of age. The total death rate was elevated as well as death rates for chronic obstructive pulmonary disease

Table 2 Effect of Acute Respiratory Conditions in the United States, 1994, Expressed per 100 Persons per Year

Condition	Number of persons[a]	Bed days[a]	Restricted activity days[a]	Lost work days[b]
Common cold	25.4	24.0	61.8	17.6
Other upper respiratory infections	11.9	12.2	28.8	8.8
Influenza	34.8	65.5	121.5	56.4
Acute bronchitis	4.7	10.8	25.9	11.0
Pneumonia	1.6	15.4	24.8	8.9
Other respiratory conditions	2.0	5.2	9.7	2.6
Total	80.5	133.1	272.5	105.3

[a] All ages.
[b] All ages 18 years and older, currently employed persons.
Source: Ref. 103.

Table 3 Prevalence of Chronic Diseases of the Respiratory Tract for All Ages, United States, 1994

Condition	Number (per 1000 persons)
Chronic bronchitis	54.0
Asthma	56.1
Hay fever or allergic rhinitis without asthma	100.7
Chronic sinusitis	134.4
Deviated nasal septum	7.8
Chronic disease of tonsils or adenoids	11.3
Emphysema	7.8
Total	372.1

Source: Ref. 103.

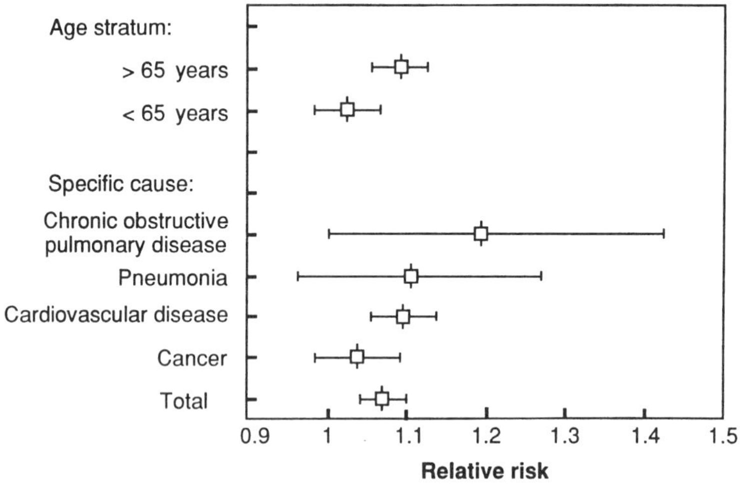

Figure 14 Relative risk of mortality in Philadelphia, 1973–1980, associated with 100 μg/m^3 of total suspended material (TSP) analyzed by age and specific cause of death (COPD, chronic obstructive pulmonary disease; pneumonia; CVP, cardiovascular disease; and cancer). (From Ref. 109.)

(COPD), pneumonia, cardiovascular disease, and cancer. For all the specific causes, the confidence intervals were very broad, and statistical significance was present only for the population older than 65 years of age and for deaths caused by cardiovascular disease.

A review by Moolgavkar and Luebeck (43) notes the difficulty in conducting and interpreting the results of epidemiological studies of air pollution. They note the difficulty of appropriately adjusting for confounding factors. They agree that the effects being attributed to particulate matter may actually be due to multiple pollutants that are all increased in many air pollution episodes. In an evaluation of data for Philadelphia from 1974 to 1988 (the data used to produce Fig. 14), Samet et al. (44) draws very similar conclusions.

Long-term studies with laboratory animals, most notably rats, involving long-term exposure to particle concentrations many times greater than those alleged to produce increased mortality in humans have uniformly failed to demonstrate differences in life span between control and particle-exposed groups until overt disease was produced. An example is the study of Mauderly et al. (45) in which the life span of even the highest diesel exhaust-exposed group, 7000 $\mu g/m^3$, 6 hr/day, 5 days/week, was no different from the control group, even when the diesel exhaust-exposed rats had an increased incidence of lung tumors. One possible explanation is that most laboratory animal studies are initiated with healthy young animals. Rarely are studies conducted using old animals with serious preexisting cardiopulmonary disease, animals that might more closely mimic the human subpopulations thought to be at increased risk from exposure to particulate material.

B. Carcinogenic Responses

Lung cancer is one of the leading causes of death in many countries, and generally the vast majority of these cases are attributed to cigarette smoking. The importance of lung cancer as a cause of death is readily apparent in Figure 15. The difference in the cancer mortality curves between men and women is generally thought to relate to men having begun smoking earlier than women, with a large number of women becoming smokers after they joined the workforce in World War II. The possible downturn in the lung cancer mortality curve for men is encouraging. For women, it is disappointing to note that the curve continues to increase in parallel with that for men, only being shifted 30 years later. This is generally attributed to women beginning to smoke at a rate comparable with men beginning with World War II. In California, lung cancer mortality for women has already begun to match that for men.

As was true for the morbidity data, most lung cancers are generally believed to be due to cigarette smoking. A small portion of the cases may be attributable to environmental tobacco smoke or residential radon. From data on the distribu-

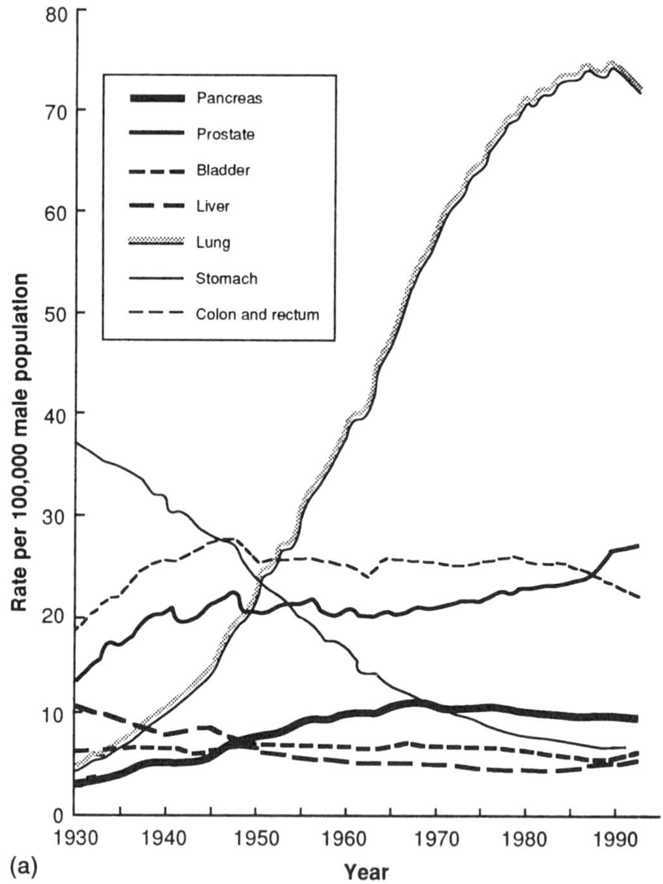

Figure 15 Age-adjusted cancer death rates for selected anatomical sites for the U.S. population, 1930–1992. Age-adjusted to the 1970 U.S. standard population. (a) males and (b) females. (From Refs. 110 and 111.)

tion of radon in U.S. single-family homes and risk factors derived from a met-analysis of data on miners, an estimated 15,000 lung cancer cases may be attributed to residential radon, with an uncertainty range of 6,000–34,000 lung cancer cases per year (10). The risk model assumed a linear increase in excess lung cancer and radon exposure. Because a relative risk model was used for extrapolation purposes, most of the excess lung cancer cases were estimated to occur in male cigarette smokers.

Even with a carcinogenic agent such as radon, the effects of cigarette smok-

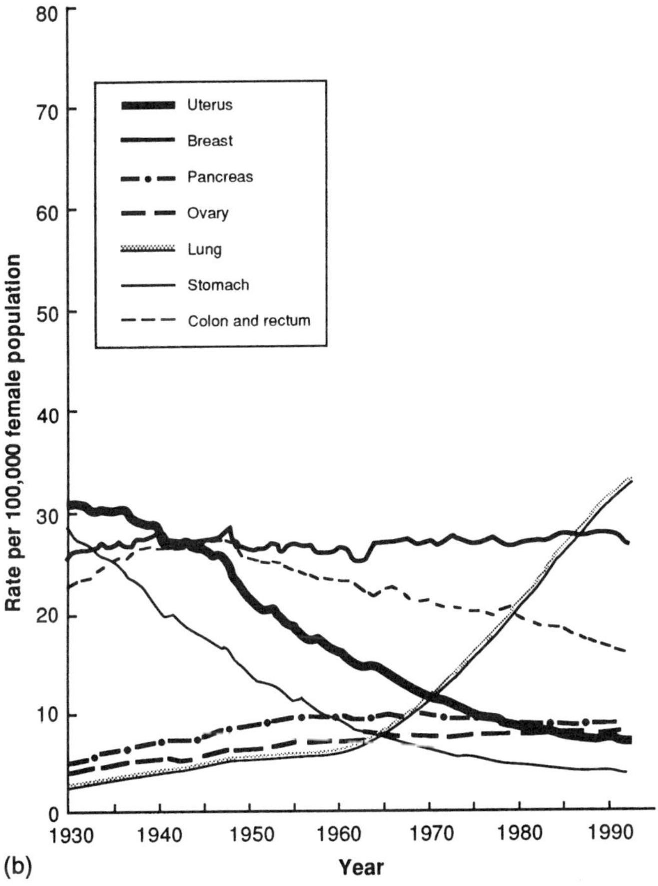

(b)

ing are so substantial that identifying excess lung cancer risk for other agents that have low carcinogenic potency, involve low levels of exposure, or both is difficult. This is illustrated by considering the lung cancer risk of exposure to diesel exhaust. The data were recently reviewed by Cohen and Higgins (46) as part of a critical analysis conducted by the Health Effects Institute (HEI; 47). The results for railroad workers, one of the populations assumed to be heavily exposed, are summarized graphically in Figure 16. Cohen and Higgins (46) concluded that ''occupational exposure to diesel exhaust from diverse sources increases the rate of lung cancer by 20% to 40% in exposed workers generally and to a greater extent among workers with prolonged or intense exposures, or both.'' The summary portion of the HEI report (48) concludes, ''The epidemiologic

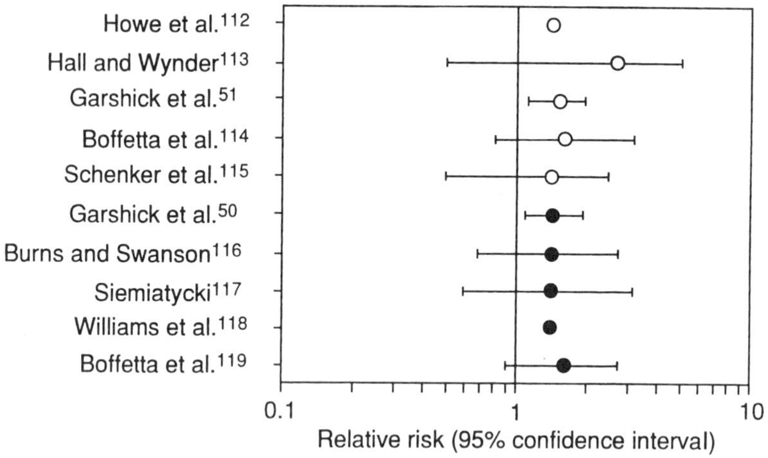

Figure 16 Lung cancer and exposure to diesel exhaust for railroad workers: solid circles, relative risk adjusted for cigarette smoking; open circles, relative risk not adjusted for cigarette smoking. For the two studies by Howe and Williams, confidence intervals were not reported and could not be calculated. (From Ref. 46.)

studies are consistent in showing a weak association between exposure to diesel exhaust and lung cancer, but vary in the strength of the statistical association; only a few studies showed elevated relative risks that were statistically significant.'' Both Cohen and Higgins (46) and Nauss and the HEI Diesel Working Group (48) call attention to the limitations of the epidemiological studies. The three major limitations are (1) the lack of control in many of the studies for confounding factors, such as cigarette smoke; (2) the lack of measurements of exposure; and (3) the lack of any characterization data on the diesel exhaust particulates for exposures that occurred decades ago. The characteristics of diesel exhaust, and especially the content of aromatic hydrocarbons, differ among locomotives, trucks, and light-duty vehicles; moreover, emissions have been steadily decreasing as engine performance and fuel quality have improved (49).

The conclusion that there is a weak association between diesel exposure and lung cancer is shaped largely by the positive findings in the two studies by Garshick et al. (50, 51; see Fig. 16). The difficulty of teasing out an effect of diesel exhaust from the substantial lung cancer risk from cigarette smoking is apparent from consideration of Table 4, which is taken from Garshick et al. (50). The odds ratio for lung cancer in the smokers extends to over 9.14 for cases of age older than 65 years and greater than 50 pack-years of smoking compared with an odds ratio of 0.91 (which was statistically significant) for diesel-exposed workers of similar age. A statistically significant increase in the odds ratio for

Table 4 Regression Results Using Diesel Exhaust Exposure as a Single Continuous Variable (Diesel-Years) Adjusted for Cigarette Smoking and Asbestos Exposure

		Odds		
Exposure category	Coefficient	Ratio	95% CI	*p* values
Case age ≤ 64				
Diesel-years	0.01719	1.41[a]	1.06, 1.88	0.02
Asbestos, Y/N	0.18111	1.20	0.87, 9.65	0.27
≤50 pack-years[b]	1.19196	3.29	1.57, 6.93	<0.01
>50 pack-years[b]	1.73606	5.68	2.73, 11.80	<0.01
Pack-years missing[b]	1.37975	3.97	1.86, 8.51	<0.01
Case age ≥ 65				
Diesel-years	−0.00461	0.91[a]	0.71, 1.17	0.47
Asbestos, Y/N	−0.01807	0.98	0.81, 1.20	0.86
≤50 pack-years[b]	1.47641	4.38	2.90, 6.60	<0.01
>50 pack-years[b]	2.21321	9.14	6.11, 13.70	<0.01
Pack-years missing[b]	1.35379	3.87	2.56, 5.84	<0.01

[a]Calculated on the basis of 20 years of exposure.
[b]Reference category of zero pack-years (nonsmokers).
Source: Ref. 50.

lung cancer and diesel exposure was observed in workers younger than 64 years of age. Individuals of similar age with greater than 50 pack-years had an odds ratio for lung cancer of 5.68. The Garshick et al. (50,51) data were recently reanalyzed (52), and the results of the reanalysis were included as an appendix to the health assessment document for diesel emissions prepared by the EPA (53). Although the reanalysis verified the higher relative risk of lung cancer among exposed workers relative to unexposed workers reported by Garshick et al. (50), it failed to demonstrate a relation between various measures of diesel exposure and lung cancer mortality. The Crump et al. (52) reanalysis suggests caution in the utilization of the Garshick and co-workers' (51) findings of a weak association and, most certainly, suggests that the data should not be used to derive quantitative estimates of lung cancer risk for diesel exhaust exposure.

C. Role of Laboratory Animal Data in Assessing Human Cancer Risks

In the absence of adequate epidemiological data to evaluate carcinogenic risks, laboratory animal studies have been used to evaluate the carcinogenic risk of various kinds of particulate matter. These studies have included the study of materials such as diesel exhaust that people have been exposed to for many years, as well as new products (54,55).

Typically such studies have been conducted using laboratory rats, with fewer studies conducted in mice and Syrian hamsters. Some serious questions have arisen concerning the interpretation of such studies, as will be illustrated using research conducted on diesel exhaust. Within a short time period in the mid-1980s, laboratories from four different countries (the United States, Germany, Switzerland, and Japan) reported that exposure of rats for 2 years or longer to high concentrations of diesel exhaust resulted in an increased incidence of lung cancer (45,56–60). The lung tumor incidence related to weekly exposure rate is shown in Figure 17, which is taken from a critical analysis conducted by the HEI (47) and Nauss and the HEI Working Group (48). In addition to the results of the initial series of investigations, data from two subsequent studies by Mauderly et al. (39); also reported in (61) and Heinrich et al. (62) are shown.

After the results of the initial round of rat studies with diesel exhaust were reported, one could readily conclude, and some did, that the story was complete: diesel exhaust was clearly a lung carcinogen in rats and probably carcinogenic to humans (63,64). However, several interrelated issues were somewhat disquieting. A major finding was the contrast between the positive lung tumor findings

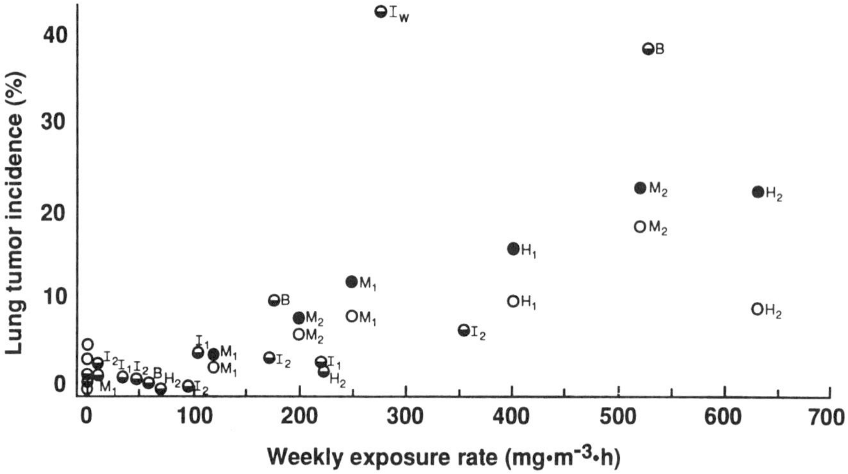

Figure 17 The relation between rat lung tumor incidence and exposure rates for diesel exhaust particulate matter: Data point code: B, Brightwell et al. (60); H_1, Heinrich et al. (56); H_2, Heinrich et al. (62); I_1 Ishinishi et al. (57); exhaust from 1.8-L engine); I_2, Ishinishi et al. (57); exhaust from 11-L engine); I_w, Iwai et al. (58); M_1, Mauderly et al. (45), M_2, Mauderly et al. (39). Solid circle, includes lesions identified by the investigator as "benign squamous tumors"; open circles, excludes these lesions. (From Ref. 48.)

in rats and the lack of clear evidence of lung tumorigenicity in mice and hamsters exposed under similar conditions (64). This dissimilarity in the responses of different species immediately raised the issue of the extent to which findings are representative of what occurs in humans.

Another significant finding was the observation that the kinetics of particle retention at the higher concentrations were quite different from the kinetics observed at the lowest exposure concentration. High-exposure concentrations impaired particle clearance, resulting in a build-up of lung burdens in excess of that predicted from particle kinetics determined for low-exposure concentrations (27,65). The findings of exposure concentration-dependent changes in the disposition kinetics of inhaled soot were paralleled by the observations on cellular and biochemical indicators of pulmonary inflammation (66), cell proliferation (67), alterations in pulmonary function (68), and lung tumor incidence (45). These data and the data of others raised the issue of the mechanisms by which the responses were produced and the nature of the exposure–dose–response relation. Concern for these matters relates to their use in extrapolating to human risks at low levels of exposure.

An outgrowth of debate over these and related findings was the concept of particle overload in the lung (33,34,65,69–72). Particle overload was a key topic of discussion at a symposium honoring Paul Morrow and subsequently published as a special issue of the *Journal of Aerosol Medicine* in 1990. In a discussion of the health effects of highly insoluble, low-toxicity particles in that issue, I defined *lung overload* as

> [A] condition characterized by (1) an overwhelming of the normal clearance processes under certain exposure conditions, (2) resulting in a lung burden greater than predicted from disposition kinetics observed at low exposure concentrations, (3) with associated pathophysiological changes, including altered macrophage function and inflammation, and (4) an uncertain association with an increased incidence of lung tumors in studies conducted in rats (33).

The overload issue has been covered in depth in a more recent conference proceedings (73).

A key aspect of the lung overload concept for the pathogenesis of lung disease, including cancer induction by chronic exposure to particles, is that the effects are caused by nonspecific mechanisms (i.e., unrelated to a unique physicochemical property of the particles). At a 1986 symposium on the health effects of diesel exhaust (74), Vostal (69) noted that the lung tumorigenic response produced by diesel exhaust in the rat was similar to that observed with a diverse array of particles: solvent-refined coal solids (75), raw spent shale (76), titanium dioxide (77), titanium tetrachloride hydrolysis products (77), and coal dust (78). He also noted that the exposure–response relation for both diesel exhaust and the other nuisance dusts exhibited a threshold. Vostal (69) argued "that the action of particles is mediated primarily by the epigenetic mechanism of carcinogenesis, can be characterized more by the promotional than the initiation stages of the carcinogenic process, and probably does not involve primary damage to the genome.'' He concluded that the threshold nature of the exposure–response relation and the findings of lung tumors in only a single species indicate that the rat results should not be extrapolated to estimate human risk of low ambient particulate matter exposures. Another report at the same symposium attracted less attention than the article of Vostal; however, it gave an indication of likely future research findings. This was the report of Kawabata et al. (79), which showed that instillation of both carbon black and diesel soot particles caused a high incidence of lung cancer.

One experimental approach to further clarify the role of the carbonaceous core of diesel soot particles relative to adsorbed polycyclic aromatic hydrocarbons (PAH) was to expose rats to inhalation of carbon black particles free of adsorbed PAH. This was performed by two research groups, and both reported results that were very similar to those observed in rats with similar lung burdens of diesel soot particles (39,61,62). Mauderly et al. (39) and Nikula et al. (61) interpreted these findings as suggesting that the organic fraction of diesel exhaust particles may not play an important role in the carcinogenicity of diesel exhaust in the rat. If the organic compounds are having an effect, it is clearly at a low level of potency and below the limits of detection in the animal bioassay.

Further insight into the mechanisms by which diesel exhaust and carbon black particles cause lung cancer are provided by additional studies (80–82). After exposing rats to various levels of carbon black for 3 months, the lung burden of particles and the inflammatory, cell proliferation, and mutagenic responses in the lungs were evaluated. The retained lung burden of carbon black increased with increased exposure concentration. At the exposure level of 1 mg/m^3, there was no indication of inflammation, as assessed by cellular and biochemical parameters in recovered bronchoalveolar lavage fluid or expression of cytokine biomarkers. Nor was there a change in epithelial cell proliferation. In contrast, a dose-dependent increase in cellular and biochemical inflammatory parameters, including neutrophils and cytokine biomarkers in lavage fluid, was observed at exposure concentrations of 7 and 53 mg/m^3. These increases in indices of inflammation were paralleled by increases in epithelial cell proliferation. Most significantly, whereas the frequency of *hprt* mutations in lung epithelial cells measured ex vivo was no different from that of controls at the lowest exposure level, it was significantly higher than the control frequency at the two highest exposure concentrations. Oberdörster (83) and Driscoll et al. (82) interpreted their findings as suggesting a threshold for particulate lung burden that must be exceeded to produce inflammation and the causally related increase in epithelial cell mutations.

The information now at hand provides a mechanistic linkage between the high lung burdens of carbon black (and indirectly diesel exhaust) and the occurrence of an increased prevalence of lung cancer in the rat. The interpretation that a threshold exists in the linkage between dose (as measured by lung burden) and the several response indicators that are putative preneoplastic events is quite compelling.

The present state of our knowledge of the pathogenesis of lung cancer induced by prolonged exposure of rats to diesel exhaust or carbon black particles is summarized in Figure 18, which is taken from a review by McClellan (84)

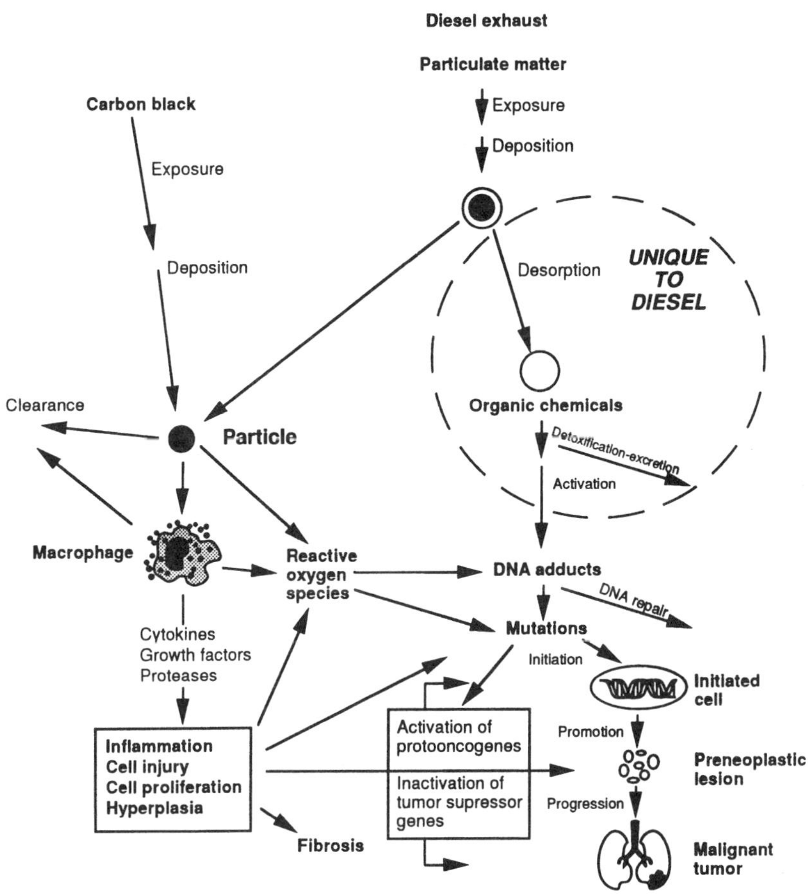

Figure 18 Schematic representation of the pathogenesis of lung cancer in rats with prolonged exposure to high concentrations of diesel exhaust or carbon black particles. (From Ref. 48.)

and adapted from an HEI report (48). The events shown are linked in a linear, unidirectional fashion. In some cases, this is an oversimplification. Repair or modulating processes are probably operative that work to counter some of the effects shown. For example, a DNA repair process is shown that influences the level of DNA adducts and, ultimately, the mutation rate. A critical issue is the modulation of reactive oxygen species and factors such as cytokines. An underlying thesis is that a threshold exists for as yet unidentified biochemical and molecular events that must be exceeded before the process progresses to lung cancer. For both diesel exhaust and carbon black particles, the process apparently begins when the quantity of particles deposited and retained exceeds the normal protective capacity of the lung. I use the term *protective capacity* to mean both clearance mechanisms that attempt to reduce the particle burden (and insult) and the cellular and molecular events that serve to counteract the effects of proteases, reactive oxygen species, and nitric oxide. These materials have all been postulated to have a role in inflammation and, most importantly, in producing mutations (41,81,83,85–91).

The role of increased cell proliferation in amplifying mutations that occur spontaneously as well as mutational events initiated by particle overload is central to the process leading to cancer (92). As shown in the diagram, certain steps are unique to diesel exhaust. If the pathway involving the adsorbed organic chemicals is operative in the rat, it must be at a much lower level of potency than the nonspecific particle effect and thus is not detectable. Lung cancer in the rat induced by the mechanisms shown schematically in Figure 18 is thought to be a threshold phenomenon, with homeostatic mechanisms able to deal with the low levels of reactive oxygen species and cytokines and other factors arising at low-exposure concentrations.

In considering the proposed scheme for pathogenesis of particle-induced disease in the rat, it is important to recognize that not all high-level particle exposures of rats yield a carcinogenic outcome. Muhle et al. (29) and Bellmann et al. (28) reported on a study in which rats were chronically exposed at concentrations of up to 16 mg/m^3 of toner (pigmented plastic powder). As with the diesel exhaust and carbon black studies, they observed a threshold with no changes in indices of pulmonary inflammation, fibrosis, or particle clearance at the lowest exposure concentration. Interestingly, they did not observe any increase in lung tumor incidence even at the highest exposure concentration, which produced a substantial lung burden of toner. This lack of a tumorigenic response may have been related to the large size of the toner particles, which had a mass median aerodynamic diameter of 4.0 μm, with a geometric standard deviation of 1.5, compared with either diesel exhaust soot or carbon black.

Again building on the HEI report (48), Table 5 illustrates the nonspecific particle effect–lung cancer paradigm observed in the rat and illustrated in Figure 18. Also shown is the extent to which the early steps in the process, inflammation

Table 5 Schematic Representation of Responses of the Lung of Laboratory Animals and Humans to Prolonged Inhalation of High Concentrations of Diesel Soot or Carbon Black Particles

Response	Rats	Mice	Hamsters	Humans
Clearance overload	+++	+++	++++	?
Inflammation	+++	+	+	?
Cell proliferation	+++	+	+	?
Fibrosis	+++	+	+	?
Mutations	+++[a]	?	?	?
Lung cancer	+++	±	−	?

[a]In the absence of information on mutation responses in other species, the rat response has arbitrarily been assigned a score of +++.
Source: Ref. 95.

and cell proliferation, are of smaller magnitude in mice and hamsters. As described earlier, mutational data are available for rats, but not for mice and hamsters, exposed to high levels of particulate material. Observations on mice and hamsters exposed to high levels of particles would be of great interest. And, finally, the column for human data contains several question marks that relate to the issue of responses to prolonged exposure to high concentrations of particles. Some of these question marks could be addressed experimentally by conducting studies in vitro using human cells or tissues and making comparisons with rodent cells or tissues. The relevance of the rat findings to human risk is an important topic that needs to be addressed if researchers continue to use rats in evaluating the carcinogenicity of new particulate materials proposed for commerce. Many individuals have hypothesized that the lung cancer findings in rats are due to the high-exposure concentration and would not be observed at low-exposure concentrations (i.e., there is a threshold exposure response phenomenon). There is urgent need for additional data to support or reject this hypothesis because the issues raised likely have an influence on how cancer risks are assessed for a broad range of particulate materials for which carcinogenicity is likely to be evaluated by studies conducted in rats.

IX. Regulatory Considerations

Many countries have government regulations intended to limit occupational or environmental exposures to particulate matter. A review of those regulations is beyond the scope of this chapter. However, I will briefly review U.S. regulations as an example of how one government has approached this matter. Occupational exposure limits will be considered first, followed by discussion of environmental exposure limits. A more detailed discussion of approaches to assessing the human health risks of airborne materials is provided in McClellan (93).

A. Occupational Exposures

In the United States, the first government regulations for particulate matter were intended to control occupational exposures to dusts. A review of the history of dust standards can be found in a paper by Morrow et al. (94), who noted the relatively undocumented basis for establishing early standards for controlling dust exposures and then argued for a downward revision of the dust standards. The earliest dust standards were evidently established on an ad hoc basis by both industrial concerns and local and state agencies. Later a volunteer national organization, the American Conference of Governmental Industrial Hygienists (ACGIH) assumed a major role in providing guidance for limiting human exposure to airborne materials.

The earliest standards recognized that some dusts, such as silica, produced rather specific toxic effects. In these cases, the ACGIH sets specific limits for the chemical. An example is aluminum, which the ACGIH elected to place in five separate subcategories; metal dust, pyropowders, welding fumes, soluble salts, and alkyls. Other examples are barium subcategorized as soluble barium and barium sulfate and coal dust.

In contrast to silica, other dusts caused transient irritation, especially of the upper respiratory tract, and no persistent effects if exposures were controlled. The latter materials were designated as nuisance dusts. The first official listing of a ''maximum allowable concentration'' (MAC) for nuisance dusts was made by the ACGIH in 1946. The MAC for ''Nuisance Dusts; . . . no free silica'' was set at 50 million particles per cubic foot (mppcf). In 1964, a threshold limit value (TLV) was recommended for ''Inert or Nuisance Particulates'' of 15 mg/m^3 or 50 mppcf. This was revised in 1971 to 10 mg/m^3 total dust or 5 mg/m^3 respirable dust and a statement provided defining ''inert or nuisance dust.''

Morrow et al. (94) credited the late Dr. Paul Gross, who had a long and distinguished association with ACGIH activities, for preparation of the ACGIH statement:

> In contrast to fibrogenic dusts which cause scar tissue to be formed in the lungs when inhaled in excessive amounts, so-called nuisance dusts have a long history of little adverse effect on the lungs and do not produce significant organic disease or toxic effect when exposures are kept under reasonable control. The nuisance aerosols have also been called biologically ''inert,'' but the latter term is inappropriate to the extent that there is no particulate which does not evoke some cellular response in the lung when inhaled in sufficient amounts. However, the lung-tissue reaction caused by the inhalation of nuisance aerosols has the following characteris-

> tics: (1) The architecture of the air spaces remains intact. (2) Collagen (scar tissue) is not formed to any significant extent. (3) The tissue reaction is potentially reversible.

Morrow et al. (94) notes the important points contained in the statement, but also calls attention to the limited documentation supporting the statement.

The 1971 revision by ACGIH was preceded by the passage of legislation creating the National Institute of Occupational Safety and Health (NIOSH) to perform research on occupational safety and health matters and the Occupational Safety and Health Administration (OSHA) to develop occupational regulations. In general, this was an era of heightened concern for occupational and environmental health. To jump-start the development of permissible exposure limits (PEL), OSHA adopted the TLV set by ACGIH as PEL. In the late 1980s, ACGIH replaced the "inert or nuisance dust" terminology with "particulates not otherwise classified" (PNOC) while retaining the 10 mg/m^3 total dust level as the TLV. In 1989, OSHA published a PEL for "particulates not otherwise regulated" (PNOR) of 15 mg/m^3 total dust (8-hr time-weighted average) and a respirable dust limit of 5 mg/m^3. The ACGIH (2) time-weighted average for PNOC is 10 mg/m^3 as inhalable particulate and 3 mg/m^3 as respirable particulate. Readers interested in more details on PNOC are referred to a recent review (95).

B. Environmental Exposures

Environmental exposure to air pollutants is regulated in the United States under authority provided by the Clean Air Act (CAA). The CAA was passed in 1967 and amended in 1970, 1974, 1977, and 1990. A major impetus to federal regulation of air quality was general recognition that many air pollution issues were natural in scope and not just local issues. The CAA is a very comprehensive piece of legislation and a review of it in detail is well beyond the scope of this chapter. Alternatively, this chapter will focus on two key provisions of the CAA as amended in 1990 because they directly involve PM; one relates to criteria pollutants and the second to hazardous air pollutants.

The original act called for what was then the Department of Health, Education, and Welfare to prepare "criteria documents" that would summarize the currently available scientific knowledge of air pollutants arising from widespread sources that were of concern across the country. The hazardous air pollutants were a second set of pollutants for which a more direct linkage could be made between specific sources and a particular air pollutant that could pose a hazard.

Criteria Air Pollutants

Amendments to the CAA in 1970 transferred authority for development of criteria documents to the U.S. Environmental Protection Agency and required the Administrator to set numerical standards, called National Ambient Air Quality Standards

(NAAQS), for the identified criteria pollutants. At that time, six ubiquitous air pollutants were designated as "criteria" pollutants: photochemical oxidants (which later became ozone), sulfur dioxide, nonmethane hydrocarbons (which was later dropped as a criteria air pollutant), nitrogen dioxides, carbon monoxide, and total suspended particulates. Lead was later added as a criteria pollutant.

The CAA calls for two types of criteria pollutant standards. The primary NAAQS are set to protect human health. Secondary NAAQS are set to protect against adverse welfare effects such as protection of plants, soiling of buildings, and visibility. The primary NAAQS are intended to protect against adverse effects, including those identified in sensitive population groups and with an adequate margin of safety to allow for uncertainties in our current knowledge. The costs of achieving the standard are not to be considered in setting the NAAQS. Although the NAAQS are supposed to be reviewed every 5 years, this has not yet been accomplished.

The actual standard-setting process is complicated and typically protracted. In current practice, key elements are the preparation of a criteria document by the EPA staff with substantial input from scientists outside the agency. The criteria document is reviewed by the Clean Air Scientific Advisory Committee (CASAC), which was created in response to congressional action in 1977. The intent of the process of review, and typically of revision, is to achieve a criteria document that CASAC views as scientifically adequate for regulatory decision making. The most recent criteria document, *Air Quality Criteria for Particulate Matter* (23), consists of three volumes about 6-in. thick. It represents an encyclopedia of current information on PM.

Preparation and acceptance of the criteria document is followed by a second step that involves another portion of the preparation, by the EPA, of a staff position paper, *Review of the National Ambient Air Quality Standards for Particulate Matter: Policy Assessment of Scientific and Technical Information* (96). This document is a distillation of the contents of the criteria document that emphasizes the information most directly relevant to the setting of a NAAQS. This document is also reviewed by CASAC. The most recent cycle of review of the NAAQS for particulate matter was done on an accelerated basis in response to a court mandate. The standard-setting process for particulate matter has recently been reviewed (97).

The first NAAQS for particulate matter was set in 1971. The standard called for a total suspended particulates metric. The primary standard specified both an annual standard (geometric mean) of 75 $\mu g/m^3$ and a maximum daily average (not to be exceeded more than once per year) of 260 $\mu g/m^3$. The secondary standard was set at 150 $\mu g/m^3$ 24-hr average, not to be exceeded more than once per year. The numerical values were selected largely on the basis of mortality associated with short-term air pollution episodes and measurements made using British Smoke Units, or Total Suspended Particulates (TSP) measurements.

In 1979, work began on revision of the particulate matter standard, which finally occurred in 1987. During this period, there was much debate and, indeed new research, that led to the adaptation of a PM_{10} metric to replace the TSP metric. The PM_{10} metric was generally felt to be more health-relevant, in that the particulate matter being sampled was that which had the highest likelihood of being inhaled and deposited in the respiratory tract. The new primary annual standard was 50 $\mu g/m^3$, and the 24-hr standard was 150 $\mu g/m^3$, with no more than one exceedance per year. The secondary standard was set equal to the primary standard. Although the regulatory compliance metric was changed to PM_{10}, much of the exposure–response data used in setting the standard was based on measurements made using the British Smoke Unit, or TSP metrics.

In 1994–1996, preparation and review of a criteria document and staff paper for the particulate matter NAAQS was carried out under a court-ordered accelerated schedule. Both documents have been completed (23,96). The criteria document and staff paper incorporate the substantial amount of new data that have become available over the last decade on the health effects of particulate matter.

The EPA revised the PM standard in 1997 (98). The new rule establishes two new $PM_{2.5}$ standards: (1) an annual standard set at 15 $\mu g/m^3$ based on the 3-year average of annual arithmetic mean $PM_{2.5}$ concentrations from single or multiple community-oriented monitors; and (2) a 24-hr standard of 65 $\mu g/m^3$ based on the 3-year average of the 98th percentile of 24-hr concentrations at each population-oriented monitor within an area. The rule revises two PM_{10} standards: (1) a 24-hour PM_{10} standard set at 150 $\mu g/m^3$ for the 3-year average of the 99th percentile of the 24-hr concentrations at each monitor within an area; and (2) an annual PM_{10} standard set at 50 $\mu g/m^3$ for the 3-year average of the annual arithmetic mean PM_{10} concentration at each monitor within an area.

There is much controversy surrounding the introduction of a new $PM_{2.5}$ metric. One point of controversy is the size cut. Some have concluded that a $PM_{1.0}$ metric would be more appropriate if the goal is to reduce the amount of the smallest particles arising from combustion. Resolution of this controversy has been stymied by the relatively modest amount of $PM_{2.5}$ and $PM_{1.0}$ data available, since most of the data have been collected for regulatory compliance purposes (i.e., TSP or PM_{10} measurements when these metrics were the standard). Another point of controversy relates to interpretation of the health effects at low concentrations of PM. The EPA has interpreted the available data as indicating a 4% increase in daily mortality for a 50 $\mu g/m^3$ increase in PM concentration with no evidence for a threshold concentration.

Hazardous Air Pollutants

The CAA also calls for the regulation of hazardous air pollutants (also called air toxics), specific chemicals, or mixtures that arise from specific sources and may pose a hazard to human health. The pre-1990 CAA required that National Emission Standard for Hazardous Air Pollutants (NESHAP) be established to protect human health with an ample margin of safety. The EPA found the NESHAP authority largely unworkable because of the presumption that there was no threshold below which exposure would be safe for cancer-causing chemicals. The EPA grappled with the problem for nearly two decades and made little progress, with only seven NESHAP promulgated by November 1990 (arsenic, asbestos, benzene, beryllium, mercury, radionuclides, and vinyl chloride). The history of the EPA assessment of cancer risks has been reviewed (99).

Frustrated by the slow rate of progress, the U.S. Congress made a radical change in the CAA provisions concerned with hazardous air pollutants in 1990. Basically, it shifted to a two-phased approach to regulating 189 hazardous air pollutants listed in the CAA Amendments of 1990. The list includes several chemicals or mixtures likely to occur as particulate matter in the atmosphere (e.g., several metal compounds). The first phase is technology-driven and requires the agency to establish a list of major sources of emissions of the various hazardous air pollutants. The agency then specifies the use of maximum achievable control technology (MACT) to reduce emissions. This can include installation of control equipment, process changes, operator training, and substitution of materials to reduce emissions of the 189 hazardous air pollutants. The second phase, which is health-risk driven, will be implemented after the MACT control phase. The health-risk phase required that if the residual risk after implementation of MACT is not sufficiently low, then more stringent standards will be placed in effect to protect the public health with an ample margin of safety. The legislation specified that for carcinogens a cancer risk be less than 10^{-6} after installation of MACT to avoid further action. Effective implementation of the hazardous air pollutant provisions requires substantial knowledge of the hazards of each of the 189 listed hazardous air pollutants, including their potency for causing cancer or other adverse effects.

To provide guidance for implementing the hazardous air pollutant provisions of the CAA Amendments of 1990, Congress requested the formation of two advisory groups. The first request was for the National Research Council (NRC) of the National Academy of Sciences (NAS) to form a committee to advise on the methods to be used in assessing risks of hazardous air pollutant exposure, especially carcinogenic risks. The committee was formed, deliberated, and issued its report, *Science and Judgment in Risk Assessment* (100,101). Congress also called for establishment of a Commission on Risk Assessment and Risk Management that was to take a broader view as implied by the title of the commission. The commission was formed, had extensive deliberations, and released a draft report in mid-1996. Both reports contain material that include recommendations highly relevant to assessing risks of exposure to particulate matter.

During the remainder of the 1990s, there should be considerable activity in regulating hazardous air pollutants. This will likely include one or more chemicals or mixtures that typically exist as particulate matter in the atmosphere. How the EPA deals with these initial cases is likely to have widespread influence on how risk assessments are conducted for other hazardous air pollutants and, potentially, on whether further research is done to improve the scientific basis for regulating hazardous air pollutants.

X. Summary

This chapter has provided an overview of the science underpinning consideration of particle–respiratory tract interactions. I have noted how the field benefited from a blending of the disciplines of physics, chemistry, and engineering with the biomedical sciences. The historical roots of the field have been reviewed with emphasis on the legacy of quantitations that came both from concern for effects of inhaled radionuclides and from the use of radioisotopic techniques. The field is now well positioned for major advances that are likely to be aided by the recent revolutionary advances in molecular and cell biology. I have advocated the use of an integrative framework that ranges from sources of particulate matter, to the exposure of persons to the dose, to critical biological targets, and ends with concern for a range of health responses. Major advances have been made and will continue to be made based on a mechanistic understanding of the linkages among these four areas. The use of this integrative framework not only encourages advances in our scientific understanding, but also provides the information that is critically needed to establish air quality standards adequately protective of health. The chapters that follow will explore in detail the general concepts outlined in this chapter.

Acknowledgments

The concepts presented in this chapter have been shaped over the years by many pleasant and valuable interactions with scientists at the Chemical Industry Institute of Toxicology, scientists at the Lovelace Inhalation Toxicology Research Institute, and those with whom I have served on numerous advisory committees such as the Clean Air Scientific Advisory Committee of the EPA and those of the National Research Council, National Academy of Science. Their input to shaping the concepts conveyed in this chapter is gratefully acknowledged. I also acknowledge the excellent assistance of Linda Smith for typing, Stan Piestrak for graphics preparation, and Dr. Barbara Kuyper for editing the manuscript.

References

1. McClellan RO, Henderson RF, eds. Concepts in Inhalation Toxicology. 2d ed. Washington, DC: Taylor and Francis, 1995:648 pp.
2. Gardner DE, Crapo JD, McClellan RO, eds. Toxicology of the Lung. New York: Raven Press, 1993.
3. Drinker P, Hatch, T. Industrial Dust: Hygienic Significance, Measurement, and Control. New York: McGraw Hill, 1936:316 pp.
4. Hatch TF, Gross P. Pulmonary Deposition and Retention of Inhaled Aerosols. New York: Academic Press, 1964:192 pp.
5. Davies CN. Dust is Dangerous. London: Farber and Farber, 1954:116 pp.
6. Stannard JN. Radioactivity and Health: A History. Springfield, VA: Office of Science and Technical Information, National Technical Information Service, 1988.
7. McClellan RO. Twenty-five years of Lovelace research in inhalation toxicology. In: Hsi D, Panitz J, eds. From Sundaggers to Space Exploration. University of New Mexico Press, 1986:330–345.
8. Fuchs NA. The Mechanics of Aerosols. Oxford: Pergamon Press, 1964.
9. Weibel ER. Morphometry of the Human Lung. New York: Academic Press, 1963.
10. Lubin JH, Boice JD Jr, Edling C, Hornung RW, Howe G, Kunz E, Kusiak RA, Morrison HI, Radford EP, Samet JM, Tirmarche M, Woodward A, Yao SY, Pierce DA. Lung Cancer and Radon: A Joint Analysis of 11 Underground Miner Studies. Report No. 94-3644. Bethesda, MD: U. S. National Institutes of Health, 1994.
11. Lubin JH, Steindorf K. Cigarette use and the estimation of lung cancer attributable to radon in the United States. Radiat Res 1995; 141:79–85.
12. U. S. Environmental Protection Agency (EPA). Technical Support Document for the 1992 Citizens' Guide to Radon. Washington, DC: U.S. Government Printing Office, 1992.
13. Mercer TT. Aerosol Technology in Hazard Evaluation. New York: Academic Press, 1973.
14. West JB. Respiratory Physiology—The Essentials. 5th ed. Baltimore, MD: Williams and Wilkins, 1994.
15. Driscoll KE. Role of cytokines in pulmonary inflammation and fibrosis. In: McClellan RO, Henderson RF, eds. Concepts in Inhalation Toxicology. 2nd ed. Washington, DC: Taylor and Francis, 1995:471–503.
16. Moss OR, Cheng Y-S. Generation and characterization of test atmospheres: particles and droplets. In: McClellan RO, Henderson RF, eds. Concepts in Inhalation Toxicology. Washington, DC: Taylor and Francis, 1995:91–126.
17. Willeke K, Baron PA, eds. Aerosol Management Principles, Techniques, and Applications. New York: Van Nostrand Reinhold, 1993.
18. Cohen BS, ed. Air Sampling Instruments for Evaluation of Atmospheric Contaminants. 8th ed. Cincinnati, OH: American Conference of Governmental Industrial Hygienists, 1995.
19. Cheng Y-S, Moss OR. Inhalation exposure systems. In: McClellan RO, Henderson RF, eds. Concepts in Inhalation Toxicology. Washington, DC: Taylor and Francis, 1995:25–66.
20. McClellan RO, Miller FJ, Hesterberg TW, Warheit DB, Bunn WB, Kane AB, Lipp-

mann M, Mast RW, McConnell EE, Reinhardt CF. Approaches to evaluating the toxicity and carcinogenicity of man-made fibers: summary of a workshop held November 11–13, 1991, Durham, NC. Regul Toxicol Pharmacol 1992; 16:321–364.
21. Warheit DB, ed. Fiber Toxicology: Contemporary Issues. San Diego, CA: Academic Press, 1993.
22. Clean Air Act Amendments of 1970, Public Law No. 91-604; 84 STAT.1676, 1970.
23. EPA. Air Quality Criteria for Particulate Matter, vol 1–3, 1996.
24. Schlesinger RB. Deposition and clearance of inhaled particles. In: McClellan RO, Henderson RF, eds. Concepts in Inhalation Toxicology. 2d ed. Washington: Taylor & Francis, 1995:191–224.
25. Miller FJ, Anjilvel S, Menache M, Asgharian B, Gerrity TR. Dosimetric issues relating to particulate toxicity. Inhal Toxicol 1995; 7:615–632.
26. Ménache MG, Miller FJ, Raabe OG. Particle inhalability curves for humans and small laboratory animals. Ann Occup Hyg 1995; 39:317–328.
27. Wolff RK, Henderson RF, Snipes MB, Griffith WC, Mauderly JL, Cuddihy RG, McClellan RO. Alterations in particle accumulation and clearance in lungs of rats chronically exposed to diesel exhaust. Fundam Appl Toxicol 1987; 9:154–166.
28. Bellmann B, Muhle H, Creutzenberg O, Dasenbrock C, Kilpper R, MacKenzie JC, Morrow P, Mermelstein R. Lung clearance and retention of toner, utilizing a tracer technique, during chronic inhalation exposure in rats. Fundam Appl Toxicol 1991; 17:300–313.
29. Muhle H, Bellmann B, Creutzenberg O, Dasenbrock C, Ernst H, Kilpper R, MacKenzie JC, Morrow P, Mohr U, Takenaka S, Mermelstein R. Pulmonary response to toner upon chronic inhalation exposure in rats. Fundam Appl Toxicol 1991; 17: 280–299.
30. Cuddihy RG, McClellan RO, Griffith WC. Variability in target organ deposition among individuals exposed to toxic substances. Toxicol Appl Pharmacol 1979; 49: 179–187.
31. Kanapilly GM. Alveolar microenvironment and its relationship to the retention and transport into blood of aerosols deposited in the alveoli. Health Phys 1977; 32:89–100.
32. Snipes MB. Species comparisons for pulmonary retention of inhaled particles. In: McClellan RO, Henderson RF. Concepts in Inhalation Toxicology. Washington, DC: Hemisphere Publishing Corporation, 1989:133–229.
33. McClellan RO. Particle overload in the lung: approaches to improving our knowledge, J Aerosol Med 1990; 3(suppl):S197–S207.
34. Morrow PE. Mechanisms and significance of "particle overload." In: Mohr U, Dungworth DL, Mauderly JL, Oberdörster G, eds. Toxic and Carcinogenic Effects of Solid Particles in the Respiratory Tract. Washingtons, DC: International Life Sciences Institute Press, 1994:17–25.
35. Stöber W, Morrow PE, Koch W, Morawietz G. Alveolar clearance and retention of inhaled insoluble particles in rats simulated by a model inferring macrophage particle load distributions. J Aerosol Sci 1994; 25:975–1002.
36. Stöber W, Morrow PE, Oberdörster G. Pulmonary retention of inhaled anatase (TiO_2) aerosols and lung tumor induction in rats simulated by a physiology-oriented model. Inhal Toxicol 1995; 7:1059–1074.

37. Stöber W, Mauderly JL. Model-inferred hypothesis of a critical dose for overload tumor induction by diesel soot and carbon black. Inhal Toxicol 1994; 6:427–457.
38. Stöber W, McClellan RO. Lung retention and clearance of inhaled aerosols: models for data reduction and models of pulmonary physiological systems. CRC Crit Rev Toxicol 1997; 27(6):539–598.
39. Mauderly JL, Snipes MB, Barr EB, Belinsky SA, Bond JA, Brooks AL, Chang L-Y, Cheng YS, Gillett NA, Griffith WC, Henderson RF, Mitchell CE, Nikula KJ, Thomassen DG. Pulmonary toxicity of inhaled diesel exhaust and carbon black in chronically exposed rats, part I, neoplastic and nonneoplastic lung lesions. Research Report Number 68, Cambridge, MA: Health Effects Institute, 1994.
40. Mauderly JL. Lung overload: the dilemma and opportunities for resolution. Inhal Toxicol 1996; 8(suppl):1–28.
41. Oberdörster G, Ferin J, Soderholm SC, Gelein R, Cox C, Baggs R, Morrow PE. Increased pulmonary toxicity of inhaled ultrafine particles: due to lung overload alone? Ann Occup Hyg 1994; 38(suppl 1):295–302.
42. Oberdörster G. Lung particle overload: implications for occupational exposures to particles. Regul Toxicol Pharmacol 1995; 21:123–135.
43. Moolgavkar S, Luebeck EG. Particulate air pollution and mortality: a critical review of the evidence. Epidemiology 1996; 7:420–428.
44. Samet JM, Zeger SC, Kelsall JE, Xu J, Kulkstein LS. Weather, air pollution and mortality in Philadelphia. 1973–1980. Report to the Health Effects Institute, 1996.
45. Mauderly JL, Jones RK, Griffith WC, Henderson RF, McClellan RO. Diesel exhaust is a pulmonary carcinogen in rats exposed chronically by inhalation. Fundam Appl Toxicol 1987; 9:208–221.
46. Cohen AJ, Higgins MWP. Health effects and diesel exhaust: epidemiology. In: Diesel Exhaust: A Critical Analysis of Emissions, Exposure, and Health Effects, A Special Report of the Institute's Diesel Working Group. Cambridge, MA: Health Effects Institute, 1995:251–292.
47. Health Effects Institute (HEI). Diesel Exhaust: A Critical Analysis of Emissions, Exposure, and Health Effects, A Special Report of the Institute's Diesel Working Group. Cambridge, MA: Health Effects Institute, 1995.
48. Nauss KM. The HEI Diesel Working Group. Critical issues in assessing the carcinogenicity of diesel exhaust: a synthesis of current knowledge. In: Diesel Exhaust: A Critical Analysis of Emissions, Exposure, and Health Effects. Cambridge, MA: Health Effects Institute, 1995:11–61.
49. Sawyer RF, Johnson JH. Diesel emissions and control technology. In: Diesel Exhaust: A Critical Analysis of Emissions, Exposure, and Health Effects, A Special Report of the Institute's Diesel Working Group. Cambridge: Health Effects Institute, 1995:66–81.
50. Garshick E, Schenker MB, Muñoz A, Segal M, Smith TJ, Woskie SR, Hammond SK, Speizer FE. A case–control study of lung cancer and diesel exhaust exposure in railroad workers. Am Rev Respir Dis 1987; 135:1242–1248.
51. Garshick E, Schenker MB, Muñoz A, Segal M, Smith TJ, Woskie SR, Hammond SK, Speizer FE. A retrospective cohort study of lung cancer and diesel exhaust exposure in railroad workers. Am Rev Respir Dis 1988; 137:820–825.
52. Crump KS, Lambert T, Chen C. Assessment of risk from exposure to diesel engine

emissions: Report to U.S. Environmental Protection Agency for Contract 68-02-4601 (Work Assignment No. 182). Washington, DC: Office of Health and Environmental Assessment, U.S. Environmental Protection Agency, 1991.
53. EPA. Health Assessment Document for Diesel Emissions: External Review Draft, EPA 600/8-90/057, Office of Research and Development, Washington, DC, 1994.
54. McClellan RO. Health effects of diesel exhaust: a case study in risk assessment. Am Indust Hyg Assoc J 1986; 47:1–13.
55. McClellan RO. Health effects of exposure to diesel exhaust. Annu Rev Pharmacol Toxicol 1987; 27:279–300.
56. Heinrich U, Muhle H, Takenaka S, Ernst E, Fuhst R, Mohr U, Pott F, Stöber W. Chronic effects on the respiratory tract of hamsters, mice and rats after long-term inhalation of high concentrations of filtered and unfiltered diesel engine emissions. J Appl Toxicol 1986; 6:383–395.
57. Ishinishi N, Kuwabara N, Nigase S, Suzuki T, Ishiwata S, Kohno T. Long-term inhalation studies on effects of exhaust from heavy and light duty diesel engines on F344 rats. In: Ishinishi N, Kozumi A, McClellan RO, Stöber W, eds. Carcinogenic and Mutagenic Effects of Diesel Engine Exhaust. New York: Elsevier, 1986: 329–348.
58. Iwai K, Udagawa T, Yamagishi M, Yamada H. Long-term inhalation studies of diesel exhaust on F344 SPF rats. Incidence of lung cancer and lymphoma. In: Ishinishi N, Koizumi A, McClellan RO, Stöber W, eds. Carcinogenic and Mutagenic Effects of Diesel Engine Exhaust. Amsterdam: Elsevier, 1986:349–360.
59. Brightwell J, Fouillet X, Cassano-Zoppi A-L, Gatz R, Duchosal F. Neoplastic and functional changes in rodents after chronic inhalation of engine exhaust emissions. In: Ishinishi N, Koizumi A, McClellan RO, Stöber W, eds. Carcinogenic and Mutagenic Effects of Diesel Engine Exhaust. Amsterdam: Elsevier, 1986:471–485.
60. Brightwell J, Fouillet X, Cassano-Zoppi AL, Bernstein D, Crawley F, Duchosal F, Gatz R, Percel S, Pfeifer H. Tumours of the respiratory tract in rats and hamsters following chronic inhalation of engine exhaust emissions. J Appl Toxicol 1989; 9: 23–31.
61. Nikula KJ, Snipes MB, Barr EB, Griffith WC, Henderson RF, Mauderly JL. Comparative pulmonary toxicities and carcinogenicities of chronically inhaled diesel exhaust and carbon black in F344 rats. Fundam Appl Toxicol 1995; 25:80–94.
62. Heinrich U, Fuhst R, Rittinghausen S, Creutzenberg O, Bellmann B, Koch W, Levsen K. Chronic inhalation exposure of Wistar rats and two different strains of mice to diesel engine exhaust, carbon black, and titanium dioxide. Inhal Toxicol 1995; 7:533–556.
63. Mauderly JL, Banas DA, Griffith WC, Hahn FF, Henderson RF, McClellan RO. Diesel exhaust is not a pulmonary carcinogen in CD-1 mice exposed under conditions carcinogenic to F-344 rats. Fundam Appl Toxicol 1996; 30:233–242.
64. International Agency for Research on Cancer (IARC). IARC Monographs on the Evaluation of Carcinogenic Risks to Humans. vol 46, Diesel and Gasoline Engine Exhausts and Some Nitroarenes. Lyon: IARC, 1989:458 pp.
65. Wolff RK, Henderson RF, Snipes MB, Sun JD, Bond JA, Mitchell CE, Mauderly JL, McClellan RO. Lung retention of diesel soot and associated organic compounds. In: Ishinishi N, Koizumi A, McClellan RO, Stöber W, eds. Carcinogenic

and Mutagenic Effects of Diesel Engine Exhaust. Amsterdam: Elsevier, 1986:199–222.

66. Henderson RF, Pickrell JA, Jones RK, Sun JD, Benson JM, Mauderly JL, McClellan RO. Response of rodents to inhaled diluted diesel exhaust: Biochemical and cytological changes in bronchoalveolar lavage fluid and in lung tissue. Fundam Appl Toxicol 1988; 11:546–567.
67. Mauderly JL, Benson JM, Bice DE, Carpenter RL, Evans MJ, Henderson RF, Jones RK, McClellan RO, Pickrell JA, Redman HC, Shami SG, Wolff RK. Lifespan study of rodents inhaling diesel exhaust: results through 30 months. In: Inhalation Toxicology Research Institute Annual Report 1982–1983, LMF-107. Springfield, VA: National Technical Information Service, 1983:305–316.
68. Mauderly JL, Gillett NA, Henderson RF. Relationship of lung structural and functional changes to accumulation of diesel exhaust particles. Ann Occup Hyg 1988; 32:659–669.
69. Vostal JJ. Factors limiting the evidence for chemical carcinogenicity of diesel emissions in long-term inhalation experiments. In: Ishinishi N, Koizumi A, McClellan RO, Stöber W, eds. Carcinogenic and Mutagenic Effects of Diesel Engine Exhaust. Amsterdam: Elsevier, 1986:381–396.
70. Lewis TR, Morrow PE, McClellan RO, Raabe OG, Kennedy GL, Schwetz BA, Goehl TJ, Roycraft JH, Chhabra RS. Contemporary issues in toxicology: establishing aerosol exposure concentrations for inhalation toxicity studies. Toxicol Appl Pharmacol 1989; 99:377–383.
71. Morrow PE. Possible mechanisms to explain dust overloading of the lungs. Fundam Appl Toxicol 1988; 10:369–384.
72. Watson AY, Green GM. Noncancer effects of diesel emissions: animal studies. In: Diesel Exhaust: A Critical Analysis of Emissions, Exposure, and Health Effects. Cambridge, MA: Health Effects Institute, 1995:141–164.
73. Mauderly JL, McCunney RJ, eds. Particle Overload in the Rat Lung and Lung Cancer, Proceedings of a Conference Held at the Massachusetts Institute of Technology on March 29 and 30, 1995. Inhal Toxicol 1996; 8(suppl):1–288.
74. Ishinishi N, Koizumi A, McClellan RO, Stöber W, eds. Carcinogenic and Mutagenic Effects of Diesel Engine Exhaust. Amsterdam: Elsevier, 1986.
75. Drozdowicz BZ, Ulrich CE, Boothe AD, Procter JE, Golberg L. Chronic inhalation toxicity and carcinogenicity study of SRC-1 (solvent refined coal) solid in rats—results from the 6- and 12-month interim sacrifices. Toxicologist 1986; 6:132.
76. Holland LM, Wilson JS, Tillery MI, Smith DM. Lung cancer in rats exposed to fibrogenic dusts. In: Goldsmith D, Winn D, Shy C, eds. Silica, Silicosis and Cancer. New York: Praeger, 1985:267–279.
77. Lee KP, Trochimowicz HJ, Reinhardt CF. Pulmonary response of rats exposed to titanium dioxide (TiO_2) by inhalation for two years. Toxicol Appl Pharmacol 1985; 79:179–192.
78. Martin JC, Daniel H, Le Bouffant L. Short- and long-term experimental study of the toxicity of coal-mine dust and some of its constituents. In: Walton WH, ed. Inhaled Particles IV. vol 1. Oxford: Pergamon, 1977:361–371.
79. Kawabata Y, Iwai K, Udagawa T, Tukagoshi K, Kazue H. Effects of diesel soot on unscheduled DNA synthesis of tracheal epithelium and lung tumor formation. In:

Ishinishi N, Koizumi A, McClellan R, Stöber, W, eds. Carcinogenic and Mutagenic Effects of Diesel Engine Exhaust. Amsterdam: Elsevier, 1986:213–222.

80. Oberdörster G, Baggs R, Gelein R, Corson N, Mercer P, Nguyen K, Pepelko W. Pulmonary effects of inhaled carbon black in rats. Fundam Appl Toxicol 1995; 15: 46 (abstr 248).
81. Oberdörster G. Extrapolation of results from animal inhalation studies with particles to humans? In: Mohr U, Dungworth DL, Mauderly JL, Oberdörster G, eds. Toxic and Carcinogenic Effects of Solid Particles in the Respiratory Tract. Washington, DC: International Life Sciences Institute Press, 1994:335–353.
82. Driscoll KE, Carter JM, Howard BW, Hassenbein DG, Pepelko W, Baggs RB, Oberdörster G. Pulmonary inflammatory, chemokine, and mutagenic responses in rats after subchronic inhalation of carbon black. Toxicol Appl Pharmacol 1996; 136:372–380.
83. Oberdörster G. Significance of particle parameters in the evaluation of exposure–dose–response relationships of inhaled particles. Inhal Toxicol 1996; 8(suppl):73–89.
84. McClellan RO. Lung cancer in rats from prolonged exposure to high concentrations of carbonaceous particles: implications for human risk assessment. Inhal Toxicol 1996; 8(suppl):193–226.
85. Cerutti, PA, Trump BF. Inflammation and oxidative stress in carcinogenesis. Cancer Cells 1991; 3:1–7.
86. Wink DA, Kasprzak KS, Maragos CM, et al. DNA deaminating ability and genotoxicity of nitric oxide and its progenitors. Science 1991; 254:1001–1003.
87. Nguyen T, Brunson D, Crespi CL, Penman BW, Wishnok JS, Tannenbaum SR. DNA damage and mutation in human cells exposed to nitric oxide in vitro. Biochemistry 1992; 285:1173–1180.
88. Maki A, Berezesky IK, Iargnoli J, Holbrook NJ, Trump BF. Role of [Ca^{2+}] in induction of c-*fos*, c-*jun* and c-*myc* mRNA in rat PTE after oxidative stress. FASEB J 1992; 6:919–924.
89. Driscoll KE, Maurer JK, Hassenbein D, Carter J, Janssen YMW, Mossman BT, Osier M, Oberdörster G. Contribution of macrophage-derived cytokines and cytokine networks to mineral dust-induced lung inflammation. In: Mohr U, Dungworth DL, Mauderly JL, Oberdörster G, eds. Toxic and Carcinogenic Effects of Solid Particles in the Respiratory Tract. Washington, DC: International Life Sciences Institute Press, 1994:177–189.
90. Driscoll KE. Role of inflammation in the development of rat lung tumors in response to chronic particle exposure. Inhal Toxicol 1996; 8:139–153.
91. Oberdörster G, Ferin J, Lehnert BE. Correlation between particle size, in vivo particle persistence and lung injury. Environ Health Perspect 1994; 102(suppl 5):173–179.
92. Ames BN, Gold LA. Chemical carcinogenesis: too many rodent carcinogens. Proc Natl Acad Sci USA 1990; 87:7772–7776.
93. McClellan RO. Health risk assessments and regulatory considerations for air pollutants. In: Swift DL, Foster WM, eds. Air Pollutants and the Respiratory Tract. New York: Marcel Dekker, Inc., 1999:289–338.
94. Morrow PE, Muhle H, Mermelstein R. Chronic inhalation study findings as a basis

for proposing a new occupational dust exposure limit. J Am Coll Toxicol 1991; 10:279–290.

95. McClellan RO. Nuisance dusts (particles not otherwise classified). In: Sipes IG, McQueen CA, Gandolfi AJ, eds. Respiratory System Toxicology in Comprehensive Toxicology. vol 8. New York: Pergamon/Elsevier Science Inc., 1997; pp. 495–520.
96. EPA Staff Position Paper. Review of the National Ambient Air Quality Standards for Particulate Matter: Policy Assessment of Scientific and Technical Information, 1996.
97. Wolff GT. The scientific basis for a particulate matter standard. Environ Manager 1996 (October):26–31.
98. EPA. National Ambient Air Quality Standards for Particulate Matter. Final Rule. Fed. Reg. 1997; 62(138):38652–38760.
99. Albert RE. Carcinogen risk assessment in the U.S. Environmental Protection Agency. Crit Rev Toxicol 1994; 24:75–85.
100. National Research Council (NRC). Committee on Risk Assessment of Hazardous Air Pollutants: Science and Judgment in Risk Assessment. Washington, DC: National Academy Press, 1994.
101. McClellan RO. A commentary on the NRC report ''Science and Judgment in Risk Assessment.'' Regul Toxicol Pharmacol 1994; 20:5142–5168.
102. Schroeder WH, Dobson M, Kane DM, Johnson ND. Toxic trace elements associated with airborne particulate material: a review. J Air Pollut Control Assoc 1987; 37:1267–1285.
103. Vital and Health Statistics. Current Estimates from the National Health Interview Survey, 1994. DHHS Publication (PHS) 96–1521, 1995.
104. Schwartz J. Air pollution and daily mortality: a review and meta-analysis. Environ Res 1994; 64:36–52.
105. Wilson WE, Spiller LL, Ellestad TG, Lamothe PJ, Dzubay TG, Stevens RK, Macias ES, Fletcher RA, Husar JD, Husar RB, Whitby KT, Kittelson DB, Cantrell BK. General Motors sulfate dispersion experiment: summary of EPA measurements. J Air Pollut Control Assoc 1977; 27:46–51.
106. Wilson WE, Suh HH. Fine and coarse particles: concentration relationships relevant to epidemiological studies. J Air Waste Manage Assoc 1997; 47:1238–1249.
107. Whitby KT. The physical characterization of sulfur aerosols. Atmos Environ 1978; 12:135–159.
108. Snipes MB. Biokinetics of inhaled radionuclides. In: Raabe OG, ed. Internal Radiation Dosimetry. Madison, WI: Medical Physics Publishing, 1994:181–204.
109. Schwartz J, Dockery DW. Increased mortality in Philadelphia associated with daily air pollution concentrations. Am Rev Respir Dis 1992; 145:600–604.
110. Wingo PA, Tong T, Bolden S. Cancer Statistics, 1995. CA Cancer J Clin 1995; 45:8–30.
111. Parker SL, Tong T, Bolden S, Wingo PA. Cancer Statistics, 1996. CA Cancer J Clin 1996; 65:5–27.
112. Howe GR, Fraser D, Lindsay J, Presnal B, Yu SZ. Cancer mortality (1965–77) in relation to diesel fume and coal exposure in a cohort of retired railway workers. J Natl Cancer Inst 1983; 70:1015–1019.

113. Hall NEL, Wynder EL. Diesel exhaust exposure and lung cancer: a case–control study. Environ Res 1984; 34:77–86.
114. Boffetta P, Harris RE, Wynder EL. Case–control study of occupational exposure to diesel exhaust and lung cancer risk. Am J Ind Med 1990; 17:577–591.
115. Schenker MB, Smith T, Muñoz A, Woskie S, Speizer FE. Diesel exposure and mortality among railway workers: result of a pilot study. Br J Ind Med 1984; 41: 320–327.
116. Burns PB, Swanson GM. The occupational cancer incidence surveillance study (OCISS): risk of lung cancer by usual occupation and industry in the Detroit metropolitan area. Am J Ind Med 1991; 19:655–671.
117. Siemiatycki J, ed. Risk Factors for Cancer in the Workplace, Boca Raton, FL: CRC Press, 1991.
118. Williams RR, Stegens NL, Goldsmith JR. Associations of cancer site and type with occupation and industry from the Third National Cancer Survey Interview. J Natl Cancer Inst 1977; 59:1147–1185.
119. Boffetta P, Stellman SD, Garfinkel L. Diesel exhaust exposure and mortality among males in the American Cancer Society Prospective Study. Am J Ind Med 1988; 14:403–415.

Part Two

PARTICLES INTERACTING WITH THE LUNG

2

Environmental Particles

ALFRED WIEDENSOHLER and FRANK STRATMANN

Institute for Tropospheric Research
Leipzig, Germany

INA TEGEN

Columbia University
New York, New York

I. Introduction

The Earth's atmosphere is a two-phase system consisting of gases and particles (solid or liquid). This means the entire atmosphere is, by definition, an *aerosol*. The number concentration and size distribution of environmental or atmospheric aerosol particles are highly variable in space (marine and continental, or boundary layer and free troposphere) and time (summer and winter). Although the total mass of these particles is small compared with the total mass of atmospheric gases, atmospheric particles play an important role in today's research on climate change, air pollution, and human health.

II. Size Distributions of Atmospheric Aerosol Particles

The particle size, volume concentration, and number are probably the most important physical properties used in describing the atmospheric aerosol. The size of atmospheric particles covers a range of five orders of magnitude, from a few nanometers up to several hundred micrometers in diameter. The total particle volume can differ from 1 to 300 $\mu m^3\ cm^{-3}$, depending on the origin of the aerosol.

Table 1 Typical Particle Number Concentration for Different Categories of Environmental Aerosols

Category	Total particle number concentration (cm^{-3})
Arctic	1–200
Background oceanic	100–400
Remote continental	100–1,000
Rural	2,000–10,000
Urban influenced	5,000–20,000
Urban polluted	10,000–1 million

Source: Refs. 1, 42.

Particle number concentrations of atmospheric aerosol vary from 1 cm^{-3} in very clean areas to 10^6 cm^{-3} in highly polluted regions (Table 1).

Atmospheric aerosol particles are principally divided into fine and coarse particles. The fine-particle–size range covers geometric particle diameters (D_P) $1 > D_P > 1000$ nm. Particles with $D_P > 1$ μm are called coarse particle. Fine particles are also defined as $D_{aP} > 2.5$ μm (e.g., by inhalation toxicologists for which D_{aP} is defined as the aerodynamic particle diameter). The entire number–size distribution can be principally described by four different aerosol particle modes (Table 2). Fine particles belong to the nucleation (ultrafine), the Aitken, or the accumulation mode (1). The fourth mode is the coarse particle mode.

The nucleation mode occurs in the atmosphere only sporadically, depending on favorable conditions for new particle formation (see under Sec. III.B) or on mixing processes (2). The Aitken mode and accumulation mode are usually always present in the boundary layer of the atmosphere. The Aitken mode

Table 2 Approximate Size Range and Origin of the Four Modes of Environmental Particles

Aerosol mode	Size range (D_P)	Origin of particles
Nucleation or ultrafine	< 20 nm	Homogeneous nucleation of aerosol gases
Aitken	20–100 nm	Particle growth of ultrafine by coagulation or diffusive mass transport
Accumulation	100–1000 nm	Growth of the Aitken particles by cloud processes; a fraction is originated from bulk-to-particle conversion
Coarse	> 1000 nm	Bulk-to-particle conversion

derives from the nucleation mode by particle growth through coagulation or diffusive mass transport (see under Sec. III.B). However, where in the atmosphere (boundary layer or free troposphere) this growth takes place is not yet well understood (3). The accumulation mode is strongly coupled to the Aitken mode. It is believed that the accumulation mode derives mainly from the Aitken mode owing to new aerosol mass production in cloud processes (4). The coarse mode is relatively independent from fine-aerosol particles because of its different origin (see Sec. III.A). However, it serves as a sink for these particles (see Sec. V).

Physical or chemical processes in the atmosphere can be related to the particle number, the available surface area of the particles, or the particle volume. The following figures will illustrate the differences between the number-size, surface area–size, and volume-size distributions of an environmental aerosol. In practice, log-normal distributions are used to simplify the description of atmospheric size distributions. Figure 1a shows an example for a typical number-size distribution of a continentally influenced marine aerosol, consisting of four log-normal aerosol modes. The geometric mean diameter of the nucleation, Aitken, accumulation, and coarse mode are assumed to be 12, 50, 200, and 1500 nm, respectively. Most particles are found in the submicrometer size range (nucleation mode: 100 cm^{-3}; Aitken mode: 400 cm^{-3}; accumulation mode: 300 cm^{-3}), whereas only a small particle fraction is usually found in the coarse mode range (3 cm^{-3}). In Figure 1b, the number-size distribution is converted to a surface–area-size distribution. Here, the surface area of the accumulation mode and coarse mode are dominating, whereas the surface area of the Aitken mode plays a minor role. The surface area of the nucleation mode is negligible. Figure 1c shows the same aerosol plotted as a volume-size distribution. The major mass fraction is found in the coarse–mode-size range, whereas the mass fraction of the accumulation mode is relatively low. The contributions to the particle mass from the nucleation and Aitken modes is unimportant for total volume.

III. Sources of Atmospheric Aerosol Particles

Sources of atmospheric aerosol particles are bulk-to-particle conversion, gas-to-particle conversion, and combustion processes. Bulk-to-particle conversion includes the formation of sea salt, dust, and biogenic particles. Gas-to-particle formation involves either new particle formation from aerosol precursor gases, or growth of preexisting particles by mass transfer processes between the gas and the particle phase. Particles derived from gas-to-particle conversion processes are also called *secondary aerosol particles.* Other particles, such as from bulk-to-particle conversion processes or combustion particles (soot, fly ash), are called *primary aerosol particles.*

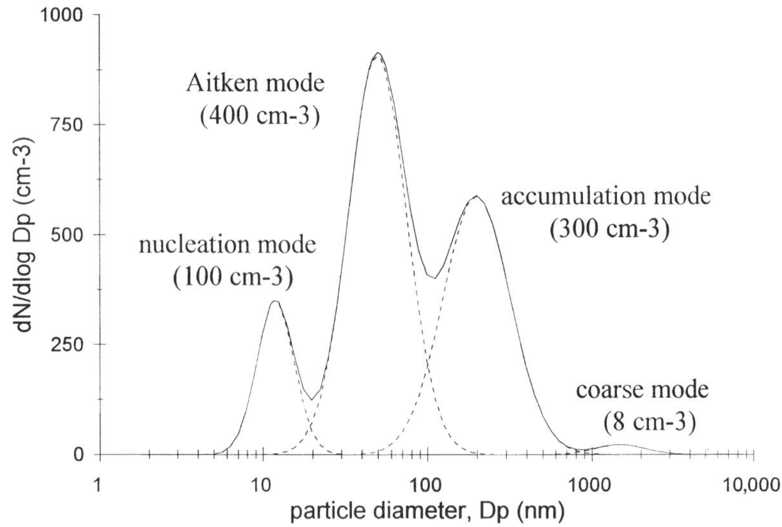

(a)

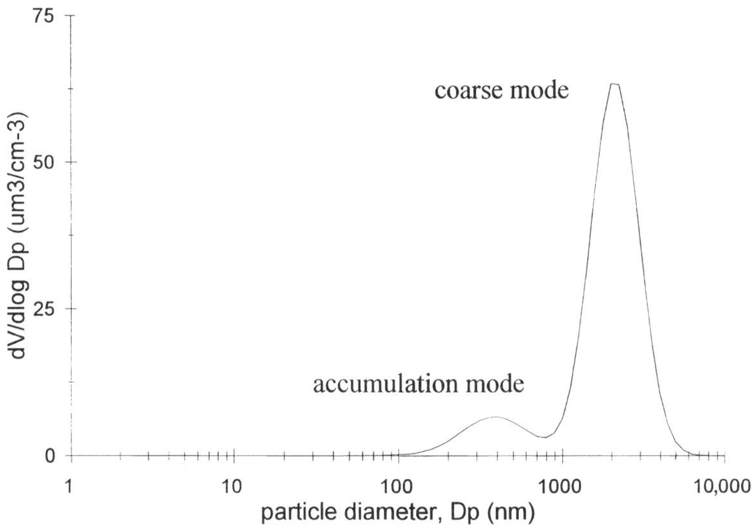

(b)

Figure 1 (a) A typical number-size distribution of a polluted marine aerosol consisting of the four atmospheric aerosol modes: (1) the nucleation or ultrafine mode, (2) the Aitken mode, (3) the accumulation mode, and (4) the coarse mode. The solid line represents the sum of log-normal distributions (dotted lines) of the ultrafine, the Aitken, the accumulation, and the coarse mode. (b) The surface–area-size distribution is calculated from number-size distribution of Figure 1a, assuming spherical particles. (c) The volume-size distribution is calculated from the number-size distribution of Figure 1a, assuming spherical particles.

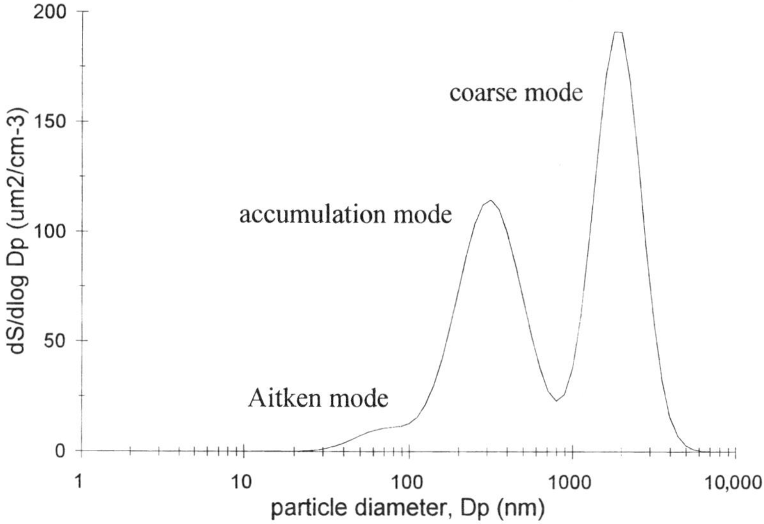

(c)

A. Bulk-to-Particle Conversion

Sea Salt Particles

Particles produced by dispersion processes occur mainly over the larger sea surfaces of the earth (oceans). The production of sea salt particles is due to the agitation of the sea surface by the wind. Wind stress on the ocean surface is a generator of air bubbles that burst, producing both film drops and jet drops (5). Bubbles are most numerous in the whitecaps associated with breaking waves, where they are formed by entrainment of air into the surface water by breaking wave motion. Whitecaps begin to appear at wind speeds of 3 m sec.$^{-1}$. Each bursting bubble produces between one and ten jet drops, and up to several hundred smaller film drops. After generation, the drops rapidly become sea salt particles or sea salt solution droplets, depending on the ambient relative humidity. Jet drops form sea salt particle (up to several tens of micrometer), whereas film drops produce mostly sea salt particle in the size range of 0.5–5 μm. In addition, there is also a production of spume droplets at high wind speeds. These droplets contribute to the large sea salt particles (6). Estimates for the global sea salt source strength range between 1,000 and 10,000 Teragram/year (Tg/yr or Tg yr^{-1}) (7–10).

Crustal Mineral Particles

Mineral dust is mostly deflated from soils in arid and semiarid regions. The emission of dust particles strongly depends on surface wind speed and gustiness as well as soil surface conditions. In wind tunnel experiments, the dust flux from the surface was dependent on the surface friction and the threshold friction velocities (11). Additionally, the friction velocity depends on the size distribution, the roughness, and the crusting of the soil surfaces. For all particle sizes, dust uplift is effected by large particles that mobilize smaller particles when they impact on the ground (12).

Mineral dust is among the coarse particles with the highest atmospheric mass loading on a global scale besides sea salt. The global source strength of mineral dust is currently estimated to be between 1000 and 5000 Tg/yr or Tg yr^{-1} (13–15).

The production of soil dust is highly variable in space and time. Changes in surface conditions caused by human activities or shifts in climatic conditions can increase dust deflation and dust storm activities in semiarid regions. An example for increased dust production are the "dust bowl" years in the 1930s and 1950s in the Midwestern United States, where large dust storms were caused not only by drought conditions, but also by inappropriate land use practices. Although many authors find that dust production is only weakly correlated with mean rainfall in the source regions (16), there is a report (17) of a strong increase in Saharan dust concentrations, measured at Barbados from the mid-1960s to the mid-1980s, which is well correlated with the rainfall deficit in the Sahel since the late 1960s (18). It has been estimated (19) that the part of the atmospheric mineral dust load that originates from disrupted soils is approximately 50% of the total dust load. The highest dust concentrations (several hundred micrograms per cubic meter) are found above source areas during dust storm conditions. Small dust particles (of a few micrometer in size) can be transported thousands of kilometres.

Biogenic Particles

Most biological particles originate from plants that release pollen and spores actively or passively into the atmosphere (20). Other sources can be found in industry (e.g., textile mills), agriculture (e.g., fertilizing), and municipal activities (e.g., sewage plants) (21). Bacteria can be released from the ocean in jet drops by bursting bubbles (22). The smallest biogenic aerosol particles, such as viruses, bacteria, protozoa, and algae are found in the accumulation mode range. Spores, pollen, plant debris, and epithelial cells from human beings and animals are usually coarse mode (tens of micrometer) particles. About 30% of the particle number in the size range $D_P > 4$ μm originates from biological sources. The number of biogenic particles in the submicron range, however, is, negligible compared with accumulation mode particles from other sources.

A study by Penner (23) estimates the source strength of biogenic material. Emissions of particles $D_{aP} < 2.5$ μm (particles from plants and submicron microorganisms) were estimated to be 56 Tg yr^{-1}. These primary emissions are estimated from the difference between other organic aerosol sources and the total source of organic matter.

B. Gas-to-Particle Conversion

Particle precursor gases are emitted into the atmosphere either directly by natural and anthropogenic sources or by oxidation processes in the atmosphere. The most prominent precursor gas is probably sulfur dioxide (SO_2). It is the precursor for particulate sulfates, such as sulfuric acid (H_2SO_4) or ammonium sulfate [$(NH_4)_2SO_4$]. Sulfur dioxide is directly emitted by natural sources (e.g., volcano eruptions). Anthropogenic sources in industrial regions are mostly associated with combustion processes (e.g., coal combustion). Additional SO_2 is derived from oxidation processes of dimethyl sulfide (DMS) over the oceans. Estimations of the global sulfur emissions from these sources are listed in Table 3.

Other particle precursor gases, such as ammonia (NH_3), hydrochloric acid (HCl), nitrogen oxides (NO_x), and organic compounds from anthropogenic sources or from vegetation also play a major role in gas-to-particle conversion processes. The most important processes are homogeneous nucleation (formation of new particles) and mass transfer to preexisting particles (e.g., condensational growth or particle mass production by aqueous-phase chemical reactions).

Homogeneous Nucleation

It is believed that particles smaller than 10 nm in diameter are formed by homogeneous nucleation from precursor gases. Random molecular collisions form molecular clusters that become stable particles if the cluster exceeds a certain size.

In remote marine areas and the free troposphere, H_2SO_4 is formed by oxidation of SO_2 in the presence of hydroxyl (OH) radicals. Ultrafine sulfuric acid particles are produced in presence of water vapor (24,25). This binary homogeneous nucleation process is strongly dependent on factors such as temperature,

Table 3 Estimates of Global Sulfur Emissions (Tg yr^{-1})

Source[a]	A	B	C	D	E	F	G
Volcanic	3–20	9.2	9.3	7.4–9.3	9	8.5	7
Terrestrial	0.1–5	1.2	0.3	3.8–4.3	1	1	7
Oceanic	12–40	19.5	15.4	19–58	12	16	36
Biomass burning	1–4	3.0	2.2	2.8	2	2.5	—
Total natural	16–69	33	27	33–75	24	28	50
Anthropogenic	70–85	92.4	76.8	—	78	70	103

[a]A, 56; B, 57; C, 58; D, 59; E, 60; F, 61; G, 62.
Source: Ref. 55.

the partial pressure of condensable material, the partial pressure of water vapor (H_2O), and the surface area of preexisting particles (26,27).

New particle formation in polluted areas is probably more complex than under remote atmospheric conditions. A host of gas precursors, such as organic compounds, HCl, HNO_3, and NH_3, may also contribute to homogeneous nucleation processes. Besides the binary homogeneous nucleation process, ternary homogeneous nucleation processes such as H_2SO_4–H_2O–NH_3, HCl–H_2O–NH_3, and HNO_3–H_2O–NH_3, may occur in the atmosphere. Modeling results (28) show that ternary homogeneous nucleation could be a viable explanation for particle production in the marine boundary layer.

There are also measurements suggesting that ultrafine particle production is associated with clouds, especially in or just above the cloud top. It is assumed that such layers, with high particle concentrations (29) or a separate ultrafine particle mode (30), are the result of in situ photochemical particle production by H_2SO_4. Other possible processes, which may occur near evaporating clouds, are the particle formation by HCl–NH_3 or HCl–H_2O–NH_3.

The influence of organic compounds on new particle formation is not well understood. However, if the total particle surface area is low, supersaturated organic compounds, such as alkanes or aromates, may also form new particles.

Particle Growth and Shrinkage Owing to Mass Transfer Processes

Once a stable particle is formed, it can grow or shrink owing to mass transfer processes between the gas and the particle phase. These processes are governed mainly by the actual particle size, by the ratio of mean free path and particle diameter (Knudsen number), by the molecular diffusion coefficient, and most importantly, by the difference between the gas phase and the particle surface equilibrium vapor pressures of the transferred chemical species. Vapor pressures in the gas phase that are higher than the equilibrium vapor pressure at the particle surface result in a net mass flux toward the particle surface (i.e., the particle gains mass and growth takes place). Gas-phase vapor pressures that are lower than the equilibrium vapor pressure at the particle surface cause a net mass flux directed away from the particle (i.e., the particle loses mass and shrinks). The most important mechanisms that influence the equilibrium vapor pressure at the particle surface are the Kelvin effect, the effect of nonvolatile solute, aqueous-phase chemical reactions, and latent heat release.

Kelvin Effect

The energy necessary to transfer a molecule from the liquid into the gas phase (i.e., to separate the molecule from the attractive forces exerted by its near neighbors) determines the vapor pressure of a liquid. It we consider small droplets of liquid, there are fewer molecules in the layers next to the surface than for a plane surface. As a consequence, the vapor pressure over a small droplet is greater than the vapor pressure over a plane surface. Therefore, it is easier for the molecules on the surface of a small droplet to escape into the vapor phase (i.e., small droplets evaporate easier than relatively larger droplets). This effect is called the Kelvin effect. It we consider a pure water droplet with a diameter of 2 μm, the equilibrium vapor pressure at the droplet surface is increased by 0.1%; that is, a relative humidity of 100.1% is needed to prevent this droplet from evaporation.

Effect of Nonvolatile Solute

If a droplet consists of a solvent (e.g., water) and a nonvolatile solute, then, depending on the nature and the concentration of the nonvolatile solute, the vapor pressure of the solvent at the droplet surface is reduced. This effect, in principle, can be understood on a purely geometric basis. If we compare a pure solvent droplet with a droplet containing the solvent and a solute, in the latter, there are relatively fewer solvent molecules in the surface layer. This leads to a vapor pressure reduction proportional to the concentration, as observed in ideal solutions (Raoult's law). Typical nonvolatile solutes found in atmospheric aerosol particles are salts, such as $(NH_4)_2SO_4$ or NaCl. Although the Kelvin effect and the effects of nonvolatile solutes are competing, the reduction of vapor pressure owing to the presence of a nonvolatile solute makes it possible for aqueous solution droplets to exist in equilibrium with air, the relative humidity of which is significantly less than 100% (haze particles). If we again consider a water droplet with a diameter of 2 μm and assume a solute—here $(NH_4)_2SO_4$—volume concentration of 20%, the equilibrium vapor pressure at the droplet surface is decreased by 10% (i.e., a relative humidity of 90% is needed to prevent this droplet from evaporation).

Absorption, Dissociation, and Aqueous-Phase Chemical Reactions

The diffusive penetration of gases or gas mixtures into a condensed phase (e.g., droplet) is called *absorption*. In equilibrium, the absorbed gas is dissolved at a certain concentration inside the droplet and the equilibrium vapor pressure over the droplet surface is proportional to the concentration at the droplet surface (Henry's law). The concentration inside the droplet itself can be influenced by dissociation or chemical reactions (sulfur production by oxidation of dissolved SO_2 to SO_4^{-2}). If these processes represent a sink for the solute, the concentration inside the droplet and, consequently, the vapor pressure at the droplet surface is decreased (i.e., mass transfer is enhanced). Typical gases that dissolve into atmospheric water droplets are CO_2, SO_2, NH_3, H_2O_2, and O_3.

Latent Heat Release

Latent heat release can play an important role, especially in water condensation. During the condensation process latent heat is released, which results in a warming of the droplet. This affects the temperature profile in the vicinity of the droplet; consequently, the equilibrium vapor pressure at the droplet surface. Latent heat release causes increasing vapor pressures at the droplet surface and reduced mass transfer.

C. Combustion

Beside the sources of primary particles from bulk-to-particle conversion and secondary particles from gas-to-particle conversion, the emissions of primary particles by combustion processes are not negligible. In principle, two types of particles are emitted into the atmosphere by combustion: carbonaceous particles (organic and black carbon), and fly ash (minerals and metals). A submicrometer number size distribution of combustion aerosol particles is shown in Figure 2. The aerosol was produced by a coal-fired power plant in Leipzig, Germany, and sampled directly from the stack on July 18, 1996. The aerosol is dominated by broad ultrafine–Aitken mode particles, probably consisting of primary carbonaceous (soot), with a geometric mean diameter of $D_P = 45$ nm (see following Sec. III.C). The accumulation mode ($D_P = 290$ nm) probably consists of fly ash particles (see following discussion on fly ash).

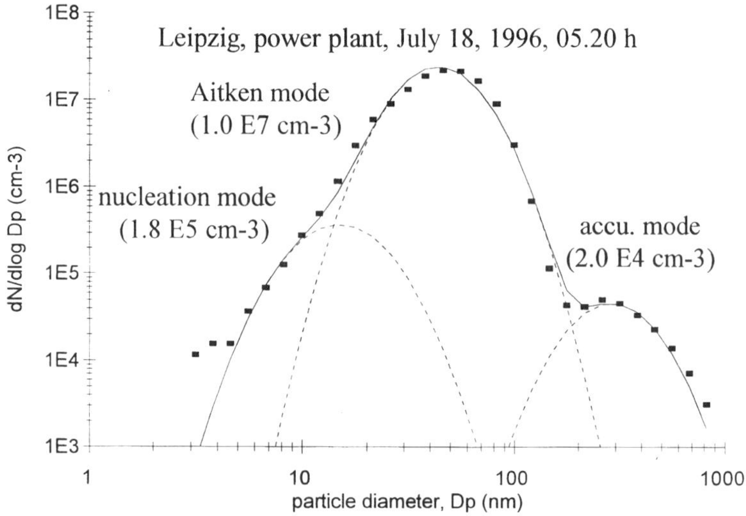

Figure 2 A number-size distribution of a primary combustion aerosol (1-hr average) measured at a coal-fired power plant in Leipzig, Germany. The measurement was performed by the Institute for Tropospheric Research in July 1996. The solid squares represent the measurement, and the solid line the sum of log-normal distributions (dotted lines) of the ultrafine, the Aitken, and the accumulation mode.

Carbonaceous Aerosols

Carbonaceous particles from combustion processes (soot) usually consist of black carbon with which some unburned hydrocarbons have become associated. The formation of such particles has often been studied in conjunction with aerosol emission from diesel engines and is described by Amann and Siegla (31) as follows: A series of rapid and incompletely understood precursory events lead to multicomponent homogeneous nucleation and to the formation of primary soot particles. Further soot mass is then added through surface growth to the nuclei. As a result of agglomeration, the resulting chains and clusters are formed. Finally, unburned hydrocarbons are adsorbed onto black carbon particles. The size of primary soot particles varies between 10 and 80 nm, although most are in the size range of 15–30 nm. Agglomerates of primary soot particles, however, can become as large as several hundred nanometers.

The global source strengths for organic and black carbon are not well known. The total strength of carbonaceous particles is commonly assumed by quantifying the ambient concentrations of total carbon and dividing them by the lifetime of carbon particles in the atmosphere (3–7 days). However, in the study by Penner (23), different source strengths from different emission categories have been estimated separately from known fuel usages and emission factors and from known volatile emissions and estimates of gas-to-particle conversion efficiencies (Table 4).

Smoke particles from biomass burning associated with savannah fires and agricultural waste burning were estimated using an emission faction of 5 g of organic matter per kilogram of biomass burned. To estimate the emissions affected by forest cleaning, an emission factor of 16 g/kg biomass was used. The sources identified with urban activities (fossil and wood fuel burning, industrial

Table 4 Sources of Fine Particle ($D_{aP} < 2.5\ \mu m$) Organic Matter and Black Carbon from Combustion Processes

Source type	Source strength ($Tg\ yr^{-1}$)
Anthropogenic	
Organic carbon from biomass burning (savannahs, forests, and agricultural waste)	50 (10–110)
Organic carbon from fossil and wood-fuel burning, industrial processes, and fugitive sources	42 (10–120)
Sources of black carbon	18 (3–30)
Natural	
Organic carbon from forest fires	4 (2–8)
Black carbon from natural fires	0.4 (0.2–0.8)

Source: Ref. 23.

processes, and fugitive emission) were assumed by scaling estimates for the total black carbon source (5–25 Tg of carbon per year, 32) and by measured ratios of organic matter to black carbon in urban areas. However, the latter estimation is very uncertain.

The estimated value of anthropogenic black carbon was derived from a study by Penner et al. (33). Approximately 6 Tg yr^{-1} results from diesel and coal and 12 Tg yr^{-1} derives from biomass burning.

The natural sources of organic carbon aerosols were estimated as follows: Smoke particles from wild fires were estimated from assumptions on the amount of fuel burned in forests wild fires using an emission factor of 16 g/kg fuel. Black carbon emission from natural fires were assumed to be about 10% of the organic emission.

Secondary organic particles from anthropogenic and natural emissions from nonmethane hydrocarbons and emissions of plants and submicron microorganisms are not included in Table 4.

Fly Ash

Pulverized coal contains typically between 3 and 20% mineral material by weight. During the combustion process, this mineral matter undergoes physical and chemical transformations and results in fly ash, with a broad distribution in size and chemical composition. Many of the mineral transformation processes occurring with coal burning are generally understood and have been briefly described (34). The inorganic constituents in coal are present either as mineral inclusions, varying in size from a fraction of a micrometer to tens of micrometers, or as atomically dispersed species. As the carbonaceous surface recedes during combustion, the imbedded inorganic materials are exposed. The ash usually grows in size as the surface of the coal particle recedes. Ash growth occurs either by the coalescence of smaller minimal inclusions, or by condensation of atomically dispersed elements (e.g., metals). The mineral matter in the coal thus forms large ash particles (tens of micrometers) as result of complete coalescence within the coal particle, or of several small ash particles (0.5–30 μm; 35), if oxidation causes the particles to break up during combustion. These processes lead to a bimodal size distribution of the fly ash particles.

IV. Physical and Chemical Properties of Particles

A. Arctic Aerosol

Numerous studies have documented both the chemistry and physics of aerosol particulates in several locations, including studies of Arctic haze in the late winter and the aerosol under much cleaner conditions in the Arctic summer. The most complete set of particle size distribution measurements is reported by Covert et al. (1). The submicrometer size distribution in the boundary layer is trimodal most of the time during the Arctic summer. The total particle number concentration varied between 1 and 400 cm^{-3}. A typical size distribution of the aerosol in Arctic summer is shown in Figure 3.

Heintzenberg and Leck (36) reported that the average total number concentration of aerosol particles observed in summer was more than twice that in winter. During winter, however, concentrations of black carbon and sea salt (Na^+) in the aerosol were higher than in summer, whereas the methanesulfonic acid (MSA; oxidation product from DMS) concentration was higher in summer.

A study by Heintzenberg et al. (37) found that the winter Arctic aerosol was dominated by anthropogenic pollution from midlatitude sources. Size-fractionated chemical measurements showed that S, Cu, Zn, and Pb were found mainly in the submicrometer particles.

B. Marine Aerosol

Marine aerosols are probably the best characterized environmental aerosols in terms of the physical and chemical particle properties. Several studies have been performed to measure the number-size distributions over the Pacific and Atlantic

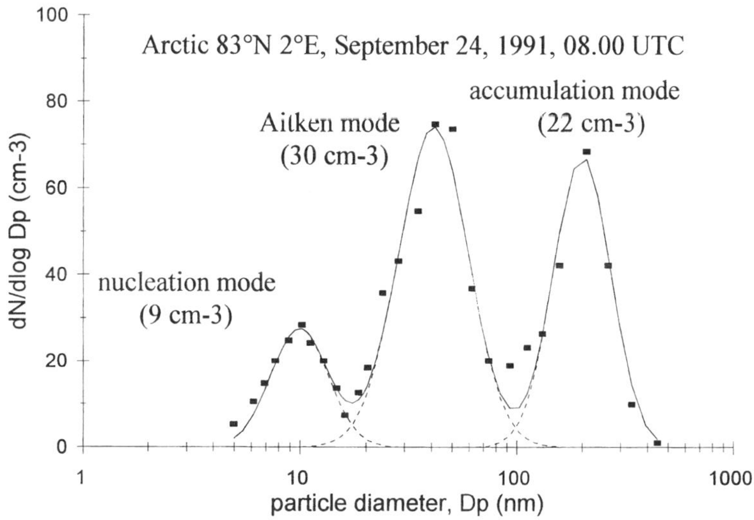

Figure 3 A trimodal number-size distribution of an Arctic aerosol measured during the International Arctic Ocean Expedition 1991 (1). The solid squares represent the measurement, and the solid line the sum of log-normal distributions (dotted lines) of the ultrafine, the Aitken, and the accumulation mode.

Oceans. Hoppel et al. (4) found, for background conditions, a double-peaked characteristic for the submicrometer particles (Aitken and accumulation mode) in the remote Atlantic. The particle number concentration varied between 200 and 300 cm^{-3}. The total particle number in the two modes for background conditions is of the same order of magnitude, whereas under continental influence, the particle number in the Aitken mode is much higher than in the accumulation mode. Under continental influence, the total particle number concentration can reach several thousands in the Atlantic.

The principal constituent of marine particles are sea salt, non–sea-salt sulfate (nss sulfate), and mineral dust (38). The nss sulfate has both a continental and marine source and is derived from homogeneous nucleation and diffusive mass transport processes of aerosol precursor gases, such as SO_2 and NH_3. Numerous studies have shown that the accumulation mode in clean marine air is predominately composed of nss sulfate. Its concentration decreases from coastal regions of the continents to the remote areas of the oceans. Single-particle analysis by electron microscopy showed that most of the particles are morphologically similar to $(NH_4)_2SO_4$ (39,40). Also a small number of H_2SO_4 particles were found.

Most particles larger than 600 nm are essentially sea salt. However, sea salt is found primarily in the coarse mode, except during episodes of continental dust transport. Sea salt concentrations are about 1–20 μg m^{-3} at surface level (40).

Mineral dust is the constituent of the marine aerosol with the highest variability. It is transported to the marine environment from semiarid and desert regions and is part of the coarse mode even under "clean" marine conditions. The mean dust concentrations vary between 0.05 and 0.5 μg m^{-3} (41). However, very high dust concentrations can occur over regions, such as the tropical and equatorial North Atlantic Ocean and northwest Indian Ocean. Saharan dust concentrations up to 27 μg m^{-3} have been reported (17) at Barbados during the summer months.

C. Continental Aerosols

Continental aerosols differ strongly from marine aerosols in terms of size distribution, particle number concentration, and chemical composition. The total particle number concentration can vary between 100 cm^{-3} in remote continental regions and several 10,000 cm^{-3} in urban-influenced regions (42). As presented by Hoppel et al. (4), the Aitken mode dominates the average continental number size distribution. Figure 4 shows an example of an average of 96 size distributions measured during a field campaign on Hoher Peißenberg, Germany, on April 11, 1994, 00.00–24.00 hr (unpublished size distribution measurements). This rural size distribution is typically bimodal and consists of an Aitken (D_P = 45 nm) and accumulation mode (D_P = 225 nm).

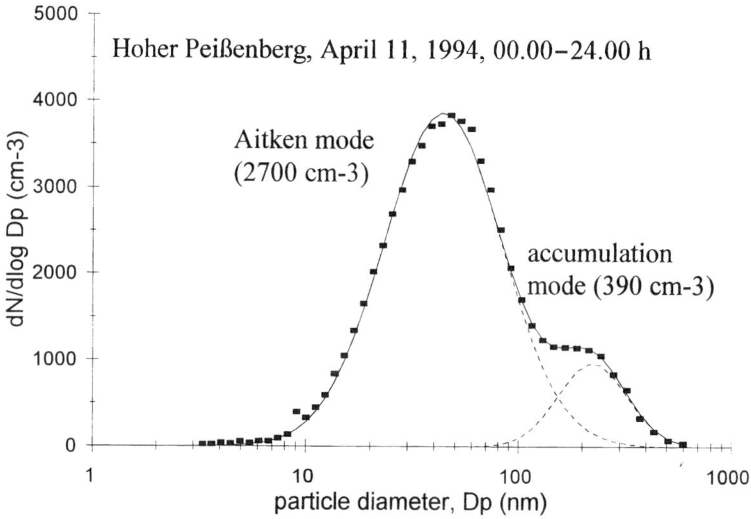

Figure 4 A typical bimodal number-size distribution of a rural aerosol (24-hr average) measured on Hoher Peißenberg, Germany. The measurements were performed by the Institute for Tropospheric Research in April 1994. The solid squares represent the measurement, and the solid line the sum of log-normal distributions (dotted lines) of the Aitken and the accumulation mode.

In polluted regions, the number concentrations often exceed 10,000 cm^{-3}, and the Aitken and accumulation mode are shifted toward larger sizes (43). The size distribution shown in Figure 5 is an average of 192 size distributions obtained during a field campaign in the highly polluted Po Valley, Italy, November 17, 1994, 00.00–24.00 hr. The distribution consists of a nucleation and an accumulation mode. However, the nucleation mode occurred only occasionally.

The most comprehensive investigation of submicrometer size distributions (3–170 nm) of urban aerosols was performed in Vienna (44; Table 5).

Three particle modes were observed in the size range investigated in this study. One mode with a geometric mean diameter of 5.5 nm was correlated with solar radiation, (i.e., with particle formation by photochemistry). Another mode (D_P = 24 nm) correlated mostly with peaks in car traffic (i.e., minimums during nights and weekends and maximums during rush hour on working days). A third mode D_P = 50 nm), however, did not show a dependency on the time of day.

Because of the manifold particle formation processes, the chemical composition of submicrometer continental aerosol particles is rather complex. The major constituents of these particles are usually sulfates, nitrates, soot, organic compounds, and soil dust. Sulfates are derived mainly from anthropogenic SO_2, ni-

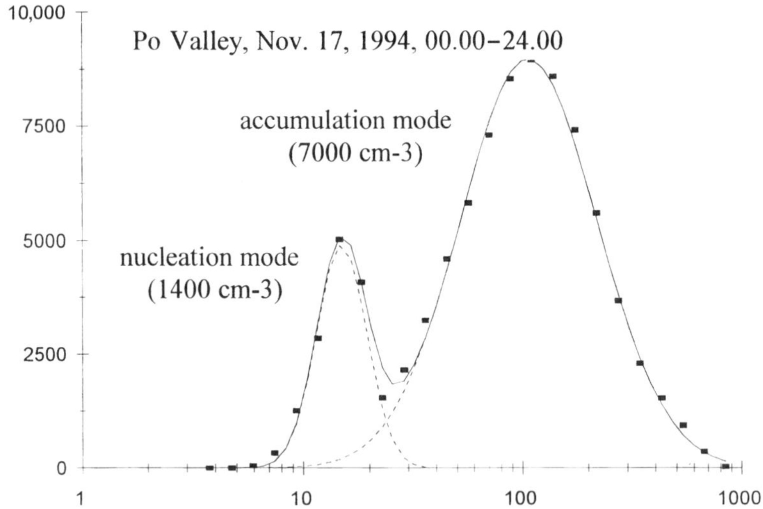

Figure 5 A typical size distribution of a highly polluted air mass consisting of a nucleation mode and a broad Aitken–accumulation mode (24-hr average). The measurements were performed by the Institute for Tropospheric Research during an intensive fog experiment in the Po Valley, Italy, November 1994. The solid squares represent the measurement, and the solid line the sum of log-normal distributions (dotted lines) of the ultrafine and the accumulation modes. (From Ref. 63.)

Table 5 Environmental Particle Number Concentration Measured During Summer and Winter 1986 in Vienna

	00.00–05.00 hr	08.00–12.00 hr
	Particle number concentration (cm^{-3})	
June–September 1996		
Average	12,000 ± 5,000	33,000 ± 11,000
Maximal	20,000	
Minimal	3,000	
November–December 1986		
Average	23,000 ± 15,000	76,000 ± 33,000
Maximal	70,000	150,000
Minimal	5,000	30,000

Source: Ref. 44.

trates from NO_x emissions, soot from combustion processes, and organic compounds from anthropogenic release, as well as emissions from plants (e.g., terpenes). In a comparison of urban and rural aerosols, Clarke et al. (45) found that particulate mass in urban sites was only 30% higher than at rural sites. The differences in sulfate and nitrates in conjunction with ammonium ions was much less (10%). The mass fraction of fine carbonaceous aerosol particles in urban atmospheres is typically 30–50%.

Continental soil dust is usually contained in the size fraction between 1 and 20 μm in diameter, with the mass median diameter about 2–4 μm. Larger particles fall out quickly because of their large sedimentation velocities, although individual dust particles of several 100 μm have been collected in South America that have been transported from the Sahara (46). The reported size spectra of mineral particles (41,47) indicate that the mass of fine clay particles is one to two orders of magnitude smaller than that of coarse silt particles (1–10 μm). Noll et al. (48) compared the composition of coarse atmospheric particles at a urban and rural site. At the rural site, the coarse particles contained predominantly crustal material (limestone 89% and silicates 6%) and biogenic material. Limestone had a mean mass diameter of about 20 μm, and silicates 12 μm. In urban samples, a significant fraction (25%) of rubber tire was found with a mean mass diameter of 25 μm.

V. Removal of Aerosol Particles from the Environment

In principle, two removal processes of aerosol particles in the atmosphere are possible: dry and wet deposition to the ground, and reduction of particle number (maintenance of particulate mass).

Dry deposition of particles to the surface of the earth is mainly by diffusive transport of fine and ultrafine particles, and gravitational settling of coarse particles. Because of the strong size dependence of the sedimentation velocity, large particles fall out close to source areas, whereas small particles are available for long-range transport. The size distribution of coarse particle shifts toward smaller sizes during transport away from their source areas into higher atmospheric layers. In terms of particle mass removal, sedimentation is predominant in dry deposition processes.

Wet deposition is the predominant process for mass removal of submicrometer particles. Particles from mainly the accumulation mode serve as condensation nuclei for cloud and fog droplets. If the droplets fall out owing to rain or drizzle, particulate material is lost to the ground and removed from the atmosphere.

Reduction of the particle number concentration is due to coagulation and coalescence: Especially the number concentration of ultrafine particle number is efficiently reduced in the well-mixed boundary layer of the atmosphere owing to coagulation with cloud droplets as well as with large particles. Coagulation reduces the total particle number; however, it maintains the total particle mass. Coalescence of cloud droplets in nonprecipitating clouds lead to a decrease of the particle number of the accumulation mode and to an increase in particle size.

VI. Summary and Outlook

Similar to trace gases, atmospheric particles go through a cycle, beginning with a multitude of sources, as described in the foregoing and, by physical and chemical transformations, lead to the particle sinks at the earth's surface. However, there are large gaps in understanding this cycle and its importance to the climate, air pollution, and human health. There is a need to better understand aerosol processes in the atmosphere, such as new particle formation, particle growth, and particle deposition. To completely describe the environmental aerosols, the concentration, particle shape, size distribution, size-resolved chemical composition, and state of mixture have to be known (49). From these parameters, aerosol dynamics during transport, radiative effects of particles, cloud and fog formation processes, and heterogeneous chemical reactions on aerosol particle surfaces, or aqueous chemical reaction inside droplets can be studied.

One present goal in environmental aerosol research is to quantify the direct and indirect effect of aerosol-forcing on the radiation balance of the earth in polluted regions, compared with atmospheric particles in remote areas. In the solar spectral range, the direct radiative-forcing of aerosol particles is due to their scattering and absorption of radiation (50). Number concentration and chemical composition of the particle fraction that serves as cloud droplet nuclei will affect the size distribution of cloud droplets and, thus, the cloud albedo (51). The indirect aerosol-forcing by cloud properties and the water cycle is much more difficult to quantify than the direct forcing, owing to the complexity of cloud processes.

It is proposed from model calculations that direct and indirect aerosol forcing of climate may lead to a negative term in the radiation balance and, thereby, to a potential cooling effect in polluted regions. However, the global geographic fields of radiative forcing by anthropogenic greenhouse gases and particles do not match; thus, there is no simple compensation (52).

Because of the large uncertainties over the problem of indirect forcing, environmental aerosol research will focus mainly on the quantification and verification of the direct forcing in the near future, and concrete results on direct forcing are expected within a few years. The understanding of indirect forcing, however, will require substantial basic research. Sensitivity studies in the field and in the laboratory must be coupled with cloud process models, including cloud microphysics and aqueous-phase chemistry.

Beyond the first step of process studies and investigations of the spatial and temporal variability of the aerosol, further research must lead to appropriate parameterization of the environmental aerosol to improve global models (53).

Another goal of present research is to understand the influence of atmospheric particles on human health. Because of the high number concentrations of fine aerosol particles (10^4–10^6 cm^{-3}) as observed in the vicinity of particle-emitting sources (especially combustion processes), these particles might have a substantial influence on human health when they are deposited in the human respiratory tract. Current research suggests that the biological effectiveness of ambient particles increase with decreasing particle size, so that even ultrafine particles may have to be considered a health risk (54). Although the total mass of these particle is low, their number concentration is relatively high. Away from particle-emitting sources total number concentrations of fine and ultrafine aerosol particles are fairly low (2,000–10,000), but even at lower concentrations these particles may have to be considered a health risk, as they may function as carrier for heavy metals and hazardous organic compounds. This is especially true for particles emitted from combustion processes. This becomes even more important because fine and ultrafine particles are not efficiently removed by state-of-the-art gas-cleaning devices used in hazardous waste combustion and coal-fired power plants.

References

1. Covert DS, Wiedensohler A, Aalto P, Heintzenberg J, McMurry PH, Leck C. Aerosol number size distributions from 3 to 500 nm diameter in the Arctic marine boundary layer during summer and autumn. Tellus 1996; 48B:197–212.
2. Wiedensohler A, Covert DS, Swietlicki E, Aalto P, Heintzenberg J, Leck C. Occurrence of an ultrafine particle mode less than 20 nm in diameter in the marine boundary layer of the Arctic summer and autumn. Tellus 1996; 48B:213–222.
3. Raes F. Entrainment of free tropospheric aerosols as a regulating mechanism for cloud condensation nuclei in the remote marine boundary layer. J Geophys Res 1995; 100(D2):2893–2903.
4. Hoppel WA, Fitzgerald JW, Frick GM, Larson RE, Mack E. Aerosol size distributions and optical properties found in the marine boundary layer over the Atlantic Ocean. J Geophys Res 1990; 95(D4):3659–3686.
5. Blanchard DC, Woodcock AH. Bubble formation and modification in the sea and its meteorological significance. Tellus 1957; 9:145–158.
6. Monahan EC, Fairall CW, Davidson KL, Jones-Boyle P. Observed interrelationships amongst 10 m-elevation winds, oceanic whitecaps, and marine aerosols. Q J R Meteorol Soc 1983; 109:379–392.
7. Hidy GM, Wolf M. Projections of trends in anthropogenic aerosol sources. In: Charlson R, Heintzenberg J, eds. Aerosol Forcing of Climate. New York: John Wiley and Sons, 1995:171–182.

8. Nriagu JO. A global assessment of natural sources of atmospheric trace metals. Nature 1989; 338:47–49.
9. Erickson DJ, Merrill JT, Duce RA. Seasonal estimates of global atmospheric sea-salt distribution. J Geophys Res 1986; 91:1067–1072.
10. Erickson DJ, Duce RA. On the global flux of atmospheric sea salt. J Geophys Res 1988; 93:14079–14088.
11. Gillette D. A wind tunnel simulation of the erosion of soil: effect of soil texture, sandblasting, wind speed, and soil consolidation on dust production. Atmos Environ 1978; 12:1735–1743.
12. Shao Y, Raupach MR, Findlater PA. Effect of saltation bombardment on the entrainment of dust by wind. J Geophys Res 1993; 98:12719–12726.
13. Schuetz L. Long range transport of desert dust with special emphasis on the Sahara. Ann N Y Acad Sci 1980; 388:515–532.
14. Duce RA, Liss PS, Merrill JT, Atlas EL, Buat-Menard P, Hicks BB, Miller JM, Prospero JM, Arimoto R, Church TM, Ellis W, Galloway JN, Hansen L, Jickells TD, Knap AH, Reinhardt KH, Schneider B, Soudine A, Tokos JJ, Tsunogai S, Wollast R. The atmospheric input of trace species into the world ocean. Global Biogeochem Cycles 1991; 5:193–259.
15. Tegen I, Fung I. Modeling of mineral dust in the atmosphere: sources, transport and optical thickness. J Geophys Res 1994; 99:22897–22914.
16. Pye K. Aeolian Dust and Dust Deposits. San Diego: Academic Press, 1987.
17. Prospero JM, Nees RT. Impact of the North African drought and El Nino on mineral dust in the Barbados trade winds. Nature 1986; 320:735–738.
18. Lamb PJ, Peppler RA, Hastenrath S. Interannual variability in the tropical Atlantic. Nature 1986; 322:238–240.
19. Tegen I, Fung I. Contribution to the mineral aerosol load from land surface modification. J Geophys Res 1995; 100:18707–18726.
20. Matthias-Maser S, Jaenicke R. Examination of atmospheric bioaerosol particles with radii > 0.2 µm. J Aerosol Sci 1994; 25:1605–1613.
21. Spendlove JC. Industrial, agricultura and municipal microbial aerosol problems. Dev Ind Microbiol 1974; 15:20–27.
22. Blanchard DC, Syzdek LD. Concentration of bacteria in jet-drops from bursting bubbles. J Geophys Res 1972; 77:5087–5099.
23. Penner JE. Carbonaceous aerosols influencing atmospheric radiation black and organic carbon. In: Charlson RJ, Heintzenberg J, eds. Aerosol Forcing of Climate. New York: John Wiley & Sons, 1995:91–108.
24. Raes F, Saltelli A, Van Dingenen R. Modelling formation and growth of H_2SO_4–H_2O aerosols: uncertainty analysis and experimental evaluation. J Aerosol Sci 1992; 23:759–771.
25. Easter RC, Peters LK. Binary homogeneous nucleation: temperature and relative humidity fluctuations, nonlinearity, and aspects of new particle production in the atmosphere. J Appl Meteorol 1994; 33:775–784.
26. Seinfeld JH. Atmospheric Chemistry and Physics of Air Pollution. New York: John Wiley and Sons, 1986.
27. Jaecker-Voirol A, Mirabel P. Heteromolecular nucleation in the sulfuric acid–water system. Atmos Environ 1989; 23:2053–2057.

28. Coffman DJ, Hegg DA. A preliminary study of the effect of ammonia on particle nucleation in the marine boundary layer. J Geophys Res 1995; 100(D4):7147–7160.
29. Hegg DA, Radke LF, Hobbs PV. Particle production associated with marine clouds. J Geophys Res 1990; 95:13917–13926.
30. Hoppel WA, Frick GM, Fitzgerald JW, Larson RE. Marine boundary layer measurements of new particle formation and the effects nonprecipitating clouds have on aerosol size distribution. J Geophys Res 1994; 99(D7):14443–14459.
31. Amann CA, Siegla DC. Diesel particulates—what they are and why. Aerosol Sci Technol 1982; 1:73–101.
32. Penner JE, Charlson RJ, Hales JM, Laulainen N, Leifer R, Novakov T, Ogren J, Radke LF, Schwartz SE, Travis L. Quantifying and minimizing uncertainty of climate forcing by anthropogenic aerosols. Bull Am Meteorol Soc 1994; 75:375–400.
33. Penner JE, Eddleman H, Novakov T. Towards the development of a global inventory for black carbon emissions. Atmos Environ 1993; 27A:1277–1295.
34. Kang SG, Kerstein AR, Helble JJ, Sarofim AF. Simulation of residual ash formation during pulverized coal combustion: bimodal ash particle size distribution. Aerosol Sci Technol 1990; 13:401–412.
35. Okazaki K. Submicron particle formation in pulverized coal combustion. J Aerosol Res Jpn 1993; 7:289–291.
36. Heintzenberg J, Leck C. Seasonal variation of the atmospheric aerosol near the top of the marine boundary layer over Spitsbergen related to the Arctic sulphur cycle. Tellus 1994; 46B:52–67.
37. Heintzenberg J, Hansson HC, Lannefors HO. The chemical composition of Arctic haze at Ny-Ålesund, Spitsbergen. Tellus 1981; 33:162–171.
38. Fitzgerald JW. Marine aerosols: a review. Atmos Environ 1991; 25A:533–545.
39. Meszaros A, Vissy K. Concentration, size distribution and chemical nature of atmospheric aerosol particles in remote oceanic areas. J Aerosol Sci 1974; 5:101–109.
40. Gras JL, Ayers GP. Marine aerosol at southern mid-latitudes. J Geophys Res 1983; 88(C15):10661–10666.
41. Prospero JM, Bonatti E. Continental dust in the atmosphere of the Eastern Equatorial Pacific. J Geophys Res 1969; 74:3362–3371.
42. Willeke K, Whitby KT. Atmospheric aerosols: size distribution interpretation. J Air Pollut Contr Assoc 1975; 25:529–534.
43. Whitby KT. Aerosol formation in urban plumes. Ann NY Acad Sci 1980; 338:258–275.
44. Winklmayr W. Untersuchung des ultrafeinen Aerosols in der urbanen Atmosphäre von Wien. Ph.D dissertation, University of Vienna, 1987.
45. Clarke AG, Willison MJ, Zeki EM. A comparison of urban and rural aerosol composition using dichotomous sampler. Atmos Environ 1984; 18:1767–1775.
46. Betzer PR, Carder KL, Merrill JT, Tindale NW, Uematsu M, Costello DK, Young RW, Feely RA, Breland JA, Bernstein RE, Greco AM. Long-range transport of giant mineral aerosol particles. Nature 1988; 336:568–571.
47. D'Almeida G, Schuetz L. Number, mass, and volume distribution of mineral aerosol and soils of the Sahara. J Clim Appl Meteorol 1983; 22:233–243.
48. Noll KE, Draftz R, Fang KYP. The composition of atmospheric coarse particles at an urban and non-urban site. Atmos Environ 1987; 21:2717–2721.

49. Heintzenberg J, Covert DS. On the distribution of physical and chemical particle properties in the atmospheric aerosol. J Atmos Chem 1990; 10:383–397.
50. Charlson RJ, Langner J, Rohde H, Leovy CB, Warren SG. Perturbation of the Northern Hemisphere radiative balance by backscattering of anthropogenic sulfate aerosols. Tellus 1991; 43AB:152–163.
51. Twomey S. The influence of pollution on the shortwave albedo of clouds. J Atmos Sci 1977; 34:1149–1152.
52. Kiehl JT, Briegleb BP. The relative roles of sulphate aerosols and greenhouse gases in climate forcing. Science 1993; 260:311–314.
53. Heintzenberg J, Graf H-F, Charlson RJ, Warneck P. Climate forcing and the physico-chemical life cycle of the atmospheric aerosol—why do we need an integrated, interdisciplinary global research programme? Contr Atmos Phys 1996; 69:261–271.
54. Peters A, Wichmann H-E, Tuch T, Heinrich J, Heyder J. Respiratory effects are associated with the number of ultra-fine particles. Am J Respr Crit Care Med 1997; 155:1376–1383.
55. Möller D. Sulfate aerosols and their atmospheric precursors. In: Charlson RJ, Heintzenberg J, eds. Aerosol Forcing of Climate. New York: John Wiley and Sons, 1995: 91–108.
56. Penner JE, Atherton CA, Graedel T. Global emissions and models of photochemically active compounds. In: Prinn R, ed. Global Atmospheric–Biospheric Chemistry. New York: Plenum, 1994:223–248.
57. Pham M, Megie G, Brasseur G, Granier C, Müller J. The global sulfur cycle in the atmosphere: a 3-dimensional model study. In: Prinn R, ed. Global Atmospheric–Biospheric Chemistry. New York: Plenum, 1994:223–248.
58. Bates TS, Lamb BK, Guenther A, Dignon J, Stoiber RE. Sulfur emissions to the atmosphere from natural source. J Atmos Chem 1992; 14:315–337.
59. Andreae MO, Jaeschke WA. Exchange of sulfur between biosphere and atmosphere over temperate and tropical regions. In: Horwarth RW, Stewart JWB, Ivanov MV, eds. Sulfur Cycling on the Continents. Chichester: Wiley 1992:27–61.
60. Spiro PA, Jacobs DJ, Logan JA. Global inventory of sulfur emissions with $1° \times 1°$ resolution. J Geophys Res 1992; 97:6023–6036.
61. Langner J, Rodhe H. A global three-dimensional model of the tropospheric sulfur cycle. J Atmos Chem 1991; 13:225–264.
62. Warneck P. Chemistry of the Natural Atmosphere. San Diego: Academic Press, 1988.
63. Yuskiewicz B, Orsini D, Stratmann F, Wendisch M, Wiedensohler A, Heintzenberg J, Martinsson B, Frank G, Wobrock W, Schell D. Changes in submircrometer particle distributions and light scattering during haze and fog events in a highly polluted environment. Contr Atmos Phys 1998; 71/1:33–45

3

Particles Inhaled in the Occupational Setting

JOE L. MAUDERLY, YUNG SUNG CHENG, MARK D. HOOVER, and HSU-CHI YEH

Lovelace Respiratory Research Institute
Albuquerque, New Mexico

NEIL F. JOHNSON

Boehringer Ingelheim Pharma KG
Biberach am Riss, Germany

I. Introduction

A. Purpose, Scope, and Organization

This chapter is intended as a summary review of the types of particles commonly inhaled in the workplace, the situations in which exposures commonly occur, and the health risks known or thought likely to result from deposition in the respiratory tract. This chapter, although lengthy, falls far short of an exhaustive description of all occupational particle exposures or their effects. The level of detail given varies considerably among classes of particles. Emphasis is given to materials, such as coal dust and diesel soot, for which there are currently widespread exposures and regulatory concern, and radionuclides, volcanic ash, and environmental tobacco smoke, which are seldom mentioned in texts and reviews. Other particles, such as most carcinogenic chemicals, are treated in less detail because the class is so diverse or because the materials are commonly described in other reviews. For example, environmental tobacco smoke is described only briefly as a workplace contaminant, because it is treated at length in other publications.

Each of the following sections contains information on the nature of the particles, the nature of typical exposures, the health effects of greatest concern, and key references to the literature. Citations of summary or recent publications are emphasized, whereas exhaustive citations are purposely avoided. The references cited provide the reader a starting point from which to explore the present information base. The reader is directed toward several reference works. For example, the *Encyclopedia of Occupational Health and Safety* (1) gives general descriptions of different industries, classes of materials handled, and inhalation and other occupational hazards. *Sax's Dangerous Properties of Industrial Materials* (2) presents brief descriptions and safety profiles of many agents. *Patty's Industrial Hygiene and Toxicology* (3) is a good series of reference materials containing information on chemical exposures and health risks. The series of International Agency for Research on Cancer (IARC) monographs published by the World Health Organization (WHO) contains reviews of the carcinogenicity of many chemicals. There are several excellent texts including information on occupational risks from different classes of inhaled particles (e.g., 4–7), as well as texts on specific classes of particles and classes of disease.

B. Particle Size Classes, Regulatory Agencies, and Exposure Limits

The hazards of inhaled particles are directly related to the amounts deposited in the respiratory tract which, in turn, are a function of the aerodynamic behavior of the particles and the amount inhaled. Although those factors are described in other chapters in this volume, it is useful to consider the general particle size ranges of the materials reviewed in this chapter. Many of the following sections mention the size of specific particle types, but Figure 1 provides a useful integration of the size ranges of particles encountered in the workplace. The document, *Evaluation of Exposure to Airborne Particles in the Work Environment* (8), presents useful information on the nature of airborne particles and international sampling recommendations and exposure limits. The text, *Particulates and Fine Dust Removal* (9), presents useful information on particle types, releases, and mitigation techniques in the industrial setting.

Government regulatory agencies and professional organizations in many countries have promulgated, recommended, or required limits for occupational exposures to particles. Most standards are based on gravimetric air concentrations, although some are based on particle number per unit volume. This chapter makes no attempt to list exposure standards for each particle type, although standards are mentioned in some sections. The American Conference of Governmental Hygienists (ACGIH) publishes handbooks listing exposure standards used in the United States and Germany (10,11). These handbooks list ACGIH threshold

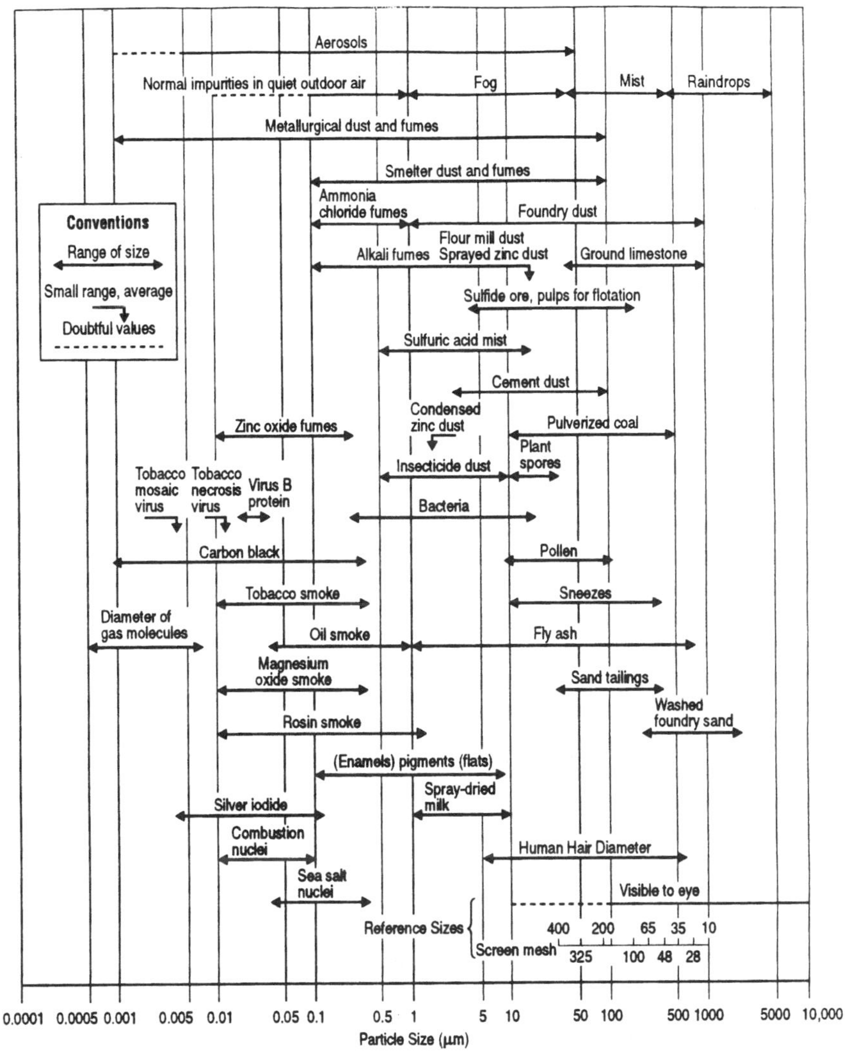

Figure 1 Size ranges of common classes of airborne particles. (Courtesy of the Mine Safety Appliances Company, Pittsburgh, PA.)

limit values (TLV), Occupational Safety and Health Administration (OSHA) permissible exposure limits, National Institute of Occupational Safety and Health (NIOSH) recommended exposure limits, and Deutsche Forschungsgemeinschaft (DFG) maximum concentration values in the workplace (MAK). These handbooks also list the current IARC, United States, and MAK classifications of carcinogens.

C. Abbreviations

Frequently used abbreviations are defined in Table 1.

Table 1 List of Abbreviations

ACGIH	American Conference of Governmental Hygienists
ALI	Annual limits on intake
AMAD	Activity median aerodynamic diameter
CWP	Coal workers pneumoconiosis
DAC	Derived air concentration
DFG	Deutsche Forschungsgemeinschaft
EPA	Environmental Protection Agency
GMAW	Gas metal arc welding
GSD	Geometric standard deviation
HBV	Hepatitis B virus
HDI	Hexamethylene diisocyanate
HIV	Human immunodeficiency virus
IARC	International Agency for Research on Cancer
ICRP	International Council on Radiation Protection
LPS	Lipopolysaccharide
MAK	Maximum concentration values in the workplace
MMAD	Mass median aerodynamic diameter
MMD	Mass median diameter
MMVF	Man-made vitreous fibers
NIOSH	National Institute of Occupational Safety and Health
OSHA	Occupational Safety and Health Administration
PCOM	Phase contrast optical microscopy
PMF	Progressive massive fibrosis
SEM	Scanning electron microscopy
SMAW	Shielded metal arc welding
STEL	Short-term exposure limit
TEM	Transmission electron microscopy
TLV	Threshold limit values
TWA	Time-weighted average
WHO	World Health Organization
WLM	Working level month

II. Review of Particles Inhaled in the Workplace

A. Nonfibrous Mineral Dusts

Silicaceous Dusts

Exposure to silicaceous dusts is a major occupational health concern in numerous industries. Much of the silicon in the earth is combined with other elements to form silicates. Various anions and cations are substituted into the crystalline silica matrix. Minerals such as kaolin, an aluminum silicate, and talc, a magnesium silicate, are silicate minerals that are used in their pure form. Many minerals of commercial importance are composed of mixtures of silica and silicates, such as feldspar and muscovite, in an infinite range of combinations. The pulmonary disease associated with silica exposure is greatly influenced by the silicate content of the material. It has been estimated that approximately 8.2 million workers in the United States are potentially exposed to crystalline silica dust each year.

Silica in Mining

Silica is the chemical term for silicon dioxide, which is a component of most minerals and rocks. Silica can exist in nature in amorphous and crystalline form. Natural glasses, such as those found in volcanic tuff, are composed of amorphous silica. Pure crystals of silicon dioxide consist of silicon–oxygen tetrahedra in various polymorphic forms. The major crystalline phases of silica are alpha-quartz, cristobalite, and tridymite. Alpha-quartz is the most abundant toxic form of silica and is the form most often of concern in industrial hygiene. Cristobalite is a high-temperature form of silica. Cristobalite is rare in the environment, but can be produced industrially by treating silica containing materials with high temperatures. It can also be formed by volcanic explosions. Tridymite is also formed at high temperatures from silica; however, its formation requires the presence of a mineralizer or flux such as sodium oxide. It is unclear whether tridymite is a low sodium silicate or an impure silica.

Silicosis is the major disease of concern following exposure to free crystalline silica. Numerous industries have the potential for exposing workers to free silica (Table 2). There are three forms of silicosis that are dependent on the nature of the silica exposure; these forms are silicotic alveolar proteinosis, accelerated silicosis, and chronic silicosis.

Alveolar proteinosis is a reaction of the lung to injury, resulting in the filling of airspace by lipoproteinaceous debris. The disease is the result of inhaling high concentrations of relatively pure silica particulates over a short time. Death can occur after a few months; however, the disease is rare in humans. In the past, workers were at risk during sandblasting, tunneling, pottery production, and quartz milling to produce abrasive soaps and silica flour. In most of these cases, no respiratory protection was worn. Although most of these cases occurred in the past, occasional clusters still occur, as happened among tombstone sandblasters,

Table 2 Occupations and Industries at Risk from Silicosis

Quarrying, mining, and dressing of sandstone, granite, and slate
Mining of tin, hematite, graphite, copper, gold, and other minerals
The pottery industry
Manufacture of refractory products, such as silica bricks
Flint crushing
Silica milling
Millstone dressing
Manufacture of abrasive soaps
Iron and steel foundries
Sand blasting
Boiler scaling
Coal mining
Vitreous enameling industry
Glass polishing
Gem polishing

reported in 1977 (12), and among silica flour workers, reported in 1981 (13). The exposures experienced by the silica flour workers were as high as 1.0 mg/m^3 which is ten times the recommended U.S. exposure limit (10).

Accelerated silicosis is a clinical term applied to a condition with intermediate progression between that of alveolar proteinosis and chronic silicosis. It develops over a period of 5–10 years after heavy exposures to fine silica particles. The condition is progressive, even in the absence of further exposure, and is frequently fatal within 10 years of the first symptoms. This condition has been reported in shipyard sandblasters (14), jade workers (15), slate pencil workers (16), and following inhalation of abrasive scouring powder (17).

Chronic silicosis occurs after prolonged exposure (10 or more years) to free silica. During long-term inhalation exposures to low concentrations of silica, particles accumulate in lymphatics and regional lymph nodes in which scattered nodules gradually develop over prolonged periods. With heavier exposure, scattered lung lesions occur. The individual nodules in simple silicosis are solitary and less than 1 cm in diameter; whereas in conglomerate silicosis, the nodules become confluent and encroach on the lung parenchyma. Progressive massive fibrosis is an uncommon lesion composed of confluent silicotic nodules.

Chronic silicosis is found in many occupations (see Table 2); however, the occurrence of silicosis is less common in the modern workplace because of improved industrial hygiene measures. However, silicosis still accounts for more than 300 deaths per year in the United States. Although many of these deaths occur in men first exposed to crystalline silica as young adults before 1950, a significant number result from more recent exposure. The Division of Respiratory

Disease Studies of NIOSH has developed a silicosis mortality surveillance system. The number of U.S. silicosis deaths in 1968 was 1157 and declined to 301 deaths in 1988. In the period from 1985 to 1990, the construction industry accounted for the highest proportion (10.8%) of silicosis deaths. The other major industries associated with deaths from silicosis were metal mining (7.9%), blast furnaces, steel works, finishing mills (6.9%), nonmetallic mineral or stone products (6.1%), coal mining (5.9%), iron and steel foundries (5.4%), and nonmetallic mining or quarrying (5.1%) (18). Respirable dust levels of between 0.01 and 0.09 mg/m^3 having silica contents of 4.8–12.2% have been reported in the granite industries in Vermont, and in iron and steel facilities, levels as high as 13.1 mg/m^3 have been reported for workers who shake out mouldings and casts (19). In four brick plants in North Carolina, only those trades associated with maintenance of the kiln experienced exposures above the OSHA standard of 0.1 mg/m^3.

Crystalline silica is recognized in most countries as toxic, and exposures are regulated by setting or mandating upper limits of exposure. Various determinants of exposure are used: particle number or mass of airborne dust, respirable dust, or fraction of free silica. Standards differ among countries and frequently differ among regulatory agencies in the same country. In the United States, the Mine Safety and Health Administration and the OSHA have set different standards for total silica that apply to general industry and underground mines. OSHA has also set a separate standard for alpha-quartz (0.1 mg/m^3), which is half the standard for cristobalite and tridymite. Both NIOSH and the ACGIH now recommend silica standards based on direct quantification of alpha-quartz, cristobalite, and tridymite. Silica can be analyzed by several methods, including optical microscopy, analytical electron microscopy, X-ray diffraction, infrared spectroscopy, differential thermal analysis, and wet chemical techniques. These techniques are used to determine total silica; infrared spectroscopy and X-ray diffraction techniques are commonly used to determine the occurrence of the various crystalline polymorphs.

In addition to the well-documented fibrogenic potential of free silica, the IARC (19) has classified silica as a possible human carcinogen. Although there is sufficient evidence for the carcinogenicity of silica in rodents, the human evidence for carcinogenicity is controversial. Studies in foundry workers consistently show increases in mortality from lung cancer; however, in addition to silica, foundry workers are exposed to a wide range of carcinogenic materials. Whereas five epidemiological studies in the stone and granite industry reported excess mortality from silicosis, one study of tunnelers showed a significant excess of lung cancer. Moderate excesses were seen in three other studies; however, smoking and radon exposure may have been confounding factors. Metal miners also have a high mortality from silicosis and frequently have lung cancer rates 20–50% above expected (19).

Nonfibrous Silicates

Many workers in occupations associated with mining and milling of talc, kaolinite, vermiculite, mica, bentonite, feldspar, Fuller's earth, and diatomaceous earth are at risk of developing lung disease (silicatosis) after extended periods of exposure to high concentrations of dust.

In some countries, exposures to talc and mica are regulated; the permissible levels are higher than for silica, reflecting their lower fibrogenic potential. In the United States silicate dusts are generally regulated as nuisance or inert dusts, with exposure limits of 5 mg/m^3 respirable dust and either 10 or 15 mg/m^3 of total dust (10).

Talc. Talc is a hydrated magnesium silicate that occurs in platy, granular, and fibrous forms. Talc crystals are made up of two sheets of silica tetrahedra, with a single layer of magnesium hydroxide sandwiched in between. Talc can be contaminated with a wide variety of other minerals, including fibrous anthophyllite and tremolite, quartz, calcite, dolomite, and magnesite. The contaminations with asbestiform minerals and quartz are potential health hazards. The talc used in the cosmetic industry contains few if any of these contaminants. Talc has a wide range of commercial applications. It is used in the manufacture of roofing products, textiles, carpets, hardwood floors, fire extinguishing powders, floor wax, water filters, and leather and rubber products. In addition, it is used as a filler and extender in paint, paper, and ceramics, and pure talc is used extensively in the cosmetic and pharmaceutical industries.

Kaolinite. Kaolinite is a leaf-like or platy mineral and is the major constituent of kaolin or china clay. Kaolin is used in the manufacture of paper products, plastics, rubber, ceramics, and refractory materials, and as a filler in paints. It is also found in inks, adhesives, insecticides, medicines, food additives, bleach, absorbents, cements, fertilizers, cosmetics, crayons, pencils, detergents, paste, floor tiles, and textiles.

Vermiculite. Vermiculite is a platy mineral derived from biotite (aluminum magnesium silicate) that may be contaminated with fibrous mineral, such as tremolite. Vermiculite is expanded at high temperatures to form products for insulation and fireproofing and as a soil conditioner in horticulture.

Mica. Micas are platy, hydrated aluminum silicates similar to talc and are common components of igneous rock. Muscovite is commonly found in clay, shale, and slate and, therefore, is a potential health hazard. Mica is extensively used as an insulator in the electrical industry. Micas are also used in drilling muds, ornaments and decorations, floor tiles, adhesives, texture paints, rubber products, and plastics.

Bentonite. Bentonite is of volcanic origin and is composed of a mixture of montmorillonite, feldspar, and biotite. Alpha-quartz and cristobalite are important contaminants. Bentonite is used in the oil industry as a catalyst and also in drilling muds. In addition, bentonite is used as an additive for paper, plastics, and paints.

Feldspar. Feldspar is found in igneous rocks and is a contaminant of many other minerals. A substantial proportion of volcanic dust released from eruptions is made up of feldspar.

Fuller's Earth. Fuller's earth is a naturally occurring material that comprises largely of montmorillonite and attapulgite, but may contain up to 20% of alpha-quartz. Fuller's earth is used to remove grease during the processing of woolens. Its absorptive properties are widely used as filtering agents, fillers in cosmetics, herbicides, and insecticides.

Diatomaceous Earth. Diatomaceous earth is a natural form of amorphous silica to which workers can be exposed during mining, calcining, and bagging. Diatomaceous earth is almost exclusively mined by open-pit methods, and exposure levels of 0.1–2.0 mg/m^3 dust of which 5% is quartz have been reported (20). When diatomaceous earth is calcined, cristobalite is formed and can account for up to 40% of the final product. Diatomaceous earth is a major substrate for filtering or clarifying solvents, pharmaceuticals, beer, whiskey, wine, and municipal and industrial water. It is also used as a filler for paints, paper, synthetic rubber, and scouring powders.

Carbonaceous Dusts

Coal

Coal is a combustible, carbonaceous, sedimentary mineral formed by the compaction and physicochemical metamorphosis of vegetation. This fossil fuel is found in large reserves and used worldwide, primarily for power production in developed countries, and for power production, heating, and cooking in less-developed areas. During 1990 in the United States, 130,000 workers in the mining industry produced over 1 billion tons of coal (21). Coal is produced by both underground and surface mining, with 59% of U.S. coal produced by surface mines in 1992 (22).

Coal is classified according to its type (material of origin), grade (purity), and rank (percentage of fixed carbon). Coal rank, and its heat value, are related to the degree of coalification of organic materials, which involves deoxygenation, followed by dehydrogenation. High-rank, or hard, coal includes anthracite and semianthracite, having approximately 90–98% fixed carbon. Intermediate-rank, or soft, coal includes low, medium, and high volatile bituminous and subbituminous coal having approximately 75–90% fixed carbon (23). Low-rank coal includes lignite, having less than 75% fixed carbon. Most coal mined in the United States is bituminous.

Coal mine dust is a heterogeneous mixture, containing as many as 50 different elements and their oxides, and varying with location, often even within the same mine. Minerals commonly associated with coal include quartz, kaolinite, illite, calcite, and pyrite. The sulfur content ranges from 0.5 to more than 10%.

Respirable dusts in underground mines range from 40–95% coal; the remainder consists of fractured rock or diesel soot (24). The toxicity of coal dust varies with rank, particle size, and mineral content, with anthracite and dusts containing high quartz contents having greater toxicities. Dust from high-rank coal contains a greater portion of silica particles than dust from low-rank coal because of the typical proximity of anthracite seams to quartzite, and also contains a greater concentration of surface oxygen radicals when the coal is crushed.

Exposures to coal dust occur during mining, preparation (crushing, screening, washing), transportation, and handling at the point of use, but the greatest exposures occur during mining. Historical underground mining exposures resulted in long-term retention of over 30 g of dust in the lungs of some career-term miners, and half that amount was common (25). Current mining practices have substantially reduced exposures. The principal approaches used to reduce exposures in underground mines are ventilation, coating of exposed surfaces, and the use of mechanical equipment at the coal face. Despite the well-known association between coal dust exposure and lung disease, masks and respirators are still not in predominant use.

The principal health risks of concern for coal dust are coal workers' pneumoconiosis (CWP) and progressive massive fibrosis (PMF), which are well-documented, thoroughly studied disorders that have been described in detail in numerous reviews (e.g., 24,26). No increased risk of lung cancer is associated with exposure to coal dust, except perhaps when accompanied by heavy exposures to quartz or other agents, and there is no synergistic interaction between cigarette smoking–induced lung cancer and coal dust exposure (reviewed in Ref. 25).

"Black lung" was recognized in British coal miners in the mid-1600s. The term, pneumokoniosis (now pneumoconiosis) was introduced in 1866, and means simply "dusty lung." CWP is defined as a parenchymal lung disease produced by deposits of coal dust in the lungs and the response to the retained dust. During long-term exposure, the dust collects into deposits termed macules, which occur primarily in first-generation respiratory bronchioles. With progression, the macules involve a local fibrotic reaction and emphysema in surrounding alveoli. By 1907, radiography using x-ray films was being used to study lungs of coal miners, and CWP is now defined largely on the basis of radiographic changes. Because pulmonary radiographic opacities are not specific to coal-dust exposure, work history is important in establishing the presence of CWP. An international convention is followed by most countries for classifying several degrees of severity of CWP according to radiographic appearance (27), but some countries, such as China (28), have different classification systems. At the most mild stages, CWP causes little or no measurable or subjective loss of function, whereas the most severe stages of CWP can be debilitating and life-threatening. In some subjects, the fibrotic reaction progresses to PMF, a large, confluent scarring of the lung that is severely debilitating and often fatal. Coal dust exposure standards in the United States and many other countries were established to prevent the progression of CWP to PMF, but they do not prevent simple CWP altogether.

Coal mine dust standards and sampling techniques were recently reviewed by NIOSH (24). International exposure standards vary, but all are based on the gravimetric concentration of respirable dust and many incorporate an adjustment for the portion of quartz. Although sampling devices vary among countries, international conventions have agreed to a broadly accepted definition of respirable dust, the size fraction that can penetrate into the respiratory tract, as having a 50% sampling cut-point of 4.0 μm (29). The WHO recommended a health-based exposure limit for respirable dust containing less than 7% quartz in the range of 0.5–4.0 mg/m^3 (30). The U.S. standard is typical, allowing exposures to 2.0 mg/m^3 respirable dust containing less than 5% silica, and 10 mg/m^3 divided by the percentage of silica for higher silica contents, measured as an 8-hr time-weighted average (TWA). NIOSH recently recommended lowering the U.S. Standard to 1 mg/m^3 TWA for a 10-hr day during a 40-hr workweek, with exposure to respirable silica not to exceed 0.05 mg/m^3 at the same TWA (24).

All aspects of occupational exposures to coal dust, including composition, sampling, U.S. and international standards, and health effects, were recently reviewed by NIOSH (24). That review serves as a good source of references containing more detail. The epidemiology and pathogenesis of coal dust–induced lung disease were reviewed in detail (26), and in lesser detail in numerous texts on occupational lung disease. Information on the amounts of dust retained in lungs of coal workers and evidence for a lack of carcinogenic effect have been reviewed (25).

Graphite

Graphite is a form of crystallized carbon that is found in geological deposits throughout the world. It is produced commercially by mining in a few countries and is also produced artificially. Naturally occurring graphite is found in lump, amorphous, and flake forms, so designated because of geological occurrence, rather than mineral configuration. Also known as black lead, mineral carbon, and plumbago, graphite is used in pencil "lead," foundry facings, crucibles, and other refractory materials, lubricants, electrodes, engine parts, nuclear reactors, and pigments, and is also used in the manufacture of carbon fibers. World production of graphite was less than 1 million tons in 1983 (1).

Most of our present information on the health effects of graphite mining comes from Sri Lanka, which is a major exporter of natural graphite. With sufficient, long-term inhalation exposure, graphite can cause a pneumoconiosis, with progressive symptoms and radiographic abnormalities. In some patients, symptoms have appeared rapidly after years of exposure. The clinical and pathological appearance of graphite pneumoconiosis resemble those resulting from exposure to coal dust and, similar to coal dust, the nature and progression of disease may be related to other minerals, such as silicates, which are often mixed with the carbon (26,31). There is little quantitative information linking graphite pneumoconiosis to measured exposure levels. The current ACGIH TLV for graphite dust is 2.0 mg/m^3 respirable dust (32).

The *Encyclopedia of Occupational Health and Safety* from the International Labour Office (1) contains a useful summary of the nature, use, and potential health effects of graphite.

Limestone and Marble

Limestone is a sedimentary rock composed largely of calcium carbonate. Various forms of limestone are contaminated with magnesium carbonate (dolomitic limestone), clay (argillaceous limestone), and sand or quartz (silaceous limestone). Marble is the crystallized form of limestone. Limestone has many uses, particularly in the construction industry where it is used as a building material, as hardcore and ballast in road and railway construction, and mixed with clay for the manufacture of cement. Limestone is extracted by quarrying, and the main health hazard is related to the silica content of the limestone. Exposure to airborne limestone dust itself appears to carry little risk (1).

Limestone is calcined to form lime which is a generic term for calcium oxide and calcium hydroxide. Calcium oxide is used as a refractory material, as a flux in steel making, as a binding agent in the building industry, in pulp and paper manufacture, sugar refining, and leather tanning. In addition, it is the raw material for chlorinated lime bleaching powder, and for soil treatment in agriculture. Calcium hydroxide is made by hydrating calcium oxide and is used in the building trade for mortars, plasters, and cements; in lubricants; as a fireproofing agent; in pulp and paper manufacture; and for dehairing hides. During lime production, workers may become exposed to lime dust; however, there are no reported cases of pneumoconiosis. Lime dust is an irritant and can affect mucous membranes, particularly those surrounding the eye. Marble is an important construction material; there are no occupational diseases specifically connected with the mining, quarrying, and processing of marble (1).

B. Natural and Man-Made Inorganic Fibers

Fibers are considered to be elongated structures with a length/diameter (aspect) ratio of greater than 3:1. Fibers also have substantially parallel sides, which distinguishes them from shards and dust. Various values of minimum length and aspect ratio have been proposed to define potentially hazardous fibers. The WHO has defined a fiber as a particle with length greater than 5 μm, among other properties (33). NIOSH (Method 7400) also proposed a minimum length of 5 μm for a fiber. Concentrations of airborne fibers can be measured on a total mass basis, by comparing weight of filters before and after sampling; however, fibers in ambient air are normally identified and counted using phase contrast optical microscopy (PCOM), scanning electron microscopy (SEM), or transmission electron microscopy (TEM). Limits of resolution that have been reported to be achievable in routine operation are 0.25–1.6 μm for PCOM, 0.05–0.2 μm for SEM, and 0.005 μm for TEM (33). SEM and TEM can be combined with X-ray elemental analysis that allows the chemical elements present in the fibers to be analyzed. In addition, TEM combined with electron diffraction can elucidate the crystalline nature of fibers.

Inhalation is the most important route of exposure to fibers. Only some fibers can be inhaled and deposited in the respiratory tract. The respirability of fibers is largely determined by two variables: density and cross-sectional area; length plays only a minor role in determining respirability. Fibers with aerodynamic equivalent diameters between 5 and 10 μm can deposit in the larger airways, and those less than 5 μm can reach the terminal bronchioles and alveoli. This latter aerodynamic diameter is equivalent to a fiber diameter of approximately 3 μm; however, density will also affect this value.

In addition to measuring airborne fibers, the dimensions of fibers retained in lung tissue can also be determined. These techniques generally involve three basic steps: dissolution and removal of the organic matrix material of the lung, recovery and concentration of the mineral fibers, and analysis of the mineral content by some form of microscopy (34). The final analytical result can be greatly influenced by the various steps in the analytical procedure. Interlaboratory comparison trials using the same sample have shown that striking differences can occur between laboratories and indicates the caution that must be taken when comparing results between laboratories. The fiber burdens are also usually measured at a time when the disease process is well advanced and may not relate to the events that occurred when the disease was actually evolving. Nonetheless, there is general agreement that the fiber burdens in the lungs are a major factor in the development of lung disease.

Inhalation of natural fibers such as asbestos is associated with the development of significant lung disease, including pulmonary fibrosis (asbestosis), primary lung cancer, and mesothelioma (invariably fatal tumor of the lining of the pleural and peritoneal cavities). However, asbestos is not a single mineral, but a group of minerals with different forms, having different abilities to induce lung disease. Fibers are ubiquitous in the environment and arise from both natural and man-made sources. Inorganic fibers have widespread uses in construction, automotive, aerospace, and filtration industries, and in some geographic areas can be found naturally in the soil and rocks. Workers can be exposed to natural fibers throughout the life cycle of the material, including extraction, milling, and processing, installation and use, and removal of the material after use. Workers in the man-made fiber industry can similarly be exposed during manufacture, use, and disposal of the material.

The factors that contribute to the pathogenicity of fibers include dose, physical dimensions, chemical composition, and durability in lung tissue. On the basis of animal studies, Stanton and Wrench (35) suggested that fibers longer than 8 μm and smaller than 0.25 μm in diameter have the greatest potential to cause mesotheliomas. Davis et al. (36) have shown that short fibers (less than 5 μm) are much less pathogenic than longer fibers by inhalation. The role of fiber dimension as a determinant of toxicity in humans is more difficult to ascertain, but Lippmann (37) suggested that asbestosis, lung cancer, and mesothelioma are related to different-sized fibers. Lippmann (37) concluded that asbestosis is most clearly related to the surface area of retained fibers, that mesothelioma is most clearly associated with the number of fibers longer than 5 μm and thinner than 0.1 μm, and that lung cancer is most clearly associated with fibers longer than 10 μm and thicker than 0.15 μm. The lesser pathogenicity of some man-made vitreous fibers compared with asbestos is thought to be due to the solubility of vitreous fibers in the lung (38).

Natural Fibers

Asbestos

The asbestos minerals are crystalline fibrous silicates, some of which have been exploited commercially, especially as an insulating material. These minerals comprise sheets, or chains of silicate tetrahedra in which oxygen is either bound to two silicon atoms or to one silicon atom, and possesses a negative charge. There are two major groups of asbestos mineral: serpentines and amphiboles. White asbestos or chrysotile is a serpentine mineral, whereas the other forms of asbestos, crocidolite (blue asbestos), amosite (brown asbestos), anthophyllite, tremolite, and actinolite, are amphiboles. Tremolite can also be found as a contaminant in other minerals, such as chrysotile, talc, and vermiculite.

The overall chemical composition of chrysotile is given in Table 3. The chemical composition of chrysotile is generally uniform, although traces of sev-

Table 3 Chemical Composition of Asbestos Minerals (typical ranges in percent)

	Chrysotile	Crocidolite	Amosite	Anthophyllite	Tremolite
SiO_2	38–44	49–53	49–53	56–58	55–60
MgO	40–43	0–3	1–7	28–34	21–26
FeO	0.8–3	13–20	34–44	3–12	0–4
Fe_2O_3	0.4–4	17–20	0–0.5	—	—
Al_2O_3	0.3–0.8	0–0.2	—	0.5–1.5	0–2.5
CaO	0.04–1	0.3–2.7	—	—	11–13
Na_2O	0–0.06	4.0–8.5	—	—	0–1.5

eral metals can occur (e.g., nickel). Chrysotile is the major commercial form of asbestos, accounting for approximately 95% of the world market. This mineral has interleaving layers of brucite (magnesium oxide-hydroxide) between sheets of polysilicate anions that are rolled up into scrolls, with their long axes parallel to the fiber. The chemical properties of chrysotile largely reflect those of the external magnesium hydroxide surface. Chrysotile is readily attacked by acid and reacts to leave a silica residue. The magnesium hydroxide surface of chrysotile results in a positive charge in solutions below pH. 11.8 (isoelectric point). These properties give chrysotile a hydrophilic surface with affinity for polar, rather than nonpolar molecules.

The overall chemical composition of the amphibole asbestos minerals is also shown in Table 3. Amphiboles have a structure that contains double chains of silicate tetrahedra, cross-linked with bridging cations attached to the hydroxyl groups. This structure allows a wide range of cation replacement, which is reflected in the chemical composition and physical properties of the amphiboles. The amphiboles are all more resistant to acid than chrysotile and have a negative charge at physiological pH because of the ionizable silanol groups on the exposed silicate surface.

All forms of asbestos may cause pulmonary fibrosis. The degree of fibrosis is primarily determined by cumulative exposure; exposures of 15–75 fibers per milliliter per year (fibers per milliliter times the years of exposure) have been reported to result in fibrotic lung disease (39). Death from asbestosis may occur in humans with cumulative exposures of 70–300 fibers per milliliter per year (40). Individuals with lung cancer almost always also have lung fibrosis. However, the relation between asbestos-induced lung cancer and pulmonary fibrosis remains controversial. All forms of asbestos, including chrysotile, which has recently been considered to be relatively inert (41), can induce pulmonary lung cancer (42). Crocidolite and amosite exposures are also associated with the induction of mesothelioma. Exposure to anthophyllite has not been associated with an increased risk of developing mesothelioma, whereas the association between chrysotile exposure and risks of mesothelioma is controversial (42).

The nature of the processes and the way in which asbestos is handled can alter the nature of the exposure and, therefore, the risk. Asbestos minerals split longitudinally when they are milled and processed so that the aerosolized fibers become thinner. The lung cancer risk among miners is lower than that observed among asbestos textile workers. Textile operations produce airborne fibers that are generally longer than fibers produced by other operations using chrysotile. Mining and milling operations produce a greater proportion of fibers less than 5 μm long compared with textile plants (43).

The IARC (19) classified asbestos as a known human carcinogen (group 1, sufficient evidence for carcinogenicity in animals and humans). Occupational exposures have been reported as high as 2700 fibers per milliliter; however, because of the known association between asbestos exposure and lung disease, exposure to asbestos has been regulated. The OSHA permissible exposure limit is 0.1 fiber per milliliter (10), and the ACGIH TLVs are 0.5 fibers per milliliter for amosite, 2 fibers per milliliter for chrysotile, 0.2 fibers per milliliter for crocidolite, and 2 fibers per milliliter for other forms of asbestos (10). The use of crocidolite has been totally banned in many European countries because of concerns for the health of exposed individuals. The German MAK for chrysotile is 0.25 fibers per milliliter (10).

Palygorskite (Attapulgite and Sepiolite)

The palygorskite group of clay minerals includes attapulgite and sepiolite, both of which are fibrous, with a crystalline structure similar to that of the amphibole group of minerals. Having similar structures, the two minerals are most readily distinguished by their chemical composition. Attapulgite has an aluminum content at least five times higher than that of sepiolite. Attapulgite is produced in greater quantities than sepiolite. The United States is the most prominent producer of attapulgite; however, deposits of the mineral occur worldwide, and the mineral is mined in Europe, Africa, and India. Commercial production of sepiolite occurs almost exclusively in Spain. Both materials have similar industrial uses as absorbent and filler materials and are marketed in granule and powder form. The most common use is as an absorbent for pet wastes and for oil and grease spills. An additional important use is in drilling muds, especially in saltwater drilling.

Attapulgite deposits are mined by open-pit techniques. Crushing, milling, and drying operations produce concentrations of total and respirable dust at the workers' breathing zone ranging from 0.05 to 2.1 mg/m^3 and 0.02 to 0.32 mg/m^3, respectively. The airborne fibers were generally short with lengths between 0.1 and 2.5 μm and diameters between 0.02 and 0.1 μm. Dust concentrations at two facilities mining and milling attapulgite were reported to be as high as 23 mg/m^3. However, the respirable dust level was lower than the 5 mg/m^3 nuisance dust level in all job categories. The dustiest jobs were those that involved crushing, screening, milling, and shipping (19). IARC (19) reported that there are inadequate data from humans to determine carcinogenicity and that the evidence from animal experiments is limited. For sepiolite, there are no data to assess potential adverse health effects in humans and inadequate data from animal experiments.

Wollastonite

Wollastonite is a naturally occurring, nondurable calcium silicate derived from metamorphosed impure limestone. It rarely occurs in pure form and is most commonly associated with calcite, quartz, garnet, and diopside. Morphologically, wollastonite can be found as a coarse-bladed, acicular or fibrous structure. Wollastonite was first mined for the production of mineral wool. Current uses of wollastonite include ceramics, for which it decreases firing times, as a filler and extender for paints and plastics, and as a replacement for asbestos. Two studies of wollastonite facilities demonstrated that the total dust level can be high (up to 99 mg/m^3), and the airborne fiber levels can range from 1 to 45 fibers. The fibers were short and fine, having median diameters of 0.2–0.3 μm and median lengths of 2–4 μm (19). A survey of 104 wollastonite workers showed no evidence of pulmonary disease, and a recently completed chronic rodent inhalation bioassay showed no evidence of fibrotic or carcinogenic response (19,44).

Zeolites (Erionite and Mordenite)

Erionite and mordenite are zeolites having a framework of aluminosilicate tetrahedra, in which each oxygen is shared between two tetrahedra. Zeolites differ from one another in the arrangement of the tetrahedra. The cavities in this framework formed by the tetrahedra are filled with calcium, magnesium, sodium, or potassium cations. Zeolites have many commercial uses, most of which are based on their ability to adsorb molecules from gases or liquids. Zeolites are mined in 16 countries; however, most of these operations are designed to mine clinoptilolite or mordenite. Erionite occurs in rocks of many types and is usually associated with other zeolites. Interest in the pathogenic potential of erionite arose from the high number of mesotheliomas associated with environmental exposures to erionite in some villages in central Cappadocia, Turkey (45). There is limited information available concerning environmental concentrations of erionite fibers. It has been reported that in villages associated with the high rates of mesothelioma, the airborne concentrations were between 0.004 and 0.175 fibers per milliliter of which the bulk were described as zeolites (45). Erionite fibers from rock samples of a zeolite deposit in Rome, Oregon, have been used in a chronic rodent inhalation study that produced mesotheliomas in 28 of the 29 exposed rats (46). This sample of erionite contained numerous fibers 0.02–0.5 μm in diameter and 0.5–60 μm in length. IARC (19) reports that there are sufficient data from humans and animals to classify erionite as a human carcinogen. There are insufficient data on the toxicity of mordenite; however, because of its fibrous nature and its relation to erionite, it may represent an inhalation hazard.

Man-Made Fibers

Man-made fibers can be amorphous, polycrystalline, or crystalline. The amorphous fibers include the man-made vitreous fibers typified by the insulation wools, which form the bulk of man-made inorganic fibers. Polycrystalline fibers include continuous carbon fibers used in composite material and specialty fibers such as Saffil. Crystalline man-made fibers include ceramic whiskers, such as silicon carbide and silicon nitride, which are used in reinforce metals and other composite materials.

Man-Made Vitreous Fibers

Man-made vitreous fibers (MMVFs) have an amorphous structure in which the constituent atoms are not arranged in a regular lattice, as in crystalline materials. The major types of MMVFs are continuous-filament fiberglass or textile fibers, glass wools, rock and slag wools, refractory ceramic fibers, and glass microfibers. Nearly 90% of continuous filaments are used to produce fiber-reinforced plastic composites. They can also be used to reinforce cement, automotive tires, and roofing materials. In addition, they can be woven into protective clothing and industrial fabrics. Glass, rock, and slag wools are used largely for thermal insulation; rock and slag wools are also commonly used in acoustic insulation. Refractory ceramic fibers have high thermal resistance and, therefore, are used mainly for high-temperature applications. These applications include furnace and kiln insulation, insulation for catalytic convertors in automobiles, filtration, and gaskets and seals for expansion joints. Glass microfibers are used in battery-separator media, for high-efficiency filtration, and as thermal and acoustical insulation in the aerospace industry.

The MMVFs are produced from liquid melts at temperatures ranging from 1000° to 1500°C. Fibers are typically made by rapid cooling of the molten material in one of the following ways: mechanical drawing, flame attenuation, blowing, wheel centrifuging, rotary spinning, or rotary disk process. Silicon dioxide is the principal constituent of most MMVFs, often composing 40–70% of the total. Lesser amounts of intermediate metal oxides or stabilizers, such as Al_2O_3, TiO_2, and ZrO_2, along with modifiers or fluxes, such as MgO, Li_2O, BaO, CaO, Na_2O, and K_2O, are also present. The composition of the material can vary considerably, depending on the chemical and physical properties required of the final product. Stabilizers increase the chemical and heat-resistant properties of the fibers, whereas the modifiers decrease fiber durability. Binders and oils are applied to the surface of most MMFVs to hold the fibers together and to suppress dust. Continuous filament glass fiber may contain a sizing agent for lubrication. Phenol formaldehyde resins are the most commonly used binders, and are cured at high temperatures to an insoluble polymer containing little formaldehyde. The binder content of most insulation wool products is generally lower than 5%.

Continuous-Filament Fiberglass. This material is also known as textile fiberglass and is produced by the continuous drawing process that makes very long fibers. In any given product, the diameter of the fiber does not differ much from the mean or average diameter. The average diameter of typical continuous-filament fiberglass ranges from 3 to 25 μm, with most products using fibers 6 μm or larger in diameter. The standard deviation of the fiber diameter of continuous-filament fiberglass is typically less than 10% of the average diameter, compared with 50% or more for the insulation wools. E-glass is the predominant glass composition (Table 4), boron oxide is a major additive, and the alkali oxides of

Table 4 Chemical Composition of Man-Made Vitreous Fibers in Weight Percent

	E-glass	Glass wool	Rock wool	Slag wool	Refractory ceramic fiber
SiO_2	52–56	55–70	41–53	38–52	48–54
Al_2O_3	12–16	0–7	6–14	5–15	43–47
B_2O_3	5–10	3–12			
Na_2O	0–2	13–18	2–3	0–1	0.5
K_2O	0–2	0–3	0.8–1	0.3–2	<0.01
MgO	0–5	0–5	8–10	4–14	<0.1
CaO	16–25	5–13	10–12	20–43	<0.1
TiO_2	0–1.5	0–0.5	2.5–3	0.3–1	2
Fe_2O_3	0–0.8	0.1–0.5	11–12[a]	0–2[a]	1

[a]In rock and slag wool produced from materials melted in a cupola with coke as fuel, all iron oxide is reduced to FeO. Typically, 8–15% of the iron is oxidized to Fe_2O_3 during the spinning process.

sodium and potassium are maintained at low levels to give acceptable electrical properties.

The very long fibers of continuous-filament fiberglass are unlikely to escape from the product and become airborne. The large diameters of continuous-filament fiberglass greatly reduce the chance of any released material being respirable. However, workers may become exposed to particles of continuous-filament fiberglass through grinding and finishing composite materials that include the filaments. The airborne dust and fiber concentrations in continuous-filament fiberglass production facilities range from 0.002 to 0.04 fibers per milliliter. There is no evidence of a relation between lung cancer mortality or incidence and duration of employment in the glass-filament industry (47).

Glass Wool. Glass wool is primarily produced by the rotary process that yields glass-fiber products of varying average diameters ranging from 1 to 10 μm. Nearly all glass-wool products have average diameters of 3–10 μm. The length of all but an extremely small fraction of the fibers is much greater than 250 μm. The fiber diameter and length are two important properties of insulation glass wool because they control most of the characteristics that make them practical for their end use. Current glass-wool compositions (see Table 4) are governed, to some extent, by the rotary process, which requires a lower temperature of formation. Rotary-process glasses have more alkaline oxides (Na_2O and K_2O) and boric oxide (B_2O_3) and less alkaline earth oxide (CaO and MgO).

Workers can be exposed to glass-wool fibers during their manufacture and use. Exposure concentrations of airborne fibers in production facilities range between 0.002 and 1.56 fibers per milliliter, with the highest exposure occurring in the production and manufacturing job categories (47). The median lengths and median diameters for airborne fibers in glass-wool production plants have been reported to be between 8 and 15 and 0.7 and 1 μm, respectively (48). During the residential installation of glass fiber by blowing the material, exposures of 12.2 mg/m^3 and 12.7 fibers per milliliter have been reported, with the fibers having a mean length of 15 μm and mean diameter of 0.6 μm (49). The standard 8-hr TWA exposures for insulation workers are reported to be as high as 3.16 fibers per milliliter (1.68 mg/m^3). Studies of glass-wool workers in European and U.S. factories show a nonsignificant increase in mortality from lung cancer that was not associated with duration of exposure (47). However, IARC has classified glass wool as a possible human carcinogen. Animal data demonstrate the carcinogenic potential of glass wool in several animal species following intratracheal instillation, or intrapleural or intraperitoneal injection (42).

Rock Wool and Slag Wool (Mineral Wool). Modern rock and slag wool are composed of calcium magnesium aluminum silicate glass (see Table 4). Both rock and slag wool are produced by melting raw materials and centrifuging, drawing, or blowing the molten matter into the desired fibrous form. Rock wool is typically produced by the melting of igneous rock containing high levels of calcium and magnesium. Rock-wool plants use basaltic rock, limestone, clay, and feldspar. Rock wool is the most commonly manufactured mineral wool. Slag wool is produced from the by-products of metal smelting, primarily the slag formed during the reduction of iron ore to pig iron. The majority of mineral wool produced in the United States is slag wool.

In general, fiber concentrations and total airborne particulate matter in rock-wool and slag-wool manufacturing facilities are higher than those in glass-wool facilities. In a slag-wool facility, the total airborne particulate ranged from 0.05 to 6.88 mg/m^3, and the fiber concentration ranged from 0.01 to 0.43 fibers per milliliter. In a rock-wool facility, the total particulate matter ranged from 0.5 to 23.6 mg/m^3, and the fiber concentration ranged from 0.2 to 1.4 fibers per milliliter. The median fiber lengths and diameters were within the ranges of 10–20 and 1.2–2.0 μm, respectively. During the installation of residential mineral wool, workers were exposed to fiber concentrations of 1.31 fibers per milliliter and 12.2 mg/m^3. The mean length of the mineral-wool fibers was 30 μm, and the mean diameter was 1.0 μm (49). The time-weighted averages for mineral-wool installers are 5.84 mg/m^3 and 0.66 fibers per milliliter. IARC (47) has classified rock wool and slag wool as possible human carcinogens; in the combined cohorts of European and U.S. workers, there was a statistically significant excess of mortality from lung cancer. The highest rates were found after more than 20 years follow-up among persons first exposed during the early technological phase, in which the estimated fiber levels were the highest. Inhalation studies with rock and slag wool in rats and hamsters show no evidence of carcinogenicity. However, intrapleural and intraperitoneal administration in rats produced mesotheliomas.

Refractory Ceramic Fiber. Refractory ceramic fibers are produced by melting a combination of Al_2O_3 and SiO_2, usually 50:50 by weight, or by melting kaolin clay. Other oxides, such as ZrO_2, B_2O_3, TiO_2, and Cr_2O_3 are sometimes added to change the fiber properties. The fibers are produced from the melt in much the same way as mineral wool, or by fiber blowing that involves attenuation of the molten stream by high-pressure air or steam. Under some conditions typical of their use, refractory ceramic fibers may crystallize, or devitrify, to mullite at temperatures above 1000°C and to cristobalite at temperatures above 1100°C. In use, it generally happens that the hot surface of a refractory ceramic furnace lining crystallizes, while the refractory ceramic fibers farther away from the hot surface remain partly or completely in the glassy state. Unlike other man-made vitreous fibers, refractory ceramic fibers are rarely used in consumer products.

Concentrations of airborne fibers and total particulate matter are generally higher in manufacturing facilities than those found in glass-wool manufacturing facilities, but are comparable with exposures in rock and slag-wool production facilities (47). To date, there is no evidence that exposure to refractory ceramic fibers can cause respiratory disease. Epidemiological investigations have included morbidity and mortality studies in cohorts from manufacturing facilities; however, because no workers have been exposed over a full working life, it may be some time before definitive human studies can be undertaken (50). IARC classifies refractory ceramic fibers as a possible human carcinogen (47).

Whiskers and Ceramic Fibers

The terms, ''whiskers'' and ''ceramic fibers,'' have been used for materials with very different physical properties and chemical compositions, including whiskers of silicon carbide, silicon nitride, tungsten oxide, and magnesium sulfate. Exposure to these materials can arise during the direct manufacture of the material or as a by-product of some other process. Whiskers of silicon carbide occur as a by-product of the production of silicon carbide abrasives, and tungsten carbide whiskers can occur during the production of hard metal. Whiskers have been produced in limited quantities and are being used to reinforce metals and plastics (silicon carbide and silicon nitride), and as replacements for asbestos (magnesium sulfate). In general, there are very few toxicological or exposure data for occupational exposures to whiskers and ceramic fibers. Sahle et al. (51) reported fiber concentrations of 0.05–0.23 fibers per milliliter and a total dust concentration of 0.22 mg/m^3 close to the reduction furnace at a hard-metal factory. The toxicity of silicon carbide whiskers has received more attention than that of the other whiskers to date. Silicon carbide whiskers are single crystals of silicon carbide grown from rice hulls or mixtures of carbon and silica using heat and a reducing atmosphere. The whiskers have a variable morphology, with varying lengths and diameters. Three samples used in an in vitro study had mean lengths of 4.5, 20.1, and 6.6 μm and mean diameters of 0.42, 0.75, and 0.32 μm, respectively (52). Workplace fiber concentrations of up to 4.9 fibers per milliliter have been measured with the fibers having a mean diameter of 0.24 μm (53), and fibers have been recovered from lung tissue of silicon carbide workers. These data and those from a limited number of cell and animal studies suggest that silicon carbide whiskers may present a health hazard to humans (52).

Carbon and Organic Fibers

Carbon Fibers. Carbon or graphite fibers are produced by high-temperature treatment of precursor fibers. Precursors used commercially include rayon, polyacrylonitrile, and pitch. The terms, ''graphite'' and ''carbon'' fibers, are frequently used synonymously; however, the term *carbon* fiber should apply specifically to carbonaceous fibrous material pyrolyzed at about 1500°C (consisting essentially of amorphous carbon), whereas *graphite* fibers are carbon fibers heated further to about 2500°C, resulting in a crystalline fiber structure. Carbon fibers made for commercial purposes are most commonly manufactured from polyacrylonitrile at nominal diameters of 7–10 μm, although smaller-diameter fibers can be made. During the manufacturing process, dust concentrations are low; mean levels for the dustiest workers are 0.39 mg/m^3 total dust and 0.16 mg/m^3 respirable dust (54). Carbon fibers are most commonly used in composite materials in which the fibers are embedded in resin or plastic. Such composite materials are used in the aerospace, automotive, sporting goods, and prosthetic industries. Workers can be exposed to material from these composites during cutting, grinding, and polishing. These processes generate a large number of small, mostly noncarbon, nonfibrous particles ranging from 0.5 to 7 μm in diameter; those larger than 7 μm consist of varying lengths of carbon fiber (54). Exposure to carbon fibers can also occur during incineration of carbon fiber composites, either during intentional incineration to remove waste, or during accidental incineration, such as in military aircraft crashes. During cleanup operations following an aircraft crash, dust levels of 0.03–0.09 mg/m^3 total dust and 0.02 mg/m^3 respirable dust, and fiber levels of up to 0.56 fibers per milliliter were reported (55).

Organic Fibers. There is widespread potential for workers to be exposed to fibrous material in the synthetic organic fiber industry; however, there are few data concerning exposures to fibrous material or their health effects. Synthetic organic fibers include polyolefin and aramid fibers.

Polyolefin fibers are made from polymers of propylene, ethylene, or other olefins. These long-chain synthetic hydrocarbon polymers are fabricated commercially by a melt extrusion technique. About 95% of polyolefin fibers are composed of polypropylene. Fiber diameter depends on the manufacturing process and can vary from more than 153 μm in monofilament yarn to an average of

1–5 μm in microfibers. Polyolefin microfibers are used in roofing and flooring felts, filters, adhesives, and joint cements, and as a substitute for asbestos (56).

Kevlar aramid fibers are used extensively for reinforcement in fabrics, rubber, and plastic products; they have also been used to replace asbestos as a reinforcement in friction material for brake shoes. The aramid pulp used generally consists of short fibers (0.5–8 mm) with fine fibrils attached to the surface. Although abrasion, cutting, machining, or grinding can break fibrils from the surface and generate fine, curled, and branched fibrils, they form mostly nonrespirable clumps. Airborne aramid fiber in manufacturing and end-user workplaces range from 0.01 to 0.4 fibrils per milliliter (8-hr TWA) with the highest short-term (1-min) peaks averaging less than 5 fibers per milliliter (57).

C. Combustion and Pyrolysis Products

Ash

Ash is the noncombustible residue remaining after the burning of any substance. Although quite variable in physical form and chemical composition, ash is typically composed of silicates, oxides, carbon, sulfur, and metals. Workers may be exposed to ash from coal and oil-fired power plants, ash from incinerators, ash from wood and other plant materials, and volcanic ash. A significant portion of most airborne ash is in the respirable size range. Fisher et al. (58) and Hatch et al. (59) described coal and oil fly ash, Fruchter et al. (60) described volcanic ash from the 1980 Mount St. Helens eruption in the United States, and Alarie et al. (61) described ash from municipal incinerators.

Ashes vary widely in toxicity, but inhaled in sufficient quantity, all ashes can cause respiratory function changes, pneumonitis, and exacerbation of other pulmonary disorders. Ash is rarely implicated in pneumoconiosis, although this could result from chronic, heavy exposures. Laboratory studies have compared the toxicities of ashes, including pulverized and fluidized bed coal ash, oil ash, and volcanic ash, and most studies included comparisons with other particles (e.g., 58,59,62,63). In general, oil fly ash is more toxic than coal fly ash, and volcanic ash is less toxic than either of the fuel ashes. The toxicity of incinerator ash would be expected to vary considerably, depending on the feedstock, but it typically has a high metal content and is irritating (61). The toxicity of ashes generally increases with decreasing particle size and increasing metal content (59).

Coal Fly Ash

Most stationery coal power plants are of the pulverized coal type, in which finely powdered coal is sprayed from a nozzle under high pressure into the combustion chamber. Ash from pulverized coal combustion is composed largely of glass-like aluminosilicate spheres, ranging in diameter from less than 0.5 to 10 μm

(58). Coal fly ash also contains metal and sulfur oxides and trace amounts of unburned carbon and condensed organic material. Ash from fluidized bed combustors has a similar composition, but is less spherical and more irregular in shape. Most coal-powered plants in developed countries use some form of ash collection and release only a small portion of the smallest particles into the environment. Workers may be exposed to the collected ash by inhalation when servicing the collection devices and the combustor, disposing of the ash, and handling ash during its use in the manufacture of other materials, such as concrete. The annual U.S. production of coal fly ash is on the order of 100 million tons.

Coal fly ash is cytotoxic to cells and fibrogenic when administered by inhalation to animals, but is less toxic than quartz (58,59,62). The potential carcinogenicity of fly ash has not been evaluated in an adequate lifetime bioassay, but exposures of several months have not produced cancer in animals. Schilling et al. (64) conducted a study of the effects of long-term occupational exposures to coal fly ash in British power plants. They found modest effects on respiratory function, but no evidence of pneumoconiosis among workers exposed long-term at concentrations up to 8 mg/m^3. Cho et al. (65) reported a case of severe acute respiratory disease following exposure of a worker, who was a smoker, to extreme concentrations of fly ash in an accident. Prolonged exposure to fly ash was thought to contribute to severe interstitial fibrosis and pneumoconiosis in a shipyard worker (66).

Oil Fly Ash

Oil fly ash consists of single and aggregated amorphous and crystalline particles of a wide range of sizes and shapes (58). Oil ash has a predominantly sulfate matrix, in contrast with the aluminosilicate matrix of coal ash, and also contrasts with coal ash by having a much higher content of metals (58,59). The general lack of removal of oil fly ash from stack gases of oil combustors also contrasts with coal combustion. Fugitive fly ash from oil combustion was estimated to contribute 125,000 tons to U.S. environmental particulate air pollution in 1992 (67), and occupational exposure concentrations as high as 6.7 mg/m^3 have been reported (68).

In comparative in vitro and in vivo studies, oil ash is typically more toxic than other ashes, and its toxicity is largely related to its high content of transition metals, particularly iron, nickel, and vanadium (63,67). Hauser et al. (68) reviewed the literature on short-term effects of exposure to oil ash among boiler workers and reported a new prospective study of the effects of working on oil boilers on respiratory function. Exposure to oil ash causes reduced function measured by spirometry, but no changes were observed in airway reactivity. There is little epidemiological information on the long-term effects of occupational exposures to inhaled oil ash.

Volcanic Ash

The composition of volcanic ash varies somewhat from location to location. The largest database on volcanic ash and its health effects is derived from studies of the 1980 eruption of Mount St. Helens in the United States. Volcanic ash comprises mostly amorphous and crystalline particles of diverse sizes and shapes of oxides of silicon, aluminum, iron, calcium, and sodium (60). Although amorphous silicates constitute a large portion of the ash, the crystalline silica content is generally 10% or less. In the Mount St. Helens ashfall, particles smaller than 10 μm in diameter constituted less than 10% of the particle mass. The greatest occupational exposures occur among workers cleaning up ashfall and engaged in logging and construction activities in heavily contaminated areas.

Comparative laboratory studies have generally shown the in vivo and in vitro toxicity of volcanic ash to be less than those of silica or oil fly ash, and approximately similar to, or less than, that of coal fly ash (59). A long-term inhalation bioassay demonstrated that extremely high (50 mg/m^3) exposures of rats to Mount St. Helens ash caused fibrosis, alveolar proteinosis, and epidermoid tumors (69), lesions commonly resulting from heavy exposures of rats to a wide range of solid particles (70). Little has been reported on long-term effects of volcanic ash inhalation in humans. Buist et al. (71) conducted a prospective 4-year study of loggers salvaging timber in areas of heavy ashfall. Measured ash exposure concentrations were generally less than 0.5 mg/m^3. Transient respiratory function effects were observed by spirometry, but there was no radiographic evidence of tissue changes.

Carbon Black

Carbon black is a generic term applied to a family of amorphous, colloidal carbon particles produced by pyrolysis of gaseous or liquid hydrocarbons. The black, odorless powder consists of spherical primary particles of elemental carbon and variably sized and shaped aggregates of primary particles. Carbon black is produced by several processes, including oil furnace (currently most prevalent), thermal decomposition, acetylene, lampblack, and channel black (72). Carbon black differs from graphite in that it is amorphous, rather than crystalline. It differs from soot and chars in that it is generally a higher-purity carbon, with less than 0.5% of its mass as solvent-extractable organic matter, in contrast with the lower purity soots and chars having higher organic contents. The wide range of carbon blacks produced under different conditions vary in their particle size, porosity, and organic chemical content, which lend themselves to a range of commercial uses. The material is used largely as a reinforcing agent in rubber. For example, automobile tires typically contain more than 2 kg each. It is also used in inks and other pigments, carbon paper, batteries, and protective coatings.

Occupational inhalation exposures to carbon black occur during its manufacture and handling as a bulk powder. The particle size of suspended carbon black is typically in the respirable range. The current OSHA, NIOSH, and ACGIH exposure limits are 3.5 mg/m^3 TWA (10). No exposure limit specific for carbon black has been set by DFG. Published data on occupational exposures are not extensive, but suggest that current exposures in the United States are well within the recommended limits.

Occupational exposures to inhaled carbon black have been reported to cause bronchitis, pneumoconiosis, and emphysema; however, this information is sketchy and derived more from case reports than from adequate epidemiological studies of morbidity (26). Epidemiological studies of workers suggest that heavy, prolonged exposures can cause reduced lung function, but there is little evidence of debilitating pneumoconiosis from contemporary exposures (72).

Renewed attention has been drawn to the potential pulmonary carcinogenicity of prolonged carbon black exposures, because of a recent review by the IARC and because of recent studies demonstrating the similar pulmonary carcinogenicities of carbon black and diesel soot in rats exposed heavily for 2 years (73). Overall, the evidence for pulmonary carcinogenicity in workers is weak and conflicting. A small excess of lung cancer was reported in a study of workers in the United Kingdom (74), but other studies have been largely negative. Carbon black is clearly a pulmonary carcinogen in heavily exposed rats (75). However, because rats respond similarly to a range of solid, weakly toxic particles under exposure conditions overloading the particle clearance capacity of the lung, this response is probably not useful for estimating human lung cancer risk (70). IARC (76) recently classified carbon black as "possibly carcinogenic to humans" (group 2B) on the basis of inadequate evidence from humans and sufficient evidence from animals.

Carbon black types, production methods, exposures, potential health effects, and international exposure limits have been reviewed (72). The carcinogenicity of carbon black was recently reviewed by IARC (76). The carcinogenicity of carbon black and other particles in rats and difficulties in extrapolating those results to humans were recently reviewed by several authors in the volume edited by Mauderly and McCunney (70).

Coke, Charcoal, and Activated Carbon

Coke and charcoal are the carbonaceous residues remaining from the dry distillation of coal and wood, respectively. Heat from another source or partial combustion of the feedstock under reducing conditions is used to drive off most of the volatile components, leaving material with a greatly increased carbon content. Activated carbon is a somewhat similar material, but is derived from soft coal by a steam process. Coke and charcoal dusts are generated by abrasion and crumbling, and particle sizes range from approximately 2 μm to the upper limit of respirability.

The world annual production of coke is approximately 400 million tons. Most coke is used as fuel in metal smelters and foundries, but it is also used in the production of graphite and other carbon materials, and in the production of calcium carbide. Charcoal is used for fuel, particularly in developing countries, and as an absorbent of gases and vapors. High-purity coke and charcoal both burn at high temperature with little smoke. Activated carbon is used as an absorbent.

Occupational inhalation exposures occur during the handling of coke, charcoal, and activated carbon, but there is little information on concentrations and sizes of the suspended particles. There are no exposure standards for these materials, aside from nonspecific dust standards, although there are standards for coal tar pitch (10). Similar to other dusts, these materials may cause transient reductions of lung function or aggravation of other respiratory symptoms on brief, high-level exposure. Pneumoconiosis from coke or charcoal dust is possible with heavy exposures, but little information has been reported. Pneumoconiosis has been reported in workers manufacturing carbon electrodes from coke (77) and from occupational exposures to activated carbon (78).

Concern for health effects of coke has largely been directed toward carcinogenesis from inhalation of the organic emissions of coke ovens, both in vapor phase and as solvent-soluble fractions of particulate. Although there is little information on exposures to the carbonaceous fraction, there have been detailed analyses of the organic emissions of coke ovens (79). There is clear epidemiological evidence of increased lung cancer from occupational exposures to coke oven emissions and coal tar pitch volatiles (e.g., 80). Although little information is available, similar effects might be expected from heavy exposure to charcoal oven organic emissions.

Descriptions of coke and charcoal and their production, use, and potential health effects are contained in the *Encyclopedia of Occupational Health and Safety* (1).

Soot

Soot is the residue from incomplete combustion of any carbon-containing material, and varies widely in composition and physicochemical properties. Soots contain variable concentrations of particulate carbon, organic tars, resins, and nonvolatile inorganic matter. Soots differ from ashes by having greater inorganic and organic carbon content. Soots differ from carbon black by a lower content of elemental carbon and higher content of volatile and solvent-extractable organic matter and inorganic ash. As a percentage of mass, the organic content of soot varies from less than 5% for soot from contemporary diesel engines to well over 50% for chimney soots from inefficient burning of wood or coal. Soot consists of agglomerates of primary particles a few nanometers in diameter. Because the degree of agglomeration can vary markedly, soot may be inhaled as particles ranging from tens of nanometers in diameter to the upper limit of respirability.

Although pneumonitis or pneumoconiosis can result from extreme inhalation exposures to soot, cancer from absorption of mutagenic and carcinogenic species among the organic compounds is the principal health concern. At present, the potential for lung cancer from inhaled diesel exhaust is the occupational soot exposure of greatest concern. Gasoline engine exhaust also contains soot, but contemporary gasoline-powered automobiles emit much less soot than diesel engines under equivalent use. Metals, and particularly metals from catalytic converters and lead from engines burning leaded fuel, are a greater concern for gasoline engines than for diesel engines. Exhaust from aircraft turbine engines contains soot, but there is little information on possible adverse effects of aircraft exhaust on civilian or military personnel at airports or on aircraft carriers. There is no present occupational exposure limit for soots, other than limits for diesel soot in some countries and limits based on nonspecific dust.

Diesel Exhaust Soot

Diesel engines are prevalent in heavy-duty applications, such as locomotives, trucks, construction, mining, and farming equipment, and marine engines. Diesel-powered automobiles comprise approximately 25% of the light-duty fleet in Europe, but only approximately 1% in the United States. Occupational exposures to diesel soot were recently reviewed by Watts (81). The highest occupational exposures were reported for underground mines using diesel equipment. Long-term mean soot concentrations ranging from 0.6 to 1.7 mg/m^3 were measured in a study of several mines, with daily averages exceeding 3.0 mg/m^3 in some locations. Measured and estimated average soot concentrations for railroad workers, heavy equipment operators, and truck drivers have generally been less than 0.1 mg/m^3.

Diesel engines ignite fuel injected into the combustion chamber by heat of compression. Incomplete combustion results in the polymerization of carbon–hydrogen units, which form spherical primary particles consisting largely of elemental carbon. As exhaust leaves the combustion chamber and cools, unburned organic hydrocarbons and volatilized sulfur and metal compounds are condensed onto the surface of the aggregating carbon particles, forming soot. Diesel engines are generally throttled by varying the mass of fuel injected into the cylinder without simultaneous adjustment of airflow. The lack of an optimized fuel–air mixture during acceleration and deceleration results in the characteristic emission of increased soot at those times. Mass emissions of soot are now quite low from well-tuned contemporary engines during steady operation.

Diesel soot particles are almost entirely of respirable size, and consist of an elemental carbon core formed of aggregated primary particles and a variable amount of adsorbed organic sulfur, and metal compounds condensed onto the surface (82,83). The solvent-extractable organic fraction typically comprises 5–40% of the particle mass, and consists of many organic species, among which are known mutagens and carcinogens. Although respiratory morbidity has been reported for some occupational exposures to diesel exhaust, the principal concern has been for the small increase in risk for lung and bladder cancer suggested by epidemiological data (82).

Concern for lung cancer was heightened during the 1980s by the report of epidemiological evidence of increased cancer risk among railroad workers, coupled with the demonstration that prolonged exposures of rats to high concentrations caused increased incidences of lung tumors. Considerable attention has been given during recent years to clarifying the lung cancer risk from diesel exhaust and extrapolating risk from occupational exposures to potential risk from environmental exposures. Although inhaled diesel soot is a pulmonary carcinogen in rats, the response is equivocal in mice and does not occur in Syrian hamsters. Present evidence suggests the rat response may not be useful for predicting human cancer risk (70,84). The weight of epidemiological evidence suggests a 20–40% increase in lung cancer risk from high occupational exposures (e.g., 100 $\mu g/m^3$ and higher); however, regulatory agencies worldwide are currently uncertain about the assignment of quantitative unit risk estimates to either occupational or environmental diesel soot exposures. IARC ranks diesel exhaust as a probable human carcinogen (class 2A). NIOSH and the EPA currently rank diesel exhaust as a potential or probable human carcinogen.

Although there are soot emission standards for diesel engines, there are now no U.S. occupational or environmental exposure limits specific for diesel soot. Exposure to diesel soot is targeted to a limited extent by Canadian mine dust standards based on respirable combustible dust. Diesel soot exposures are limited in Germany to 0.6 mg/m^3 in underground noncoal mines and construction sites, and 0.2 mg/m^3 in other occupational settings (81).

The most recent review of the nature of diesel soot, current exposures, known and suspected health effects, and regulatory issues was published by the Health Effects Institute (85). Mauderly (82) reviewed both the animal and human carcinogenicity databases. The volume by Mauderly and McCunney (70) contains summaries of issues surrounding the extrapolation of carcinogenicity in rats to cancer risks in humans.

Smoke

Smoke is a heterogeneous mixture of particulate and nonparticulate products of the incomplete combustion of any material. The most common high-level occupational exposures to smoke occur in firefighters attempting to control structure or wildland fires. There are approximately 80,000 full-time or seasonal wildland firefighters in the United States, and a much greater number of municipal firefighters. Occupational exposures to biomass fires also occur seasonally in agricultural areas in which crop residues (predominantly sugarcane, rice, and wheat) are destroyed by burning. Old grass is burned to promote new growth, or trees and brush are burned to clear land for planting. Involuntary exposure to environmental tobacco smoke can also present a hazard in workplaces, such as restaurants, bars, aircraft, and nonsmoking areas contaminated by fugitive emissions from designated smoking areas.

The composition of smoke is highly variable, depending on both the feedstock and conditions of combustion, and generally contains a range of particle sizes. Smoke from structural fires contains soot, ash, and a range of highly toxic agents, including hydrogen cyanide, ammonia, halogen acids, acrolein, and isocyanates. Exposures of structural firefighters to particulate matter have been measured to range from 4 mg/m^3 to 20 g/m^3 (86). Smoke from wildland fires also contains ash, soot, and other materials, including the irritants aldehydes and acrolein, in concentrations that often exceed permissible occupational exposure limits (87). Biomass smoke has a somewhat characteristic composition (88); however, the organic content varies with the efficiency of combustion, and the silica content is higher in smoke from burning silicaceous plants, such as rice, wheat, and sugarcane. The composition of environmental tobacco smoke differs slightly from that of mainstream smoke, but contains most of the same irritants and carcinogens (89,90). Coultas et al. (91) measured nicotine concentrations from 3 to 53 $\mu g/m^3$ and respirable particulate levels from 4.0 to 146 $\mu g/m^3$ by personal samplers on workers in restaurants, offices, and hospitals. Drake and Johnson (92) measured concentrations of 10 and 38 $\mu g/m^3$ nicotine and respirable particulate, respectively, in smoking sections of aircraft on international flights, and approximately one-third those values in nonsmoking sections.

Inhalation of structural and wildfire smoke can cause acute, cross-shift, cross-season, and long-term effects. Acute effects, including suffocation, airway constriction, bronchitis, and airway injury can limit activity and can even be fatal. Structural firefighters have decreased airway function and increased airway responsiveness after workshifts involving exposure (93). Similar effects have been observed in wildland firefighters by cross-season measurements (94). A 10-year follow-up of Danish firefighters demonstrated an increased cancer incidence, including a threefold increase in risk for lung cancer (95). Other cancers, but not lung cancer, were increased in a mortality study of firefighters in the northwestern United States (96). Exposure to environmental tobacco smoke can cause irritating effects, and slight increases in lung cancer risk are thought to result from chronic, heavy exposures (reviewed in 90).

D. Natural Organic Particles

Organic dusts originate from vegetables, animals, or microbes, such as bacteria and fungi (Committee on Organic Dust, cited in 97). Whereas inorganic dusts are derived from mineral sources, organic dusts are carbon-based. Organic dusts are ubiquitous, and significant exposures to these materials occur in agricultural, industrial, and indoor environments. Exposures to organic dusts occur in farming, grain silos, cotton mills, and saw mills and consist largely of grains, parts from the plant material or wood, and microbes existing in these materials. Dusts from animals, feed material, and microorganisms are common on dairy farms and in poultry and swine houses. In hospitals, health-care facilities, and laboratories, pathogens originate from patients, workers, and sometimes tissue samples derived from patients. In agricultural and industrial environments, dusts are suspended in air by mechanical processes, such as airflow or dispersion, and by movements of people and animals. In health-care facilities and laboratories, pathogens can be dispersed from people by coughing or wheezing, or from surgical procedures. Health consequences from occupational exposures to organic dusts have long been recognized and studied extensively (98–100). The major health effects are (1) irritation and inflammation of the upper airways, (2) chronic bronchitis, (3) allergic alveolitis or hypersensitivities, (4) byssinosis, and (5) nasal cancer.

Dusts generated in agricultural, forestry, and livestock industries and the processing of raw materials or commodities are complex mixtures consisting of raw material, animal dander, feces, fungal spores, bacteria, pollens, and soil components. The composition of inorganic dusts varies greatly depending on the location, and activity at the time of study. Some components of organic dusts are more biologically active than others. Because of the variability in dust components and their biological activities, the agents responsible for some occupational diseases, including byssinosis, are difficult to elucidate and confirm. Detailed physical, chemical, and biological characterizations of organic dusts are necessary for understanding the etiology of the corresponding lung diseases and for monitoring the exposure environment for compliance and prevention. Extensive reviews on several aspects of organic dusts are available (101–107). The following sections describe organic dusts of biological origin commonly found in occupational settings and give the characteristics of the dusts that are particularly important.

Bioaerosols

Bioaerosols are defined as airborne particles composed of, or derived from, living organisms (108,109). Bioaerosols comprise viruses, bacteria, fungal spores, pollens, mites, and parts derived from microorganisms, such as toxins. Bioaerosols can be found in most atmospheres; the following descriptions pertain to those significant to occupational environments.

Viruses

Viruses are tiny, simple forms of microbes that require living cells to reproduce. They are classified as DNA or RNA viruses, depending on the genetic material they carry (106). The particle size of viruses ranges from 0.01 to 0.25 μm. Common diseases such as cold, influenza, smallpox, polio, chickenpox, and measles are transmitted from airborne viruses (106). They are spread by talking, singing, and coughing, from patients carrying the pathogens. Hospitals, clinics, schools, and child-care facilities are occupational environments in which both workers and patients can be exposed to these pathogens. There are increasing concerns that medical and dental personnel may be at increased risk of infection from contaminated airborne particles produced by oral operations, laser smoke, dermabrasion, or surgical procedures (110–115). Airborne particles produced in these processes include debris of blood, cells, and tissues, with particle sizes ranging from 0.7 to 20 μm. The particles typically have bimodal distributions with a fine-size mode $\leq$1 μm and a coarse-size mode of $\geq$5 μm (111,115–117). Potential risks of acquiring bloodborne viral diseases, such as hepatitis B virus (HBV) and human immunodeficiency virus (HIV) in dental, surgical, and laser procedures have been investigated both in simulated procedures (113) and in actual surgical settings (111,115,116).

Lasers are used for dermal treatments, including removing verrucae and warts. Smoke generated from applying CO_2 lasers to tissues contain carbonized particles and damaged or intact cells (118). Intact human papillomavirus DNA was detected in smoke produced from CO_2 laser therapy for treatment of human warts (110). Aerosols produced by orthopedic surgical procedures have been measured (115,117). The concentration and size distribution varied depending on the instruments and procedures used in the surgery. The aerosol concentration was highest when the surgical site was opened by a scalpel and when electrocautery, and irrigation and suction were used. Some of the particles contained hemoglobin. The time-averaged concentrations were 0.031–0.064 mg/m^3 for a hip replacement, knee replacement, or back fusion. Whether or not blood aerosols could contain HIV has not been determined directly. However, in a laboratory experiment, several common surgical power instruments used to generate aerosols from HIV-inoculated blood in culture medium showed that HIV could be cultured from aerosols generated by a spinning router and bone saw (119).

Dental operations, especially those requiring the use of a handpiece or syringe, produce aerosols that may include enamel, dentin, blood, saliva, water, and other debris expelled from the patient's mouth (120). Saliva and dental plaque are the principal sources of microorganisms, and blood may contain pathogens such as HIV and HBV. In a laboratory simulation, aerosols generated from dental procedures using handpieces and syringes had bimodal size distributions, with a fine particle mode of about 0.3 μm and a coarse mode of 13 μm (114). Fine particles were plasma spheroids that contained no detectable hemoglobin or red blood cell fragments, whereas coarse particles contained both. All particles could contain 0.042-μm HBV and could be inhaled. These findings lend support to the hypothesis of an airborne route for HBV infections reported for dental professions. However, in one study, air samples, taken in a dental clinic where HBV-positive patients were treated, did not show positive results for HBV surface antigen (121).

Bacteria

Bacteria are procaryotic cells without internal membranes. Depending on the structures of the cell wall or envelope, they can be classified as gram-positive bacteria, gram-negative bacteria, mycoplasmas, and archaebacteria (122). Bacteria range in size from 0.1 to 10 μm. Most bacteria fall into one of three groups, depending on their shape: spherical (cocci), rod-like (bacilli), or spiral (spirilla), although other shapes may exist. Respiratory diseases that may have been transmitted by airborne bacteria particles include whooping cough, pneumonia, diphtheria, tuberculosis, and legionellosis (106). Again, health-care and day-care workers are likely to be exposed to these pathogens, which are spread from patients in hospitals, clinics, or child-care centers. In a controlled experiment, airborne bacteria produced from various oronasal activities showed a range of production rates: sneezing and brushing teeth produced the highest rate (>500 colony-forming units (cfu) per minute) of bacteria, whereas singing, shouting, and coughing produced fewer (10–36 cfu/min). During some dental procedures, bacteria counts exceeded those produced during coughing or sneezing (123). Of the aerosols that people generated, a significant portion were smaller than 5 μm and, therefore, were respirable. *Legionella pneumophilia* (Legionnaires' disease) is thought to be spread by droplets aerosolized from showers or air-conditioning units contaminated with the bacteria (106). Airborne samples taken in a patient waiting room showed bacteria concentrations between 80 and 630 cfu/m^3 with most bacteria being cocci and bacilli (124). Bacteria, especially gram-negative, are commonly found in agricultural environments (98,107), in the transport and processing of agriculture material, and in waste-treatment and composting plants (125–127).

Endotoxin

Endotoxin is a class of compounds called lipopolysaccharide (LPS) found only in the outer envelope of gram-negative bacteria (106). Endotoxin is a complex molecule, with a lipid A at one end and a polysaccharide at the other end (122). The polysaccharide portion of the molecule varies widely, depending on the bacterial species, and to a lesser extent on the composition of the lipid A. Endotoxin is present in the environment as whole cells, large membrane fragments, or macromolecular aggregates. LPS is relatively heat-stable at 110°C. Airborne endotoxins are found in farming, industrial, and waste-treatment environments associated with high concentrations of gram-negative bacteria. Clark et al. (125) measured airborne concentrations of gram-negative bacteria and endotoxin in poultry and swine-confinement buildings. The bacteria and endotoxin concentrations were 9×10^4 cfu/m^3 and 0.12 μg/m^3 for swine-confinement units and 4×10^4 cfu/m^3

and 0.31 μg/m^3 for poultry-confinement units, respectively (125). The level of airborne endotoxin in poultry-processing houses was between 0.044 and 0.92 μg/m^3, with a measured bacteria concentration of 10^3–10^6 cfu/m^3 (128,129). The endotoxin concentration correlated well with total dust concentration (129). In cotton mills, the endotoxin level was 0.01–5.6 μg/m^3 (130–132). Most endotoxins were associated with particles in the size range of 2.9–5.9 μm (130). In solid waste-composting plants, gram-negative bacteria and endotoxin concentrations were 10^2–10^4 cfu/m^3 and 0.001–0.014 μg/m^3, respectively (126).

Inhalation of particles containing endotoxin causes fever, cough, airway inflammation, and acute airflow obstruction (131,133). Recent studies have demonstrated that endotoxin in cotton dust accounted for acute bronchoconstriction (131,132). It has been suggested that endotoxin in cotton dust may be the causative agent for byssinosis.

Fungi

Fungi consist of yeast, mushrooms, and molds. They are eukaryotic and do not photosynthesize. Fungi obtain nutrients through the decomposition of dead and decaying organic material, and they are ubiquitous in rural areas, forests, grain storage, and waste-processing facilities (105). Fungi normally reproduce through the formation of spores that may result from either sexual or asexual processes. Spores contain one to many cells and differ greatly in size, shape, and color. They normally range in size from 0.7 to 9 μm, and are usually shaped to maximize airborne dispersion (134). Spores are released into the air by air movement or the mechanical action of raindrops, animals, or humans. Some are actively discharged into the air (106). Spore concentrations are usually higher outdoors, and are in the concentration range of 10^3–10^4 cfu/m^3, with *Cladosporium* and *Alternaria* species predominant (105). Higher concentrations have been found in farming environments. Fungal spore concentrations at mushroom farms have been measured at 10^4–10^8 cfu/m^3 (105). The concentration of viable fungal spores ranged from 10^3 to 10^4 cfu/m^3 in poultry-confinement buildings (135), 10^3–10^5 cfu/m^3 in swine-confinement houses (136), and 10^6–10^8 cfu/m^3 in dairy barns where hay and straw were being chopped (137). The viable concentrations of fungal spores were in the range of 10^1–10^3 cfu/m^3 in cow barns, but the total concentration (including nonviable spores) was 10–100 times higher (134). In this study, the major species were *Aspergillus* sp., *A. umbrosus, A.* fumigatus, and *Penicillium*. The geometric size of these spores was between 1.5 and 3 μm. Inhalation exposure to dusts containing fungal spores can cause a range of respiratory symptoms. Allergic rhinitis and asthma have been reported to occur in susceptible agriculture workers during harvest and animal husbandry, and in workers at municipal waste-treatment facilities (105). The most frequently identified species were *Cladosporium* and *Alternaria. Aspergillus* and *Penicillium* species have been implicated in allergic alveolitis (105).

Pollens

Pollen grains are large, near spherical particles, with extremely resistant walls. They contain male reproductive cells and are produced by seed plants. There are two general types of pollens: anemophilous (wind-pollinated) and entomophilous (insect-pollinated) (106). Entomophilous plants produce pollens that are often sticky and can be quite large (up to 250 μm), whereas anemophilous pollens tend to be small (10–50 μm). The production of pollens depends on the stage of the plant life cycle, soil conditions, and the weather. The outdoor airborne concentration of pollens is generally higher than the indoor concentration because large pollens settle rapidly. The major health effect associated with inhaled pollens is allergic rhinoconjuctivitis in the upper airways, where large pollens deposit. An allergic reaction to pollens may also be a significant risk factor for asthma (106). These allergic reactions affect large numbers of susceptible members of the general population. Occupational allergy and asthma have occasionally been documented in farm workers exposed to sunflower (138) and palm pollens (139).

Mites

House dust mites and storage mites are tiny insects of the Acarina order of the Arachnida class. House dust mites feed on detritus of animals and are ubiquitous in homes in temperate and tropical climates. They are 250 and 500 μm in size. Several groups of mite allergens have been identified (106). Known house mite reservoirs include bedding, carpeting, and upholstered furniture. Mite allergens have been measured in house dusts collected from these places. Although, airborne concentrations of mite allergens are very low or nondetectable under most conditions, occupational exposures can occur in persons cleaning rooms. Some mite allergens are found in mite fecal particles in the size range of 10–20 μm. Storage mites rely on decaying vegetation as a food source and are found in farm houses and grain storage areas. They occur in large numbers in grain, hay, straw, and dust in farm buildings (140,141). Storage mites also constitute a part of mite fauna in house dust (141). Exposure to dust and storage mites has been associated with asthma, allergic rhinitis, and atopic dermatitis (106). Occupational exposures of grain workers and farmers have also been documented (141,142).

Agricultural and Commodity Dusts

Agriculture and other environments involved in the production and handling of grain, food, and raw materials; livestock husbandry; storage and transport of materials; and the processing of raw materials are often dusty. Concentrations of dust are usually high and sometimes exceed the nuisance level. These dusts are typically mixtures of organic dusts and inorganic soil particles, and contain active components that can cause respiratory diseases in heavily exposed workers. Because of the complex nature of these dusts, it is sometimes difficult to determine the etiology of the diseases and to identify the causative agents. Organic dusts originate from different sources and are generated by different mechanical processes in different environments, which affect dust composition, concentration, and particle size distribution. Respiratory diseases such as farmers' lung, silo fillers' disease, byssinosis, and bakers' asthma have been associated with these dusts.

Agricultural Dusts

Agriculture workers can be exposed to dusts during various activities including harvesting, transporting, storing grains, milling grains, or preparing feed (143). Animal-related dusts are inhaled during routine animal care, including feeding, cleaning, handling animals, milking dairy cows, or replacing the bedding. All dusts are especially problematic when generated in an enclosed structure, such as a barn, silo, or livestock-confinement house. Agriculture dusts are very heterogeneous; they may include (1) particles of agriculture products or plants, feed grain, hay, and silage; (2) animal dander, feathers, hair, urine, and feces; (3) bioaerosols such as bacteria, pollens, fungal spores, mites, and endotoxins; and (4) mineral components from soil sources (98,144).

Characterization of outdoor aerosols in two farming areas of Alberta, Canada, demonstrated seasonal patterns with peak levels of total suspended particle concentrations (140–160 $\mu g/m^3$) in the spring and fall, corresponding with specific farming activities, as compared with concentrations of 40–80 $\mu g/m^3$ in other seasons (144). The mean organic fractions of airborne particles measured in cereal grain and forage crop areas were 4.5 and 28%, respectively. The rest appeared to be mineral particles from suspension of soils, consisting largely of silicate minerals, with a small portion of free silica (1–17%). The particle mass median aerodynamic diameter (MMAD) measured with cascade impactors was 2.5–3.4 μm with a large geometric standard deviation (GSD) of 2.6–4.7. In the field, much higher dust concentrations (70–180 mg/m^3) were sampled outside of agricultural tractors during seeding, fallowing, spraying, and baling operations (145). However, inside the cabs of enclosed tractors, the dust concentration was reduced to 0.03–2.5 mg/m^3 by filtering air and by pressurizing the cab. Fruit in the central valley of California is often harvested manually. During the harvest season, high dust concentrations of 13, 21, and 31 mg/m^3 were measured in peach orchards, vineyards, and citrus groves, respectively (146). These concentrations far exceeded the recommended limit of exposure, 10 mg/m^3 for nuisance particulate matter (11). The measured size distribution had MMADs between 2 and 4 μm.

Starting in the 1950s and 1960s in Western Europe and North America, many farmers intensified their livestock production by using semiautomated structures called confinement buildings (98). Confinement operations can involve poultry, beef, swine, dairy cattle, or veal calves. The dusts and gases associated with livestock production are concentrated in these buildings and can pose severe health hazards to workers. Airborne dusts collected from swine-confinement buildings had mean total concentrations of 6.3 and 4.6 mg/m^3 in the United States and Sweden, respectively. The particle size had a MMAD of 9.6 μm (143). The main constituents of this dust included animal feed components (starch granules and trichomes) and swine fecal material (bacteria, gut epithelium, and undigested feed). Other identified components of the dust included swine dander, mold spores, insect parts, and mineral ash. Gram-positive bacteria predominated the microbial flora, but gram-negative bacteria and fungal spores were also present. The total and viable bacterial particle concentrations were 1.8×10^7 and 1.4×10^6/m^3, respectively. The endotoxin level averaged 0.12–0.2 μg/m^3. Dust concentrations in poultry-confinement buildings were somewhat lower with mean mass concentrations near 2.3–4.5 mg/m^3 (125,135). The particle size had a MMAD of 15 μm and a GSD of 2.2 (135). The concentrations of airborne bacteria and fungal spores were 1.5×10^5 and 1.0×10^4/m^3, respectively (135). The endotoxin concentration ranged from 0.001 to 0.061 μg/m^3.

On a dairy farm, preparation of feed and bedding produces dust. Silage, grain, hay, and straw contain large amounts of microorganisms. Kotimaa et al. (147) found that on dairy farms in Finland, baled hay and straw released the greatest amount of airborne bacteria and fungal spores, ranging from 6.3 to 18×10^4 cfu/g of material. In central New York, airborne samples, taken while hay or straw was being chopped, had a mean total concentration of 12 mg/m^3 and an MMAD of 10 μm (137). Major constituents of the dust included starch grain, plant parts, mineral particles, fungal spores and hypha, and bacteria. Viable fungal spores and bacteria concentrations were 5.0×10^6 and 4×10^6 cfu/m^3, respectively.

Grain Dust

Handling and processing grains during harvest, as well as the storage, transport, and transfer of grains, produce dusts to which workers are exposed during these processes. Grain dusts released in ambient air can be a major source of air pollution (148). In grain elevators, dust constitutes about 0.2–0.5% of the total grain mass (148,149). The primary constituents of grain dust are derived from the parent grain and plant, but the dust may also include soil, seeds, pollen, fungal spores, bacteria, and animal and insect fecal material (149). The organic content of grain dust is typically between 60 and 75%, and the balance is inorganic content, which may include quartz (148,149). Grain dust is released into the air by abrasion and attrition of grain kernels each time the grain mass is handled. The concentration and size distribution of particles in a grain dust cloud are strongly related to the type of grain handled and the mechanical processes involved. For example, inside grain elevators in Canada, mean mass concentrations of total suspended particles ranged from 0.3 to 192 mg/m^3 (148,150). The dust concentrations often reached levels constituting potential fire and explosion hazards. The particle size distribution had MMADs between 3.8 and 8.5 μm (148). The particle sizes of corn dust appeared to be larger than those of wheat and barley (150). Airborne fungal spore concentrations found in Canadian grain elevators had a particle range of 1×10^4 to $3.6 \times 10^6/m^3$ (149).

Cotton Dust

Cotton dust is defined as dust generated into the atmosphere as a result of the processing of cotton fibers combined with any naturally occurring material that may have accumulated on the fibers during growing and harvest (151). Prolonged exposures of workers to cotton dusts or other vegetable fibers, such as flax and hemp, can cause an occupational respiratory disease called byssinosis. Cotton dust contains fibers, leaf, bract, and other plant debris, soil particles, and microorganisms. These materials are released during ginning, spinning, and other processes (152). The chemical composition of some cotton dusts consisted of 30% cellulose, 25% noncellulose organic, 27% inorganic, a 13% water-soluble component, a 2% alcohol-soluble component, and 3% moisture (152,153). Dust concentrations in cotton gins ranged from 0.5 to 6.5 mg/m^3 for total dust and 0.07 to 4.1 mg/m^{-3} for respirable dust (152). In a carding operation, dust concentrations ranged from 0.5 to 2.2 mg/m^3 (130,131). The particle size distribution included particles between 0.7 and 20 μm, with a median diameter between 2 and 3 μm (154,155). The endotoxin level was 0.01–5.6 $\mu g/m^3$ (130–132). Most endotoxins were associated with particles in the size range of 2.9–5.9 μm (130).

Epidemiological studies have suggested that the prevalence of byssinosis can be correlated with averaged concentrations of lint-free dust (as measured by the vertical elutriator cotton dust sampler with a 50% cut-off diameter of 15 μm). The current threshold value for occupational exposure is 0.2 mg/m^3 (11). Many components in cotton dust have been proposed as the potential causative agent of byssinosis (97). Several studies have recently demonstrated a dose–response relation between airborne endotoxin or gram-negative bacteria and chest tightness or changes in 1-sec forced expiratory volume (FEV_1, 131,132).

Flour and Sugar Dusts

Occupational exposures to flour and sugar dusts in the confectionery industry cause rhinitis and asthma (156). Deposition of sugar particles on tooth surfaces during respiration can also cause dental diseases (157). Measurements of inhalable dusts in Swedish bakeries showed high concentrations ranging from 5.5 mg/m^3 for doughmakers to 0.5 mg/m^3 for packers (156). Impactor samples showed mean sizes larger than 10 μm, with 19% in the respirable fraction. The percentages of total protein had a mean value of 9% in these samples. Measurements conducted in the Finnish confectionery industry showed a 20–48 mg/m^3 dust concentration during the addition of sugar and a 0.01 mg/m^3 or lower concentration during biscuit packing (157). The ranges of sugar dust and flour dusts were between 0.03 and 20.5 mg/m^3 (mean of 0.1 mg/m^3) and 0.01 and 8.1 mg/m^3 (mean of 1.7 mg/m^3), respectively.

Wood Dust

Wood is one of world's most important renewable resources and is used for fuel as well as for industrial materials (102). Trees are classified as deciduous—hardwoods, or coniferous—softwoods (102). Wood dusts are produced by many processes, including sawing, sanding, planing, shaping, turning, carving, cutting, and chipping. Workers may be exposed to wood dust in many industries, including a sawmill operation, furniture manufacturing, carpentry, construction, or manufacture of plywood and particle board. The health effects associated with exposure to wood dust include skin and eye irritation, rhinitis, asthma, and cancer of the nasal cavity and paranasal sinus (158). Comprehensive reviews and summaries of the physical and chemical characterization, exposure assessment, and health effects of wood dust are available (102,103,159).

Wood dusts comprise irregularly shaped particles that are slightly elongated (160,161). The bulk of the dust represents shattered cells with main components of lignin, cellulose, and polyoses (102). Wood dust has either single or bimodal size distributions, with a primary mode of 20–40 μm and a secondary mode of 0.7–1.5 μm (160). The MMAD is between 5 and 20 μm (160,161). With most of the mass (>80%) consisting of particles larger than 10 μm, wood dust deposits mainly in the nasal cavity (158,160–162). It is likely that the risk of nasal cancer is increased by direct deposition of inhaled wood dust. Airborne dust also contains chemical agents other than wood components, such as chlorophenol for antistaining, phenol–formaldehyde plywood adhesives, solvents from coating materials, and pesticides. Microorganisms may also be suspended during wood processing. The number of fungi and bacteria in wood increases during storage and drying. In Finnish sawmills, airborne bacteria and fungal spore concentrations were 1.4×10^4 and 1.1×10^4 cfu/m^3, respectively (102).

Airborne concentrations of wood dust in sawmills and planing mills range from 0.1 to over 100 mg/m^3, with mean values close to 1 mg/m^3 (102). The highest concentration often occurred in the vicinity of chippers, saws, and planers. Mean concentrations of wood dust in plywood, particle board, and other wood-based panel mills were often close to 1 mg/m^3. The heaviest exposure usually occurred in the finishing department where plywood is sawed and sanded. Furniture industries, including manufacturers of cabinets, have reported mean values higher than in sawmills and plywood mills. The mean concentration often exceeded 1 mg/m^3. The highest exposures occurred in wood-machining and cabinet-making processes. Limits on occupational exposures to wood dusts have been set at 5 and 1 mg/m^3 for softwood and hardwood, respectively (102). These limits are based on epidemiological studies showing a clear association between exposures to hardwood dust and nasal cancer, whereas exposures to softwood dust cause elevated, but lower risks for nasal cancer (102,159).

E. Metal Particles

Occupational exposures to metal particles occur during smelting, refining, and production of primary metals; during preparation of metals by abrading, degreasing, cleaning, grinding, polishing, or buffing; during fabrication of metal products involving foundry operations, machining, welding, and heat treating; during metal finishing by electroplating or metal spraying; and in industries, such as electronics, during soldering of metals, fabrication of microelectronics, and production and use of batteries. Occasionally, exposures to inert particles such as iron oxide, titanium dioxide, and zirconium compounds are considered nuisance exposures at low concentrations (<5 mg/m^3) and are of little health concern. Frequently, however, exposures to airborne metals can cause health effects ranging from local irritation to acute or chronic disease. Even relatively inert materials, such as iron oxide, are not always benign. Inhalation of excessive concentrations of iron oxide, particularly fumes from welding operations, causes siderosis, involving symptoms such as chronic bronchitis and shortness of breath.

A comprehensive review of the materials, processes, and health hazards of metal handling in industrial activities was compiled by Burgess (6). Vincoli (165) also presents a useful review of metals encountered in the workplace and their health effects. Benson and Zelikoff (166) have reviewed the neoplastic and non-neoplastic changes in the respiratory tract from exposures to metals, including discussions of three metals (Be, Cr, and Ni) that primarily affect the respiratory tract and five metals (Al, As, Cu, Pb, and Zn) that affect other organ systems as well as the respiratory tract.

Concerns for occupational exposures of workers to metals are not limited to individuals directly involved in their processing. Secretaries have contracted chronic beryllium disease from infrequent contacts with beryllium-handling areas (163). Incidental exposures can occur to maintenance or janitorial workers. Garage, agricultural, and other general business workers frequently create exposure situations by manipulation or modification of metals or metal-containing compounds. In addition, not all exposures are confined to the workplace. As noted by Piacitelli et al. (164) in a study of lead contamination in the automobiles of lead-exposed bridge workers, paraoccupational or ''take-home'' exposures have been documented for workers at lead smelters, battery factories, radiator shops, and electronics plants, when workers carry contamination away from the workplace on their skin, hair, shoes, or dirty work clothes. Although subsequent exposures of workers and family members are primarily by ingestion, inhalation exposures can occur, especially in areas where dirty work clothes are stored and laundered.

Physicochemical Characteristics of Metal Aerosols

Metal aerosols include a wide range of vapors, fumes, smokes, mists, droplets, and dusts; thus, particle sizes range from 0.001 to 1000 μm. Most fumes and smokes contain ultrafine particles, ranging in diameter from about 0.01 to about 0.3 μm. Dusts from smelting operations involve fumes, droplets, and dusts, with particle diameters from about 0.1 to 100 μm. Powder sprays, such as zinc oxides, are somewhat larger and can range from a few micrometers to more than 300 μm in diameter. Dusts from foundry operations range from 1 to 1000 μm in diameter. *Vapors* are formed when normally liquid or solid materials are heated (e.g., mercury vapors); *fumes* consist of small, solid particles from condensation of vaporized metals (such as zinc oxides from welding); *smokes* result from incomplete combustion or combustion residues of carbon-containing materials (such as arsenic from pyrotechnics); *mists* are liquid droplets from condensation of evaporated or vaporized liquids (such as lead-containing gasoline); *droplets* can also be created by splashing, foaming, bursting of bubbles, or atomization (such as chrome salts in plating operations); and *dusts* are solid particles from handling, crushing, grinding, rapid impact, detonation, or other abrasive action of any type solid material. Metal aerosols can also exist in fiber form, as discussed earlier in the section on man-made metal whiskers.

The physical dispersion of aerosols frequently provides the mechanism for transfer of material to skin or eyes, at which dermal absorption can occur. Such dispersion also provides a pathway for ingestion when heavy metals are deposited on or in vegetation and water. Arsenic and lead from smelters, molybdenum from steel plants, and mercury from chlorine-caustic plants are dispersed in this way (167).

The level of concern for health hazards frequently depends on the chemical form of the metal compounds. This is primarily because the critical influence of chemical form on the uptake of inhaled, ingested, or skin-deposited materials, and can result in substantially different exposure limits for different compounds. For example, the ACGIH TWA TLV for exposure to chromium compounds is most restrictive for insoluble hexavalent chromium compounds (0.01 mg/m^3), which are poorly removed from lung following inhalation; less restrictive for water-soluble hexavalent compounds (0.05 mg/m^3), which are more readily absorbed into the bloodstream following inhalation; and least restrictive for the less-reactive trivalent chromium compounds and chromium metal (0.5 mg/m^3) (11). Chromic acid and chromate aerosols can be caustic to mucous membranes, and some water-insoluble chrome IV compounds are carcinogens. In addition, exposures to chromium compounds can cause skin ulcerations, dermatitis, perforation of the nasal septa, and kidney damage (165). Water-soluble hexavalent salts (sodium, potassium, and others) of chromium are absorbed into the bloodstream through inhalation, and exposure to some chromite dusts may cause lung diseases such as pneumoconious and pulmonary fibrosis.

A similar dependence on chemical form exists for mercury, which can be absorbed through the skin as well as taken in by inhalation. The TLV is most restrictive for alkyl compounds (0.01 mg/m^3); less restrictive for inorganic forms, including metallic mercury (0.025 mg/m^3); and least restrictive for aryl compounds (0.1 mg/m^3). Mercury compounds can cause bronchitis, pneumonitis, coughing, chest pain, respiratory distress, salivation, and diarrhea (165). Central nervous system effects include tremor, insomnia, depression, and irritability. Inhalation of vapors can also damage the liver and kidneys.

Characteristics of Metal Exposures

The following sections describe the characteristics of several typical, and some unusual, exposures to metals. Where possible, the examples include information on the particle size distributions measured in the workplace, along with discussions of the variables, such as the type of material and dispersion process, that influence the resulting particle size. Note, however, that most published studies report only the airborne concentrations of metals, but fail to provide information on the particle size distributions. This is largely due to the difficulties and expense of obtaining size-selected samples, especially personal air samples in the breathing zone. In addition, when data on particle size distributions are provided, they may not represent the true particle size distribution to which workers may be exposed. For example, large particles may be unable to enter the sampling inlet or may be trapped on the internal surfaces of the inlet; the sampler may be located outside the plume from a highly directional source, such as a grinding operation; or the timing of the size-selected sample may not be synchronized with the significant periods of aerosol release. Frequently, a general knowledge of the physical form of the airborne metal (e.g., vapor, fume, or dust) is sufficient to estimate the magnitude of inhalation risks and design an adequate control program. However, when it is important to know the true particle size distribution of an aerosol, care should be taken to understand the reliability and limitations of the sampling procedures.

Primary Production of Metals

Workers in mines and smelters can be exposed to a wide range of metal aerosols, including metals that are only present in trace amounts (168). For example, cadmium is a by-product of zinc and lead mining and smelting, with workplace concentrations generally 0.05 μg/m^3 or less (168). The ACGIH TLV for cadmium is 10 μg/m^3 for inhalable (total) dust and 2 μg/m^3 for the respirable fraction of airborne particles (11). Inhalation of high concentrations of cadmium oxide fumes from some silver solders and metal coatings can be fatal. Acute symptoms from exposure to cadmium are nausea, vomiting, diarrhea, headache, abdominal pain, muscular ache, salivation, and shock (165). Inhalation of cadmium fumes or dusts can cause cough, tightness of chest, respiratory distress, lung congestion, and bronchopneumonia. Cadmium is a poison that accumulates in the liver and kidneys, and it is also thought to cause certain diseases in bone. Absorption of cadmium through the digestive system is low.

Exposures to arsenic are also of concern in primary smelting of copper, zinc, and lead. Not all exposures are to particulate forms of arsenic. Arsine gas is formed by the reaction of hydrogen with arsenic during refining of nonferrous metals. In addition to concerns for cancer, exposure to arsenic can cause fever, gastrointestinal disturbances, irritation of the respiratory tract, ulceration of the nasal septum, and dermatitis. Prolonged exposure can produce pigmentation of the skin, peripheral neuropathy, and degeneration of the liver and kidneys (165).

Inhalation of freshly formed zinc oxide fume is the most common cause of metal fume fever, and cases involving magnesium oxide, copper oxide, and other metallic oxides have also been reported (169). Exposure to these oxides in aged powder form does not cause metal fume fever. Inhalation of mercury, nickel, and selenium can also cause fever. Nickel is a respiratory tract carcinogen in workers in the nickel-refining industry, especially when inhaled as a nickel carbonyl (168).

The air-sampling history from the primary reduction of metals was reviewed comprehensively by IARC (19,170), and individual studies showed great variability in the severity of exposures. Primary production of iron and steel involves exposures to ore and coal dust, iron oxide dusts and fumes, coke oven emissions, silica dust, and silica sand (6). Production of specific steel alloys to achieve improved mechanical properties involves addition of metals such as copper, vanadium, chromium, molybdenum, aluminum, and nickel. Production of hard steels for cutting tools involves addition of metals such as cobalt, niobium, and tungsten. Workers can be exposed to the raw materials during handling and mixing or to fumes and dusts during furnace and casting operations. Inhalation of dusts, fumes, and mists of copper can cause irritation of the eyes and mucous membranes, and perforation of the nasal septa (165). Symptoms such as cough, dry throat, muscle ache, and chills may be produced, and skin contact can result in dermatitis.

Inhalation exposures of workers in the metals industries frequently involve a range of other chemicals. For example, in the "potrooms" conducting electrolytic reduction of aluminum, workers are exposed to sulfur dioxide, polynuclear aromatic hydrocarbons, coal tar pitch volatiles, CO and CO_2 from the consumable petroleum coke and pitch anode; to fluoride compounds from the cryolite

(Na_3AlF_6) used to dissolve the alumina, from the fluorspar (CaF_2) added to control the melting point of the mixture, and from the aluminum fluoride (AlF_2) used to increase the efficiency of the reduction pot; and to dusts from the finely ground bauxite ore and from handling the alumina and other granular materials (6). In a study by Eduard and Lie (171), total particulate concentrations in the workplace were 5.4 mg/m^3 when the pots were charged with fresh alumina and were 7.6 mg/m^3 when the pots were charged with alumina recovered from the process exhaust dry scrubbers. The ACGIH TLV for alumina is 10 mg/m^3 of total particulate matter containing no asbestos and less than 1% crystalline silica (11). Repeated inhalation of high concentrations of aluminum may result in aluminosis or lung fibrosis (165). Inorganic fibers can be formed during reduction of alumina (6). Studies in Norwegian potrooms (172) identified airborne fibers of sodium aluminum tetrafluoride having a diameter of less than 0.01 μm and lengths less than 5 μm.

Preparation, Fabrication, and Finishing of Metal Products

Preparation of metals involves abrading, degreasing, cleaning, grinding, polishing, and buffing. Abrasive blasting is widely used to remove surface coating, scale, rust or oxidation, or fused sand in preparation for subsequent finishing operations. As noted earlier in this chapter, there is major concern for inhalation of the primary sandblasting media, especially for media involving free silica, which can cause silicosis. Although entrainment of toxic metals into the sandblasting media can pose additional inhalation concerns, indoor occupational exposures can generally be controlled by use of containment enclosures (abrasive blasting cabinets or rooms), with proper ventilation, and by modifying handling techniques. In contrast, outdoor occupational exposure of workers to lead during removal of lead-based paints from large structures remains a concern, and has been addressed in several alerts and standards, including NIOSH (173) and OSHA (174). Acute symptoms of exposures to lead include ataxia, vomiting, headache, stupor, hallucinations, tremors, convulsions, and coma (165). Lead concentrations can exceed 10,000 μg/m^3 during removal of lead-based paint by abrasive blasting, and some efforts to protect the environment by enclosing the abatement activities have caused increased exposures of workers (164).

Degreasing operations remove grease, oil, wax, and other surface contaminants. Burgess (6) reviewed the history of this technology. In general, exposures during degreasing are primarily to the solvents themselves, rather than to the metals being processed. Following degreasing, metal parts are frequently treated with acid or alkaline solutions to prepare the surfaces for electroplating or other surface finishing. Releases of the metals themselves in these processes are generally secondary concerns.

Conroy et al. (175) measured workplace emissions during hexavalent chromium plating of pistons. The electrical current that reduces the hexavalent chromium to metal also causes hydrolysis of water in the bath. The hydrogen gas bubbles released at the cathode and the oxygen gas bubbles released at the anode entrain chromic acid, causing a mist, which can be released to the workplace. During chrome plating of engine pistons, average hourly concentrations of airborne chromium were 37 $\mu g/m^3$ in the local process exhaust line and were 3.2, 2.5, and 0.8 $\mu g/m^3$ at distances of 50, 137, and 249 in. from the plating operation. These values are less than the ACGIH TLV of 50 $\mu g/m^3$ for soluble compounds of hexavalent chromium (11), although concentrations as high as 85 $\mu g/m^3$ were sometimes noted in the exhaust duct. Airborne concentrations of chromium were correlated with the total area plated per hour, which is a function of the rate of electrical current usage (amp-h/h). Such relations between release rates and production variables provide a systematic basis for control of emissions.

Grinding, polishing, and buffing create significant airborne concentrations of metal particles. Without citing any specific exposure concentrations or particle size distributions, Deadman et al. (176) noted that mechanics in hydroelectric-generating stations were exposed to chromium- and nickel-containing dusts during grinding operations to repair pitting (cavitation) damage on turbine blades. Linnainmaa (177) studied the influence of local enclosures and ventilation on exposures of Finnish workers to cobalt during grinding of hard metal blades. Concentrations of cobalt in air ranged from 0.006 to 0.160 mg/m^3 before improvement of enclosures and exhausts at three grinding stations and, after improvements, were less than 0.003 mg/m^3 during semiautomatic grinding and 0.011–0.015 mg/m^3 during manual grinding. No particle size distributions were reported. Cobalt is carcinogenic in laboratory animals, and the ACGIH TLV for cobalt was recently reduced from 0.05 mg/m^3 to 0.02 mg/m^3 (11). Linnainmaa also studied the influence of replacing the standard grinding coolant with a coolant developed for hard metal grinding. The new coolant, which dissolves very little cobalt, reduced the airborne concentrations of cobalt, but did not reduce urinary concentrations of cobalt in the workers, suggesting that exposures were dominated by sources other than dispersed coolant.

The concentration and aerodynamic size of the particles depend on both the mechanical machining or grinding process and the hardness of the metal itself. The following case studies illustrate this point for beryllium and its alloys. Beryllium causes cancer in laboratory animals and causes an immunologically mediated granulomatous lung disease following inhalation of beryllium aerosols by genetically susceptible persons. In a comparison of sawing and milling of beryllium metal, copper–beryllium alloy, and nickel–beryllium alloy, peak concentrations in the ventilation shroud exceeded 7 mg/m^3 during the machining of beryllium metal, compared with the ACGIH TLV of 2 $\mu g/m^3$ (11), but were more than a factor of 10 lower when using the less-brittle alloys of copper and nickel

(178). Taking into account the mass fraction of beryllium in the alloys, the overall airborne beryllium production rate for the alloys was more than a factor of 500 lower than for the metal. When the coarse particles from sawing and milling were examined visually, particles from the alloys were plate-like turnings typical of machining softer metals, whereas particles from the beryllium metal had smaller, more compact shapes that appeared to have been fractured, rather than peeled, from the work piece. This difference in hardness influenced the mass median sieve diameter of the particles from identical sawing operations: 300 μm with GSD 2.8 for the nickel–beryllium alloy, 280 μm with GSD 2.4 for the copper–beryllium alloy, and only 130 μm with GSD 2.0 for beryllium metal. When milling was done at a depth of 50 μm, turnings from the alloys had mass median diameters (MMDs) three times greater than the depth of the mill cut (150 μm and 170 μm for the nickel and copper alloys, respectively), whereas the beryllium metal particles had a MMD equivalent to the depth of the cut (50 μm). Geometric standard deviations of about 1.6 were associated with each of these size distributions. Less than 0.01% of the mass of displaced material from milling the alloys had an aerodynamic diameter less than 5 μm, whereas 9% of the displaced mass of beryllium metal had an aerodynamic diameter less 5 μm. The brittle behavior of beryllium metal was further confirmed when the depth of milling was increased by a factor of 10 (to 500 μm); the MMD of the resulting particles was increased to only 175 μm with GSD 2.1, and the mass of aerosol smaller than 5 μm aerodynamic diameter was decreased to only 4%.

In contrast with normal machining operations, such as grinding, sawing, or drilling, it appears that the fine polishing and buffing operations created particles of significantly smaller particle size and, therefore, of greater risk from inhalation. For example, in a current study of wet polishing of beryllium metal and oxide compounds in a commercial toxic metals shop, we are finding that nearly 100% of the airborne release of beryllium to the workplace is associated with particles having an aerodynamic diameter less than 10 μm.

In a retrospective study of the beryllium-processing industry, Seiler et al. (179,180) reviewed beryllium exposure measurements collected from 1950 through 1978 at five different facilities. More than 35 job titles were identified, with beryllium exposure concentration estimates based on job titles ranging from 0.12 $\mu g/m^3$ for nurses at one facility to 22 $\mu g/m^3$ for leach mill operators at another facility (compared with the 8-hr TWA exposure limit of 2 $\mu g/m^3$). However, the authors noted that only 58% of the plant-specific job titles had at least two exposure measurements. In addition, sufficient information on individual plant processes was not available to fully characterize the potential reductions in exposure by engineering controls over time. In their analysis of 643 individual daily weighted average exposure values from 1972 to 1975, 67% of the mean breathing zone values exceeded 2 $\mu g/m^3$, and 73% of the maximum exposures exceeded 2 μg/m^3. In contrast, only 18% of the general area mean exposures exceeded 2 μg/m^3.

Exposures to Metal Aerosols in Other Industries

Workers in industries, such as glass manufacturing, can be exposed to metals, such as antimony, arsenic, nickel, and lead, when they are added as raw materials to the manufacturing process (181). For example, arsenic trioxide is used as a decolorizing agent in the manufacturing of uncolored glass. Inhalation and ingestion of arsenic trioxide are associated with cancer in humans (165). In one study (182), results suggested that the high urinary arsenic concentrations were probably more closely related to oral intake from contaminated hands than to uptake by inhalation. Exposures of construction workers to chromium in contaminated soils were estimated to be a small occupational hazard when chrome–ore-processing residues were used to fill low-lying areas (183). Most of the chromium airborne particles were assumed to come from disruption of soil by heavy truck traffic at unpaved industrial sites. Incidental ingestion of chromium-contaminated soils was estimated to pose a negligible health hazard.

Exposures to metal aerosols in industries, such as electrical utilities and electronics, can result from soldering of metals, fabrication of microelectronics, production and use of batteries, general construction, maintenance, welding, and dispersion of metals from electronic components. Krochmalnyckyj (184) described a case in which 13 workers were exposed to mercury at estimated concentrations ranging from 31 to 1091 μg/m^3 during overheating of thermocouple seals in a metallurgical sintering furnace operation. The 8-hr TWA concentrations before the accident were between 8 and 54 μg/m^3; the ACGIH TLV is 25 μg/m^3 (11). Each seal contained about 5 lb (2.25 kg) of mercury to isolate the hydrogen atmosphere within the furnaces. The accident occurred when the furnace operating temperatures rose to 2550°F (1399°C) (from a normal range of 2150–2300°F; 1177°–1260°C) after insulation was added around the furnaces, and coolant flow to the furnaces was lowered to reduce employee risks for heat stress on the furnace deck. The accident was discovered when several workers experienced ''flu-like'' symptoms of dyspnea, sweating, shaking, and coughing after work. Employee urine concentrations of mercury ranged from 38 to 1331 μg/g creatinine, which exceeded the ACGIH Biological Exposure Index for mercury of 35 μg/g of creatine (11).

Automobile mechanics and other transportation-related workers can be at risk from inhalation hazards, such as metal fume fever, from inhalation exposures to manganese, which is released in automobile exhaust from combustion of manganese antiknock additives in nonleaded gasoline. According to the EPA (185), 30% of the manganese in gasoline is released from the automobile exhaust pipe. The size of manganese particles emitted to the atmosphere varies from 0.25 to

0.4 μm (186,187). Zayed et al. (188) estimated that garage mechanics were exposed to concentrations about ten times higher than taxi drivers (0.250 $\mu g/m^3$ vs. 0.024 $\mu g/m^3$). Sierra et al. (189) compared exposures of mechanics (0.010–6.673 $\mu g/m^3$, with a mean of 0.45 $\mu g/m^3$) with those of nonautomotive workers (0.011–1.862 $\mu g/m^3$, with a mean of 0.04 $\mu g/m^3$). These concentrations are small compared with the ACGIH TLV of 200 $\mu g/m^3$ for manganese as elemental or inorganic compounds (11). The ACGIH TLV for the antiknock agent itself (manganese cyclopentadienyl tricarbonyl) is 100 $\mu g/m^3$ (11).

Trace-metal contaminants in commercial-grade chemicals can also cause exposures of workers. Sánchez-Ocampo et al. (190) measured selenium levels in the serum of workers at a rubber tire repair shop. Selenium is present as a contaminant of sulfur compounds used in the vulcanizing process, and selenium compounds are sometimes used as additives in the rubber industry. Selenium concentrations were 70–300 μg/L in the serum of tire repair workers and 70–130 μg/L in a control group. Although inhalation of dust generated during the scraping of tire surfaces may be a factor responsible for the elevated serum levels of selenium, it was noted that there is a lack of specific data on the amount of dermal contact and absorption of selenium in the tire-handling process. Selenium is toxic to the respiratory tract, liver, kidneys, blood, skin, and eyes (165). Symptoms of excessive exposure to selenium include headache, fever, chills, sore throat, and bronchitis. Prolonged exposure can cause loss of hair, teeth, and nails; depression; nervousness; giddiness; blurred vision; and a metallic taste.

In a retrospective estimation of exposures to confirmed or suspected carcinogens in the electrical utility industry, Deadman et al. (176) listed concerns for exposures to arsenic compounds during application of wood preservatives and handling of pretreated poles or cross-pieces; exposures to beryllium compounds, cadmium compounds, and chromium VI compounds during electroplating, welding, and metallization of surfaces; exposures to lead during fabrication of enamel parts and during tinning with lead at metal-splicers school and during construction of lead splices; and exposure to lead chromate and zinc chromate during spray painting. However, in a summary of exposures by job and metal, only one exposure of an electrician to beryllium was listed as being greater than 200% of the ACGIH TLV. Six exposures to arsenic were documented in electricians, welders, and generation station workers, with four below 10% of the TLV, one between 10 and 25% of the TLV, and one between 25 and 100% of the TLV. Twelve exposures to chromium were documented for electricians, electrician helpers, a machinist apprentice, a mechanic, a utility man, and a welder, with ten exposures less than 10% of the TLV, one between 10 and 25% of the TLV, and one between 25 and 100% of the TLV. Two exposures of welders to nickel were less than 10% of the TLV. Three exposures to lead were documented in electricians and generating station workers, with only one being greater than 25% of the TLV. Various lead–tin solder amalgams were commonly in use, and the amount of lead volatilized depended on the equipment used and the degree of caution taken when melting the solder.

Worker exposures to welding fumes have been widely documented. Aerosols consist primarily of branched-chain ultrafine aggregates with aerodynamic diameter less than 1 μm, but also include larger spherical particles that are ejected as molten droplets. A large number of variables can affect the composition and concentration of the welding fumes. A recent study (191) compared worker exposures in a shipyard as a function of the degree of confinement (open or enclosed), direction of welding (on an overhead ceiling, horizontal, vertical, and welding on a ledge), type of welding (automatic vs. manual), type of electrode, use of air extraction, and ventilation. No personal samples of the worker breathing zone exceeded the TLV when welding was done on the ceiling, but during horizontal welding 50% of samples exceeded the TLV for particulates, 16% exceeded the TLV for iron, and 11% exceeded the TLV for manganese. Results for vertical and ledge welding were somewhat lower than for horizontal welding. It was suggested that horizontal welding is more hazardous because the worker's airways are more closely exposed to the welding fumes. Some results were counterintuitive. For example, samples collected in the presence of ventilators were higher than those obtained in their absence. This was attributed to the possibility that ventilators are only used in extreme cases and that, when used, they are inadequate.

The characteristics of welding fumes and the associated inhalation risks depend on the welding method and the composition and size of the consumable welding wire or rod. Hewett (192) measured the particle size distributions, densities, and specific surface areas for welding fumes from mild steel and stainless steel consumables using two welding processes, and estimated the regional pulmonary deposition fraction for each fume (193). Shielded metal arc welding (SMAW) uses a flux-coated welding rod, which melts and fuses with the base metal during welding. The flux prevents oxidation of the molten metal. Gas metal arc welding (GMAW) uses machine-fed wire, either uncoated stainless steel or copper-coated mild steel, with an inert shield gas (argon) providing protection of the molten metal from the ambient oxidizing atmosphere until the molten metal has cooled and hardened. Process type had a substantial influence on the fume characteristics, with relatively minor influences from the type of consumable. For example, bulk densities of fume materials were 3.4 g/cm^3 for the SMAW processes and about 5.8 g/cm^3 for the GMAW processes. For SMAW, specific surfaces areas were about 20 m^2/g using both mild and stainless steel. For GMAW, specific surface areas were about 30 m^2/g using mild steel and about 40 m^2/g using stainless steel. Particle size distributions had MMAD of about 0.5 μm with GSD about 1.7 for SMAW, and MMAD of about 0.25 μm with GSD about 1.6 for GMAW. These size distributions are consistent with historical values reported by the American Welding Society (194) that nearly 100% of SMAW fumes have aerodynamic equivalent diameters less than 1 μm, and nearly 100% of GMAW fumes have aerodynamic equivalent diameters less than 0.5 μm. Based on the smaller size distribution of the GMAW fumes, total lung deposition for GMAW fumes was estimated to be 60% greater than for SMAW fumes, assuming equal exposures on a milligram per cubic meter basis.

F. Mists and Droplets

A *mist* is defined as a liquid particle aerosol. Mists can be formed by condensation of supersaturated vapors or by the physical shearing of liquids, such as in atomization (nebulization), spraying, or bubbling (195,196). A visible mist is called a *fog*. Particle sizes for mists generally range from submicrometer to about 20 μm. Larger liquid particles are generally referred to as *droplets*, which include mists. The particle shape of mists and droplets is spherical owing to the surface tension of the liquid. However, liquid particles may contain impurities, such as metals or volatile components, and they may become irregularly shaped after evaporation and deposition on surfaces. Based on industrial applications and mist-formation mechanisms, potential occupational exposures to mists and droplets can generally be divided into four categories. These will be described in the following.

Acid Mists

Strong acids that are manufactured or used in a manufacturing process can be released as mists, vapors, or gases into work environments. These industries include pickling and other acid treatment of metals, the manufacture of isopropanol, synthetic ethanol, sulfuric acid, soap, detergent, nitric acid, phosphate fertilizer, lead–acid batteries, and various petroleum and chemical products (197). The degree of mist and droplet formation varies with the process employed, such as acid splashing owing to handling or chemical reactions, mist produced by gas bubbles bursting at the surface of an acid solution (185,198), or condensation of vapors. Millions of workers worldwide may be exposed to acid mists.

Sulfuric acid is the most widely used of the strong inorganic acids. Exposure to sulfuric acid may occur in the manufacturing of lead–acid batteries, the acid itself, or in pickling, electroplating, and other acid treatment of metal. Workers can also be exposed to sulfuric acid during the production of phosphate fertilizer, isopropanol, synthetic ethanol, and detergents. Exposures to hydrochloric, nitric, and phosphoric acids are also important. Exposures to hydrochloric acid may occur in industries that involve acid treatment of metals, during synthesis of the acid, or in numerous other industrial processes. Pickling and other acid treatment of metal may entail occupational exposures to nitric and phosphoric acids. Exposure to nitric acid also occurs when it is manufactured, and exposure to phosphoric acid can occur in production of phosphate fertilizer.

An IARC working group reviewed occupational exposures to acid mists in various industries (197), and their findings are summarized briefly as follows: In the plating and pickling industries, average air concentrations of sulfuric acid mists in work environments were found to range from less than 0.01 to 5.6 mg/m^3. Average concentrations of hydrochloric acid ranged from less than 0.2 to 13.6 mg/m^3 in Finnish and American studies; 59 mg/m^3 in a Chinese study; 0.2 to 49.8 mg/m^3 in French, German, and Russian studies; and 1.8 to 12.4 mg/m^3 in a Dutch study. Air concentrations of nitric acid and phosphoric acid were measured at 0.01–0.4 mg/m^3, and less than 0.67 mg/m^3, respectively; ACGIH has recommended TWA exposure limits for sulfuric, hydrochloric, nitric, and phosphoric acids. These limits are 1, 7.5 (7 OSHA), 5.2 (5 by OSHA), and 1 mg/m^3, respectively.

Sulfuric acid causes respiratory irritation, bronchitis, and death (199–201). Dental erosion has been observed among workers exposed to acid mists (202,203). Acute symptoms of bronchoconstriction have been observed following human exposures to high levels (>500 μg/m^3) of sulfuric acid (204), whereas mild throat irritation and increased airway responsiveness were noted after exposure to 450 μg/m^3 for 4 hr during moderate exercise (205). An excess of nasal sinus, laryngeal, and lung cancer among workers exposed to sulfuric acid has been reported, and the IARC working group concluded that occupational exposure to strong inorganic acid mists containing sulfuric acid is carcinogenic to humans (197).

There is a little information on the particle size distribution of acid mists in occupational settings. Van Dusen and Smith (198) reported particles ranging in size from 0.5 to 39 μm in their study on electrowinning of metals. Gamble et al. (206) measured mean exposures to sulfuric acid of 0.18 mg/m^3 at an average MMAD of close to 5 μm in their study of health effects of sulfuric acid in lead–acid battery plants.

Machining Fluids and Oil Mists

Machining fluids are used for lubrication and cooling in many metalworking operations, such as drilling, milling, turning, grinding, boring, and broaching. Several types of these fluids have been used in industry, the most common being (1) petroleum-based mineral oils (straight cutting oils), (2) emulsions of mineral oils (soluble mineral oils), and (3) synthetic fluids. During machining or grinding operations, oil mists are generated because of splashing or spraying from components moving at high speeds, or evaporation and condensation owing to the high heat generated. In the operation of a high-speed newsprint press, an oil (ink) mist aerosol is often released into the pressroom (207,208).

The composition of these oils varies depending on the source of the oil, the manufacturing process, and the additives present. Machining fluids contain numerous chemical additives that improve their physical characteristics or prolong their usable life. These additives include biocides, surfactants, corrosion inhibitors, extreme-pressure agents, water conditioners, antifoaming agents, glycols, ethanolamines, and occasionally fluorescein and petroleum azo dyes (209). The emulsified oils also become contaminated with bacteria during use (210). Some of these agents or bacteria can cause acute pulmonary inflammation or airway sensitization (211,212).

Data on occupational exposures to mineral oils before 1984 were reviewed by an IARC working group (213). They reported that air concentrations of oil mist in major U.S. industries (including automobile, steel products, and hardware manufacturing, brass and aluminum production, copper mining, and newspaper pressroom) ranged from 0.8 to 56.5 mg/m^3, and that the average exposure concentrations were probably less than 15.0 mg/m^3. In their study of automobile workers exposed to aerosols of machining fluids, Kennedy et al. (209) reported that the total aerosol exposure concentrations for assembly workers ranged from 0.07 to 0.44 mg/m^3, and for machinists from 0.16 to 2.03 mg/m^3. Menichini (214) found oil mist concentrations produced by mold lubrication to range from 0.1 to 1.3 mg/m^3. Woskie et al. (215), using a two-stage personal cascade impactor plus a backup filter, measured a mean total exposure concentration of 706 μg/m^3 for workers in machining and grinding operations in the automobile manufacturing industry.

Because of the nature of the mechanisms that produce mists from machining fluids, workers are subjected to both dermal and inhalation exposures. Thus, the lungs and skin are the major sites in humans affected by the toxicity of machining fluids. Skin tumors are reported to result from exposures to various types of mineral oils (213). Inhalation of white oils and petrolatums can lead to lipid pneumonia and lipid granuloma (213). Mists of machining fluids cause chronic cough, chronic phlegm, expectoration, or dyspnea in machine shop workers (216,217). Cases of occupational asthma were also reported (210,212). IARC reviewed the results of three cohort mortality studies of printing pressman for excess lung cancer and cancers of the buccal cavity and pharynx, and concluded that mineral oils (containing various additives and impurities) are carcinogenic to humans (213).

Only a few studies have measured the particle size or size distributions of machining fluid mists. Kennedy et al. (209) used two-stage impactors to measure aerosols of machining fluids in three size fractions: smaller than 3.5 μm, 3.5–9.8 μm, and larger than 9.8 μm in aerodynamic diameter. Relatively even distribution among three mass fractions was observed for aerosols from three types of machining fluids. Lippmann and Goldstein (207) reported an average median droplet diameter of 14 μm (range, 9–30 μm) for ink-mist particles in a pressroom. No GSD was given. Menichini (214) measured particle size distributions of four different oil types used for lubricating molds in concrete and glass manufacturing.

The cumulative size distributions were bimodal, and count median diameters ranged from less than 0.5 μm to about 10 μm. Woskie et al. (215) used both six-stage and two-stage Marple Personal Cascade Impactors to measure metal-working fluid aerosols released from various machine types, including grinding, boring/milling/turning, drilling/tapping/reaming, lapping, screw machines, large multioperation transfer machines, gear cutting, and broaching. They reported MMDs to range from 1.6 to 8.2 μm with GSDs ranging from 2.4 to 4.4.

Pesticide and Herbicide Spray

Chemicals have been used to control insects and plants for centuries, but have come into widespread use only within the past century, with the development of a variety of synthetic pesticides and herbicides. Insecticides are used on several crops important in world agricultural production. Herbicides are used mainly in corn and soya bean fields, insecticides mainly on cotton and horticultural crops, and fungicides mainly on horticultural crops and wheat. Pesticides are also used by the greenhouse industry. Of the several hundred chemicals that have been applied for insecticidal purposes, fewer than 100 have been used extensively.

The principal classes of compounds that have been used as pesticides and herbicides are organochlorine, organophosphorus, carbamate and pyrethroid compounds, and various inorganic compounds. Insecticides constitute a higher proportion of the total pesticide usage in developing countries than in developed countries.

Pesticides and herbicides are applied by aerial spraying and by various ground-based techniques, ranging from handheld sprayers and dusters to vehicle-mounted sprayers, foggers, and power dusters. The volume of liquid spray applied is determined by the size of the target and by whether the intent is to deposit discrete droplets or a complete film on the target. Optimal droplet sizes can range from 10 to larger than 500 μm.

Occupational exposures may occur during the manufacture and processing of pesticides and herbicides, as well as during their use. Inhalation and dermal exposures can occur in the mixing and loading of equipment and in the spraying and application of pesticides or herbicides. Because pesticides and herbicides used in spray are usually highly soluble and absorbable, the relative importance of the routes of occupational exposure is usually in the following order: dermal exposure > respiratory exposure > oral exposure (218,219). Inhalation and dermal exposures may also occur among workers engaged in recycling pesticide containers, during which metal is washed and shredded (220).

Barthel (221) reported an increased incidence of lung cancer in workers repeatedly exposed to various types of pesticides, but no carcinogenic effect could be attributed to specific individual pesticides. Cases of acute poisoning from pesticide spraying have been reported (222,223). Disorders of the skin, cardiovascular system, nervous system, sensory organs, respiratory system, and reduced lung function have been reported following exposure to pesticides (218,224).

Abbott et al. (225) studied workers exposed to a 2,4-dichlorophenoxyacetic acid (2,4-D) that was applied with five types of ground sprayers. During spraying, the dermal exposure ranged from 40 to 142 mg/hr, whereas the airborne concentration ranged from 10.6 to 30.5 $\mu g/m^3$. They concluded that the hands were the most highly exposed part of the body during mixing, and that the inhalation exposure was negligible compared with dermal exposure. A study of the use of the herbicide alachlor demonstrated exposures ranging from 0.32 to 6.4 $\mu g/m^3$ (226),

Archibald et al. (227) studied the potential pesticide exposure of greenhouse workers using high- and low-volume application methods with two types of pesticides. The average concentration of pirimicarb ranged from 2840 to 4300 $\mu g/m^3$ and 1100 to 2100 $\mu g/m^3$ for high- and low-volume applications, respectively. The deltamethrin concentration ranged from 142 to 454 $\mu g/m^3$ and 86 to 215 $\mu g/m^3$ for high- and low-volume applications, respectively. Aerosol size was not measured.

Fenske et al. (228) studied the occupational exposure to fosetyl-Al fungicide during spraying of ornamentals in a greenhouse using commercial backpack sprayers; the air concentration of the fungicide ranged from 4 to 132 $\mu g/m^3$ during mixing and spraying. They concluded that dermal exposure was much higher than inhalation exposure, with inhalation exposure contributing only 7–9% of total exposure,

Jauhiainen et al. (229) studied the occupational exposure of forest workers to glyphosate during brush saw spraying and reported that the air concentration of glyphosate was less than 15.7 $\mu g/m^3$.

Leonard and Yeary (230) studied the occupational exposure to four insecticides and two fungicides among workers using handheld equipment when spraying pesticides on trees and shrubs. They reported concentrations of 0.01–0.07, 0.001–0.04, and 0.001–0.007 mg/m^3 for carbaryl, diazinon, and dicofol, respectively. These levels were well below the acceptable ACGIH exposure limits of 5.0, 0.1, and 1.0 mg/m^3 for these pesticides, respectively.

Libich et al. (231) studied the exposure of herbicide applicators to three herbicides while using handheld spray guns or mist blowers. They reported that the mean air concentrations ranging from 1.3 to 55.2 $\mu g/m^3$, well below the TLV of 10 mg/m^3 for 2,4-D and picloram (231).

Because of the highly absorptive characteristic of pesticides and herbicides, and the various spraying equipment and methods used, most studies did not report particle size measurements. The useful information on chronic illness resulting from exposure to insecticides is limited because of the highly variable exposures, the wide variety of compounds used, the presence of many confounding factors, and the lack of sensitive, specific endpoints for toxicity (218).

Paints and Coatings

Spray painting and coating are used to finish chassis and drive-train components in the automobile industry. Other industries, such as wood and metal furniture, transportation equipment (nonautomotive), appliance, and heavy machinery, also use spray painting to finish products. A spray-painting gun or other types of atomizers atomize the paint into droplets, some of which impact on the surface to form a coating of paint. These droplets that do not impact on the surface being painted or break up and bounce off the surface owing to the high velocity of the spray are called paint overspray aerosols. The painter is exposed to these overspray aerosols and solvent vapors that evaporate from both the overspray and the painted surface. Some paints contain toxic chemicals and metals, such as isocyanates, epoxy-curing agents, lead, or chromium. Exposure to organic solvents can affect the central nervous system (232). Exposures to isocyanates (including polyisocyanates) are reported to cause skin and eye irritation, respiratory sensitization, asthma, and reduced lung function (233,234).

Chan et al. (235) evaluated the efficiency of a scrubber attached to a spray-painting booth in the automobile industry and measured the size distributions of paint overspray aerosols inside the booth before the scrubber and in the exhaust after the scrubber. Their results indicated that, inside the painting booth, the MMAD from air-atomized spray guns ranged from 4 to 12 μm (GSD ranged from 2.1 to 3.5), depending on atomization pressure. The MMAD from rotary atomizers ranged from 20 to 35 μm (GSD ranged from 2.4 to 3.1), depending on rotational speed. In the exhaust after the scrubber, the MMAD ranged from 1.30 to 1.65 μm (GSD ranged from 1.8 to 2.3; mass concentrations ranged from 3.0 to 18.9 mg/m^3), and 2.41 μm (GSD 2.7; mass concentration ranged from 5.9 to 6.7 mg/m^3) for the spray gun and rotary atomizer, respectively. In an evaluation of a newly developed, high-velocity oxyfuel thermal metal spray gun for coating power train components, Chan et al. (236) reported that the size distribution of highly polydisperse aerosols ranged from 0.2 to 5 μm and that a concentration of 34.7 mg/m^3 was measured at the exhaust duct. The chemical compositions of size-classified, high-solid paint overspray aerosols were studied by D'Arcy and Chan (237). Their results indicated that the chemical composition can be nonuniform among different particle sizes. Zhuang and Myers (238) observed that the ambient paint overspray aerosol concentration in an aircraft paint-spraying operation ranged from 0.38 to 10.7 mg/m^3, but did not measure particle size.

Heitbrink et al. (233) studied worker exposures in auto body repair shops for three types of spray-painting booths using a lapel sampler. They reported a mean particulate overspray concentration ranging from 1.9 to 30 mg/m^3, depending on the type of the booth and booth flow rate. No particle size information was given. About one third of the total concentration was hexamethylene diisocyanate (HDI)-based-polyisocyanates. Using this one-third factor, the Oregon short-term exposure limit (STEL) of 1.0 mg/m^3 for HDI-based polyisocyanates was exceeded frequently. Similar HDI polyisocyanate concentrations (ranging from 0.25 to 3 mg/m^3) were also observed by Maître et al. (239). This STEL is being proposed in a few countries and recommended by manufacturers of polyisocyanates. Rosenberg and Tuomi (240) reported values of 0.006–0.12 mg/m^3 for the HDI monomer, and 0.28–3.6 mg/m^3 for the HDI oligomer for two-component polyurethane paint. Similar results were also obtained by others (241,242). A hygienic limit value for the HDI monomer of 0.07 mg/m^3 was set by the National Board of Labour Protection in Finland (240), and a TLV of 34 μg/m^3 has been recommended by ACGIH (242). No exposure limit has been set for HDI oligomer.

In their review and evaluation of control technology for spray painting, O'Brien and Hurley (243) observed that mean paint mist concentrations for selected, manual-finishing operations ranged from 0.1 to 39.2 mg/m^3. No particle size information was available.

A complete hazard evaluation of paint overspray aerosols would require a comprehensive physical and chemical characterization of the various chemical components in the overspray. A nonuniform distribution of chemical components in different particle-sized fractions can exist. Using the size distribution of the total overspray aerosol alone to estimate the lung burden, which may differ from lung burdens based on the chemical distribution of the species in different particle sizes, can introduce significant errors in lung burden estimates (237).

G. Radioactive Particles

Occupational exposures to radioactive particles can result from encounters with natural or man-made radioactivity. Of primary concern for inhaled particles are alpha-, beta-, and gamma-radiation, and neutrons and positrons can be of concern in some special circumstances. Alpha-radiation is the least penetrating, but most highly ionizing type of radiation. The alpha-particles consist of two neutrons and two protons, carry two positive charges, are identical with a helium nucleus, and are created spontaneously during the radioactive decay of high atomic number elements, such as radium, uranium, or plutonium. Alpha-emitting radionuclides can be identified by the characteristic energy of their emissions. They are of special concern when they are inhaled and deposited in the respiratory tract. If inhaled in large quantities, damage to cells in the lung or in other organs to which the material is translocated can cause acute health effects, such as inflammation, and long-term health effects, such as fibrosis and cancer (see, e.g., 244).

Beta-radiation is more penetrating than alpha-radiation and consists of negatively charged particles that are identical with electrons. Beta-radiation can penetrate the skin, and, similar to alpha-radiation, is of concern when large amounts of beta-emitting radionuclides are deposited in the body. The energy spectrum of beta-emissions covers a broad range up to a characteristic maximum. Iodine 131, cesium 137, and strontium 90 are beta-emitting radionuclides that are of special concern for accidents involving nuclear reactors. In some cases, the radioactive emissions of radioactive decay products are of greater biological concern than the emissions of the parent radionuclide. For example, although strontium 90 has a relatively long half-life (28.8 years) and emits beta-radiation at a relatively low energy (0.54 MeV), its progeny radionuclide yttrium 90 has a short half-life (64.2 hr) and is a high-energy beta-emitter (2.28 MeV).

Gamma-rays are penetrating quanta of electromagnetic energy. They are not charged particles, but they can cause ionization in materials and biological damage in tissues. Gamma-radiation originates in the nucleus of atoms during radioactive decay. Gamma-radiation is emitted at discrete, characteristic energies for each radionuclide. Many alpha- and beta-emitting radionuclides also emit gamma-radiation.

Radioactive particles can exhibit all the physical and chemical properties of nonradioactive aerosols. Depending on their origin, they can range from ultrafine dusts, mists, or metal fumes, to large solid particles or liquid droplets. An extensive compilation of the airborne release fractions and respirable fractions (smaller than 10-μm aerodynamic diameter) for spills, explosions, combustion, impaction stressing, and other disruption of radioactive materials was prepared for the U.S. Department of Energy (245). Parameters can range from an airborne release fraction of 1.0 and a respirable fraction of 1.0 for volatile radionuclides, such as iodine, to an airborne release fraction of 3×10^{-4} and a respirable fraction of 0.01 for free-fall spills of a coarse powder. Methods for characterizing radioactive aerosols include traditional techniques for determining physical and aerodynamic size, in combination with radioactivity counting and radiochemistry techniques for determining parameters such as specific activity (radioactivity per unit mass) and solubility in biological media (246). A wide range of radiation detection systems are available for use in worker protection. The ease of detecting the presence of radioactive materials in real time is a major facilitator of maintaining worker exposures well below acceptable limits.

The specific activity and biological behavior of materials are considered in determining acceptable annual limits on intake (ALIs) for workers exposed to radioactive aerosols (see 247 and its addendums). A related concept is the derived air concentration (DAC). A DAC is the calculated air concentration to which a worker could be exposed 8 hr/day, 5 days/week, for 50 weeks (an entire work year of 2000 hr), without exceeding the ALI for the radionuclide. The worker is assumed to breathe at the rate of 20 L/min as given for the ICRP Reference Man (248). Thus, the DAC is the ALI divided by the volume of air inhaled during the working year (2400 m^3).

Particle number concentrations for three radioactive materials at their DAC are listed in Table 5 as a function of particle size. These materials include $^{238}PuO_2$, $^{239}PuO_2$, and enriched uranium. Specific activity is of practical concern for radioactive materials because it determines the amount of radioactivity that will be present in a sample of a given mass, and the mass or number of particles that will be associated with a sample of a given activity. Insoluble ^{238}Pu has a specific activity of 6.44×10^{11} Bq/g and a DAC of 0.3 Bq/m^3. Insoluble ^{239}Pu has a specific activity of 2.26×10^9 Bq/g and a DAC of 0.2 Bq/m^3. For enriched uranium, the specific activity is 2.35×10^6 Bq/g (dominated by the contribution from ^{234}U, which is present at 1% by mass), and the DAC for the insoluble material is 0.6 Bq/m^3. This example demonstrates that the number of particles of concern for different radionuclides covers a broad range. It also illustrates that the particle number concentration for high-specific–activity materials such as ^{238}Pu can be very low at the DAC. This means that the probability of actually inhaling a particle might be very low, which can result in the overestimation of the worker intake of radioactivity (249).

Natural Radioactivity

A myriad of radioactive and nonradioactive materials was created at the inception of the universe, with every element in the periodic table existing as a mixture

Table 5 Number of Particles per Cubic Meter as a Function of Monodisperse Particle Size for Three Radioactive Materials[a] at Their Derived Air Concentration (DAC)

Particle diameter (mm)	$^{238}PuO_2$	$^{239}PuO_2$	Enriched uranium
10	0.0001	0.02	54
5	0.0008	0.15	433
3	0.004	0.7	2007
1	0.1	19	54,180
0.5	0.8	150	433,443

[a]Insoluble ^{238}Pu has a specific activity of 6.44×10^{11} Bq/g and a DAC of 0.3 Bq/m^3. Insoluble ^{239}Pu has a specific activity of 2.26×10^9 Bq/g and a DAC of 0.2 Bq/m^3. For enriched uranium, the specific activity is 2.35 $\times 10^6$ Bq/g (dominated by the contribution from ^{234}U, which is present at 1% by mass), and the DAC is 0.6 Bq/m^3.

of stable and radioactive isotopes. The current concentration of a radionuclide in the earth's crust depends on the half life of that radionuclide, the time for half of the atoms present to undergo a spontaneous nuclear transformation. Nearly all of the original radionuclides in the earth's crust have long since decayed to stable elements. A few, such as radioisotopes of uranium, thorium, radon, and potassium, have long enough half-lives to remain of radiological concern. Occupational exposures to these radionuclides typically occur during mining and extraction. Risks from occupational exposures to these radionuclides may be augmented by smoking or other lifestyle or environmental factors. For example, tobacco contains minute amounts of uranium and thorium decay products in its plant matrix and in residual soil and phosphate fertilizer contamination on leaf surfaces. Lead 210, a beta-emitting radionuclide, is taken up naturally from the soil by tobacco plants because lead behaves similarly to calcium. Polonium 210, the alpha-emitting progeny of lead 210, is responsible for most of the radioactivity inhaled as a part of cigarette smoke. It has been postulated that polonium 210 in cigarette smoke contributes to lung cancer in smokers (see, e.g., 250).

Radioactive aerosols also occur naturally in our environment from the interaction of cosmic rays with our atmosphere producing radionuclides such as carbon 14 and beryllium 7. These exposures are measurable, but not biologically significant. Coal, oil, and natural gas also contain radioactivity that is released during combustion. Based on the amounts of radioactive aerosol routinely released per unit of electrical energy produced, coal combustion may provide a higher cancer risk for people than nuclear power (see, e.g., 251). However, the radiation doses to individual workers or members of the public are small and may not be biologically significant.

Workers who mine and process mineral sands containing tin and associated trace metals can also be exposed to uranium and thorium dusts from the sands (252). In a United Nations-sponsored study of radiological exposures in the tin by-product industry in Southeast Asia, Hewson found that many of these exposures are above occupational exposure limits, but could easily be reduced by use of standard radiation protection practices involving ventilation and respiratory protection. Implementation of such practices may be difficult, however, because most of the estimated 2000 workers employed in this industry work in plants that employ fewer than 20 workers, with many plants employing fewer than 5 workers.

Although thoriated tungsten electrodes are frequently used in industry to provide easier arc starting, greater stability, and reduced weld metal contamination, Crim and Bradley (253) found that exposures of workers during grinding and welding with these electrodes were below the DAC.

Installers of phosphogypsum plaster board can also be exposed to radium 226 and other radionuclides from the uranium 238 decay series in radioactive dusts from the plaster board. O'Brien et al. (254) estimated potential doses to workers and occupants from higher-radium–content gypsum board. At dust concentrations equal to the ACGIH nuisance dust limit of 10 mg/m^3 (10), the annual effective dose to workers would be 0.5 mSv if particles had an activity median aerodynamic diameter of 5 μm, and 1.5 mSv if particles had an activity median aerodynamic diameter of only 1 μm. The occupational exposure limit corresponds to 50 mSv. Reasonable work practices, including respiratory protection and ventilation, would lower exposures substantially. Most of the radiation exposure from the radium-containing plaster board is from the emanation of radon gas.

Radon gas and the decay products of radon are naturally ubiquitous in the environment, and they can be of occupational concern in poorly ventilated underground mines or in buildings constructed from or on uranium-bearing materials. The half lives of radon and its decay products are typically short (3.8 days for ^{222}Rn, 3.05 min for ^{218}Po, 26.8 min for ^{214}Pb, 19.9 min for ^{214}Bi, and 164 μsec for ^{214}Po), but their concentrations are constantly replenished by the decay of long-lived isotopes of uranium and radium. Lead 210, the final radionuclide from decay of ^{222}Rn, has a half-life of 10.2 years and can accumulate in the body to significantly measurable levels. Most radon progeny (typically more than 90%) are attached to other airborne particles. This prolongs their presence as an aerosol and increases their availability for inhalation. In environmental settings, the activity median particle diameter of the attached mode is on the order of 0.125 μm, and the average activity median diameter for the unattached fraction is about 0.001 μm (255). In mine atmospheres, the activity median particle diameter of the attached mode is on the order of 0.25 μm, with a GSD of 2.5 (256).

Concentrations of radon progeny in the workplace are generally measured in working levels, and cumulative exposures over time are measured in working level months (WLM), based on a work month of 170 hr. The *working level* is defined as any combination of the short-lived radon progeny in 1 L of air that results in the ultimate release of 1.3×10^5 MeV of potential alpha-energy (257). This amount is approximately equal to the amount of alpha-energy emitted by the short half-life progeny in equilibrium with 100 pCi of radon. The health effect of concern from exposure to radon progeny is lung cancer, especially in workers who smoke. The effects of combined exposures to cigarette smoke and radon progeny are believed to be multiplicative rather than additive (257). The lifetime risk of lung mortality caused by lifetime exposure to radon progeny is estimated to be 350 cancer deaths per 10^6 person WLM, but this depends on factors such as gender, age at exposure, and smoking history (257). The current standard for radon progeny exposure in underground mines limits the annual total exposure to 4 WLM. The average lifetime risk of lung cancer mortality for males of unspecified smoking status sustaining 4 WLM annually from age 20 through age 50 is 13.1% (257). This is about twice the baseline risk for all males, which is 6.7%. If miners are smokers, the lifetime risk for this exposure situation is 22.6%, compared with 12.3% for unexposed male smokers.

Industrial and Medical Uses of Radioactivity

Several industrial and medical processes use radioactive materials. These include production and use of radioactive particles for diagnosis or treatment of disease, manufacture and use of thickness gauges that use attenuation of beta- or gamma-emissions to determine or monitor the density and thickness of materials or soils, and manufacturing of smoke alarms that use attenuation of alpha-emissions, from small americium 241 sources, to detect the presence of smoke particles in the air. Most of these products are produced and used without risk or mishap. For example, the National Council on Radiation Protection (258) has determined that firefighters face negligible risks from dispersion of the americium in smoke detectors during industrial or residential fires. In addition, increased awareness and improved work practices have removed many historical exposure situations from current concern. Routine use of glovebox enclosures and respiratory protection means that large, repeated exposures of workers are unlikely. Such exposures occurred before World War II when workers producing luminous dial devices inhaled radium paint dusts in poorly ventilated workrooms and ingested radium by using their tongues to ''tip'' their brushes to provide a fine point for applying the radium paint. In addition, recent efforts have been made to replace radioactive materials, such as thorium phosphors in lantern mantles, with inert substitutes. However, aerosol releases during manufacturing, handling, and disposal of radiation sources have occasionally occurred. In 1957, iridium 192 dust was released from a work enclosure during opening of a container of iridium pellets in a commercial laboratory engaged in the preparation of encapsulated sources for gamma cameras (259). Particle size distributions and air concentrations were not reported. Employees dressed in street clothing inadvertently spread the dust beyond the laboratory to homes and automobiles.

O'Grady et al. (260) reported on work procedures and worker protection during decontamination of the hoppers in a steel mill following the inadvertent inclusion of a ^{137}Cs radiography source in a consignment of scrap metal. An attempt was made to use heavy-duty mechanical vibrators to dislodge contaminated dusts from the inside walls of the hoppers, but this was unsuccessful. Workers in protective clothing had to enter the hoppers and clean them using mobile vacuum units. Without proper precautions, exposures of the workers could have been substantial. Although relatively rare events, these incidents are likely to continue as a potential source of worker exposures to radioactive materials.

Production of Nuclear Power

The use of nuclear fission power for energy production involves exposures of uranium miners to radon gas and radon progeny. Lung cancer has been observed in uranium miners and other hard rock miners, especially those who smoked and those who were exposed to radon progeny at high levels in poorly ventilated mines. Use of nuclear fission power also involves exposures of uranium-milling workers to small amounts of aerosol during the extraction of uranium from ore. Concentrations of airborne uranium during drum-filling operations at four uranium mills ranged from 0.04 to 0.34 μg/L, with a broad range of aerodynamic size distributions, such that between 24 and 86% of the airborne uranium mass was associated with aerodynamic particle diameters less than 12 μm (261). Workers may also be exposed to aerosols during fabrication of nuclear fuel (see, e.g., 262), where typical particle size distributions have been on the order of 5-μm–activity median aerodynamic diameter with a GSD of 2. However, such work is typically done within glovebox enclosures, and exposures are generally limited to failures in procedures or engineered controls.

Dorrian and Bailey (263) compiled values from 52 publications for the activity median aerodynamic diameter of radioactive aerosols in a wide variety of industries and workplaces. Their survey was done to assist in selecting a realistic default activity median aerodynamic diameter (AMAD) value for evaluation of occupational exposures using the International Council on Radiation Protection Task Group on Human Respiratory Tract Models reference (as in comments). Reported values of AMAD ranged from as small as 0.12 μm from an oxide burner operation in a uranium plant, to as large as 25 μm from breakup of ^{226}Ra-contaminated concrete floor with pneumatic hammers in a luminizing factory. Both nuclear power and nuclear fuel-handling industries gave median values of approximately 4 μm. Uranium mills gave a median value of 6.8 μm with AMADs frequently greater than 10 μm. High-temperature and arc–saw-cutting operations generated submicrometer-sized particles and occasionally, bimodal log-normal particle size distributions. Most particle size distributions were well fitted by a log-normal distribution with a median value of 4.4 μm. Thus, a default AMAD value of 5 μm with a GSD of 2 was selected as the default value for respiratory tract models by the ICRP (264). In view of the wide range of AMADs found in the survey, it was recommended that greater emphasis be placed on air sampling to characterize aerosol particle size distributions for individual work practices.

A search for inhalation exposure incidents among licensees of the U.S. Nuclear Regulatory Commission revealed almost no cases. One reason for the very low rate of inhalation exposures in the U.S. nuclear power industry has been a management and regulatory mindset that viewed internal dose as preventable through the use of respiratory protection and engineering controls, such as ventilation and decontamination, but has viewed radiation dose from external exposure as a fact of the job that must be reduced where practical (265). This attitude is changing because of recent changes in the Nuclear Regulatory Commission requirements for worker protection (266), which updated approaches to treat internal and external exposures with equal concern. Recent experience at a commercial boiling water reactor power plant involved reducing the number of respirators used from almost 15,000 per maintenance outage period to only 350, with little increase in inhalation exposure, but substantial reduction in external exposure. This was enabled, in part, by a tenfold reduction in the square footage of ''contamination area'' within the plant (265). In general, the desire to reduce respirator use is an incentive to maintain cleaner plant areas.

Nuclear power plant workers and emergency response personnel can face inhalation risks during reactor accidents and as part of the ensuing cleanup activities. However, inhalation exposures of workers were negligible in the 1979 accident at Three Mile Island. Radioactive releases from the damaged reactor involved the noble gases xenon 133 and krypton 85, which were quickly dispersed in the environment. Radioiodine releases were much smaller than noble gas releases. Inhalation exposures of workers were prevented during the cleanup process by extensive use of remote-cleaning techniques and respiratory protection.

Airborne dispersion of ^{131}I and ^{137}Cs particles over Europe was a consequence of the 1986 accident at Chernobyl, but external radiation exposure was the cause of death for emergency response workers involved in fighting the fire itself. Apparently much of the radiation injury resulted from protracted contact of beta-emitting particles with the skin of the firefighters. Workers in the immediate area around the reactor are still being exposed to resuspended ^{137}Cs particles (see, e.g., 267).

Fabrication and Testing of Nuclear Weapons

National programs to produce, test, and deploy nuclear weapons have both knowingly and accidentally released radioactive aerosols into the workplace and the environment. Eisenbud (259) summarized these releases, including those from a chemical explosion in a plutonium-processing pilot plant at the Oak Ridge National Laboratory in Tennessee, from a major fire at the Rocky Flats weapons manufacturing plant in Colorado, and from atmospheric testing in the South Pacific. Atmospheric fallout of radioactive aerosols from the tests was measured and documented in a series of reports by the U.S. Atomic Energy Commission's Health and Safety Laboratory, which is now the U.S. Department of Energy's Environmental Measurements Laboratory (see, e.g., 268). Human radiation exposures related to the nuclear weapons industries have been reviewed (269). Data from direct measurements of particle size distributions are not generally available. Accidental nuclear detonation of a weapon is unlikely, but accidental detonation of the high explosive has occurred during accidents such as plane crashes or fires. Such detonations of the high explosives disperse the fissile material. Because of the pyrophoric nature of metallic plutonium or uranium, a very fine oxide aerosol (less than 10-μm–aerodynamic diameter) can be formed.

Current workers at former sites of weapons testing, such as the Nevada Test Site in the United States, remain at risk for inhalation exposures to resuspended radionuclides from contaminated soils. In a study on setting secondary standards for cleanup of radionuclides in soil, Anspaugh and Daniels (270) developed a scientific basis for establishing ''posting criteria'' for contaminated soils in areas of the Nevada Test Site where ''unrestricted casual access'' would be allowed. This would involve areas where no earth-moving or construction activities would cause substantial disturbance of soil. Radionuclides of concern include long-lived fission and neutron activation products and residual materials, such as tritium and plutonium. Concerns for external radiation exposures control the recommended limits for nearly all the radionuclides, with only the beta-emitting radionuclides $^{90}Sr/^{90}Y$ and the alpha-emitting radionuclides ^{238}Pu, $^{239,240}Pu$, and ^{241}Am being of concern for inhalation following resuspension of particles by wind or casual activities. Long-term average values for air concentrations of total suspended material at the Nevada Test Site were reported to be between 16 and 71 $\mu g/m^3$, with concentrations greater than 100 $\mu g/m^3$ being possible during brief periods of severe soil disturbance.

A substantial body of information is now becoming available on worker exposures in the nuclear facilities of the former Soviet Union (see, e.g., a case–control study of 500 workers; 271). Worker exposures involved gamma-irradiation over a wide dose range and exposures to airborne ^{239}Pu. Particle size distributions of alpha-emitting radionuclides included a large dispersive component with an AMAD of 60–70 μm, a middle dispersive component with an AMAD of 11–14 μm, and a small component with an AMAD of 0.5 μm. Tokarskaya et al. (271) reported that 162 persons in the 500-person case–control study had contracted lung cancer. Some of these workers were employed before the introduction of special respiratory protection in 1957.

Radioactive Waste and Environmental Remediation

In spite of, or perhaps because of, the concern for potential exposures of workers to radioactive aerosols, few cases of inhalation exposure have occurred. Among those that have occurred, many have involved handling or processing of wastes. The following reports illustrate the nature of potential exposure scenarios. In a 1976 incident at a waste-treatment facility in Hanford, Washington, a 64-year-old nuclear chemical operator was injured by a chemical explosion of an ion-exchange column used to recover americium (see 272,273). Based on sodium iodide detector measurements, about 3000 μCi of americium was deposited on the face, and 300 μCi was embedded in facial tissue. About 40 μCi of ^{141}Am was measured in the lung on day 3 after the accident.

In a 1991 material storage incident at the Savannah River Site in Aiken, South Carolina, a worker opened what was thought to be an empty ^{238}Pu shipping container (274), which had been in storage for 7–20 years. After opening the container, the worker walked approximately 7 ft to a count rate meter to survey the container for contamination. The survey meter alarmed, and almost simultaneously, the continuous air monitor in the room exhaust duct alarmed. The exhaust duct was approximately 10 ft away near the floor. The worker replaced the lid on the container, and all individuals immediately evacuated the room. Other individuals in the room at the time of the incident included a second worker, who was standing nearby, a separations chemist and an observer who were standing toward the back of the room, and a health protection inspector, who was standing in the airlock. The 4-ft × 4-ft area of floor under the container measured 60,000 dpm. This corresponds to a value of 400 dpm/100 cm^2, which is greater than the U.S. Department of Energy limit of 20 dpm/100 cm^2 for removable surface contamination involving transuranium radionuclides, but less than the limit of 500 dpm/100 cm^2 for total fixed and removable (275). An air concentration of 84,000 DAC was calculated from the air monitor planchet, and 64 DAC was measured with a grab sample 15 min after the incident. A fixed air sampler in the airlock measured 3.4 DAC. The worker had 10,000 dpm of alpha-contamination on her right rubber glove and 260 dpm nasal contamination. The observer at the back of the room had 260 dpm nasal contamination, and case 835 had 50 dpm nasal contamination. Both individuals were treated with chelation therapy.

In a 1971 material damage inspection incident at Los Alamos National Laboratory (Lawrence, unpublished), seven workers were disassembling and inspecting a ^{238}Pu heat source. The material consisted of PuO_2-Mo cermet disks that had been broken apart, producing a moderate amount of powered material. Disassembly and inspection operations were carried out in dry-box enclosures inside shielded hot cells. The remote manipulators that extended into the dry boxes were enclosed in polyvinylchloride plastic boots. During the operation, a hole occurred in a plastic boot. The pumping action of the manipulators is believed to have forced some of the airborne PuO_2 outside of the dry-box system into the area occupied by workers. A continuous air monitor alarm occurred in an adjacent room about 30 min after the start of the inspection operation. The alarm was reset on the belief that it was a false alarm caused by a nearby lightning strike. Checks for surface contamination revealed low levels of activity in the vicinity of the air monitor. A second continuous air monitor alarm occurred 20 min after the first alarm. At this time the alarm would no longer accept being reset. Personnel donned respirators to complete essential tasks and vacated the area. The total exposure time was 20–50 min. Nose swipes ranged from 60 dpm to 5050 dpm, indicating that minor inhalation of airborne plutonium had occurred. Estimates of the actual level of internal contamination were considered unreliable.

In a routine work incident in a plutonium-handling facility (276), a worker was exposed to a small amount of plutonium dioxide while performing a routine pressing, sintering, and density measurement of plutonium dioxide pellets in a glovebox. Because of a fatigue crack in a glove, a small amount of plutonium dioxide powder was released to the room when the worker removed his arm from the port. Contamination was detected on the worker's right hand, nostrils, and protective clothing, as well as on the room floor and the exterior surface of the glovebox. Preliminary in vivo measurements of 1.3 nCi ^{241}Am in the upper thorax indicated an internal deposition of plutonium. Although plutonium was detected in urine samples collected immediately after the exposure incident, samples obtained several hours later were negative. This implied that some or all of the initial plutonium activity may have been caused by external contamination. The concentration of plutonium in the first fecal sample, which was collected the day after the incident, was approximately 30 pCi/g.

It is generally considered that the greatest current opportunities for worker inhalation exposures to radioactive materials are posed by remediation of contaminated sites. Although a large number of radioactivity-contaminated sites exist in the former Soviet Union and within the United States, few definitive data are available describing the particle size distributions that are being or might be encountered. In a generic dose and risk assessment for intrusion into mixed-waste disposal sites, Kennedy and Aaberg (277) simply projected that particle size distributions would range from 0.1- to 10-μm–activity median aerodynamic diameter. In general, the composition and distribution of radioactive materials in buried wastes or historically contaminated sites are unknown.

H. Other Chemical Particles

All particles consist of ''chemicals.'' However, workers are exposed by inhalation during the manufacture, packaging, transport, and end use of a wide range of droplets and solid particles of chemicals not described in other sections of this chapter. The range of chemicals, exposure scenarios, and potential health effects is far too broad to describe in detail in this chapter; thus, only general descriptions are given. The reader is referred to published studies, reports, and reference materials for information on individual chemical compounds, classes, and products. Some key reference materials containing information about chemicals are listed in the Introduction.

The *Encyclopedia of Occupational Health and Safety* (1) gives a general description of the chemical industry, classes of chemicals handled, and occupational hazards. Chemicals generally fall into two classes: organic and inorganic. Organic chemicals have a basic structure of carbon atoms, and 90% of contemporary organic chemicals are derived from petroleum and natural gas. Inorganic chemicals may contain carbon, but do not have a basically carbonaceous structure, and are derived largely from minerals. Chemicals encountered by workers fall generally into three groups. Base chemicals are typically produced in large quantity and used in producing other compounds. Intermediates are derived from base chemicals, and represent mostly intermediate compounds in the production of finished products. Finished chemical products are sold to consumers or to other manufacturers. The primary sectors of the chemical industry are: basic inorganics; basic organics; fertilizers and pesticides; plastics, resins, and synthetics; pharmaceuticals; paints and finishes; soaps, cleaners, cosmetics, and toiletries; and miscellaneous, such as explosives, adhesives, inks, and photographic materials.

The known and potential health risks from inhaled chemicals are nearly as diverse as the chemicals themselves. Effects in the respiratory tract may include irritation, airway constriction, airway sensitization, impairment of clearance, inflammation, tissue destruction, edema, pneumoconiosis, fibrosis, emphysema, and cancer. For soluble chemicals, the respiratory tract may serve primarily as a portal of entry, and the toxic effects may be manifested elsewhere. In such instances, there may be little difference in effect between inhalation and other routes of exposure except for effects that might occur in the respiratory tract as the chemicals pass through it. Inhaled chemicals may also be metabolized in the respiratory tract, giving rise to toxic metabolites that manifest their effects either in the respiratory tract or elsewhere.

References

1. International Labour Office (ILO). Encyclopedia of Occupational Health and Safety. 3rd rev. ed. Parmeggiani L, ed. Vol 1 A–K. Geneva: ILO, 1983.
2. Lewis RJ. Sax's Dangerous Properties of Industrial Materials. 8th ed. vols. 1–3. New York: Van Nostrand Reinhold, 1992.
3. Patty's Industrial Hygiene and Toxicology. In: Clayton GD, Clayton FE, eds. Toxicology. Vol 2, part A. New York: John Wiley and Sons, 1993.
4. Muir DCF, ed. Clinical Aspects of Inhaled Particles. London: William Heinemann Medical Books, 1972.
5. Morgan WKC, Seaton A, eds. Occupational Lung Diseases. Philadelphia: WB Saunders, 1975.
6. Burgess WA. Recognition of Health Hazards in Industry: A Review of Materials and Processes. 2d ed. New York: John Wiley and Sons, 1995.
7. Harber P, Scheneker M, Balmes J. Occupational and Environmental Respiratory Diseases. Boca Raton; FL: Mosby-Yearbook Publishers, 1995.
8. World Health Organization (WHO). Evaluation of Exposure to Airborne Particles in the Work Environment. Publication No. 80. Geneva: WHO, 1984.
9. Sittig M. Particulates and Fine Dust Removal: Processes and Equipment. Park Ridge, NJ: Noyes Data Corporation, 1977.
10. American Conference of Governmental Industrial Hygienists (ACGIH). Guide to Occupational Exposure Values–1995. Cincinnati: ACGIH, 1995.
11. ACGIH. Threshold Limit Values (TLVs) for Chemical Substances and Physical Agents and Biological Exposure Indices (BEIs). Cincinnati: ACGIH, 1995.
12. Suratt PM, Winn WC, Brody AR. Acute silicosis in tombstone sandblasters. Am Rev Respir Dis 1977; 115:521–529.

13. Banks DE, Morring KL, Boehlecke BA. Silicosis in silica flour workers. Am Rev Respir Dis 1981; 124:445–450.
14. Ziskind M, Weill H, Anderson AE. Silicosis in shipyard sandblasters. Environ Res 1976; 11:237–243.
15. Ng TP, Allan WGL, Tsin TW. Silicosis in jade workers. Br J Ind Med 1985; 42: 761–764.
16. Saiyed HN, Chatterjee BB. Rapid progression of silicosis in slate pencil workers. Am J Ind Med 1985; 8:135–142.
17. Gong H, Tashkin DP. Silicosis due to intentional inhalation of abrasive scouring powder. Am J Med 1979; 67:358–362.
18. Bang KM, Althouse RB, Kim JH, Game SR, Castellan RM. Silicosis mortality surveillance in the United States, 1968–1990. Appl Occup Environ Hyg 1995; 10: 1070–1074.
19. International Agency for Research on Cancer (IARC). Monographs on the Evaluation of the Carcinogenic Risk of Chemicals to Humans, Overall Evaluations of Carcinogenicity: An Updating of IARC Monographs. Vols. 1–42, suppl 7. Lyon: IARC, 1987.
20. IARC. Monographs Evaluation on the Carcinogenic Risks to Humans. 65. IARC Working Group on the Evaluation of Carcinogenic Risks to Humans. Lyon, France, Oct 10–17, 1995.
21. Energy Information Administration (EIA). Coal data: a reference. Washington: U.S. Department of Energy, Energy Information Administration, Office of Coal, Nuclear, Electric and Alternate Fuels, Publication DOE/EIA-0064(90), 1991.
22. EIA. Coal production. Washington: U.S. Department of Energy, Energy Information Administration, Office of Coal, Nuclear, Electric and Alternate Fuels, Publication DOE/EIA-0118(92), 1993.
23. Parkes RW. Pneumoconiosis due to coal and carbon. In: Occupational Lung Disorders. 2nd ed. London: Butterworths, 1982:175–232.
24. National Institute for Occupational Safety and Health (NIOSH). Criteria for a Recommended Standard: Occupational Exposure to Respirable Coal Mine Dust. Cincinnati: NIOSH, 1995.
25. Mauderly JL. Contribution of inhalation bioassays to the assessment of human health risks from solid airborne particles. In: Mohr U, Dungworth DL, Mauderly JL, Oberdörster G, eds. Toxic and Carcinogenic Effects of Solid Particles in the Respiratory Tract. Washington, DC: International Life Sciences Institute (ILSI), 1994:43–55.
26. Merchant JA, Taylor G, Hodous TK. Coal workers' pneumoconiosis and exposure to other carbonaceous dusts. In: Occupational Respiratory Disease. Washington, DC: US Department of Health and Human Services Publication, Center for Disease Control, NIOSH, US Government Printing Office, 1986:329–384.
27. ILO. Guidelines for the use of ILO international classification of radiographs of pneumoconiosis. rev. ed. Occupational Safety and Health Series No. 22. Geneva: ILO, 1980.
28. Yi Q, Zhang Z. The survival analyses of 2738 patients with simple pneumoconiosis. Occup Environ Med 1996; 53:129–135.

29. ISO. Air quality-particle size fraction definitions for health-related sampling. Geneva: ISO Report ISO 7708, 1993.
30. WHO. Recommended health-based limits in occupational exposure to selected mineral dusts (silica, coal). Geneva: WHO, Technical Report Series 734, 1986:3–82.
31. Morgan WKC. Other pneumoconioses. In: Morgan WKC, Seaton A, eds. Occupational Lung Diseases. Philadelphia: WB Saunders, 1975:216–250.
32. ACGIH. Threshold Limit Values (TLVs) for Chemical Substances and Physical Agents and Biological Exposure Indices (BEIs). Cincinnati: ACGIH, 1994.
33. WHO/EURO Technical Committee for Monitoring and Evaluating Airborne MMMF. Reference Methods for Measuring Airborne Man-Made Mineral Fibers. Copenhagen: WHO, 1985.
34. Roggli VL. Human disease consequences of fiber exposures: a review of human lung pathology and fiber burden data. Environ Health Perspect 1990; 88:295–303.
35. Stanton MF, Wrench C. Mechanisms of mesothelioma induction with asbestos and fibrous glass. J Natl Cancer Inst 1972; 48:797–821.
36. Davis JMG, Addison J, Bolton RE, Donaldson K, Jones AD, Smith T. The pathogenicity of long versus short fibre samples of amosite asbestos administered to rats by inhalation and intraperitoneal injection. Br J Exp Pathol 1986; 67:415–430.
37. Lippmann M. Asbestos exposure indices. Environ Res 1988; 46:86–106.
38. Eastes W, Hadley JG. Dissolution of fibers inhaled by rats. Inhal Toxicol 1995; 7: 179–196.
39. Berry G, Gilson JC, Holmes S, Lewinsohn HC, Roach SA. Asbestosis: a study of dose–response relationships in an asbestos textile factory. Br J Ind Med 1979; 36: 98–112.
40. Hughes JM, Weill H, Hammad YY. Mortality of workers employed in two asbestos cement manufacturing plants. Br J Ind Med 1987; 44:161–174.
41. Mossman BT, Bignon J, Corn M, Seaton A, Gee JB. Asbestos: scientific developments and implications for public policy. Science 1990; 247:294–302.
42. Johnson NF. An overview of animal models for assessing synthetic vitreous fibers (SVFs) safety. Regul Toxicol Pharmacol 1994; 20:S7–S21.
43. Dement JM, Brown DP, Okun A. Follow-up study of chrysotile asbestos textile workers: cohort mortality and case–control analyses. Am J Ind Med 1994; 26:431–447.
44. McConnell EE, Hall L, Adkins B. Studies on the chronic toxicity (inhalation) of wollastonite in Fischer 344 rats. Inhal Toxicol 1991; 3:323–337.
45. Baris I, Simonato L, Artvinli M, Pooley F, Sarraci R, Skidmore J, Wagner J. Epidemiological and environmental evidence of the health effects of exposure to erionite fibers: a four-year study in the Cappadocian region of Turkey. Int J Cancer 1987; 39:10–17.
46. Wagner JC, Skidmore JW, Hill RJ, Griffiths DM. Erionite exposure and mesotheliomas in rats. Br J Cancer 1985; 51:252–269.
47. IARC. Evaluation of Carcinogenic Risks to Humans, Man-Made Mineral Fibers and Radon. Lyons: IARC, 1988.
48. Cherrie J, Dodgson J, Groat S, Maclaren W. Environmental surveys in the European

man-made mineral fiber protection industry. Scand J Work Environ Health 1986; 12(suppl):18–25.
49. Lees PSJ, Breysse PN, McArthur BR, Miller ME, Rooney BC, Robbins CA, Corn M. End user exposures to man-made vitreous fibers: 1. Installation of residential insulation products. Appl Occup Environ Hyg 8: 1993; 1022–1030.
50. Glass LR, Brown RC, Hoskins JA. Health effects of refractory ceramic fibers: scientific issues and policy considerations. Occup Environ Med 1995; 52:433–440.
51. Sahle W, Laszlo I, Krantz S, Christensson B. Airborne tungsten oxide whiskers in a hard-metal industry: preliminary findings. Ann Occup Hyg 1994; 38:37–44.
52. Johnson NF, Hoover MD, Thomassen DG, Cheng YS, Dalley A, Brooks AL. In vitro activity of silicon carbide whiskers in comparison to other industrial fibers using four cell culture systems. Am J Ind Med 1992; 21:807–823.
53. Bye E, Eduard W, Gjonnes J, Sorbroden E. Occurrence of airborne silicon carbide fibers during industrial production of silicon carbide. Scand J Work Environ Health 1985; 11:111–115.
54. Jones HD, Jones TR, Lyle WH. Carbon fiber: results of a survey of process workers and their environment in a factory producing continuous filament. Ann Occup Hyg 1982; 26:861–868.
55. Mahar S. Particulate exposures resulting from the investigation and remediation of a crash site of an aircraft containing carbon composites. Am Ind Hyg Assoc J 1990; 51:459–461.
56. Hesterberg TW, McConnell EE, Miller WC, Hamilton R, Bunn WB. Pulmonary toxicity of inhaled polypropylene fibers in rats. Fundam Appl Toxicol 1992; 19: 358–366.
57. Lee KP, Kelly DP, O'Neal FO, Stadler JC, Kennedy GL. Lung response to ultrafine Kevlar aramid synthetic fibrils following 2-year inhalation exposure in rats. Fundam Appl Toxicol 1988; 11:1–20.
58. Fisher GL, McNeill KL, Prentice BA, McFarland AR. Physical and biological studies of coal and oil fly ash. Environ Health Perspect 1983; 51:181–186.
59. Hatch GE, Boykin E, Graham JA, Lewtas J, Pott F, Loud K, Mumford JL. Inhalable particles and pulmonary host defense: in vivo and in vitro effects of ambient air and combustion particles. Environ Res 1985; 36:67–80.
60. Fruchter JS, Robertson DE, Evans JC, Olsen KB, Lepel EA, Laul JC, Abel KH, Sanders RW, Jackson PO, Wogman NS, Perkins RW, Van Tuyl HH, Beauchamp RH, Shade JW, Daniel JL, Erikson RL, Sehmel GA, Lee RN, Robinson AV, Moss OR, Briant JK, Cannon WC. Mount St. Helens ash from the 18 May 1980 eruption: chemical, physical, mineralogical, and biological properties. Science 1980; 209: 1116–1125.
61. Alarie Y, Iwasaki M, Stock MF, Pearson RC, Shane BS, Lisk DJ. Effects of inhaled municipal refuse incinerator fly ash in the guinea pig. J Toxicol Environ Health 1989; 28:13–25.
62. Benson J, Bice DE, Carpenter RL, Hanson RL, Henderson RF, Hobbs CH, Mauderly JL, Pickrell JA. Comparative inhalation toxicity of quartz and coal combustion fly ash. In: Goldsmith DF, Winn DM, Shy CM, eds. Silica, Silicosis, and Cancer. New York: Praeger Scientific, 1985:117–123.
63. Ghio AJ, Stonehuerner J, Pritchard RJ, Piantadosi CA, Quigley DR. Humic-like

substance in air pollution particulates correlate with concentrations of transition metals and oxidant generation. Inhal Toxicol 1996; 8:479–494.

64. Schilling CJ, Tams IP, Schilling RSF, Nevitt A, Rossiter CE, Wilkinson B. A survey into the respiratory effects of prolonged exposure to pulverised fuel ash. Br J Ind Med 1988; 45:810–817.
65. Cho K, Cho YJ, Shrivastava DK, Kapre SS. Acute lung disease after exposure to fly ash. Chest 1994; 106:309–311.
66. Golden EB, Warnock ML, Hulett LD Jr, Chrug AM. Fly ash lung: a new pneumoconiosis? Am Rev Respir Dis 1982; 125:108–112.
67. Dreher KL, Jaskot RH, Lehmann JR, Richards JH, McGee JK, Ghio AJ, Costa DL. Soluble transition metals mediate residual oil fly ash induced acute lung injury. J Toxicol Environ Health Feb. 21, 1997, 50(3), 285–305.
68. Hauser R, Elreedy S, Hoppin JA, Christiani DC. Airway obstruction in boilermakers exposed to fuel oil ash: a prospective investigation. Am J Respir Crit Care Med 1995; 152:1478–1484.
69. Wehner AP, Dagle GE, Clark ML, Buschbom RL. Lung changes in rats following inhalation exposure to volcanic ash for two years. Environ Res 1986; 40:499–517.
70. Mauderly JL, McCunney RJ, eds. Particle Overload in the Rat Lung and Lung Cancer: Implications for Human Risk Assessment. Proceedings of a conference held at the Massachusetts Institute of Technology, March 29, 30, 1995. Washington: Taylor and Francis, 1996.
71. Buist AS, Vollmer WM, Johnson LR, Bernstein RS, McCamant LE. A four-year prospective study of the respiratory effects of volcanic ash from Mt. St. Helens. Am Rev Respir Dis 1986; 133:526–534.
72. Robertson JM, Smith RG. Carbon black. In: Clayton GD, Clayton FE, eds. Patty's Industrial Hygiene and Toxicology. Vol 2. 4th ed. part C. New York: John Wiley and Sons, 1994:2395–2423.
73. McClellan, RO. Lung cancer in rats from prolonged exposure to high concentrations of carbonaceous particles: implications for human risk assessment. In: Mauderly JL, McCunney RJ, eds. Particle Overload in the Rat Lung and Lung Cancer: Implications for Human Risk Assessment. Proceedings of a conference held at the Massachusetts Institute of Technology, March 29, 30. Washington: Taylor and Francis, 1995; 193–226.
74. Hodgson JT, Jones RD. A mortality study of carbon black workers employed at five United Kingdom factories between 1947 and 1980. Arch Environ Health 1985; 40:261–268.
75. Nikula KJ, MB Snipes, Barr EB, Griffith WC, Henderson RF, Mauderly JL. Comparative pulmonary toxicities and carcinogenicities of chronically inhaled diesel exhaust and carbon black in F344 rats. Fundam Appl Toxicol 1995; 25:80–94.
76. IARC. Printing Processes, Printing Inks, Carbon Black, and Some Nitro Compounds. Lyon: IARC, 1996.
77. Petsonk EL, Storey E, Becker PE, Davidson CA, Kennedy K, Vallyathan V. Pneumoconiosis in carbon electrode workers. J Occup Med 1988; 30:887–891.
78. Wehr KL, Johanson WG Jr, Chapman JS, Pierce AK. Pneumoconiosis among activated-carbon workers. Arch Environ Health 1975; 30:578–582.

79. Davies GM, Hodkinson A, DiVetta P. Measurement and analysis of occupational exposures to coke oven emissions. Ann Occup Hyg 1986; 30:51–62.
80. Dong MH, Redmond CK, Mazumdar S, Costantino JP. A multistage approach to the cohort analysis of lifetime lung cancer risk among steelworkers exposed to coke oven emissions. Am J Epidemiol 1988; 128:860–873.
81. Watts WF Jr. Assessment of occupational exposure to diesel emissions. In: Diesel Exhaust: A Critical Analysis of Emissions, Exposure, and Health Effects. Cambridge: Health Effects Institute (HEI), 1995:109–123.
82. Mauderly JL. Diesel exhaust. In: Lippmann M, ed. Environmental Toxicants—Human Exposures and Their Health Effects. New York: Von Nostrand–Reinhold, 1992:119–162.
83. Sawyer RF, Johnson JH. Diesel emissions and control technology. In: Diesel Exhaust: A Critical Analysis of Emissions, Exposure, and Health Effects. A Special Report of the Institute's Diesel Working Group. Cambridge: HEI, 1995:67–81.
84. Nikula KJ, Avila KJ, Griffith WC, Mauderly JL. Lung tissue responses and sites of particle retention differ between rats and cynomolgus monkeys exposed chronically to diesel exhaust and coal dust. Fundam Appl Toxicol 1997; 37:37–53.
85. HEI. Diesel Exhaust: A Critical Analysis of Emissions, Exposure, and Health Effects. A Special Report of the Institute's Diesel Working Group. Cambridge: HEI, 1995.
86. Brandt-Rauf PW, Fallon LF Jr, Tarantini T, Idema C, Andrews L. Health hazards of fire fighters: exposure assessment. Br J Ind Med 1988; 45:606–612.
87. Materna BL, Jones JR, Sutton PM, Rothman N, Harrison RJ. Occupational exposures in California wildland firefighting. Am J Ind Hyg 1992; 53:69–76.
88. Smith KR, Liu Y. Indoor air pollution in developing countries. In: Samet JM, ed. Epidemiology of Lung Cancer. New York: Marcel Dekker, 1994:151–184.
89. Aviado DM. Complex mixtures of tobacco smoke and the occupational environment. In: Clayton GD, Clayton FE, eds. Patty's Industrial Hygiene and Toxicology. New York: John Wiley and Sons, 1993:107–148.
90. Pershagen G. Passive smoking and lung cancer. In: Samet JM, ed. Epidemiology of Lung Cancer. New York: Marcel Dekker, 1994:109–130.
91. Coultas DB, Samet JM, McCarthy JF, Spengler JD. A personal monitoring study to assess workplace exposure to environmental tobacco smoke. Am J Public Health 1990; 80:988–990.
92. Drake JW, Johnson DE. Measurements of certain environmental tobacco smoke components on long-range flights. Aviat Space Environ Med 1990; 61:531–542.
93. Sherman CB, Barnhart S, Miller MF, Segal, MR, Aitken M, Schoene R, Daniell W, Rosenstock L. Firefighting acutely increases airway responsiveness. Am Rev Respir Dis 1989; 140:185–190.
94. Liu D, Tager IB, Balmes JR, Harrison RJ. The effect of smoke inhalation on lung function and airway responsiveness in wildland fire fighters. Am Rev Respir Dis 1992; 146:1469–1473.
95. Hansen ES. A cohort study on the mortality of firefighters. Br J Ind Med 1990; 47:805–809.
96. Demers PA, Heyer NJ, Rosenstock L. Mortality among firefighters from three northwestern United States cities. Br J Ind Med 1992; 49:664–670.

97. Jacobs RR. Sampling environments containing organic dust. Am J Ind Med 1994; 25:3–11.
98. Donham KJ. Hazardous agents in agriculture dusts and methods of evaluation. Am J Ind Med 1986; 10:205–220.
99. Rylander R. Lung diseases caused by organic dusts in the farm environment. Am J Ind Med 1986; 10:221–227.
100. Raffle PAB, Adams PH, Baxter PJ, Lee WR. Hunter's Diseases of Occupations. 8th ed. London: Edward Arnold, 1994.
101. Montalvo JG. Cotton Dust: Controlling an Occupational Health Hazard. Washington, DC: American Chemical Society, 1982.
102. IARC. Wood Dust and Formaldehyde. vol 62. Geneva: WHO 1995.
103. IARC. Wood, Leather and Some Associated Industries. vol 25. Geneva: WHO, 1985.
104. Rylander R, Donham KJ, Peterson Y. Health effects of organic dusts in the farm environment. Am J Ind Med 1986; 10:193–335.
105. Lacey J, Crook B. Fungal and actinomycete spores as pollutants of the work and occupational allergens. Ann Occup Hyg 1988; 32:515–533.
106. Burge HA. Bioaerosols. Boca Raton, FL:Lewis Publishers, 1995.
107. Rylander R, Peterson Y. Causative agents for organic dust related disease. Am J Ind Med 1994; 25:1–146.
108. Cox CS, Wathes CM. Bioaerosols Handbook. Boca Raton, FL: CRC Press, 1995.
109. Macher JM, Chatigny MA, Burge HA. Sampling airborne microorganisms and aeroallergens. In: Cohen BS, Herring SV, eds. Air Sampling Instruments for Evaluation of Atmospheric Contaminants. Cincinnati: ACGIH, 1995:589–618.
110. Garden JM, O'Banion MK, Sheinitz LS, Pinski KS, Bakus AD, Reinchmann ME, Sundberg JP. Papillomavirus in the vapor of carbon dioxide laser-treated verrucae. JAMA 1988; 259:1199–1202.
111. Wentzell JM, Robinson JK, Wentzell JM Jr, Schwartz DE, Carlson SE. Physical properties of aerosols produced by dermabrasion. Arch Dermatol 1989; 125:1637–1643.
112. Tokars JI, Chamberland ME, Schable CA, Culver DH, Jones M, McKibben PS, Bell DM. A survey of occupational blood contact and HIV infection among orthopedic surgeons. JAMA 1992; 268:489–491.
113. Heinsohn P, Jewett DL. Exposure to blood-containing aerosols in the operating room: a preliminary study. Am Ind Hyg Assoc J 1993; 54:446–453.
114. Miller RL. Characteristics of blood-containing aerosols generated by common powered dental instruments. Am Ind Hyg Assoc J 1995; 56:670–676.
115. Yeh HC, Turner RS, Jones RK, Muggenburg BA, Lundgren DL, Smith JP. Characterization of aerosols produced during surgical procedures in hospitals. Aerosol Sci Technol 1995; 22:151–161.
116. Heinsohn P, Jewett DL, Balzer L, Bennett CH, Seipei P, Rosen A. Aerosol created by some surgical power tools: particle size distribution and qualitative hemoglobin. Appl Occup Environ Hyg 1991; 6:773–776.
117. Yeh HC, Muggenburg BA, Guilmette RA, Snipes MB, Turner RS, Jones RK, Smith JP. Characterization of aerosols produced during total hip replacement surgery in dogs with ^{51}Cr-labeled blood. J Aerosol Sci 1995; 26:511–518.

118. Oosterhuis JW, Verschueren RCJ, Eibergen R, Oldhoff J. The viability of cells in the waste products of CO_2-laser evaporation of Cloudman mouse melanomas. Cancer 1982; 49:61–67.
119. Johnson GK, Robinson WS. Human immunodeficiency virus-1 (HIV-1) in the vapors of surgical power instruments. J Med Virol 1991; 33:47–50.
120. Liu DP, Zambito RF. Aerosols and cross infection in dental practice—a historical view. Gen Dent 1981; 29:136–142.
121. Petersen NJ, Bond WW, Favero MS. Air sampling for hepatitis B surface antigen in a dental operatory. J Am Dent Assoc 1979; 99:465–467.
122. Ingraham JL, Ingraham CA. Introduction to Microbiology. Belmont, CA: Wadsworth, 1995.
123. Micik RE, Miller RL, Mazzarella MA, Ryge G. Studies on dental aerobiology: I. Bacteria aerosols generated during dental procedures. J Dent Res 1969; 48:49–56.
124. Macher JM, Alevantis LE, Chang YL, Liu KS. Effect of ultraviolet germicidal lamps on airborne microorganisms in an outpatient waiting room. Appl Occup Environ Hyg 1992; 7:505–513.
125. Clark CS, Rylander R, Larsson L. Airborne bacteria, endotoxin and fungi in dust in poultry and swine confinement buildings. Am Ind Hyg Assoc J 1983; 44:537–541.
126. Clark CS, Rylander R, Larsson L. Levels of gram-negative bacteria, *Aspergillus fumigatus*, dust, and endotoxin at compost plants. Appl Environ Microbiol 1983; 45:1501–1505.
127. Weber S, Kullman G, Petsonk E, Jones WG, Olenchock S, Sorenson W, Parker J, Maecelo-Baciu R, Frazer D, Castranova V. Organic dust exposures from compost handling: case presentation and respiratory exposure assessment. Am J Ind Med 1993; 24:365–374.
128. Olenchock SA, Lenhart SW, Mull JC. Occupational exposure to airborne endotoxins during poultry processing. J Toxicol Environ Health 1982; 9:339–342.
129. Hagmar L, Schutz A, Hallberg T, Sjoholm A. Health effects of exposure to endotoxins and organic dust in poultry slaughter-house workers. Arch Occup Environ Health 1990; 62:159–164.
130. Olenchock SA, Mull JC, Jones WG. Endotoxins in cotton: washing effects and size distribution. Am J Ind Med 1983; 4:515–521.
131. Rylander R, Haglind P, Lindholm M. Endotoxin in cotton dust and respiratory function decrement among cotton workers in an experimental cardroom. Am Rev Respir Dis 1985; 131:209–213.
132. Castellan RM, Olenchock SA, Kinseley KB, Hankinson JL. Inhaled endotoxin and decreased spirometric values. N Engl J Med 1987; 317:605–610.
133. Sandstrom T, Bjermer L, Rylander R. Lipopolysaccharide (LPS) inhalation in healthy subjects increases neutrophil, lymphocytes and fibronectin levels in bronchoalveolar lavage fluid. Eur Respir J 1992; 5:992–996.
134. Heikkila P, Kotimaa M, Tuomi T, Salmi T, Louhelainen J. Identification and counting of fungal spores by scanning electron microscope. Ann Occup Hyg 1988; 32: 241–248.
135. Jones W, Morring K, Olenchock SA, Williams T, Hickey J. Environmental study of poultry confinement buildings. Am Ind Hyg Assoc J 1984; 45:760–766.

136. Crook B, Robertson JF, Glass SAT, Botheroyd EM, Lacey J, Topping MD. Airborne dust ammonia microorganisms and antigens in pig confinement houses and the respiratory health of exposed farm workers. Am Ind Hyg Assoc J 1991; 52: 271–279.
137. Jones WG, Dennis JW, May JJ, Whitmer MP, Siegel PD, Sorenson WG, Schwegler-Berry D, Kullman GJ. Dust control during bedding chopping. Appl Occup Environ Hyg 1995; 10:467–475.
138. Jimenez A, Moreno C, Martinez J, Martinez A, Bartolome B, Guerra F, Palacios R. Sensitization to sunflower pollen: only an occupational allergy. Arch Allergy Immunol 1994; 105:297–307.
139. Blanco C, Carrillo T, Quirate J, Pascual C, Esteban MM, Castillo R. Occupational rhinoconjunctivitis and bronchial asthma due to *Phoenix canariensis* pollen allergy. Allergy 1995; 50:277–280.
140. Griffiths DA, Wilkin DR, Southgate BJ, Lynch SM. A survey of mites in bulk grain stored on farms in England and Wales. Ann Appl Biol 1976; 82:180–184.
141. Iversen M, Korsgaard J, Hallas T, Dahl R. Mite allergy and exposure to storage mites and house dust mites in farmers. Clin Exp Allergy 1990; 20:211–219.
142. van Hage-Hamsten M, Johansson E, Wiren A, Johansson SGO. Storage mites dominate the fauna in Swedish barn dust. Allergy 1991; 46:142–146.
143. Donham KJ, Popendorf W, Palmgren U, Larsson L. Characterization of dusts collected from swine confinement buildings. Am J Ind Med 1986; 10:294–297.
144. Green FHY, Yoshida K, Fick G, Paul J, Hugh A, Green WF. Characterization of airborne mineral dusts associated with farming activities in rural Alberta Canada. Int Arch Occup Environ Health 1990; 62:423–430.
145. Casterton RM. Enclosed environments on agricultural tractors. Am Conf Gov Ind Hyg 1982; 2:121–127.
146. Popendorf WJ, Pryor A, Wenk MR. Mineral dust in manual harvest operations. Ann Am Conf Gov Ind Hyg 1982; 2:101–115.
147. Kotimaa MH, Oksanen L, Koskela P. Feeding and bedding materials as sources of microbial exposure on dairy farms. Scand J Work Environ Health 1991; 17:117–122.
148. Yoshida K, Maybank J. Physical and environmental characteristics of grain dust. In: Occupational Pulmonary Disease Focus on Grain Dust and Health. New York: Academic Press, 1980:477–504.
149. Farant JP. Assessment of dust nature and levels in the grain. In: Principles of Health and Safety in Agriculture. Boca Raton, FL: CRC Press, 1989:178–181.
150. Farant JP, Moore CF. Dust exposures in the Canadian grain industry. In: Occupational Pulmonary Disease Focus on Grain Dust and Health. New York: Academic Press, 1980:477–504.
151. Wakelyn PJ, Greenblatt GA, Brown DF, Tripp VW. Chemical properties of cotton dust. Am Ind Hyg Assoc J 1976; 37:22–31.
152. Griffin AC, Columbus EP. Dust in cotton gin: an overview. In: Montalvo JG, ed. Cotton Dust: Controlling an Occupational Hazard. Washington, DC: American Chemical Society, 1982:27–36.
153. Brown DF, McCall ER, Piccolo B, Tripp VW. Survey of effects of variety and

growing location of cotton on cardroom dust composition. Am Ind Hyg Assoc J 1975; 38:107–114.
154. Bethea, RM, Morey, PR. Effect of operational parameters on vertical elutriator performance for cotton dust sampling. In: Cotton Dust. Cincinnati: ACGIH, 1975: 285–327.
155. Wesley RA, Hatcher JD, McCaskill OL, Cocke JB. Dust levels and particle-size distributions in high-capacity cotton gins. Am Ind Hyg Assoc J 1978; 39:368–377.
156. Burdorf A, Lillienberg L, Brisman J. Characterization of exposure to inhalable flour dust in Swedish bakeries. Ann Occup Hyg 1994; 38:67–78.
157. Masalin KE, Degerth RK, Murtomaa HT. Airborne sugar and flour dust in the Finnish confectionary industry. Appl Ind Hyg 1988; 3:231–235.
158. Hinds WC. Aerosol Technology: Properties, Behavior, and Measurement of Airborne Particles. New York: John Wiley and Sons, 1982.
159. Nylander LA, Dement JM. Carcinogenic effects of wood dust: review and discussion. Am J Ind Med 1993; 24:619–647.
160. Darcy FJ. Physical characteristics of wood dust Ph.D. dissertation. St. Paul: University of Minnesota, 1982.
161. McCammon CS, Robinson C, Waxweiler RJ, Roscoe R. Industrial hygiene characterization of automotive wood model shops. Am Ind Hyg Assoc J 1985; 46:343–349.
162. Whitehead LW, Freud T, Hahn LL. Suspended dust concentration and size distributions, and qualitative analysis of inorganic particles, from wood working operations. Am Ind Hyg Assoc J 1981; 42:461–467.
163. Eisenbud M, Lisson J. Epidemiological aspects of beryllium-induced nonmalignant lung disease: a 30-year update. J Occup Med 1983; 25:196–202.
164. Piacitelli GM, Whelan EA, Ewers LM, Sieber WK. Lead contamination in automobiles of lead-exposed bridgeworkers. Appl Occup Environ Hyg 1995; 10:849–855.
165. Vincoli JW. Basic Guide to Industrial Hygiene. New York: Van Nostrand Reinhold, 1995.
166. Benson JM, Zelikoff JT. Respiratory toxicology of metals. In: Chang LW, ed. Toxicology of Metals. New York: Lewis Publishers, 1996:929–937.
167. Stern AC, Boubel RW, Turner DB, Fox DL. Fundamentals of Air Pollution. 2nd ed. New York: Academic Press, 1984.
168. Goyer RA. Toxic effects of metals. In: Klaassen CD, ed. Casarett and Doull's Toxicology: The Basic Science of Poisons. New York: McGraw-Hill, 1995:691–736.
169. Hogan TJ. Particulates. In: Plog BA, ed. Fundamentals of Industrial Hygiene. Itasca, IL: National Safety Council, 1996.
170. IARC. Monographs on the Evaluation of the Carcinogenic Risk of Chemicals to Humans. vol 34, part 3, 1984.
171. Eduard W, Lie A. Influence of fluoride recovery alumina on the work environment and the health of aluminum potroom workers. Scand J Work Environ Health 1981; 7:214–222.
172. Gylseth B, Bjorseth O, Dugstad O, Gujonnes J. Occurrence of fibrous sodium aluminumtetrafluoride particles in potrooms of the primary aluminum industry. Scand J Work Environ Health 1984; 10:189–195.

173. NIOSH Alert: Preventing Lead Poisoning in Construction Workers. DHHS (NIOSH) Publ. 91–116. Cincinnati: NIOSH, 1991.
174. OSHA. Lead Exposure in Construction: Interim Final Rule. Title 10 Code of Federal Regulations Part 1926. Washington, DC: US Department of Labor, 1993.
175. Conroy LM, Wadden RA, Scheff PA, Franke JE, Keil CB. Workplace emission factors for hexavalent chromium plating. Appl Occup Environ Hyg 1995; 10:620–627.
176. Deadman JE, Church G, Bradley C, Armstrong B, Thériault G. Retrospective estimation of exposures to confirmed or suspected carcinogens in an electrical utility. Appl Occup Environ Hyg 1995; 10:856–871.
177. Linnainmaa MT. Control of exposure to cobalt during grinding of hard metal blades. Appl Occup Environ Hyg 1995; 10:692–697.
178. Hoover MD, Finch GL, Mewhinney JA, Eidson AF. Release of aerosols during sawing and milling of beryllium metal and beryllium alloys. Appl Occup Environ Hyg 1990; 5:787–791.
179. Seiler DH, Rice C, Herrick RF, Hertzberg VS. A study of beryllium exposure measurements, part 1: estimation and categorization of average exposures from daily weighted average data in the beryllium industry. Appl Occup Environ Hyg 1996; 11:89–97.
180. Seiler DH, Rice C, Herrick RF, Hertzberg VS. A study of beryllium exposure measurements, part 2: evaluation of the components of exposure in the beryllium processing industry. Appl Occup Environ Hyg 1996; 11:98–102.
181. IARC. Beryllium, cadmium, mercury, and exposures in the glass manufacturing industry. Evaluation of Carcinogenic Risks to Humans 3. IARC Monogr 1993: 58.
182. Roels H, Buchet J-P, Truc J, Croquet F, Lauwerys R. The possible role of direct ingestion on the overall absorption of cadmium or arsenic in workers exposed to CdO and As_2O_3 dust. Am J Ind Med 1982; 3:53–56.
183. Paustenbach DJ, Meyer DM, Sheehan PJ, Lau V. An assessment and quantitative uncertainty analysis of the health risks to workers exposed to chromium contaminated soils. Toxicol Ind Health 1991; 7(3):159–196.
184. Krochmalnyckyj R. Exposure to mercury from a metal furnace. Appl Occup Environ Hyg 1995; 10:730–732.
185. EPA. Comments on the Use of Methylcyclopentadienyl Manganese Tricarbonyl in Unleaded Gasoline. Washington, DC: EPA, 1990:1–56.
186. Ter Haar GL, Griffing ME, Brandt M, Oberling GD. Methylcyclopentadienyl manganese tricarbonyl as an antiknock: composition and fate of manganese exhaust products. J Air Pollut Control Assoc 1975; 25:858–860.
187. Waldron HA. Metals in the Environment. London: Academic Press, 1980:214–215.
188. Zayed J, Gérin M, Loranger L, Sierra P. Occupational and environmental exposure of garage workers and taxi drivers to airborne manganese arising from the use of MMT (methylcyclopentadienyl manganese tricarbonyl) in unleaded gasoline. Am Ind Hyg Assoc J 1994; 55:53–58.
189. Sierra P, Loranger S, Kennedy G, Zayed J. Occupational and environmental exposure of automobile mechanics and nonautomotive workers to airborne manganese

arising from the combustion of methylcyclopentadienyl manganese tricarbonyl (MMT). Am Ind Hyg Assoc J 1995; 56:713–724.
190. Sánchez-Ocampo A, Torres-Pérez J, Jiménez-Reyes M. Selenium levels in the serum of workers at a rubber tire repair shop. Am Ind Hyg Assoc J 1996; 57:72–75.
191. Bellido-Milla D, Hernandez-Artiga MP, Hidalgo-Hidalgo de Cisneros JS, Muñoz-Leyva JA. Analytical study of hygiene hazards involved in naval industry welding processes. Appl Occup Environ Hyg 1995; 10:921–942.
192. Hewett P. Estimation of regional pulmonary deposition and exposure for fumes from SMAW and GMAW mild and stainless steel consumables. Am Ind Hyg Assoc J 1995; 56:136–142.
193. Hewett P. The particle size distribution, density, and specific surface area of welding fumes from SMAW and GMAW mild and stainless steel consumables. Am Ind Hyg Assoc J 1955; 6:128–135.
194. American Welding Society. The Welding Environment, a Research Report on Fumes and Gases Generated during Welding Operations. Miami: American Welding Society, 1973.
195. Hinds WC. Basis for particle size-selective sampling for wood dust. Appl Ind Hyg 1988; 3:67–72.
196. Baron PA, Willeke K. Bridging science and application in aerosol measurement. In: Willeke K, Baron PA, eds. Aerosol Measurement: Principles, Techniques, and Applications. New York: Van Nostrand Reinhold, 1993:8–22.
197. IARC. Occupational exposures to mists and vapours from sulfuric acid and other strong inorganic acids. In: Evaluation of Carcinogenic Risks to Humans. IARC Monogr 1992; 54:41–130.
198. Van Dusen J, Smith JW. Comparison of the effectiveness of bubble coalescence and foamed surfactant in controlling the acid mist formed by electrowinning cells. Am Ind Hyg Assoc J 1989; 50:252–256.
199. WHO. Working Group. Health impact of acidic deposition. Sci Total Environ 1986; 52:157–187.
200. WHO. Air quality guidelines for Europe. Copenhagen: Regional Office for Europe, 1987:338–360.
201. American Thoracic Society. Health effects of atmospheric acids and their precursors. Am Rev Respir Dis 1991; 144:464–467.
202. Bruggen Cate HJT. Dental erosion in industry. Br J Ind Med 1986; 25:249–266.
203. Remijn B, Koster P, Houthuijs D, Boleij J, Willems H, Brunekreef B, Biersteker K, van Loveren C. Zinc chloride, zinc oxide, hydrochloric acid exposure and dental erosion in a zinc galvanizing plant in the Netherlands. Ann Occup Hyg 1982; 25: 299–307.
204. Balmes JR, Fine JM, Gordon T, Sheppard D. Potential bronchoconstrictor stimuli in acid fog. Environ Health Perspect 1989; 79:163–166.
205. Utell MJ. Effects of inhaled acid aerosols on lung mechanics: an analysis of human exposure studies. Environ Health Perspect 1985; 63:39–44.
206. Gamble J, Jones W, Hancock J. Epidemiological–environmental study of lead acid battery workers. II. Acute effects of sulfuric acid on the respiratory system. Environ Res 1984; 35:11–29.

207. Lippmann M, Goldstein DH. Oil-mist studies, environmental evaluation and control. Arch Environ Health 1970; 21:591–599.
208. Pasternack B, Ehrlich L. Occupational exposure to an oil mist atmosphere. Arch Environ Health 1972; 25:286–294.
209. Kennedy SM, Greaves IA, Kriebel D, Eisen EA, Smith TJ, Woskie SR. Acute pulmonary responses among automobile workers exposed to aerosols of machining fluids. Am J Ind Med 1989; 15:627–641.
210. Hendy MS, Beattie BE, Burge PS. Occupational asthma due to an emulsified oil mist. Br J Ind Med 1985; 42:51–54.
211. Jarvholm B. Cutting oil mist and bronchitis. Eur J Respir Dis 1982; 63(suppl 118): 79–83.
212. Robertson AS, Weir DC, Burge PS. Occupational asthma due to oil mists. Thorax 1988; 43:200–205.
213. IARC. Mineral oils (lubricant based oils and derived products). In: Evaluation of Carcinogenic Risks of Chemicals to Humans IARC Monogr 1984; 33:87–168.
214. Menichini E. Particle size distribution of oil mist in the workplace. Ann Occup Hyg 1986; 30:349–363.
215. Woskie SR, Smith TJ, Hallock MF, Hammond SK, Rosenthal F, Eisen EA, Kriebel D, Greaves IA. Size-selective pulmonary dose indices for metal-working fluid aerosols in machining and grinding operations in the automobile manufacturing industry. Am Ind Hyg Assoc J 1994; 55:20–29.
216. Drasche VH, Finzel L, Martschei H, Meyer R. Arbeitsmedizinische Erhebungen bei ölnebelexponierten Personen. Zentralbl Arbeitsmed Arbeitsschutz 1974; 24: 302–312.
217. Oxhøj H, Andreasen H, Henius UM. Respiratory symptoms and ventilatory lung function in machine shop workers exposed to coolant-lubricants. Eur J Respir Dis 1982; 63(suppl 118):85–89.
218. IARC. Occupational exposures in spraying and application of insecticides. In: Evaluation of Carcinogenic Risks to Humans IARC Monogr 1991; 53:45–92.
219. Freed VH, Davies JE, Peters LJ, Parveen F. Minimizing occupational exposure to pesticides: repellency and penetrability of treated textiles to pesticide sprays. Residue Rev 1980; 75:159–167.
220. Guidotti TL, Yoshida K, Clough V. Personal exposure to pesticide among workers engaged in pesticide container recycling operations. Am Ind Hyg Assoc J 1994; 55:1154–1163.
221. Barthel E. High incidence of lung cancer in persons with chronic professional exposure to pesticides in agriculture. Z Erkrank Atm-Org 1976; 146:266–274.
222. Jeyaratnam J, Premawardewa LDKE, de Silva DGH, Wijeratne U, Seneviratne KN. Occupational pesticide poisoning. Proceedings of the 10th Asian Conference on Occupational Health, vol 1. Singapore, September 1982:204–207.
223. Peoples SA, Maddy KT, Peifer WR, Edmiston S. Occupational exposures to pesticides containing organoarsenicals in California. Vet Hum Toxicol 1979; 21:417–421.
224. Nagle G, Woodbury MA, Zenz C. Occupational health aspects of pesticides: clinical and hygienic principles. In: Zenz C, ed. Developments in Occupational Medicine. Chicago: Year Book Medical, 1980:259–311.

225. Abbott IM, Bonsall JL, Chester G, Hart TB, Turnbull GJ. Worker exposure to a herbicide applied with ground sprayers in the United Kingdom. Am Ind Hyg Assoc J 1987; 48:167–175.
226. Sanderson WT, Ringenburg V, Biagini R. Exposure of commercial pesticide applicators to the herbicide alachlor. Am Ind Hyg Assoc J 1995; 56:890–897.
227. Archibald BA, Solomon KR, Stephenson GR. Estimation of pesticide exposure to greenhouse applicators using video imaging and other assessment techniques. Am Ind Hyg Assoc J 1995; 56:226–235.
228. Fenske RA, Hamburger SJ, Guyton CL. Occupational exposure to fosetyl-Al fungicide during spraying of ornamentals in greenhouses. Arch Environ Contam Toxicol 1987; 16:615–621.
229. Jauhiainen A, Räsänen K, Sarantila R, Nuutinen J, Kangas J. Occupational exposure of forest workers to glyphosate during brush saw spraying work. Am Ind Hyg Assoc J 1991; 52:61–64.
230. Leonard JA, Yeary RA. Exposure of workers using hand-held equipment during urban application of pesticides to trees and ornamental shrubs. Am Ind Hyg Assoc J 1990; 51:605–609.
231. Libich S, To JC, Frank R, Sirons GJ. Occupational exposure of herbicide applicators to herbicides used along electric power transmission line right-of-way. Am Ind Hyg Assoc J 1984; 45:56–62.
232. NIOSH Organic Solvent Neurotoxicity. Curr Intell Bull 48—DHHS/NIOSH Pub. 87–104, Washington, DC: Government Printing Office, 1987.
233. Heitbrink WA, Wallace ME, Bryant CJ, Ruch WE. Control of paint overspray in autobody repair shops. Am Ind Hyg Assoc J 1995; 56:1023–1032.
234. Séguin P, Allard A, Cartier A, Malo JL. Prevalence of occupational asthma in spray painters exposed to several types of isocyanates, including polymethylene polyphenylisocyanate. J Occup Med 1987; 29:340–344.
235. Chan TL, D'Arcy JB, Schreck RM. High-solid paint overspray aerosols in a spray painting booth: particle size analysis and scrubber efficiency. Am Ind Hyg Assoc J 1986; 47:411–417.
236. Chan TL, Rouhana SW, Mulawa PA, Reuter RJ. Occupational health assessment of the high velocity Oxy-fuel thermal metal spray process. Appl Occup Environ Hyg 1995; 10:482–487.
237. D'Arcy JB, Chan TL. Chemical distribution in high-solid paint overspray aerosols. Am Ind Hyg Assoc J 1990;51:132–138.
238. Zhuang Z, Myers WR. Field performance measurements of half-facepiece respirators—paint spraying operations. Am Ind Hyg Assoc J 1996; 57:50–57.
239. Maître A, Leplay A, Perdrix A, Ohl G, Boinay P, Romazini S, Aubrun JC. Comparison between solid sampler and impinger for evaluation of occupational exposure to 1,6-hexamethylene diisocyanate polyisocyanates during spray painting. Am Ind Hyg Assoc J 1996; 57:153–160.
240. Rosenberg C, Tuomi T. Airborne isocyanates in polyurethane spray painting: determination and respirator efficiency. Am Ind Hyg Assoc J 1984; 45:117–121.
241. Goyer N. Performance of painting booths equipped with down-draft ventilation. Am Ind Hyg Assoc J 1995; 56:258–265.
242. Rudzinski WE, Dahlquist B, Svejda SA, Richardson A, Thomas T. Sampling and

analysis of isocyanates in spray-painting operations. Am Ind Hyg Assoc J 1995; 56:284–289.
243. O'Brien DM, Hurley DE. An evaluation of control technology for spray painting. Am Ind Hyg Assoc J 1982; 43:695–703.
244. Hobbs CH, McClellan RO. Toxic effects of radiation and radioactive materials. In: Klaassen CD, Amdur MO, Doull J, eds. Casarette and Doull's Toxicology: The Basic Science of Poisons: 3rd ed. New York: MacMillan Publishing, 1986:497–530.
245. US DOE. Airborne Release Fractions/Rates and Respirable Fractions for Nonreactor Nuclear Facilities. DOE-HDBK-3010-94. Prepared by Mishima J, Pinkston D. Washington, DC, US Department of Energy, 1994.
246. Hoover MD, Newton GJ. Radioactive aerosols. In: Willeke K, Baron P, eds. Aerosol Measurement: Principles, Techniques, and Applications. New York: Van Nostrand Reinhold, 1993:768–798.
247. International Commission on Radiological Protection (ICRP). Limits on Intakes of Radionuclides by Workers. ICRP Publication 30 and addendums. Oxford: Pergamon Press, 1979.
248. ICRP. Reference Man: Anatomical, Physiological and Metabolic Characteristics. ICRP Publication 23. Oxford: Pergamon Press, 1975.
249. Scott BR, Hoover MD, Newton GJ. On evaluating respiratory tract intake of high-specific–activity alpha-emitting particles for brief occupational exposure. Radiat Prot Dosim 1997; 69:43–50.
250. Martell EA. Tobacco radioactivity and cancer in smokers. Am Sci 1975; 63:404–412.
251. Cuddihy RG, McClellan RO, Hoover MD, Dugan VL, Chapman LD, Wayland JR. Radiation risks from plutonium recycle. Environ Sci Technol 1977; 11:1160–1165.
252. Hewson GS. Overview of radiation safety in the tin by-product (Amang) industry of South East Asia. Health Phys 1996; 71:225–234.
253. Crim EM, Bradley TD. Measurements of air concentrations of thorium during grinding and welding operations using thoriated tungsten electrodes. Health Phys 1995; 68:719–722.
254. O'Brien RS, Peggie JR, Leith IS. Estimates of inhalation doses resulting from the possible use of phospho-gypsum plaster-board in Australian homes. Health Phys 1995; 68:561–570.
255. NCRP. Evaluation of Occupational and Environmental Exposures to Radon and Radon Daughters in the United States. Report 78. Bethesda, MD: NCRP, 1985.
256. NAS. Comparative Dosimetry of Radon in Mines and Homes. Washington, DC: National Academy Press, 1991.
257. NAS. Health Risks of Radon and Other Internally Deposited Alpha-Emitters (BEIR IV). Committee on the Biological Effects of Ionizing Radiations, Board on Radiation Effects Research, Commission on Life Sciences, National Research Council. Washington, DC: National Academy Press, 1988.
258. NCRP. Radiation Exposure of the U.S. Population from Consumer Products and Miscellaneous Sources. Bethesda, MD: NCRP, 1987.
259. Eisenbud M. Environmental Radioactivity from Natural, Industrial, and Military Sources. San Diego: Academic Press, 1987.

260. O'Grady J, Hone C, Turvey FJ. Radiocesium contamination at a steel plant in Ireland. Health Phys 1996; 70:568–572.
261. Eidson AF, Damon EG. Predicted deposition rates of uranium yellowcake aerosols sampled in uranium mills. Health Phys 1984; 46:165–176.
262. Hoover MD, Newton GJ, Yeh HC, Eidson AF. Characterization of aerosols from industrial fabrication of mixed-oxide nuclear reactor fuels. In: Marple VA, Liu BYH, eds. Aerosols in the Mining and Industrial Work Environments. Ann Arbor: Ann Arbor Science, 1983:533–548.
263. Dorrian M-D, Bailey MR. Particle size distributions of radioactive aerosols measured in workplaces. Radiat Prot Dosim 1995; 60:119–133.
264. ICRP. Human Respiratory Tract Model for Radiological Protection. ICRP Publication 66. Oxford: Pergamon Press, 1994.
265. Michal R. Respirators, internal dose, and Oyster Creek. Nucl News 1996; 39:27–28.
266. Code of Federal Regulation, Title 10, Part 20. Standard for Protection Against Radiation. Washington; DC: Office of Federal Register, January 1, 1993.
267. Garger EK, Hoffman FO, Miller CW. Model testing using Chernobyl data: III. Atmospheric resuspension of radionuclides in Ukranian regions impacted by Chernobyl fallout, Health Phys 1996; 70:18–24.
268. HASL. Final Tabulation of Monthly ^{90}Sr Fallout Data: 1954–1976. HASL-329. New York: HASL, 1977.
269. Cuddihy RG, Newton GJ. Human Health Exposures Related to Nuclear Weapons Industries. LMF 112. Lovelace Biomedical and Environmental Research Institute. Springfield: National Technical Information Services, 1985.
270. Anspaugh LR, Daniels JI. Bases for secondary standards for residual radionuclides in soil and some recommendations for cost-effective operational implementation. Health Phys 1996; 70:722–734.
271. Tokarskaya ZB, Okladnikova ND, Belyaeva ZD, Drozhko EG. The influence of radiation and nonradiation factors on the lung cancer incidence among the workers of the nuclear enterprise Mayak. Health Phys 1995; 69:356–366.
272. Heid KR, Breitenstein BD, Palmer HE, McMurray BJ, Wald N. The 1976 Hanford Americium Accident. Richland: Pacific Northwest Laboratory Report TID-28938. UC-48, 1979.
273. Toohey RE, Kathren RL. Overview and dosimetry of the Hanford americium accident case. Health Phys 1995; 69:310–317.
274. Westinghouse Savannah River Company. Evaluation of Savannah River Site Internal Dosimetry Registry Case 664 (U). Report ESH-HPT-920178. Health Protection Department. Aiken: Westinghouse Savannah River Company, Savannah River Site, 1992.
275. Code of Federal Regulation. Title 10, Part 835. Occupational Radiation Protection. Washington, DC: Office of Federal Register, December 14, 1993.
276. Spitz HB, Robinson B. Deposition of plutonium in the lungs of a worker following an accidental inhalation exposure. In: Proceedings of the Snowbird Actinide Workshop on Actinides in Man and Animal, October 15–17, 1979, Radiobiology Division. Salt Lake City: University of Utah Press, 1981.
277. Kennedy WE Jr, Aaberg RL. Dose and risk assessment for intrusion into mixed-waste disposal sites. Appl Occup Environ Hyg 1996; 11:404–409.

4

Medicinal Particles

MAGNUS SVARTENGREN

Karolinska Institute
Stockholm, Sweden

KATHARINA SVARTENGREN

Karolinska Institute
Huddinge University Hospital
Stockholm, Sweden

I. Use of Aerosols in Medicine (Diagnostics and Therapy)

The area of the adult lung that is exposed to the environment ranges from 40 to 120 m^2. The conducting airways have a total area of less than 1 m^2. An increased interest of use of the inhalation route has been seen over the years. For example, with beta-adrenergic agonists, used in treating asthma, inhaled material is at least tenfold more effective in the lung than an equivalent oral dose (1). Major groups for uses of inhaled pharmaceuticals are given in Table 1, possible future uses under experimental investigation in Table 2, and diagnostic uses of aerosols in Table 3.

Inhaled aerosols are widely used in diagnosis of lung disease; for example, as nonspecific provocation tests with histamine and methacholine and specific provocation tests for different allergens. Comparison of data between research centers is hampered by differences in the methods used. Aerosols of hypertonic saline have been used in induction of sputum for test of bronchial responsiveness (3–5). Analysis of sputum samples seems to be an interesting possibility as an alternative to bronchoalveolar lavage.

Aerosol bolus dispersion technique has been used for studying airway di-

Table 1 Major Uses of Inhaled Pharmaceuticals: Primary Current Uses

Use	Class of agent	Example
Asthma	β-Agonists	Albuterol
		Metaproterenol sulfate
	Long-acting β-agonists	Salmeterol
		Formoterol
	Anticholinergics	Ipratropium bromide
	Corticosteroids	Beclomethasone
		Flunisolide
		Triamcinolone
	Mast cell stabilizers	Cromolyn sodium
Infectious disease	Antibiotics	Gentamicin
		Tobramycin
		Pentamidine
	Antifungals	Amphotericin B
	Antivirals	Ribavirin
Prolonged labor	Hormone	Oxytocin
Diabetes insipidus	Antidiuretic hormone	Vasopressin (arginine)
Anesthetics	Halogenated hydrocarbons	Halothane
		Isoflurane

Table 2 Major Uses of Inhaled Pharmaceuticals: Future Uses Under Experimental Investigation

Use	Class of agent	Example
Asthma	Leukotriene D antagonists	Zafirlukast (ICI 204,219)
		Sulukast (LY170680)
Cystic fibrosis	Gene therapy	Cystic fibrosis gene
	Gene products	α_1-Antitrypsin, CFTR
		DNase
	Ion transport regulations	Amiloride
Respiratory distress syndrome	Surfactant	Dipalmitoyl phosphatidylcholine
Systemic diseases	Proteins and peptides	Insulin
		Growth hormone
		Leuprolide acetate
Lung transplantation	Immune suppression	Cyclosporine

Source: Ref. 2.

Table 3 Diagnostic Uses of Aerosols

Disease	Test	Example agent
Asthma	Nonspecific provocation test	Histamine or methacholine
	Specific provocation test	Occupational and environmental allergens
Several inflammatory airway diseases	Sputum induction for cell analysis	Hypertonic saline
Healthy and obstructive airway diseases	Airway dimensions using bolus inhalation volumetric depth	Inert test particles
Inflammatory changes	DTPA clearance as a measure of damage and airway permeability	^{99m}Technetium-labeled DTPA particles
Primary ciliary dyskinesia	Mucociliary clearance	Insoluble, labeled test particles, iron, Teflon, polystyrene

mensions. Here, too, there are difficulties comparing results obtained from different laboratories owing to differences in the methods used (6–10).

Other diagnostic uses of aerosols are, for example, measurements of mucociliary transport and airway permeability, the latter with pentetic acid (diethylenetriamine pentaacetic acid; DTPA) clearance.

II. Factors Influencing Aerosol Dose

A. Deposition Mechanisms of Major Importance

The main physical mechanisms for deposition of aerosol particles are impaction, sedimentation, diffusion, and electrostatic attraction. Impaction is a flow–rate-dependent mechanism for particles larger than 1-μm–aerodynamic diameter (AD). The probability of impaction increases with increasing AD of the particles and increasing velocity of the airflow (Fig. 1). This mechanism is important for deposition in the nasal and oral cavities and in the large bronchi. Deposition by impaction can be described by the parameter AD^2F, where AD is the aerodynamic diameter and F is the flow rate (Figs. 2–4). This parameter can be used for normalizing for different flow rates and particle sizes. All particles with densities exceeding that of air experience a downward force due to gravity. The distance covered by gravitational sedimentation increases with increasing AD of the particles and increasing residence time in the airways (Fig. 5). Thus, breath-holding enhances deposition by sedimentation. This mechanism is important for deposi-

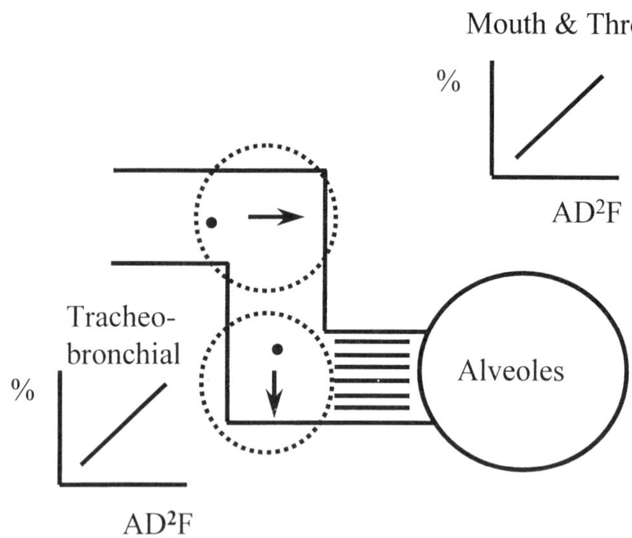

Figure 1 Deposition by impaction: A schematic drawing of the respiratory tract, which can be seen as three filters in line, to protect the fragile alveoli from particles. The first two filters, mouth and throat and tracheobronchial airways, work by impaction (i.e., particles tend to continue forward and deposit when the gas flow changes direction). Impaction is the most important deposition mechanism for medical aerosols in the upper airways and in larger bronchus, and correlates well with the impaction parameter AD^2F. In the last filter, the bronchioles, impaction is insignificant owing to the large total cross-sectional area, leading to low velocities.

tion of particles larger than 0.5 μm (AD) in the small bronchi, bronchioles, and alveoli, where airflow rates are low. The probability of brownian diffusion increases with decreasing geometric diameter of the particles and increasing residence time. This mechanism is important for particles smaller than 0.5 μm. The probability of deposition by electrostatic attraction increases with an increasing number of electrical charges and decreasing size of the particles. This mechanism may be important in the small airways for 0.1- to 1.0-μm particles that are charged.

B. Factors Determining Deposition

There are several factors determining the site of deposition of an inhaled aerosol. (1) The aerodynamic diameter (AD) of the particles; for a spherical particle, it can be calculated as $D \times P^{0.5}$, where D is the geometric diameter, and P is the particle density; (2) breathing pathway; compared with nose-breathing, mouth-

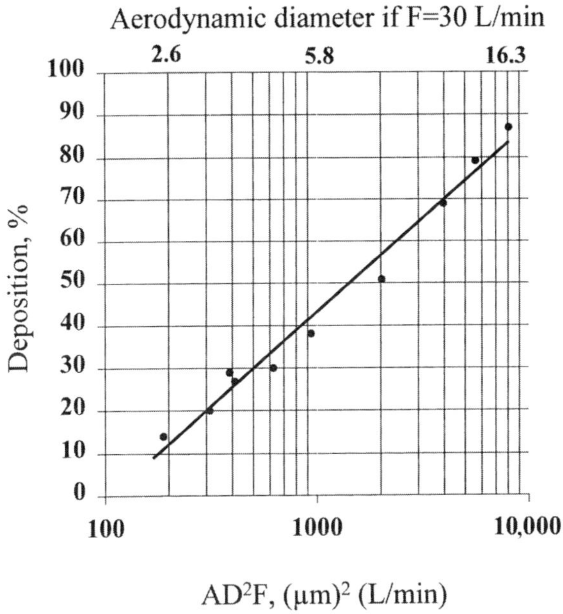

Figure 2 Relation between the parameter AD^2F and particle deposition in mouth and throat: Each point represents a mean from six to ten healthy adults (median age 27, range 19–54 years and 15% women). On the lower x-axis the AD^2F values are shown, and on the upper, the corresponding particle sizes at an inhalation flow of 30 L/min. The formula of the regression line is $y = -90.1 + 19.3(ln x)$; $r = 0.99$.

breathing results in an enhanced tracheobronchial deposition; (3) breathing pattern: a slow and deep inhalation, with a breath-holding pause, will favor deposition in the lung periphery; (4) the geometry of the respiratory tract: the geometry of the larynx may be important for the velocity profiles in the trachea and the bronchi. The vocal folds act as an aperture and the sudden increase in the downstream area leads to turbulence (11). The intensity and persistence of this turbulence is dependent on the ventilatory flow rate through the larynx. Studies on fluid dynamics in computational models of the human airways indicate that the glottic aperture may influence the velocity profile beyond the carina (12). In diseased airways, airflow diverts to nonobstructed segments and, at sites of obstruction, turbulence is expected to increase particle deposition (13,14). (5) Hygroscopic growth: this is important for aerosols composed of water-soluble particles, for instance sodium chloride crystals.

Descriptions of clinical responses to inhaled drugs are of little value in the absence of accurate measurements of the dose, preferably at the site of action.

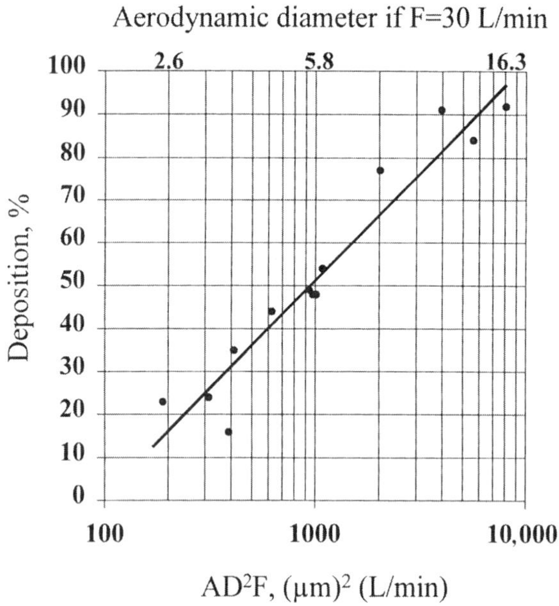

Figure 3 Relation between the parameter AD^2F and tracheobronchial deposition in percentage of particles entering the trachea. Each point represents a mean from six to ten healthy adults (median age 27, range 19–54 years and 15% women). On the lower x-axis the AD^2F values are shown, and on the upper, the corresponding particle sizes at an inhalation flow of 30 L/min. The formula of the regression line is $y = -99.3 + 21.8\ (lnx)$; $r = 0.96$.

Consequently, aerosol delivery presents a special problem, because the actual retained dose is often difficult to determine. Furthermore, the precise site within the lungs to which therapeutic aerosols should be delivered is not clear, and probably varies according to the type of drug being inhaled. However, in general, it is desirable to reduce the amount of aerosol deposited by impaction in the oropharynx and to increase the amount reaching the lungs. To increase the quantity reaching the peripheral airways, it is necessary to consider the mode of inhalation, the aerosol characteristics, and the subject inhaling the aerosol. The inhalation flow rate is an important feature of the inhalation mode. A slow and deep inhalation, with a period of breath-holding favors penetration to the lung periphery (15). Particle size is the single most important factor determining the site of aerosol deposition. Therapeutic aerosols are heterodisperse, and the droplets cover a range of sizes. The aerodynamic behavior of these aerosols can be approximately described by their mass median aerodynamic diameter (MMAD). In prac-

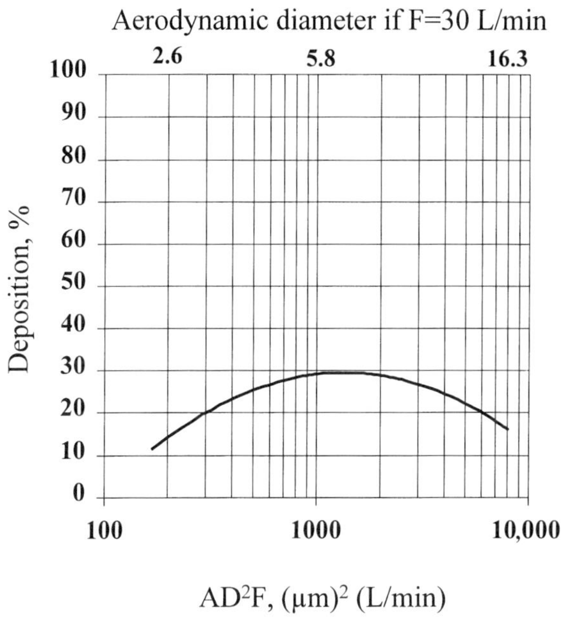

Figure 4 The relation between AD^2F and tracheobronchial deposition in percentage of all inhaled particles, calculated from the regression lines in Figures 2 and 3: The curve has its maximum, 30% tracheobronchial deposition of all inhaled particles, at a AD^2F of 1365 μm^{2}* L/min, which corresponds to an aerodynamic particle size of 6 μm at an inhalation flow rate of 30 L/min.

tice, changes in aerosol deposition can be brought about by changing the mode of inhalation, the particle size, airway dimensions, or combinations of these factors. In estimating lung deposition experimentally, however, use of well-defined monodisperse aerosols simplifies the interpretation of the results.

In healthy subjects, a maximal tracheobronchial deposition has been found for 6 μm (AD) particles inhaled by mouth-breathing at 0.5 L/sec (see Fig. 4; 16). Smaller particles (1–5 μm) will be deposited mainly in the alveolar region, or exhaled, owing to reduced deposition by impaction and sedimentation in central and peripheral bronchial airways, and larger particles will deposit mainly in the oropharynx and central airways of the tracheobronchial region. Changing the mode of inhalation, on the other hand, represents another possibility for influencing the amount of aerosol delivered to the lungs. For instance, it is possible to increase the aerosol mass delivered to the peripheral airways of the tracheobronchial region, with minimum losses, by inhaling rather large particles (6 μm) at an extremely slow flow (0.05 L/sec) (see Fig. 5; 17). A spacer is sometimes

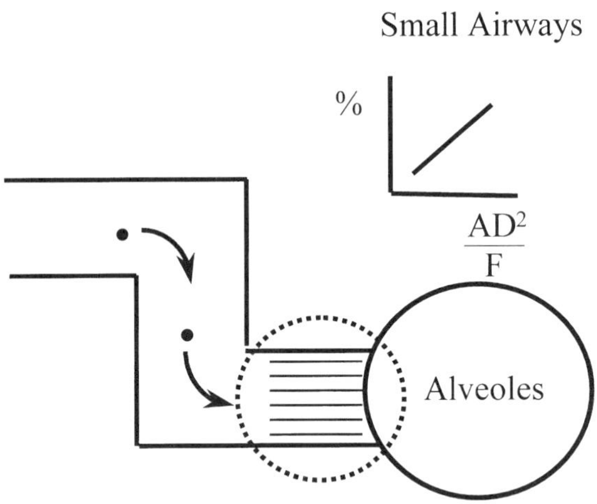

Figure 5 Deposition at extremely slow inhalations: Here deposition in mouth and throat as well as large bronchi will be low. On the other hand, when particles reach the small airways, where the total cross-sectional area is large, sedimentation is more important. Similar to impaction, sedimentation has a positive correlation to the square of the aerodynamic diameter (AD^2), but will increase with lower flow rates, owing to longer residence time.

recommended for patients treated with metered-dose inhalers (MDI). In such situations, mean deposition in the oropharynx may be reduced at least tenfold, but delivery of aerosol to the lungs remains unchanged with values of about 10–15% (18,19). This finding is explained by the collection of large and high-velocity particles by the spacer and evaporation of the remaining suspended particles, resulting in a selective delivery of small particles to the lungs.

Alderson and co-workers (20) have studied patients with suspected pulmonary emboli after imaging with both DTPA aerosols and radioactive gas. They observed that patients studied in an upright position, have markedly uneven apex-to-base gradients of deposited DTPA that were not explained by the distribution of regional ventilation by radioactive gas. In contrast, these marked apex-to-base gradients were not observed in patients who had inhaled the DTPA aerosol in a supine position. There are increasing apex-to-base gradients for both ventilation and particle deposition. There are, however, different processes governing ventilation and deposition, that might explain the lack of correlation found in their work. Studies of Baskin et al. and O'Doherty et al. (21,22) illustrate a possible role for manipulation of body position in optimizing the regional delivery of pharmaceutical aerosols. More studies need to be performed to show that it is clinically relevant.

There are very limited data on deposition of particles in children. Knight and Gilberg (23) performed calculations, using deposition models and lung models (24), and age adjustment for respiratory frequency and tidal volume, according to Hoffman (25). These estimates indicate that, in the proximal lung generations 1–12, the deposition is double in a child of 6 months of age, compared with a 25-year-old adult, for small, 1.3-μm–aerodynamic mass median diameter, particles.

Although many factors affect total and regional deposition, the underlying disease process in the lungs may be a major determinant of the final deposition pattern, for stiffened or obstructed parts will receive little or no drug owing to uneven ventilation (26,27). Frequently, it is the diseased parts of the lungs that are most in the need of therapeutic intervention. Whether the clinical efficacy of an aerosolized drug is dependent on the local dose remains to be clarified.

III. Individual Deposition Variability (Nose, Mouth, and Lung)

A. Deposition in the Nose

The nose acts as a filter, more efficient than the oral route, for inhaled particles. There is no advantage in using the nasal route for treatment of lung disease; consequently, it is rarely used in clinical situations except for local treatment. The nasal route might also be used for systemic treatment.

Becquemin and co-workers (28) have studied nasal deposition of particles in adults and in children older and younger than 12 years of age. Total resistance in the nose was about twice that of adults for the children. The percentage deposition was equal or higher in adults than in children, for both resting ventilation and moderate exercise ventilation.

Nasal mucociliary transport of a local dose of saccharine decreased after 8–10 km of fast jogging. This might possibly be an effect of increased ventilation on nasal mucociliary transport (29).

B. Deposition in the Oropharynx

Studies of oropharyngeal deposition in healthy subjects (30–32), as well as in patients with asthma (33) have shown wide interindividual variations. For instance, deposition in the oropharynx of inhaled 3.6-μm test particles varied between 10 and 70% in asthmatics. This implies that the dose of a therapeutic aerosol in the lungs is difficult to predict and is sometimes suboptimal. Furthermore, adverse effects of inhaled corticosteroids, such as oral candidiasis (34), dysphonia (35), and osteoporosis (36), may arise locally and systematically. It is evidently important to reduce a high oropharyngeal deposition.

In our studies, monodisperse Teflon particles are aerosolized into a glass bulb and the inhalation procedure is well standardized. In spite of this optimal situation, there are wide variations in oropharyngeal deposition among patients.

These findings are well reproducible in patients with asthma (33,37) and in those with chronic bronchitis (38), strongly indicating individual factors affecting deposition. Furthermore, about one-fourth of the patients with asthma seem to have extensive oropharyngeal deposition (33,37,39). Fiberoptic examination revealed great differences in behavior of the pharyngeal and laryngeal regions among patients with asthma, but the behavior was consistent on an individual basis (37,39). A marked functional constriction at the tongue base–epiglottic level was related to extensive oropharyngeal deposition.

Deposition in the oropharynx can be influenced by using a spacer (18,19), or by adding an external resistance during inhalation (37), and can probably also be influenced by the design of the mouthpiece that is used (40,41). The spacer collects, among other things, large and high-velocity particles from a metered-dose inhaler, thereby reducing oropharyngeal deposition. However, because the airways are comparable to two serial filters, a decrease in the size of the particles reduces deposition not only in the oropharynx, but also in the tracheobronchial region (see Figs. 2–4). An added external resistance, on the other hand, not only reduces a high oropharyngeal deposition, but also correspondingly increases lung deposition of particles of the same size (37). Furthermore, it does not adversely affect oropharyngeal or lung deposition in patients with an already low oropharyngeal deposition. Dolovich collected data from different studies and found an indication with a positive correlation between lung deposition and resistance in the device (42). Thus, inhalations of aerosols using a resistance device could be beneficial for patients with extensive oropharyngeal deposition, with a possible exception of certain patients who experience difficulties in inhaling with increased resistance. Despite a thorough fiberoptic examination of the pharynx and larynx, we are unable to provide simple criteria for the identification of patients who would benefit from an increased resistance. There are obviously factors other than the shape of pharynx and larynx that are important in determining this deposition. Extensive oropharyngeal deposition might possibly be related to symptoms of local adverse effects, such as candidiasis or dysphonia or, perhaps more importantly, to suboptimal effects of aerosol therapy. Further clinical and experimental studies are needed to permit an appropriate identification of patients with inhalation problems.

Changes in pharyngeal and laryngeal shape may also influence regional lung deposition. For instance, we have found lower lung retention values at 24 hr for patients who have a narrowing of their laryngeal and pharyngeal spaces (37,39). This finding may be explained by the narrowing causing a turbulence in the airflow that is propagated down into the trachea and larger bronchi, leading to an increased deposition in the central airways (12).

In general, during normal inhalation flow rates, deposition in the oropharynx may be estimated by the impaction factor AD^2F (see Fig. 2). In the future, it would be desirable to develop methods for clinical use in evaluating oropharyngeal, as well as lung deposition of inhaled drugs.

C. Tracheobronchial Deposition

Lippmann et al. (43) showed the effects of particle size on the regional deposition of inhaled aerosols in the human respiratory tract. There are wide variations in lung deposition among healthy subjects (44,45). For instance, tracheobronchial deposition may vary by a factor of 5 (46), but within the same subject, results are fairly well reproducible (45,46). Gerrity et al. (47) studied deposition variability owing to particle size in experiments and compared this with theoretical data using the lung model of Weibel (24). The differences in regional lung deposition among healthy subjects are mainly explained by variations in airway dimensions, indicating that lung deposition may be estimated by lung function measures. Lung retentions are closely correlated with airway resistance in healthy subjects (48–50); thus, the deposition in the tracheobronchial region may be generally estimated by the parameter AD^2F using normal inhalation flow rates (see Fig. 3).

Therapeutic aerosols play a prominent role in the treatment of diseases of the lower conducting airways, such as bronchial asthma and chronic bronchitis. An increased tracheobronchial deposition of the inhaled aerosols for this purpose is probably to be desired. Studies of regional lung deposition in healthy subjects, using different normal inhalation flow rates (0.4–1.2 L/sec) and particle sizes (2.5–16.4 μm), show a maximal tracheobronchial deposition of 30% for 6-μm particles inhaled at 0.5 L/sec (see Fig. 4; 16). Impaction in the large bronchi is normally the most important mechanism for deposition of 6-μm particles. However, when inhaled at an extremely slow flow (0.05 L/sec), impaction should be insignificant for these particles, whereas deposition by sedimentation ought to dominate in the small bronchi owing to the prolonged transit time (24). This hypothesis was tested in healthy subjects (17). The tracheobronchially deposited fraction of 6-μm particles inhaled at 0.05 L/sec could be increased to 50%, compared with maximally 30% inhaled at 0.5 L/sec. Another possibility to influence deposition in the oropharynx and lung may be by using carrier gases, such as helium–oxygen mixture. Because of reduced turbulent flow, deposition in the oropharynx may be lowered, and lung deposition may be enhanced in asthma, suggesting that inhalation of drugs in helium–oxygen might be of therapeutic value in treating patients with severely obstructed airways (51). Still, another possibility of enhancing tracheobronchial deposition would be to apply the, technically rather complicated, bolus inhalation technique. The deposition results with this technique, however, are still conflicting.

D. Alveolar Deposition

Measurements of whole-lung clearance in healthy subjects using inhaled radiolabeled test aerosols show a rapid clearance phase, which is completed within 24 hr (44,45,52). The rapidly cleared fraction has generally been equated with tracheobronchial deposition, and the retained fraction with alveolar deposition. Recently, results from studies using a shallow bolus technique indicate that particles deposited in the conducting airways of healthy subjects may be retained for days (53,54). The underlying mechanism is unclear, but the geometric particle diameter has been proposed to be a major determinant (55). Surfactant has been reported to displace particles, smaller than 6 μm in diameter, from air to the aqueous phase in hamsters' conducting airways, driven by the low surface tension of surfactant (56,57). Bennett et al. (58) have studied clearance between 24 and 48 hr in ten young, normal subjects using technetium Tc99m-labeled iron oxide particles. Albuterol given immediately after particle exposure increased clearance significantly. A corresponding stimulation after 24 hr did not affect clearance compared with control. These data do not support the hypothesis that a significant number of particles are accessible to clearance by the mucociliary system at 24 hr. An alternative explanation of the bolus results, however, may be penetration of the particles into the alveoli (59). Deposition in the bronchioles, from which mucociliary clearance may be less effective, could be another possibility (54,59,60).

The alveolar elimination of insoluble particles is slow and may take years (61,62), with wide interindividual variations in clearance rates of identical particles (63). Philipson and co-workers (64) studied long-term clearance using 5.3-μm (AD) Teflon particles labeled with ^{195}Au. Retention by the thorax was followed for 900 days using two separate detector systems. Gold 195 activity in feces could be measured as long as activity in the thorax could be measured. For a 7–250 days, the half-lives were similar for the two detector systems, 740 and 680 days, respectively. The average half-lives, estimated from about 250 to 900 days, were 1750 days with the NaI detectors and 880 days with the Ge detectors. The Ge detectors cover a smaller area of the thorax and the measurements with the two detector systems indicate that translocation within the thoracic region occurred. This might be explained by transportation of particles from the lung parenchyma to the regional lymph nodes.

Recent studies in healthy subjects have suggested that a sizeable fraction of particles deposited in the bronchiolar region is retained for more than 72–96 hr, and that these particles clear more similarly to alveolarly deposited particles. An increased deposition with retentions in the smallest ciliated airways is supported by the similarity in the clearance patterns from these airways, by healthy subjects, for particles inhaled by bolus and particles inhaled extremely slowly (0.05 L/sec), with an intermediate phase of continued clearance between 24 and 96 hr (17,54). From these studies, clearance in the smallest ciliated airways seems to be incomplete, with retentions of about 40% of the particles assumed to have been deposited in the tracheobronchial region, probably because of ineffective mucociliary transport and cough clearance in small airways. Clearance from the bronchiolar region may have features in common with alveolar clearance (65). This region may thus constitute a vulnerable zone in which small airway diseases eventually may arise after repeated exposures to noxious agents.

Dust overload mechanisms have been studied by Oberdörster et al. (66)

using intratracheal instillation of radioactively labeled plastic microspheres of 3.3 and 10.3 μm in diameter in Fischer rats. Microscopic assessments revealed that essentially all of the particles were phagocytosed by alveolar macrophages within 24 hr postinstillation. The measured pulmonary retention half-lives for the small and large particles were 86–109 days and 870–1020 days, respectively. The results support the volumetric overload hypothesis.

IV. Airway Receptor Distribution

There is very limited information about longitudinal distribution of receptors in humans. Barnes and coworkers (67) have studied receptor distribution in ferrets. The results indicated that beta-adrenergic receptors were present in high density throughout the airways, with highest density in the bronchioles. Alpha receptors were sparse in large airways, but numerous in small bronchioles, whereas cholinergic receptors were numerous in bronchial smooth muscle, sparse in proximal bronchioles, and almost absent from distal bronchioles. This study has been frequently cited.

At least three subtypes of muscarinic receptors have been found in human lung, M_1–M_3 (68). Mak and Barnes (69) found that in human lung and lung from guinea pigs, muscarinic receptors have a different distribution from that reported in the ferret. Airway smooth muscle was distributed with M_3-receptor subtype, and there was a more peripheral distribution of receptors than was expected from the studies on ferret.

V. Bronchial Circulation

Blood flow to the airways varies greatly among species. The entire airway blood flow constitutes less than 3% of the cardiac output (70). The bronchial circulation is part of the systemic circulatory system and supplies extrapulmonary and pulmonary airways with oxygen and nutrients. The bronchial circulation is also involved in air-conditioning (i.e., warming and humidifying the inspired air). Furthermore, the bronchial circulation has been proposed to participate as a defense mechanism through a plasma exudation that washes away toxins (71). The extrapulmonary and pulmonary airways down to the terminal bronchioles are supplied from bronchial arteries that originate directly from the aorta or from intercostal arteries. There are at least two vascular plexus along the bronchial tree: one submucosal and one adventitial. There is also a potentially important anastomosis between the bronchial and pulmonary circulation, beyond the terminal bronchioles. The venous blood flow from the extrapulmonary airways, supporting structures, and extraparenchymal airways returns to the right atrium of the heart; the pulmonary circulation is supplied from the right ventricle and drains into the left atrium.

This complex circulation system has been proposed to be important for distribution of soluble components of particles deposited in the conducting airways (72; Fig. 6). Particles and drugs deposited in the extrapulmonary airways are absorbed into the bronchial circulation, are drained into the right atrium, and are then delivered back to the lung by the pulmonary circulation, diluted in venous blood coming from the systemic circulation. Drugs can possibly also reach the

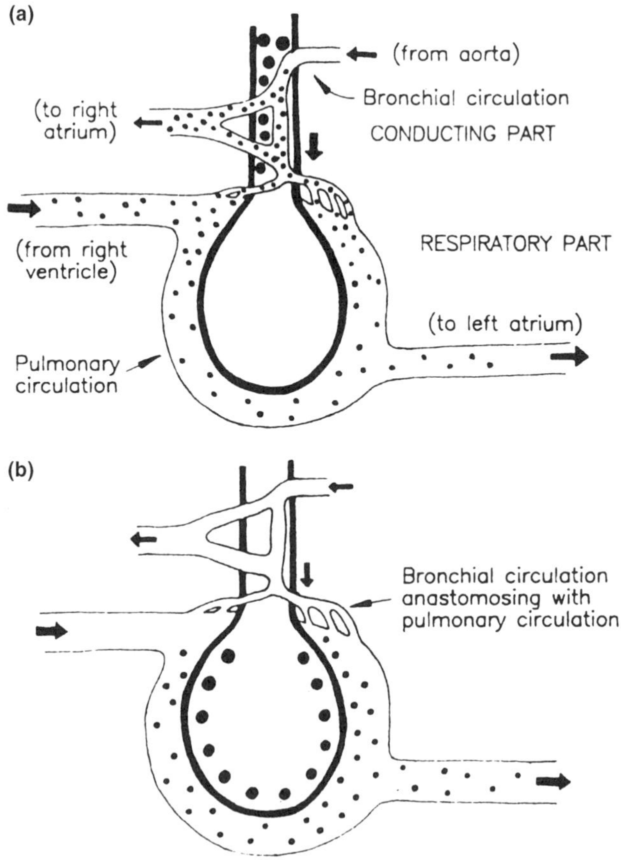

Figure 6 Schematic drawing of the bronchial and pulmonary circulation: (a) Aerosol particles deposited in the conducting parts (e.g., trachea, bronchi, bronchioles) of the lung; (b) aerosol particles deposited in the respiratory part (mainly alveolar region) of the lung; ● inhaled drug particles, • solute drug. (From Ref. 72.)

pulmonary region directly from the anastomosis between the bronchial and pulmonary circulation. Particles or drugs deposited in the pulmonary region are absorbed into the systemic circulation and become tremendously diluted by tissue distribution, and age eliminated by metabolism and biliary–renal excretion. Particles and drugs deposited in the pulmonary region, therefore, will probably have marginal effects only on other areas of the lung. The amount of particles or drugs returning to the lung through the pulmonary circulation is often insignificant. Ryrfeldt (72) proposed that the bronchial circulation with anastomosis and blood plexus might be very important for distribution of drugs, especially in a disease, such as obstructive lung disease, which includes constriction and hypertrophy of smooth muscles, hypertrophy of mucous glands, edema of the bronchial wall, and infiltration of various white blood cells. This mechanism provides a potential explanation for the good effect of inhaled drugs, with the bronchial circulation distributing drugs and particles evenly to parts that cannot be reached by the airway lumen. The importance of the airway circulation, as a local distribution system during inhalation, would be dependent on the ability of the aerosol to traverse the airway fluid lining and the epithelial layer and be absorbed by the submucosal vessels, the perfusion pattern of the capillary bed, and the stability of the inhaled agent (73). Experimental data in support of this interesting hypothesis is, however, scarce.

Information on the importance of absorption into the blood for the effect of local treatment within the lung is limited. Wollmer et al. (74), used the bronchial dilator terbutaline in aerosol form and reported data supporting the importance of the bronchial circulation. They found no difference in effect whether the aerosol was deposited centrally or peripherally in the lung of asthmatic patients. Dahlbäck et al. (75) presented a study using the tritiated glucocorticoid budesonide in rat lung. They found that owing to the high lipophilicity, the local concentration in the airways was much higher after inhalation than after systemic administration. Miller-Larsson et al. (76) presented interesting results from an animal model using rats. They studied uptake and dwell time of glucocorticoids in the airway tissue. Glucocorticoids were administered in three ways: by in situ superfusion, by intratracheal instillation, and by inhalation. They used budesonide, fluticasone propionate, and beclomethasone dipropionate. In all three models, the drugs had similar high topical uptake into the airway tissue 10–20 min after administration. The uptake of hydrocortisone was 50–100 times lower. The dwell time in the airway tissue was much higher for budesonide and fluticasone propionate, compared with beclomethasone dipropionate and hydrocortisone. The authors concluded that all of the inhaled types of glucocorticoids have a high topical uptake, but there are differences in retention in the airway tissue, and the prolonged release of glucocorticoids from the tissue may promote their topical anti-inflammatory action in the airways. Intracellular formation of an ester conjugate has been proposed as an explanation for the long retention of budesonide. Provided that local retention is important for the duration of clinical drug effect, then these studies illustrate the importance of topical treatment and regional deposition. The influence in distribution of the deposited steroid drug through the bronchial circulation is not fully understood. A consequence of the bronchial and pulmonary circulation systems would be that in diseases in the conducting airways the possibilities for redistribution of drugs deposited in the alveolar region back up to the airways is very limited; conversely, for diseases localized in the alveolar region, deposition in the conducting airways might be sufficient. Lipophilic drugs, for instance, may stay localized where they deposit. For insoluble particles, the airway circulation may influence particle clearance mainly by an indirect effect on the mucociliary system (73).

For lung diseases, it is also important to know that inflammation can increase bronchial flow (77–81). The importance of this for treatment of respiratory diseases with inhaled drugs is still unproved. Kuwano et al. (82) showed that the vascular area as a fraction of the airway wall was increased in asthmatic airways, probably owing to distension of existing vessels. Chronic inflammation causes extensive vascular remodeling in sheep airways (83). The bronchial circulation interacts with the pulmonary circulation and under conditions of acute lung injury, can attenuate edema formation and permeability changes (84). Also after pulmonary artery obstruction, bronchial blood flows markedly through to the obstructed region, presumably providing nutrient flow to the ischemic region (85). Bronchial circulation influences recovery from intravenous histamine challenge (86). Also, in a sheep model, recovery from challenge with methacholine through the bronchial artery was influenced by bronchial circulation (87). Bronchoconstrictor agents are less effective when mucosal blood flow is enhanced, presumably because the blood removes the agents more rapidly. In sheep, the magnitude and duration of the airway response to aerosol antigen challenge was increased by vasoconstriction (88).

Lorino et al. (89) studied the effects of intensive prolonged exercise on the pulmonary clearance rate of aerosolized ^{99m}Tc-labeled pentetic acid (^{99m}Tc-DTPA) in seven healthy nonsmoking volunteers. Clearance was measured before and after 75 min of constant-load exercise performed on a treadmill, corresponding to 75% of maximal oxygen uptake. Both measurements were made during similar conditions of pulmonary blood flow, respiratory rate, and tidal volume. After exercise, total, apical, and basal clearance were significantly increased; there were no changes in pulmonary mechanics. The results show that prolonged intensive exercise induces an increase in epithelial permeability, possibly by an alteration in the intercellular tight junctions, rather than from a surfactant deficiency, because no changes were evidenced in pulmonary volumes or in lung elasticity. Technegas might provide an alternative to ^{99m}Tc-DTPA in measurement of epithelial permeability (90). Thus, both methods can be used to test for increased airway permeability caused by inflammatory changes in the airways.

VI. Pulmonary Diseases Attributed to Aerosol Therapy

A. Obstructive Airway Diseases

Asthma and Chronic Bronchitis: Pathophysiological Changes

Bronchial asthma is characterized by an increased responsiveness of the trachea and bronchi to various stimuli and is manifested by a widespread narrowing of the airways that changes in severity either spontaneously or as a result of therapy (91). *Chronic bronchitis* is defined as a condition with chronic or recurrent bronchial hypersecretion, cough and expectoration during at least 3 months for at least 2 successive years (92). Chronic bronchitis is often associated with chronic airways obstruction with minimal reversibility; it is then called *chronic obstructive pulmonary disease* (COPD). Chronic airways obstruction in COPD is believed to be caused by either emphysema or irreversible obstructive changes in the peripheral airways, or both. There is an overlap between asthma and COPD, and many patients may have features of both diseases (93). Asthma is considered an important risk factor for the development of COPD. Bronchial hyperresponsiveness is a hallmark of asthma, whereas its importance in COPD is more obscure. Airway inflammation is a key factor for the development of bronchial hyperresponsiveness (94). Table 4 shows the main pathophysiological features of airways obstruction in asthma, chronic bronchitis, and emphysema.

In chronic bronchitis, the very first morphological change to occur in the peripheral airways are squamous cell metaplasia of the epithelium, associated with a progressive inflammatory reaction, leading to fibrosis of the airway walls and emphysema (95). Goblet cell metaplasia and mucosal ulceration appears with progress of the disease. With clinical progress of the disease, hypersecretion of mucus and cough become prominent symptoms. The epithelial mucus-secreting cells increase in number and extend down to the terminal bronchioles, where they replace the Clara cells (96). This results in production of mucus at a site

Table 4 Pathophysiological Features of Airway Obstruction

Bronchial asthma	Chronic bronchitis	Emphysema
Bronchial hyperresponsiveness	Mucus hypersecretion	Loss of alveolar walls
Airway inflammation (eosinophilia)	Mucous gland hypertrophy	Bronchiolitis
Smooth-muscle hypertrophy	Mural thickening	Normal clearance
Mucosal edema	Loss of cilia	
Hypersecretion or plugging	Impaired clearance	
Epithelial sloughing		
Normal or impaired clearance		

that may not easily be cleared by cough and in an instability of these airways, leading to early airway closure. Furthermore, the excessive secretion in the airways causes airflow obstruction. In bronchial asthma, smooth-muscle hypertrophy does not seem to be distributed uniformly throughout the lung. In states of nonfatal disease, the most pronounced changes may be found in the small bronchi and the bronchioles (97).

Mucociliary clearance is impaired in chronic bronchitis, even in the absence of apparent airways obstruction (98,99), as well as in symptom-free smokers (100). Impaired mucociliary transport may be an important pathogenic factor for the development of COPD. The association between impaired clearance and asthma is less clear. The impairment in asthma has been suggested to be a sign of airway inflammation and epithelial damage (101).

Emphysema

Morphological Changes

Emphysema is a condition of the lung characterized by an abnormal increase in size of the respiratory portion of the lung distal to the terminal bronchioles, either from dilation or from distraction of their walls. The bronchioles supplying emphysematous spaces are often inflamed, and neutrophil leukocytes are seen in the alveoli. The early respiratory bronchiolitis is followed by partial destruction and distension of respiratory bronchioles to the final appearance of emphysema. Tobacco smoking and environmental air pollution are causal factors, and the disease is rare at ages younger than 40 years. A second type of human emphysema is the familiar emphysema with α_1-antitrypsin deficiency. This type of emphysema often appears before the age of 40 years and involves predominantly the lower lobes. α_1-Antitrypsin is believed to neutralize proteolytic enzymes released from circulating leukocytes. In its absence, the enzymes are free to digest connective tissue of the lung. In nonsmoking patients with emphysema associated with α_1-antitrypsin deficiency, mucociliary clearance may be normal in the large airways (102).

Influence of Obstructive Airway Diseases on Aerosol Deposition

Most data concerning aerosol deposition have been obtained from healthy subjects; however, the deposition pattern may be quite different in patients with lung diseases (103). In patients with asthma or bronchitis, the airways may be narrowed by bronchospasm, edema, or mucous hypersecretion, which may increase impaction in the central airways of the lungs, thereby reducing aerosol penetration to the lung periphery (44,104–106). For instance, with noxious substances, an increased concentration of the substance may occur in a part of the lung that is already damaged. Furthermore, in patients with airway diseases, tracheobronchial clearance may be delayed, and the rapid clearance phase may not be completed within 24 hr (38,52,107,108). However, patients with asthma, chronic bronchitis, and immotile cilia syndrome, overall clear larger fractions of inhaled particles than healthy subjects owing to central deposition in obstructive airways (104,106,108). Studies of tracheobronchial clearance in subjects with immotile cilia syndrome provide unique possibilities for investigating other mechanisms behind tracheobronchial clearance than mucociliary transport (e.g., coughing). These subjects can effectively clear their airways by spontaneous or voluntary coughing, provided the particles are deposited in the central airways of the tracheobronchial region (108–110). Clearance of particles deposited in the small ciliated airways, however, is incomplete, probably owing to ineffective cough clearance in this region (111).

In previous studies, we found significant correlations between lung deposition and lung function measures for different respiratory diseases using a normal inhalation flow. Deposition is, for instance, correlated with R_{aw}, $FEF_{75-85\%}$ and N_2-delta in patients with asthma (39,112,113) and immotile cilia syndrome (108). In patients with chronic bronchitis, we have found that specific airway resistance (SR_{aw}) is slightly better correlated with lung retentions than with R_{aw} (38). In these patients, particles are more centrally deposited in the tracheobronchial region than in healthy subjects with induced bronchoconstriction, even at corresponding R_{aw} values. One tentative explanation for this discrepancy could be that changes in small airways are also important for the tracheobronchial deposition. Another explanation could be a generally more turbulent flow in diseased than in healthy airways, resulting in increased deposition in the tracheobronchial region (14,32). Lung retentions, considered to represent alveolarly deposited particles, have been normally distributed in asthma (39), as well as in chronic bronchitis (38). The relations found between R_{aw} and alveolar deposition for particles inhaled at a normal flow rate, in healthy subjects and in patients with obstructive airway diseases, exist because large airway anatomy controls penetration through the tracheobronchial tree, with an increased effect of impaction in larger airways when the diameters are diminished.

Inhaled aerosols are widely used as nonspecific provocation tests with histamine and methacholine and with specific provocation tests for different allergens. Comparison of data between research centers is hampered by differences in the methods used. Results are often given as concentration of the test substance in the nebulizer, giving rise to an effect such as 15 or 20% decrease in FEV_1 (PC_{20}) or 100% increase in specific airway resistance from baseline. The use of the corresponding provocation dose gives information on dose to the mouth, but without information on the nebulizer used or of particle size distribution, comparability cannot be ascertained. Aerosols of hypertonic saline have been used in induction of sputum for test of bronchial responsiveness (3,4). Analysis of sputum samples seems to be an interesting possibility as an alternative to bronchoalveolar lavage. Iredale and co-workers (5) found, however, no correlation between bronchial inflammation and bronchial responsiveness to inhaled hypertonic saline.

Therapeutic aerosols play a prominent role in the treatment of diseases of the lower airways, such as bronchial asthma and chronic bronchitis. It has been proposed that an increased deposition in the peripheral airways would be of value, in particular for treatment with inhaled corticosteroids. In patients with asthma, tracheobronchial deposition could be increased, practically independent of airway dimensions, by inhaling large aerosol particles extremely slowly (17,114). This could be a potentially useful approach of therapeutic importance, particularly in the treatment of patients with airways obstruction. Still, another possibility to enhance deposition of therapeutic aerosols in asthmatics could be the use of carrier gases such as helium–oxygen mixture (113).

B. Infectious Diseases of the Lung

Bacterial Pneumonia

Morphological Changes

Lobar pneumonia results from intralobular spread of infected edema fluid through aveoli, infection being halted only by the pleural membrane. Such infected fluid may flow through the bronchi from one lobe to another, resulting in multilobular involvement. Bronchopneumonia is due to inhalation of microorganisms into the bronchial tree, and localization of infection is due to a rapid neutrophil leukocyte response in the alveoli immediately surrounding the bronchiole or alveolus, in which the organisms lodge. At an early stage, the alveoli are filled with proteinaceous edema fluid in which bacteria can be detected. The capillaries surrounding the alveolar walls are densely congested. The zone of edema spreads rapidly to reach the hilum and pleura. At later stages, the alveoli become filled with macrophages, which remove the intra-alveolar cellular debris that results from disintegration of neutrophils and the remaining bacteria. The fluid exudate is absorbed into alveolar capillaries, or is cleared by lymphatics, and the lung again becomes fully aerated. If complications arise, there may be nonresolution, with the parenchyma undergoing fibrosis or carnification. Abscess formation and pleural effusion or emphysema may also complicate the pneumonic process.

Aerosol Therapy

The use of antibiotics in aerosol form has been reviewed by several authors, among them Stout and Derendorf (115). Several factors affect the penetration of antibiotics into sputum following systemic administration, among these are chemical properties, such as the molecular weight, lipophilicity, and protein binding. Also bronchial inflammation might cause alteration in tissue barriers. Intratracheal and aerosol administration of gentamicin resulted in low serum concentrations and high local levels (116). For penicillins and cephalosporins the penetration into bronchial secretions after systemical administration is limited. Ilowite et al. (117) presented a very nice review of the use of inhaled antibiotics. Topical treatment with aerosolized antimicrobial agents might be a solution for problems with poor penetration of many antibiotics into the lung and the high systemic toxicity for broad-spectrum antimicrobials. It is possibile to obtain a high local concentration of antibiotics and to overcome poor penetration into the lung, with less systemic absorption of certain antimicrobials and, consequently, less side effects and also to target specific areas of the lung. There are, however, several drawbacks, among them difficulties in determining the dose delivered to the lung and variable regional distribution in the lung, that are partly dependent on individual factors and partly on aerosol factors. Furthermore, emergence of resistant organisms may be a problem. Ilowite and co-workers (118) concluded that aerosol antibiotics, given as prophylactics, are extremely effective in altering the normal bacterial flora of the throat, but there is very little data in support on reduction in mortality. A general flaw in most of the studies is that too little attention has been paid to the choice of nebulizer, dose administered, and the pharmacokinetics of the inhaled agents. Drugs that have been used are polymyxin B, gentamicin, tobramycin, penicillins, and cephalosporins and, last but not least, pentamidine (see section on *Pneumocystis carinii* pneumonia). The authors conclude that treatment of chronic pulmonary infections and gram-negative pneumonias with a variety of agents has produced mixed results, and there is little consensus among physicians for the role, if any, of aerosol antibiotics for treatment of bacterial infections in the lung.

Viral Pneumonia

Morphological Changes

The virus attacks the ciliated respiratory epithelium of the airways, with necrosis of the epithelium. Usually, these changes affect mainly the upper conducting airways, but in severe and fatal cases, they extend down to the level of the terminal bronchioles, and the alveoli become filled with protein-containing edema fluid, red cells, and desquamated alveolar epithelial cells. Following alveolar epithelial cell necrosis, hyaline membranes are often prominent. With recovery from initial infection, the respiratory epithelium regenerates. During this period, however, the mucociliary defense mechanism is defective, and the respiratory tract is particularly prone to attack by secondary invaders.

Slauson et al. (119) have studied deposition, retention, and clearance of inhaled cobalt oxide particles from the lungs of calves with acute inflammatory lung injury induced by parainfluenza-3 virus. Typical parainfluenza-3 virus pulmonary lesions were found 7 days after virus infection. The animals were exposed to an aerosol of particulate cobalt oxide (geometric mean 0.6 μm) before onset of the infection. The animals were sacrificed at 0, 7, and 25 days after aerosol exposure. Control animals had a typically biphasic clearance pattern, with rapid initial clearance of 50% of the initial lung burden, followed by slower prolonged clearance. Clearance was significantly retarded in calves with viral-induced acute inflammatory lung injury. Ninety percent of the initial lung burden was retained at 7 days following exposure. Essentially all cobalt particles recovered by bronchoalveolar lavage were intracellular within pulmonary alveolar macrophages in both experimental and control groups.

Of special interest for inhalation therapy is the respiratory syncytial virus (RSV) infection in infants and young children. Two patterns of disease are present: acute bronchiolitis and interstitial pneumonia. The inflammatory edema of bronchiolitis will have serious effects on luminal diameter. In the early stages, there is necrosis of the lining epithelial cells. Later there is peribronchiolar lymphocytic infiltration and edema. In the fully developed case, the bronchiolar lumen is plugged by cellular debris and mucus. This plugging of small airways may result in collapse or acute overdistention of lung parenchyma. As the ciliated bronchiolar epithelium is destroyed, infection may penetrate to the distal parts of the lung. The parenchymal response to viral infections tends to be interstitial reaction, rather than an intra-alveolar exudation of inflammatory cells, which is more typical of bacterial infections. The inflammatory cell infiltration with lymphocytes occurs mainly within alveolar walls.

Aerosol Therapy

Aerosol treatment with ribavirin, 60 mg/mL for 2-hr periods, three times a day up to 5 days, has been used in children with suspected RSV infection (120). This high-dose, short-duration treatment was well tolerated by all patients. The concentration of ribavirin in lung secretion was rapidly cleared, but mean peak ribavirin triphosphate levels in erythrocytes were 15- to 300-fold higher than plasma ribavirin by the end of therapy. No adverse health effect was noted. There was more than a 98% reduction of viral load. The study, however, was not designed to evaluate the effect of drugs, but primarily the safety and efficacy. The authors concluded that this is a safe model to treat children. They also found tendencies toward higher concentrations in respiratory secretions for those who received the aerosolized drug by an endotracheal tube, compared with administration using an oxygen hood. Smith et al. (121) tested ribavirin against RSV infection in a study on 28 infants, age 1.4 ± 1.7 months. Among the 14 children receiving ribavirin, mean duration of mechanical ventilation was 4.9 days, compared with 9.9 days for placebo. Also, the duration of oxygen administration and mean length of hospital stay were significantly shorter for those receiving active treatment.

Inhaled beclomethasone dipropionate, 100 μg, has been tried in the treatment of 100 patients with acute tracheitis, tracheobronchitis, or bronchitis (122). There was no evidence that inhaled drug conferred any benefit or detriment on the progress of the conditions, as assessed by daily symptom scores and weekly clinical visits for up to 2 weeks.

Mycoplasmal Pneumonia

Patients with *Mycoplasma pneumoniae* infection have impaired mucociliary transport as measured 1–2 weeks after onset of the disease (123). Clearance improved significantly within 3 weeks. Tracheobronchial clearance was studied in 17 nonsmokers who had suffered from a serologically verified *M. pneumoniae* pneumonia 5–15 months earlier (124). The subjects inhaled 6-μm–Teflon particles tagged with ^{99m}Tc. The retention of particles in the lung was measured for 2 hr. The retention in this group was significantly higher than in a control group of healthy nonsmokers. This result suggests that some impairment persists 5–15 months after the infection, or that persons with slow clearance contract a mycoplasmal pneumonia more easily than do those with fast clearance. Aerosol therapy has, so far, no place in the treatment of pulmonary infection with *m. pneumoniae*.

Pneumocystis carinii *Pneumonia*

Morphological Changes

Pneumocystis pneumonia occurs in patients with congenital or acquired immunodeficiency, for instance transplant patients and others who are receiving immunosuppressive therapy. Not infrequently, *Pneumocystis* pneumonia coexists with other pulmonary infections. The infection may be diffuse or focal, with a propensity to affect the lower lobes. In contrast with several other forms of pneumonia, there is no fibrinous pleurisy. The alveolar septa are increased in thickness and infiltrated with plasma cells and lymphocytes. The characteristic feature is the intra-alveolar exudate. This is foamy and strongly periodic acid–Schiff (PAS) positive, being composed of parasitic cysts. An intra-alveolar cellular reaction to the exudate is absent, and a few areas of hyaline membrane formation may be found. The diagnosis may be obtained by lung biopsy material. The organism may also be seen in sputum. In some instances, diffuse interstitial fibrosis may be the end result.

Aerosol Therapy and Prophylaxis

Over the last decade there has been much interest in the possibility of using inhaled antibiotics. Virtually all of the studies that have been performed have been with pentamidine treatment or prophylaxis against *P. carinii* pneumonia (PCP) in patients suffering from either human immunodeficiency virus (HIV) infection or other immune deficiency syndromes. Use of the inhalation route can be an advantage for drugs that have low gastrointestinal absorption and low absorption from the lung. Lidman et al. (125) demonstrated that aerosolized pentamidine, 300 mg initially and then 60 mg twice every month, was as good as intravenous dosages of 200–300 mg biweekly. They concluded that pentamidine for secondary prophylaxis might be useful either way. Among 78 patients, 25 deaths were recorded, and recurrent PCP contributed to death in only 1 case. The authors conclude that PCP is not the most serious problem in immunodeficient patients. Lidman et al. (126) also demonstrated that aerosolized pentamidine has significant prophylactic efficacy, but they could not detect any major effect on mortality and morbidity. The overall mortality and morbidity were not markedly influenced by *P. carinii* pneumonia. The authors conclude that pentamidine can be a justified alternative for treatment in selected patients.

Nybo Jensen et al. (127) investigated the efficacy of a biweekly dose of 60 mg aerosolized pentamidine for PCP prophylaxis. Pentamidine was administered by a System 22 nebulizer. There were 15 cases of *Pneumocystis* pneumonia among 105 patients (13%) in the prophylaxis group and 32 cases among 104 control patients (30%) during the 18-month study ($p = 0.002$). During the study period 19 patients (18%) in the prophylaxis group died, and 24 patients (23%) in the control group died ($p = 0.28$). There was no difference in survival between the groups, suggesting that pentamidine prophylaxis has an influence on morbidity only. Guinet et al. (128) followed 456 patients with HIV. Pentamidine was given as primary prophylaxis at 300 mg/month, or as secondary prophylaxis at 300 mg twice a month, which was well tolerated. The authors concluded that aerosolized pentamidine is of prophylactic value second to trimethoprim–sulfamethoxasol. Side effects are acceptable.

Ng et al. (129) reported that in prophylactic treatment with aerosolized pentamidine, there was no difference in the diagnostic yield from induced sputum specimens in *Pneumocystis* pneumonia. Katial and co-workers (130), however, reported a case of PCP in a patient with acquired immunodeficiency while receiving aerosolized pentamidine prophylaxis. The authors found that there was an underlying ventilatory abnormality and that the aerosolized pentamidine might not have reached the region in which *P. carinii* pneumonia started. This might support the importance of topical distribution of pentamidine.

Since the introduction of aerosolized pentamidine prophylaxis, the incidence of PCP has decreased significantly (131,132). In normal subjects, the upper lobes receive relatively less ventilation than the lower lobes (133). It has also been proposed that patients receiving aerosolized pentamidine prophylaxis develop pneumonia in the upper lobes, as read from chest radiographs (134). O'Riordan et al. (135) performed a study on 51 HIV-positive patients. Bronchoalveolar lavage (BAL) was performed, using a bronchoscope, in the right middle lobe and the apical segment of the right upper lobe, or if predominantly left-sided disease, BAL was performed in the lingula and the apical-posterior segment. There were very similar concentrations of pentamidine in the BAL supernatant and the cell pellet of BAL from PCP-negative patients. For PCP-positive patients ($n = 32$), the concentration differed: 37.8 ng/mL in the cell pellet of BAL for upper lobe, versus 57.5 ng/mL for the middle lobe. This difference, however, was not significant owing to the large standard deviations. The authors concluded that regional differences in pentamidine dose did not significantly contribute to failure of pentamidine prophylaxis. It still remains a possibility that the concentration could be important. Other possible reasons for not detecting a ''true'' difference could be method variations in the BAL technique. Treatment was further carried on over several months and recidivism might be due to earlier low levels of pentamidine. We have no information on what the least effective concentrations are as measured by BAL method. Smaldone and co-workers (136) compared subjects receiving PCP prophylaxis with aerosolized pentamidine using AeroTech II nebulizer. They found no differences in the deposited amount of pentamidine among failures, 8.18 ± 4.74 mg, compared with protected patients, 6.39 ± 3.07 mg. Most of the variability in deposition was accounted for by variability in nebulizer output.

O'Riordan and Smaldone (137) have studied the influence of ventilation on regional deposition. They studied ten male subjects with HIV-infection. Pentamidine in solution was labeled with technetium bound to human serum albumin. By superimposing deposited ^{99m}Tc on ventilation distribution of ^{81m}Kr, information on the influence of regional ventilation on deposition was obtained. The ratios of upper to lower lobe deposition were less than predicted from regional ventilation and were fairly constant. The upper/lower lobes ratios were not significantly influenced by particle size for the Respirgard II jet nebulizer (small particles) 0.83 ± 0.05 (mean ± SE) and a little higher for ultrasonic Fisoneb device (0.86 ± 0.04; large particles). Fisoneb gave a more central deposition than did the Respirgard II. Finally, the authors could not demonstrate a positive effect of the bronchodilator agent albuterol, either in lung function or in the distributions, central to peripheral, in those HIV patients who had FEV_1/FVC of more than 80%. One possible way to predict if bronchodilator pretreatment has a potential beneficial effect could be to measure simple pulmonary function reversibility.

Thomas et al. (138) studied pulmonary deposition by different nebulizers, using ^{99m}Tc human serum albumin (HSA) as an indirect marker of pentamidine. Alveolar retention was estimated by scans after 24 hr. Pulmonary deposition in milligrams, from an inhaled dose of 300 mg pentamidine, ranged from 2.9 to 14.3 mg. The nebulizers giving the largest particles also had a significantly higher central/peripheral ratio. The ventilation-corrected ratios between upper and lower lobes ranged from 0.61 to 0.76 for the different nebulizers. Alveolar deposition was estimated using 24-hr retention and ranged from 53 to 71%. The validity of alveolar deposition is dependent on unsubstantiated assumptions about the fate of ^{99m}Tc HSA marker and that mucociliary clearance from the airways is normal after *P. carinii* infection. The nebulizer producing the largest particles also caused significantly lower FEV_1 values in the patients. There was a relation between side effects and nebulizer and particle size. This study illustrates the importance of a knowledge about equipment characteristics in the administration of drugs.

Ilowite and co-workers (118) compared equipment for administration of pentamidine to HIV patients. They studied the Respirgard II, Aero Tech II, Portasonic, and Fisoneb nebulizers. The mass median aerodynamic diameter was 0.9, 1.3, 1.4, and 3.9 μm, respectively. They used inhalations of 60 mg pentamidine in 3 mL of sterile water and 1 mL of ^{99m}Tc bound to HSA. Deposition in the lung expressed as percentage of amount placed in the nebulizer was 5.3, 15.7, 17.3, and 26.4%, respectively. Extrapulmonary deposition in percentage of dose in the nebulizer was 0.4, 2.7, 4.4, and 4.9%, respectively. There was a clear correlation between side effects and extrapulmonary deposition. The nebulizers used in the study were all slightly modified. In this study, patient factors influenced the regional distribution at least as much as aerosol particle size. In the choice of nebulizer, one has to take advantages and disadvantages for specific situations into account. For patients who easily develop bronchospasm, a nebulizer producing the least amount of side effects, in this case the Respirgard II, could be of advantage. On the other hand, if the dose to the lung and time to nebulize is important, then the Fisoneb nebulizer could be the appropriate choice.

O'Doherty et al. (139) showed that the incidence of adverse airway effects were related to deposition in the large airways, or to larger particles. These authors have compared different inhalation systems for particle size distribution. They studied nine male patients receiving 150 mg pentamidine labeled with ^{99m}Tc-Sn-colloid in 4 mL of water. Respirgard II system with baffles delivered 73 ± 12% alveolar deposition, compared to 47 ± 8% for Acorn 22 nebulizer, and 53% ± 13% for Respirgard system without an inspiratory baffle. Alveolar deposition was defined as 24-hr retention as a percentage of the initial lung deposition. Respirgard II system with baffle had a mass median diameter of 1.0 μm and 99% of the particles were smaller than 5 μm compared with a MMD of 3.4 μm for Acorn 22 and 1.7 μm for Respirgard II without battle. This report also provides data for droplet sizes produced by different commercially available nebulizers, illustrating that most nebulizers give a higher fraction of larger particles than Respirgard II. The target for pentamidine should be the alveolar region.

There are quite a number of studies on inhalation treatment of *P. carinii* pneumonia. They show that pentamidine might be useful for selected patients in addition to oral treatment with antibiotics. Side effects are dependent on aerosol particle size, and the treatment should be targeted toward the alveolar region.

Fungal Infections

Morphological Changes

Some fungal infections may be treated by inhalation therapy, for instance, aspergillosis. The respiratory tract is the main portal of entry for this fungus and the lung is the most frequent site for infection. *Aspergillus* infections may be divided into noninvasive aspergillosis, with allergic reaction or the formation of fungus balls in preexisting bullae or cavities, and invasive aspergillosis, with necrotizing bronchopneumonia. The allergic form usually presents as asthma, with identical histological findings. The invasive form is most often encountered in patients whose defense mechanisms are compromised. The pneumonic areas are characterized by an edematous hemorrhagic exudation into alveoli, accompanied by numerous polymorphonuclear cells. Fungal hyphae can be seen in these zones.

Aerosol Therapy

Antifungal agents, such as amphotericin B and nystatin, have been administered by aerosols or intratracheal instillations (140–143). Diot et al. (144) investigated inhaled labeled amphotericin B (5 mg) by either Fisoneb, or DP100 (ultrasonic), or Respirgard II (jet) nebulizers in three patients suffering from pulmonary aspergilloma. Inhaled mass of the three nebulizers, assessed as percentage drug caught in inspiratory filters in duplicate experiments, were 5.8 and 3.6% for Respirgard II, 26.5 and 28.3% for Fisoneb, and 5.9 and 6.3% for DP100. Mass median aerodynamic diameters were given as 10.3 μm for Respirgard II, 4.8 μm for Fisoneb, and 2.3 μm for DP100. Amphotericin B serum concentrations correlated with pulmonary deposition and remained lower than 25 mg/mL. No untoward effects were reported by the patients during the 4-week trial. This study demonstrates that amphotericin B suspension can be administrated by a variety of nebulizers. The study was extremely limited in size, and the results indicated quite large differences between combinations of patients and the nebulizers used. The allergic form of *Aspergillus* bronchopulmonary ''infection'' should be treated with systemic steroids.

C. Other Diseases

Sarcoidosis

Morphological Changes

Sarcoidosis is a systemic disease of unknown etiology. It is characterized by noncaseating epitheloid granuloma in several organs or tissues. Intrathoracic disease is the most common manifestation. Histological examination of tissues is of prime importance in establishing the diagnosis. In the active stage, typical epithelioid granulomas, with giant cells, are present in alveolar and interlobular septa, in subpleural regions, and in lymph nodes, but there are none to be seen within alveolar spaces. Ulceration of bronchial mucosa is uncommon, but deeper regions of the bronchial wall may be involved in the disease, and this can be reflected in disturbances of airway function. The granuloma have a proclivity for peribronchiolar and perivascular sites. There is a predominant venous involvement. Smaller sarcoid lesions may undergo complete resolution. Larger granuloma heal by fibrosis, which may be followed by pulmonary hypertension.

Aerosol Therapy

Treatment of pulmonary sarcoidosis using inhaled budesonide has been reported in a few studies (145–147). Spiteri et al. (147) found that 21.2% of the dose of 3-μm (AD) Teflon particles from MDI and Nebuhaler spacer reached the lung. Alberts and co-workers (148) studied the effect of budesonide on newly diagnosed pulmonary sarcoidosis in a double-blind placebo-controlled design. Inclusion criteria were age 20–65 years, diagnosis of pulmonary sarcoidosis within 6 months before entering the study, biopsy-proved histology, and chest radiographic stages I, II, or III, abnormal lung function, with decreased inspiratory vital capacity (IVC) below 79%, or transfer factor for carbon monoxide (TLCO) below 77% of predicted. Patients without lung function impairment could also be included if they had chest radiographic stage II or III and more than 20% lymphocytes in BAL fluid. Treatment consisted of budesonide 1.2 mg (six puffs of 0.2 mg) once daily for 6 months. Patients global clinical impression score showed a significant difference in favor of the budesonide, when compared with nontreatment. Inspiratory vital capacity (IVC) showed a significant difference of 7.9% predicted between the two groups during active treatment and during follow-up. Transfer factor for carbon monoxide (TLCO) remained unchanged over time. Improvement in chest radiographic appearance and change in serum angiotensin-converting enzyme (ACE) were similar for both groups. The authors concluded that inhaled corticosteroids in pulmonary sarcoidosis may reduce deterioration and postpone a need for systemic corticosteroids.

Adult Respiratory Distress Syndrome and Acute Lung Injury

Morphological Changes

Patients in the intensive care units, with a variety of conditions, often unconnected with the thorax and lungs, may develop a syndrome of acute respiratory failure. This is called shock lung, as it was first noticed in patients who suffered from trauma followed by an initial period of shock and hypotension. The initiating processes are many, for instance high-level oxygen delivery, burns, influenza, hemorrhagic shock, drowning, and septic shock. Almost all patients had at some stage had mechanical ventilation accompanied by oxygen therapy. Histological examination reveals diffuse alveolar damage with collapse, congestion, interstitial and alveolar edema, desquamation of lining epithelium, and hyaline membrane formation. Necrotic alveolar epithelium is replaced by an amorphous eosinophilic mass. This mass comprises the hyaline membranes, which form the characteristic findings of this condition. They are particularly prominent in alveolar ducts and respiratory bronchioles. The hyaline membranes may be seen after 24 hr, but usually they are found between 4 and 7 days after onset of respiratory distress. Following this acute alveolar damage is a prominent cellular lining of alveoli of type II pneumonocytes. Their hyperplasia is at a maximum at 14 days.

Many of these patients die, but some may recover completely. Recovery, however, can be impaired or delayed by intensive oxygen therapy, by pulmonary edema caused by overtransfusion, or by secondary infections. After 14 days, fibroblasts become increasingly prominent in the alveolar walls and often the end result is severe interstitial fibrosis. This progressive alveolar duct fibrosis may also account for death in patients.

The precise mechanism whereby the changes following traumatic shock are initiated is not understood. In many patients there may be a period of profound pulmonary hypoperfusion, leading to endothelial damage with interstitial and intra-alveolar edema. This may be accompanied by decreased or absent surfactant synthesis owing to functional impairment of type II cells. The surfactant that is present will be inactivated by the edema fluid, resulting in the alveolar collapse and decreased compliance observed clinically. The changes may further be aggravated by administration of high concentrations of oxygen, which is very toxic to alveolar epithelium. The necrosis of alveolar epithelium and hyaline membrane formation, together with type II cell hyperplasia and thickening of the alveolar capillary barrier, gives rise to further difficulty in oxygenation of the blood. Increasing the oxygen concentration further worsens the situation, creating a vicious cycle, eventually leading to death.

Aerosol Therapy

Treatment of both underborn children with immature lungs lacking surfactant and adults with adult respiratory distress syndrome (ARDS), with suspensions of exogenous surfactant, most often as a bolus instillation, has shown promising results (149–154). A drawback with bolus instillation has been the risk of adding excess liquid to the lungs in early stages of ARDS, causing negative effects on blood gas levels.

Several studies have compared the administration of aerosols with bolus instillation of exogenous surfactant. For example, Li et al. (155) compared administration of 250 mg surfactant as an aerosol with instillation of about 25 mg in rats. Lung damage was induced initially by repeated lung lavage to deploy the animals' own surfactant. Surfactant aerosol was generated by the ultrasonic nebulizer and the droplet diameter was 3.4 ± 1.2 μm. Fresh surfactant was added to the nebulizer every 15 min to avoid changes in surface properties of the surfactant.

Determination of phospholipid revealed 35–45% of aerosolized surfactant in the filter of the nebulizer circuit and 50–60% in the expiratory tubing as condensed liquid. Less than 10% of the total amount of the aerosolized preparation had a possibility to reach the animal lung. Both groups showed improvement in blood gas values. There was no better effect using the aerosol route. Improved administration seems necessary to make inhalation a competitive way to administer surfactant. The advantage will possibly be that one can avoid initial addition of liquid to the lung. However, in this study, no acute effect of administration of a liquid bolus was seen (155). Lewis and McCaig (156) used an adult sheep model to evaluate aerosol versus instilled exogenous surfactant. In this study, aliquots of hydrochloric acid were bronchoscopically instilled into selected lobes. Thereafter, the whole lung underwent repetitive saline lavage to induce diffuse lung injury. Surfactant was administered either by instillation of 4 g surfactant or as a nebulized aerosol of about 500 mg during a total of 3 hr. Initially 10 mL of surfactant at concentrations of 25 mg/mL of phospholipid given to the nebulizer, thereafter aliquots of 5 mL as needed. Animals treated with aerosolized surfactant had significant increases in $Pa{O_2}$ values, starting at 60 min after treatment through 180 min, compared with pretreatment values. Animals treated with the instilled surfactant had significant increases in values from 90 min after treatment versus pretreatment. Ventilatory parameters such as $Pa{CO_2}$ were significantly lower for the nebulized surfactant group throughout the treatment period. For the group getting instilled surfactant, there were significant increases in $Pa{CO_2}$ after 15 min. Distribution of the surfactant was more uneven for the instilled surfactant compared with nebulizer administration. Approximately 50% of the total amount instilled surfactant, compared with 8% for the total aerosolized surfactant deposited, could be recovered from the most severely damaged lung lobes.

Cystic Fibrosis

Morphological Changes

Cystic fibrosis is a recessive genetic disease reflecting mutations in gene coding for CF transmembrane regulator protein, which normally functions as a cyclic adenosine monophosphate (cAMP)-regulated chloride channel. Functional abnormalities include thick airway secretions, resulting from defective chloride secretion and its related defect in excessive sodium absorption. Changes in the lungs are plugging of small bronchi and bronchioles by mucoid exudate. Secondary infections with bronchitis and bronchiolitis result in mucosal ulceration and fibrosis, frequently followed by true obliterative bronchiolitis, leading to collapse and fibrosis of pulmonary parenchyma. The airways are filled with infected debris. The infection spreads through all layers of the bronchial wall and bronchiectasis may be the result from a combination of obstructive collapse and severe inflammatory changes. A notable feature is alveolar distension, which alternates with the zones of collapse and fibrosis. The increased viscosity of sputum in cystic fibrosis is often due to the high DNA content brought about by secondary pyogenic infection, usually by *Staphylococcus aureus* or *Pseudomonas aeruginosa*. There are great advantages to treating these patients with aerosols.

Aerosol Therapy

Patients suffering from cystic fibrosis are often treated with aerosolized drugs; for example, antibiotics, such as aminoglycosides (gentamicin, tobramycin, and others), and drugs to treat the functional abnormalities caused by abnormal ion transport to diminish excessive sodium absorption, using amiloride and possibly also triphosphate nucleotides, preferably uridine triphosphate (UTP), to induce chloride secretion by non–cystic fibrosis transmembrane regulator (CFTR) channels (157). Virtually all patients with cystic fibrosis develop chronic obstructive airway disease. There are studies (9,158,159), suggesting that the obstructive lung disease has considerable influence on drug administration. This is also in accordance with our own studies, showing very close relations between lung deposition and airway dimensions, measured by airway resistance, and lung function measures reflecting small airway changes (39,108,112,113). Martonen et al. (160) performed calculations using different airway dimensions in a computed model. They concluded that airway caliber enhances the dose delivered to the tracheobronchial tree by a factor of 2–3, relative to controls. A tendency toward shallow breathing might also influence aerosol administration. The need for more experimental and modeling studies on patients, rather than healthy subjects, is also pointed out.

Antibiotic Treatment

Aerosol antibiotics in controlled studies improved lung function and reduced the number of acute hospital admissions in patients with cystic fibrosis. Minimal drug hypersensitivity has been reported, and there is no solid evidence that the small increase in resistance to some antibiotics, associated with the use of aerosol antibiotics, is in any way detrimental to the patients (for review, see 161). The drugs used are, for example, tobramycin, carbenicillin, and gentamicin.

Nebulization of antibiotics in cystic fibrosis has also been reviewed (162). For β-lactams, an improvement in pulmonary function was demonstrated with carbenicillin (163). For polymyxin, colistin alone (164), or in conjunction with oral ciprofloxacin (165), there was a decrease in the rate of decline in pulmonary function and in the frequency of *P. aeruginosa* recovered from respiratory tract secretions. Antibiotics of this class have been reported to cause bronchospasm and respiratory failure (166). Aminoglycosides have been administered as aerosols since 1950, and they have demonstrated improvement of pulmonary function, decreased sputum bacterial density, no ototoxicity or renal toxicity, and according to Smith and Ramsey (162), they are of clinical benefit for patients with cystic fibrosis. Treatment by inhaled antibiotics has been reviewed by Touw et al. (167). They found eight placebo-controlled studies, six of them showing significant improvement of lung function in the treatment groups of patients with cystic fibrosis. Four studies showed a reduction in the number of hospital admissions. Studies with antibiotic aerosols as adjuncts to intravenous therapy in patients with cystic fibrosis with an acute exacerbation, showed no enhancement of the clinical effects of the intravenous antibiotic by the aerosol. However, sputum colony counts were lower. Toxicity studies carried out have as yet shown no renal or ototoxicity. There is still a need for long-term toxicity studies to be performed. Selection of resistant bacteria is relatively rare, but remains a matter of concern. The authors conclude that treatment with an appropriate antibiotic in high enough dosages can be recommended for patients with cystic fibrosis who are chronically infected with *P. aeruginosa*.

Zach (168) has shown a relation between peak serum levels of gentamicin and inhaled dose in children with cystic fibrosis. The children inhaled 120 mg of gentamicin from a jet-type nebulizer that produces particles of 0.5 and 5.5 μm at 0.38 mL/min. Inhalation of repeated doses with 360 and 600 mg of gentamicin were given. Peak gentamicin serum levels were measured with a high correlation with the given dose. After a 600-mg dose by inhalation, serum levels were between 1.5 and 4.2 mg/mL, with the average 2.5 mg/mL. Steinkamp et al. (169) investigated 14 patients with cystic fibrosis, ages 8–19 years, receiving tobramycin aerosol therapy for a mean duration of 20 months. Eighty milligrams of tobramycin were inhaled twice daily after physiotherapy with a Pariboy or Pari-Privat jet-nebulizer, using slow and deep inhalations. After 1 year, weight-for-height increased significantly by 2.9% of predicted normal. Clinical score improved, and the frequency of hospital admissions decreased from 2.0 to 1.3 per patient during the years before and after the study onset. No evidence of ototoxicity or renal damage was observed. The highest serum level of tobramycin was 0.4 mg/L. Systemic absorption seems to be the exception to the rule.

Mucolytic Treatment

Tomkiewicz et al. (170) have studied treatment in cystic fibrosis using amiloride inhalation. Prolonged, 25-week therapy significantly increased the sputum sodium and chloride content. The sputum potassium content was unaltered. An index of sputum rigidity decreased during treatment, corresponding to a threefold decrease in viscoelasticity. There was no corresponding change in mucous solids contents. There are indicative results that aerosolized UTP treatment increase mucociliary clearance (171).

VII. Aerosols for Systemic Treatment

Aerosols might be used for systemic treatment, and this has been reviewed (172). Systemic treatment might be valuable for drugs (e.g., polypeptides) to bypass the enteral route because of its proteolytic activity and first-pass metabolism. Inhalation applications using insulin, heparin, ergotamine, ribavirin, and aminoglycosides have not revealed any relevant allergic reactions (173–182). For insulin, uptake into the blood was increased for smokers, compared with nonsmokers (174).

Heparin seems to be a most promising substance, and its effects have been shown for more than 24 hr, and also on postmyocardial survival rate and on atherosclerosis (180,182). A general problem with the inhalation route can be as illustrated for insulin in that transport of the drug from the lung into the blood can be increased by cigarette smoking and by different lung diseases, such as sarcoidosis, allergic alveolitis, ARDS, infections, and possibly asthma (87,88, 174,181,183–188).

Metered-dose propellant-driven aerosols of an antigenically reactive protein have been produced by combining bovine gammaglobulin with surfactants soluble in freon or dimethylether propellants (189). Propellants for delivering protein aerosols need further development. In this study, dimethylether was most effective, but this propellant is not approved by the US Food and Drug Administration (FDA) for respiratory aerosols.

Weissman and co-workers (190) have studied the effect of localized deposition of antigen in the human lung. They used a well-characterized, highly immunogenic, soluble antigen, keyhole limpet hemocyanin (KLH), in ten healthy nonsmoking volunteers. Follow-up BALs were performed, 10–14 days after immunization, in the immunized, superior lingular segment and the contralateral, unimmunized, medial segment of the right middle lobe. There were greater albumin concentrations and cell recoveries in the immunized segments than in the control segments, suggesting local inflammation. The total number of cells was increased; however, the proportion of alveolar macrophages, lymphocytes, and neutrophils were similar. CD4/CD8 ratios were greater in the immunized segments and anti-KLH IgG and IgA concentrations were higher. The IgA/albumin ratios were higher in the immunized segments than in serum, suggesting local production, or active transport of serum-derived anti-KLH IgA. The results support the importance of local deposition and also the important role for $CD4^+$ to T cells and secretory IgA in respiratory tract responses to exogenous soluble antigen.

Immunization might also become a problem, for instance, when using viral vectors in gene therapy.

VIII. General Types of Devices and Aerosol Administration

There are several possibilities for administration of drugs to the lung. One would be instillation of liquid directly through a bronchoscope, or corresponding type instrument. Other ways that are commonly used in treatment are metered-dose inhalers (MDI) using a jet-discharge. These can be combined with spacers. Several years ago, the use of chlorinated fluorocarbons (CFC) as propellants in MDI have been banned in Sweden. Alternative propellants, fluorinated hydrocarbons (HFA), have been developed and more countries have taken action against CFCs in MDIs. New propellants might change aerosol characteristics, which might influence the dose to the lung. Lung deposition, for example, is much improved with HFA (191,192) for beclomethasone dipropionate per MDI compared with the corresponding CFC formulation. It is important to evaluate the full combination of an inhalation device and the drug. Aerosols can also be delivered as a dry powder, single-dose or multidose equipment, and these have a widespread use, especially in the Scandinavian countries. There is also a possibility to use nebulization primarily by jet or ultrasonic nebulizers.

A. Metered-Dose Inhaler and Spacer

There are studies showing an improved clinical effect in bronchodilation in asthmatic patients when MDIs are combined with auxiliary devices (see, e.g., 193–196). These auxiliary devices provide extra space between the actuator and the mouth, diminishing impaction. There is also a possibility, to some extent, for large-volume spacers to dry out the particles. Kim et al. (197) have, in a laboratory setup, compared four different kinds of auxiliary devices, one open-end straight tube and three commercially available spacers; namely, the Aerochamber, Nebuhaler, and InspirEase. In essence, at oropharyngeal deposition of MDI aerosols of different kinds ranged from 33 to 71% at 0.33 L/sec, slightly higher at higher airflows. With auxiliary devices, the oropharyngeal deposition was drastically reduced to less than 6% at the low airflow and slightly higher at an increased airflow. The loss in the spacers corresponded highly with the diminished oropharyngeal deposition. The total amount reaching the lung with spacer in this model was slightly lower or similar for all spacers except Nebuhaler, which had a similar or higher dose to the lung, compared with the actuator alone. The improved lung depositions for Nebuhaler only, are most probably due to its large size.

The foregoing results do not explain why MDI and auxiliary devices give greater bronchodilation than MDI alone, with the possible exception for Nebuhaler. On the other hand, one can conclude that oropharyngeal deposition does not add substantially to bronchodilator effect. The potentially greatest advantage using spacer would probably be that the inhalation technique would be less important. The spacers are useful to avoid oropharyngeal deposition, but are sometimes perceived as bulky by the patients.

Newman and co-workers (198) compared deposition of particles, with and without an open spacer device. Distribution of labeled drug and unlabeled drug and radioactivity was similar using an impinger system. Inhalation using a spacer resulted in slightly higher whole-lung deposition, 16.1 versus 11.0%. There was a corresponding decrease in oral deposition. Vidgren and co-workers (199) showed a positive effect on the fraction of the dose reaching the lungs using the InspirEase spacer device compared with conventional aerosol actuator. The main effect, however, is, to reduce deposition in the upper airways. This was studied using labeled disodium cromoglycate and gamma camera imaging. Barry and O'Callaghan (200) studied the effect of electrostatic field strength for new spacers. They found that there is a large reduction in delivered dose from a spacer yield owing to an electrostatic field. For new spacers, 19.3 μg was delivered from an actuation of 100 μg with a 20-sec delay, only 3.3 μg was delivered. In a used spacer, the corresponding figures were 54.2 μg delivered without delay and 40.8 μg delivered after a 20-sec delay. The output from the Volumatic spacer was also reduced by multiple actuations, 20.7 μg/100 μg after five actuations compared with 42.4 μm/100 μg actuation after two actuations. Callaghan and co-workers (201) determined the amount of cromolyn sodium (sodium cromoglycate) particles smaller than 5 μm available for inhalation from Fisonair spacer devices 0.5 mg of particles smaller than 5 μm were delivered from a 5-mg actuation directly from the MDI. After one actuation with spacer, 0.59 mg was delivered. After three actuations, 0.26 mg/actuation was delivered. Also, 10-sec delay before inhalation decreased the amount from 0.59 to 0.23 mg. Antistatic lining increased the amount of particles available to 1.44 mg, or 244%, immediately before inhalation and 0.52 mg at a 20-sec delay before inhalation. This study illustrates the problem with losses from electrostatic fields and also that multiple actuations into the spacer before inhalation should be avoided, and finally, that inhalation should be performed immediately after actuation.

Drug delivery from holding chambers with attached facemask has been studied (202). The authors used a model to simulate respiratory pattern of individuals and determination of deposition on a filter. The dose delivered to the filter was dependent on the combination tidal volume and size of spacer device. The dose deposited on the filter ranged from less than 1% up to maximum 5.3%. The authors could also show that the introduction of a large dead space decreased drug delivery.

Newman et al. (203) compared different methods to estimate total lung deposition. They compared radiolabeled, pressurized pMDIs, and a pharmacokinetic technique (charcoal-block), to determine whole-lung deposition. Regional distribution of drug within the lung and deposition in the oropharynx was assessed by gamma scintigraphy, but not by charcoal-block method. Whole-lung deposition was 11.2% using the charcoal-block method for pMDI at 30 L/min, compared with 10.7% for gamma scintigraphy. A decrease in pulmonary deposition of increased flow to 180 L/min was detected using the charcoal-block method—7.2% lung deposition—but not by gamma scintigraphy, 10.4%. Using pMDI and nebuhaler spacer, deposition increased up to 33.8% for charcoal-block method and 31.6% for gamma scintigraphy. Inside surfaces of the spacer were treated using benzalkonium chloride before use.

B. Dry Powder Inhalers

Patients, especially young children, might have difficulties in using pMDI inhalers, unless a spacer device is used. To overcome this problem, inspiratory flow-driven dry powder inhalers might be advantageous. Powder devices have generally larger output variability compared with MDIs, but there is no evidence that this should be of clinical importance compared with the great intersubject variability for aerosol deposition. There are a wide variety of powder inhalation devices available; however, there are limited deposition data for several of them, and the efficacy varies substantially between them.

Oldaeus et al. (204) compared the efficacy and safety of the two powder inhalers—Bricanyl Turbuhaler (terbutaline sulfate 0.5 mg tid) and Ventoline Rotahaler (salbutamol 0.4 mg tid)—in 20 children, 2–6 years old, with mild to moderate asthma. Peak expiratory flow increased significantly ($p < 0.01$) after both treatments. There were no statistically significant differences, indicating that enough drug reached the patients. Borgström et al. (205) investigated deposition for an inspiratory flow-driven, multidose, powder inhaler (Turbuhaler, Astra Draco AB) in ten healthy volunteers. The radionuclide ^{99m}Tc was used to label drug particles, and radioactivity indicating drug deposition, was measured using a gamma camera. Budesonide was inhaled at a normal flow of 58 L/min and at a slow flow of 36 L/min. At the faster flow, 27 ± 9.5% (mean ± SD) of the metered dose was deposited in the lung, and at the slower flow 15 ± 3% was deposited ($p < 0.001$). Mean lung deposition of terbutaline sulfate inhaled at 57 L/min was highly similar (27 ± 8%). Vidgren and co-workers (206) compared deposition of ^{99m}Tc-labeled particles of disodium cromoglycate using two dry powder inhalers, Rotahaler (Gloxo, U.K.) and Chiesi powder inhaler (Chiesi Farm, Italy). Whole-lung deposition of the drug was similar for both devices. The coefficient of variation was about 50%. Each subject inhaled with both inhalers. There was, however, no correlation in lung deposition between the two inhalers, $r = -0.30$. Dolovich (42) has put together data from different studies and found an indication with a positive correlation between lung deposition and resistance in the device. Increased resistance within the device might be an advantage, provided that inhalation flow is unaffected (37).

C. Nebulizers

There are two dominating principles used in nebulizing therapy: ultrasonic nebulization and jet nebulization. Ultrasonic nebulizers are based on a piezoelectric converter. The transducer vibrates at megahertz frequency and, in contact with liquids, can give high output of reasonably sized particles into a reservoir. Output and particles size depend on the frequency; solution or suspension, and solution—transducer interface area; and different baffle constructions used to eliminate large particles. There are several portable, single-patient, models developed that are easy to handle. However, the transducers and reservoirs are generally small, and the particles produced tend to be larger compared with similar priced jet nebulizers.

Most of the nebulizers developed for therapy during recent years apply compressors and the jet–venturi principle. The particle size produced is dependent on the pressure from the compressor. The particle size distribution to the patient is further dependent on the different baffle constructions used to eliminate large particles and on inhalation flow. Time needed to nebulize a certain amount of drug is often perceived as very important by the patients considering regular use of nebulizer therapy. For most jet nebulizers there is need for regular control of output because the characteristics might change over time, often owing to improper maintenance and cleaning.

Köhler (207) discusses problems with reproducibility of an inhaled dose with a Pari Provocation test Device I nebulizer as an example. The author concludes that up to 50% of the volume loss in a nebulizer is due to vapor losses and, from this, it is clear that the intrabronchial dose cannot be calculated according to the weight loss of the nebulizer. It is also clear that evaporation of the nebulized solution leads to an increase in the concentration of the test substance, especially toward the end of the evaporation process. Köhler also concludes that, for the Pari inhalation device, a slower inhalation maneuver gives better reproducibility, and that reservoirs that store the aerosol before inhalation increase reproducibility, for they stabilize the aerosol by vapor saturation.

Everard et al. (202) discuss different technical factors, such as driving gas force and the effect of aerosol output. They also conclude that at high tidal volume, drug delivery is dependent on the aerosol concentration and volume of available aerosol, but essentially independent of tidal volume. This is consistent with the relations between the AD^2F and oropharyngeal and tracheobronchial deposition (see Figs. 2 and 3). At low tidal volume, the influence of tidal volume is important. Equipment dead space, consequently, is especially important in treatment of small children.

Clay and Clarke (209) compared administration of ^{99m}technetium in 0.9% saline using three different nebulizers, one with a particle size of 1.8, the other with one of 4.6, and the third with 10.3 μm. Lung deposition were 79, 59, and 44%, of the aerosol released from the nebulizer and deposited in the body, respectively. Methodological errors might have been introduced in that the radioaerosol released from the nebulizer was determined using weight measurements before and after inhalation.

Nebulization of suspensions demands that the nebulizer produces particles large enough to contain the drug. Dahlström and Larsson (210) found average lung deposition of nebulized budesonide to be 14–16% of nominal dose for Pari Inhalerboy, Pari LC Jet Plus, and Maxim MA-2, giving droplet sizes of 7, 5, and 3 μm, respectively. The lung dose in relation to systemic dose was 0.82 for Inhalerboy and 0.92 for LC Jet Plus and Maxim.

Nebulizers are often chosen when a patient cannot comply with demands of other inhalation devices. They have gained a reputation as inhalation devices not requiring adaptation by the patient. The amount of drug from a nebulizer, however, is strongly dependent on the breathing pattern and patient–device interface (i.e., mouthpiece or facemask). Several breath-synchronized jet nebulizers have been developed to overcome the problem of waste of drug during exhalation. Another possibility might be inhalation from a standing cloud. Even so, there might still be considerable problems to deliver an exact dose. Recent attention has focused on development of adaptive aerosol delivery devices. These devices deliver drug as a timed pulse during the inspiratory phase and the pulse can be timed according the patient's breathing pattern.

When choosing a nebulizer for therapy, one has to consider the combination of drug, equipment, and patient adaptation.

D. Liposomes

Microencapsulation of drugs in phospholipid vesicles (liposomes) for site-targeted delivery of compounds is a novel area of drug delivery. It is still in its infancy, but could be a promising method for conferring sustained release and prolonged duration of action of drugs in the lung (211). When phospholipids are agitated in aqueous medium, they spontaneously form microscopic vesicles, either as single lipid bilayer spheres or as multilayered vesicles, called liposomes. The liposomes are in the nanometer range, but their deposition is determined by the droplet size from the nebulizer. Administration of liposomes has been reviewed (212,213). Liposomes have been studied both in short- and long-term studies and are well tolerated (214–218). Most studies have used intratracheal administration, but cromolyn sodium has been nebulized (214), as has beclomethasone (219). For liposomal cromolyn, a more prolonged retention was observed for the encapsulated drug than for drug in solution. Also Martin (218) presented preliminary information on a liposomal beta-adrenergic agonist; liposomal metaproterenol (orciprenaline), 30 mg, given by nebulization was tolerated without adverse effects.

Vidgren and co-workers (219) studied six normal volunteers who inhaled 20 breaths of beclomethasone dipropionate liposomes labeled with ^{99m}technetium in the presence of $SnCl_2$ as a reducing agent. Particles were inhaled from each of two nebulizers; Aerotech II nebulizer and Spira nebulizer. Pulmonary deposition was 17 ± 7% for Aerotech II and 14 ± 3% for Spira nebulizer. At 3 hr, 93% of the deposited activity was detected in the volunteers breathing from the

Aerotech II, whereas it was 82% following inhalation from the Spira nebulizer. The measured exhaled activity from the Spira was 48% and from the Aerotech II 57%. The differences in clearance rate might possibly be due to the larger aerosol particles produced by the Spira nebulizer. The authors conclude that liposomal formulations are generally retained within the lung longer than most soluble drugs.

Schreier and co-workers (220) have produced a dry liposome powder formulation for aerosolization, with a particle size range of 5–6 μm, activated from a Spinhaler dry powder inhaler. The in vivo performance of the system remains to be demonstrated. In conclusion, it seems possible to nebulize liposomal antiasthmatic drugs. Also a dry liposome powder technology may be available. The selection of compounds and the prospect of developing liposomal carriers for antiasthmatic drugs needs further investigation. Gonzalez-Rothi and Schreier (211) propose, for example, new leukotriene receptor antagonists and 5-lipoxygenase inhibitors the chemical properties of which might make them suitable for liposomal delivery.

IX. Aerosol Administration and Mechanical Ventilation

Thomas and co-workers (221) have studied deposition of technetium-labeled human serum albumin particles, administered through a Siemens Servo 945 nebulizer system and a system 22 Acorn nebulizer unit. Total pulmonary deposition by percentage of the dose in the nebulizer was on the average 2.2%. There was considerable variability between subjects, with a coefficient of variation of 46%, but within subjects reproducibility was close, with a coefficient of variation of 15%.

Manthous and Hall (222) have reviewed the use of therapeutic aerosols by mechanically ventilated patients. For patients who need mechanical ventilation there are several problems. Still, bronchodilators are frequently used in intubated patients. Also, aerosolized surfactant and antibiotics have been administered. There are some problems in this situation. For example, (1) airway mucosal function and drug absorption might be altered during critical illness; (2) the endotracheal tube and ventilator circuit may trap aerosolized drug before it reaches the patient; (3) ventilator settings may unpredictably and adversely affect aerosol delivery; and (4) the patients airway anatomy, or artificial airway geometry may limit distribution of aerosol. For patients undergoing mechanical ventilation, a wide variety of techniques are employed to provide delivery of aerosolized drugs to the inspiratory limb of the ventilator at the appropriate time point in the respiratory cycle. O'Doherty et al. (223) studied deposition of nebulized radioactive albumin and found a drug delivery of 3.1–5.4% of initial dose. Low flow rate, low respiratory rates, and higher inspiratory times improved delivery of the nebulized particles. The greater fill volume of the nebulizer improved aerosol delivery, as did slower respiratory rates (224), whereas endotracheal tube size did not affect delivery. Several studies have proved that a combination of MDI plus spacer is more effective than MDI alone or nebulizer (225–227). Most studies that have shown an effect of either nebulized or MDI-distributed drug in adults have used physiological endpoints for treatment of bronchospasm with $beta_2$-agonists (225,228–238). Fernandez et al. (232) showed an effect for MDI-inhaled ipratropium bromide.

One special problem for intubated, ventilated patients is the often long distances between aerosol production and the endotracheal tubing. In conclusion, it seems that the nebulizer does not outperform a combination of spacer and MDI (222). Nebulizer treatment seems to give low-efficacy in this setting, but there are still several questions to be answered. Furthermore, other possibilities for specially selected cases can be of value; for example, treatment using helium–oxygen gases for aerosols (14,32,113). For treatment with aerosols in mechanically ventilated children, even more needs to be done. From other data it is clear that for small children a more centralized deposition might be expected if care is not taken to change the ventilatory pattern (24,160). Everard and co-workers (239) have demonstrated that 1–5% of MDI cromolyn sodium could be delivered by a spacer in a ventilator lung model, and Grigg et al. (240) found an average of 1.7% with spacer and MDI, a little more effective than with an ultrasonic nebulizer (1.3%). Treatment with bronchodilator in infants decreased airway resistance in all patients (241). There are several ongoing studies using aerosolized surfactant and also ribavirin treatment. The efficacy of these treatments remains to be proved (153). Also, mucolytics have been inhaled (242,243), but the clinical merits of this treatment are still uncertain.

Durbin (244) concludes that many questions remain to be answered relative to aerosol therapy in mechanically ventilated patients: Among them, what are the optimal ventilation parameters and what is the optimal delivery device or circuit for intubated patients? He argues that both physiological- and deposition-driven endpoints must be used.

X. Bioequivalence of Inhaled Medication

Wong and Hargreave (245) have written an excellent review about the bioequivalence of metered-dose inhaled medications. The article is written for comparisons of generic drugs with the original. It is, however, also relevant for comparison between different administration systems. The authors discuss the criteria for equivalence of medications in in vitro studies: it should be close to 15% of the innovator. They also discuss the different main types of inhalation drugs (e.g., bronchodilators, steroids, and antiallergic aerosols).

In the evaluation of bronchodilators, one must consider not only the ability to produce bronchodilation, but also the ability to protect against bronchoconstriction to nonallergic stimuli, such as methacholine, histamine, AMP, exercise, and eucapnic hyperventilation (246–248). There is evidence that the commonly used doses of beta$_2$-agonists that are currently available may be higher than required to produce a maximal effect (246); i.e., they reach a plateau, and no difference will be detected between different types of administration or different drugs, even if there is one). This problem could possibly be overcome by using several doses and by examining the duration of action in addition to the magnitude.

Wong and Hargreave (245) also discuss the problems in evaluating steroid aerosols. A potential model could be inhibition of the allergen-induced late asthmatic response and of the increase in histamine or methacholine airway responsiveness (249,250). Investigation of safety should be included; for example, measurement of 24-hr urinary cortisol in subjects receiving regular medication, to monitor possible systemic absorption. For the newer steroids, the major part of the systemic dose comes from the dose deposited in the lung.

For antiallergic aerosols, it is unclear which stimulus will be the most appropriate. One proposal was the shift in the dose response curve for AMP (251).

References

1. Jenne JW, Ahrens RC. Pharmacokinetics of beta-adrenergic compounds. In: Jenne JW, Murphy S, eds. Drug Therapy for Asthma. New York: Marcel Dekker, 1987: 213.
2. Wolff RK, Dorato MA. Toxicological testing of inhaled pharmaceutical aerosols. Crit Rev Toxicol 1993; 23:343–369.
3. Pin I, Gibson PH, Kolendowicz R, Girgis-Gabardo A, Denburg JA, Hargreave FE, Dolovich J. Induced sputum cell characteristics in normal (N) and asthmatics (A) subjects. Thorax 1992; 47:25–29.
4. Smith CM, Anderson SD. Inhalation provocation tests using nonisotonic aerosols. J Allergy Clin Immunol 1989; 84:781–790.
5. Iredale MJ, Wanklyn SAR, Phillips IP, Krausz T, Ind PW. Non-invasive assessment of bronchial inflammation in asthma: no correlation between eosinophilia of induced sputum and bronchial responsiveness to inhaled hypertonic saline. Clin Exp Allergy 1994; 24:940–945.
6. Keefe MJ, Bennett WD, Dewitt P, Seal E, Strong AA, Gerrity R. The effect of ozone exposure on the dispersion of inhaled aerosol boluses in healthy human subjects. Am Rev Respir Dis 1991; 144:23–30.
7. Heyder J, Blanchard JD, Feldman HA, Brain JD. Convective mixing in human respiratory tract: estimates with aerosol boli. J Appl Physiol 1988; 64:1273–1278.
8. McCawley M, Lippmann M. Development of an aerosol dispersion test to detect early changes in lung function. Am Ind Hyg Assoc J 1988; 49:357–366.
9. Anderson PJ, Blanchard JD, Brain JD, Feldman HA, McNamara JJ, Heyder J. Ef-

fect of cystic fibrosis on inhaled aerosol boluses. Am Rev Respir Dis 1989; 140: 1317–1324.
10. Blanchard JD, Anderson PJ, Brain JD, McNamara J, Heyder J. Deposition and Clearance of Aerosols in the Human Respiratory Tract. Vienna: Facultas-Universitatsverlag 1987:151–156.
11. Martonen TB. Measurement of particle dose distribution in a model of a human larynx and tracheobronchial tree. J Aerosol Sci 1983; 14:11–22.
12. Martonen TB, Yang Y, Xue ZQ, Zhang Z. Motion of air within the human tracheobronchial tree. Particle Sci Technol 1994; 12:175–188.
13. Goldberg IS, Lourenço RV. Deposition of aerosols in pulmonary disease. Arch Intern Med 1973; 131:88–91.
14. Svartengren M, Anderson M, Philipson K, Camner P. Human lung deposition of particles suspended in air or in helium/oxygen mixture. Exp Lung Res 1989; 15: 575–585.
15. Pavia D, Thomson ML, Clarke SW, Shannon HS. Effect of lung function and mode of inhalation on penetration of aerosol into the human lung. Thorax 1977; 32:194–197.
16. Anderson M, Svartengren M, Dahlbäck M, Nerbrink O, Philipson K, Camner P. Human tracheobronchial deposition and effect of two cholinergic aerosols. Exp Lung Res 1993; 19:653–669.
17. Anderson M, Philipson K, Svartengren M, Camner P. Human deposition and clearance of 6-μm particles inhaled with an extremely low flow rate. Exp Lung Res 1995; 21:187–195.
18. Dolovich M, Ruffin R, Corr D, Newhouse MT. Clinical evaluation of a simple demand inhalation MDI aerosol delivery device. Chest 1983; 84:36–41.
19. Chua HL, Chambers CB, Newhouse MT. Upper respiratory tract salbutamol deposition following MDI or MDI + Aerochamber: effect of mouth rinsing on oropharyngeal clearance. J Aerosol Med 1995; 8:89.
20. Alderson PO, Biello DR, Gottschalk A, Hoffer PB, Kroop SA, Lee ME, Ramanna L, Siegel BA, Waxman AD. Tc-99m-DTPA aerosol and radioactive gases compared as adjuncts to perfusion scintigraphy in patients with suspected pulmonary embolism. Radiology 1984; 153:515–521.
21. Baskin M, Abd A, Ilowite JS. Regional deposition of aerosolised pentamidine: effects of body position and breathing pattern. Ann Intern Med 1990; 113:677–683.
22. O'Doherty MJ, Thomas SH, Bradbeer C, Nunan TO, Bateman NT. Does inhalation in the supine position increase deposition in the upper part of the lung? Chest 1990; 97:1343–1348.
23. Knight V, Gilbert BE. Aerosol treatment of respiratory viral disease. Lung 1990; suppl: 406–413.
24. Weibel ER. Morphometry of the Human Lung. New York: Academic Press, 1963: 136–143.
25. Hoffman W. Mathematical model for the post natal growth of the human lung. Respir Physiol 1982; 49:115–129.
26. Itoh H, Ishii Y, Maeda H, Todo G, Torizuka K, Smaldone GC. Clinical observations of aerosol deposition in patients with airways obstruction. Chest 1981; 80:837–840.

27. Sweeney TD, Brain JD, Leavitt SA, Godleski JJ. Emphysema alters the deposition pattern of inhaled particles in hamsters. Am J Pathol 1987; 128:19–28.
28. Becquemin MH, Swift DL, Bouchikhi A, Roy M, Teillac A. Particle deposition and resistance in the noses of adults and children. Eur Respir J 1991; 4:694–702.
29. Cederlund A, Camner P, Svartengren M. Nasal mucociliary transport before and after jogging. Phys Sportsmed 1987; 15:93–98.
30. Stahlhofen W, Gebhart J, Heyder J. Biological variability of regional deposition of aerosol particles in the human respiratory tract. Am Ind Hyg Assoc J 1981; 42: 348–352.
31. Yeates DB, Pitt BR, Spektor DM, Karron GA, Albert RE. Coordination of mucociliary transport in human trachea and intrapulmonary airways. J Appl Physiol 1981; 51:1057–1064.
32. Anderson M, Svartengren M, Philipson K, Camner P. Deposition in man of particles inhaled in air or helium–oxygen at different flow rates. J Aerosol Med 1990; 3: 209–216.
33. Svartengren M, Anderson M, Bylin G, Philipson K, Camner P. Mouth and throat deposition of 3.6 μm radiolabelled particles in asthmatics. J Aerosol Med 1991; 4: 313–321.
34. Vogt FC. The incidence of candidiasis with use of inhaled corticosteroids. Am Allergy 1979; 43:205–210.
35. Williams AJ, Baghat MS, Stableforth DE, Cayton RM, Shenoi PM, Skinner C. Dysphonia caused by inhaled steroids: recognition of a characteristic laryngeal abnormality. Thorax 1983; 38:813–821.
36. Smith BJ, Phillips PJ, Pannall PR, Cain HJ, Leckie WJH. Effect of orally administered beclomethasone dipropionate on calcium absorption from the gut in normal subjects. Thorax 1993; 48:890–893.
37. Svartengren K, Lindestad PÅ, Svartengren M, Philipson K, Bylin G, Camner P. Added external resistance reduces oropharyngeal deposition and increases lung deposition of aerosol particles in asthmatics. Am J Respir Crit Care Med 1995; 152: 32–37.
38. Ericsson CH, Svartengren K, Svartengren M, Mossberg B, Philipson K, Blomquist M, Camner P. Repeatability of airway deposition and tracheobronchial clearance rate over three days in chronic bronchitis. Eur Respir J 1995; 8:1886–1893.
39. Svartengren K, Lindestad PÅ, Svartengren M, Bylin G, Philipson K, Camner P. Deposition of inhaled particles in the mouth and throat of asthmatic subjects. Eur Respir J 1994; 7:1467–1473.
40. Bowes SM, Swift DL. Deposition of inhaled particles in the oral airway during oronasal breathing. Aerosol Sci Technol 1989; 11:157–167.
41. Svartengren K, Anderson M, Svartengren M, Philipson K, Camner P. Oropharyngeal deposition of 3.5-μm particles inhaled through an elongated mouthpiece. Eur Respir J 1996; 9:1556–1559.
42. Dolovich M. Characterisation of medical aerosols: physical and clinical requirements for new inhalers. Aerosol Sci Technol 1995; 22:392–399.
43. Lippmann M, Albert RE. The effects of particle size on the regional deposition of inhaled aerosols in the human respiratory tract. Am Ind Hyg Assoc J 1969; 30: 257–275.

44. Lippmann M, Albert RE, Peterson HT. The regional deposition of inhaled aerosols in man. In: Walton WH, ed. Inhaled Particles III. Old Woking, UK: Unwin Bros 1971:105–120.
45. Camner P, Philipson K. Human alveolar deposition of 4 μm Teflon particles. Arch Environ Health 1978; 33:181–185.
46. Svartengren M, Linnman L, Philipson K, Camner P. Regional deposition in human lung of 2.5 μm particles. Exp Lung Res 1987; 12:265–279.
47. Gerrity TR, Lee PS, Hass FJ, Marinelli A, Werner P, Lourenço RV. Calculated deposition of inhaled particles in the airway generations of normal subjects. J Appl Physiol 1979; 47:867–873.
48. Palmes ED, Lippmann M. Influence of respiratory air space dimensions on aerosol deposition. Inhal Particles 1975; 4(1):127–136.
49. Svartengren M, Philipson K, Linnman L, Camner P. Airway resistance and deposition of particles in the lung. Exp Lung Res 1984; 7:257–269.
50. Svartengren M, Philipson K, Camner P. Individual differences in regional deposition of 6-μm particles in humans with induced bronchoconstriction. Exp Lung Res 1989; 15:139–149.
51. Anderson M, Svartengren M, Bylin G, Philipson K, Camner P. Deposition in asthmatics of particles inhaled in air or helium–oxygen. Am Rev Respir Dis 1993; 147: 524–528.
52. Smaldone GC, Perry RJ, Bennett WD, Messina MS, Zwang J, Ilowite J. Interpretation of "24 hour lung retention" in studies of mucociliary clearance. J Aerosol Med 1988; 1:11–20.
53. Stahlhofen W, Gebhart J, Rudolf G, Scheuch G. Measurement of lung clearance with pulses of radioactive-labelled aerosols. J Aerosol Sci 1986; 17:333–336.
54. Scheuch G, Philipson K, Falk R, Anderson M, Svartengren M, Stahlhofen W, Camner P. Retention of particles inhaled in boli with and without induced bronchoconstriction. Exp Lung Res 1995; 21:901–916.
55. Scheuch G, Kreyling W, Haas F, Stahlhofen W. The clearance of polystyrene particles from human intrathoracic airways. J Aerosol Med 1993;6(suppl):47.
56. Schurch S, Gehr P, Im Hof V, Geiser M, Green F. Surfactant displaces particles toward the epithelium in airways and alveoli. Respir Physiol 1990; 80:17–32.
57. Gehr P, Geiser M, Im Hof V, Schurch S, Waber U, Baumann M. Surfactant and inhaled particles in the conducting airways: structural, stereological and biophysical aspects. Microsc Res Technol 1993; 26:423–436.
58. Bennett WD, Chapman WF, Lay JC, Gerrity TR. Pulmonary clearance of inhaled particles 24 to 48 hours post deposition: effect of beta-adrenergic stimulation. J Aerosol Med 1993; 6:53–62.
59. Kreyling WG, Blanchard JD, Godleski JJ, Häusermann S, Heyder J, Schulz H, Sweeney TD, Takenaka S. Shallow aerosol bolus inhalation in beagle dogs: sites of retention and clearance. J Aerosol Med 1995; 8:82.
60. Wolff RK, Tillquist H, Muggenburg BA, Harkema JR, Mauderly JL. Deposition and clearance of radiolabeled particles from small ciliated airways in beagle dogs. J Aerosol Med 1989; 2:261–270.
61. Bohning DE, Atkins HL, Cohn SH. Long-term particle clearance in man: normal and impaired. Ann Occup Hyg 1982; 26:259–271.

62. Kreyling WG, Schumann G, Ortmaier A, Ferron GA, Karg E. Particle transport from the lower respiratory tract. J Aerosol Med 1988; 1:351–370.
63. Philipson K, Falk R, Camner P. Long-term lung clearance in humans studied with Teflon particles labeled with chromium-51. Exp Lung Res 1985; 9:31–42.
64. Philipson K, Falk R, Gustafsson J, Camner P. Long-term lung clearance of ^{195}Au-labeled Teflon particles in humans. Exp Lung Res 1996; 22:65–83.
65. Brain JD. Lung macrophages. How many kinds are there? What do they do? Am Rev Respir Dis 1988; 137:507–509.
66. Oberdörster G, Ferrin J, Morrow PE. Volumetric loading of alveolar macrophages (AM): a possible basis for diminished AM-mediated particle clearance. Exp Lung Res 1992; 18:87–104.
67. Barnes PJ, Basbaum B, Nadel JA. Autoradiographic localisation of autonomic receptors in airway smooth muscle. Am Rev Respir Dis 1983; 127:758–762.
68. Barnes PJ. Muscarinic receptor subtypes in airways. Life Sci 1993; 52:521–527.
69. Mak JC, Barnes PJ. Autoradiographic visualisation of muscarinic receptor subtypes in human and guinea pig lung. Am Rev Respir Dis 1990; 141:1559–1568.
70. Deffebach ME, Charan NS, Lakshminarayan S, Butler J. The bronchial circulation. Small, but a vital attribute of the lung. Am Rev Respir Dis 1987; 135:463–481.
71. Persson CGA, Erjefält I, Alkner U, Baumgarten C, Greiff L, Gustafsson B, Luts A, Pipkorn U, Sundler F, Svensson C, Wollmer P. Plasma exudation as a first line respiratory mucosal defence. Clin Exp Allergy 1991; 21:17–24.
72. Ryrfeldt Å. The bronchial circulation—a significant local distribution system in the lung, in inhalation therapy? J Aerosol Med 1990; 3:165–168.
73. Wagner EM. The role of the tracheobronchial circulation in aerosol clearance. J Aerosol Med 1995; 8:1–5.
74. Wollmer P, Hultquist C, Jonson B, Eklund G. Relationship between the site of deposition and efficacy of inhaled terbutaline studied with radioactive aerosols. J Soc Nucl Med 1987; 26:270–271.
75. Dahlbäck M, Mattsson H, Prytz M, Hjertberg E, Tunek A, Miller-Larson A, Brattsand R. Uptake of a glucocorticoid budesonide, in rat airways and lung after inhalation and intravenous infusion. Eur Respir J 1994; 7:(S18):381.
76. Miller-Larsson A, Mattsson H, Ohlsson S, Hjertberg E, Tunck A, Dahlbäck M, Brattsand R. Prolonged release from the airway tissue of glucocorticoids budesonide and fluticasone propionate as compared to beclomethasone dipropionate and hydrocortisone [abstr]. Am J Respir Crit Care Med 1994; 149:A466.
77. Parsons GH, Kramer GC, Link DP, Lantz BMT, Gunter RA, Green JF, Cross CE. Studies of reactivity and distribution of bronchial blood flow in sheep. Chest 1985; 87(suppl 5):182s.
78. Deffebach M, Agostoni P, Lakshminarayan S, Kirk W, Butler J. Prostacyclin (PGI_2) increases bronchial blood flow in the dog. Am Rev Respir Dis 1986; 133:A162.
79. Lakshminarayan S, Jindal SK, Kirk W, Butler J. Increases in bronchial blood flow following bronchoconstriction with methacholine and prostaglandin $F_2\beta$ in dogs. Chest 1985; 87(suppl 5):183s–184s.
80. Long WM, Sprung CL, El Fawal H, Yerger LD, Eyre P, Abraham WM, Wanner A. Effects of histamine on bronchial artery blood flow and bronchomotor tone. J Appl Physiol 1985; 254–261.

81. Deffebach ME, Lakshminarayan S, Kirk W, Butler J. Bronchial circulation and cyclooxygenase products in acute lung injury. J Appl Physiol 1987; 63:1083–1988.
82. Kuwano K, Bosken CH, Paré PD, Bai TR, Wiggs BR, Hogg JC. Small airways dimensions in asthma and in chronic obstructive pulmonary disease. Am Rev Respir Dis 1993; 148:1220–1225.
83. Charan NB, Turk GM, Dhand R. The role of bronchial circulation in the lung abscess. Am Rev Respir Dis 1985; 131:121–124.
84. Pearse DB, Wagner EM. Role of the bronchial circulation in ischemia–reperfusion lung injury. J Appl Physiol 1994; 76:259–265.
85. Michel RP, Hakim TS, Petsikas D. Segmental vascular resistance in postobstructive pulmonary vasculopathy. J Appl Physiol 1990; 69:1022–1032.
86. Kelly L, Kolbe J, Mitzner W, Spannhake EW, Bromberger-Barnea B, Menkes H. Bronchial blood flow affects recovery from constriction in dog lung periphery. J Appl Physiol 1986; 60:1954–1959.
87. Wagner EM, Mitzner WA. Bronchial circulatory reversal of methacholine-induced airway constriction. J Appl Physiol 1990; 69:1220–1224.
88. Csete ME, Chediak AD, Abraham WM, Wanner A. Airway blood flow modifies allergic airway smooth muscle contraction. Am Rev Respir Dis 1991; 144:59–63.
89. Lorino AM, Meignan M, Bouissou P, Atlan G. Effects of sustained exercise on pulmonary clearance of aerosolised ^{99m}Tc-DTPA. Am Physiol Soc 1989; 67:2055–2059.
90. Monaghan P, Provan I, Murray C, Mackey DWJ, Van der Wall H, Walker BM, Jones PD. An improved radionuclide technique for the detection of altered pulmonary permeability. J Nucl Med 1991; 32:1945–1949.
91. American Thoracic Society. Standards for the diagnosis and care of patients with chronic obstructive pulmonary disease (COPD) and asthma. Am Rev Respir Dis 1987; 136:225–244.
92. Medical Research Council. Definition and classification of chronic bronchitis for clinical and epidemiological purposes. Lancet 1965; 1:775–781.
93. Burrows B, Bloom JW, Traver GA, Cline MG. The course and prognosis of different forms of chronic airways obstruction in a sample from the general population. N Engl J Med 1987; 317:1309–1314.
94. Barnes PJ. New concepts in the pathogenesis of bronchial hyperresponsiveness and asthma. J Allergy Clin Immunol 1989; 83:1013–1026.
95. Cosio M, Ghezzo H, Hogg JC, Corbin R, Loveland M, Dosman J, Macklem PT. The relations between structural changes in small airways and pulmonary-function tests. N Engl J Med 1977; 298:1277–1281.
96. Eberg RV, Terracio MJ. Observation of the secretion on the surface of the bronchioles with the scanning electron microscope. Am Rev Respir Dis 1972; 111:4–11.
97. Green FHY, Harji S, Butt JC, Li F, Ruff M, Karkhanis A, Hessel P, Perry S. Regional distribution of airway smooth muscle in asthma. J Aerosol Med 1995; 8:94.
98. Camner P, Mossberg B, Philipson K. Tracheobronchial clearance and chronic obstructive lung disease. Scand J Respir Dis 1973; 54:272–281.
99. Mossberg B, Strandberg K, Philipson K, Camner P. Tracheobronchial clearance and chronic obstructive lung disease. Scand J Respir Dis 1976; 57:281–289.

100. Camner P, Philipson K. Tracheobronchial clearance in smoking discordant twins. Arch Environ Health 1972; 25:60–63.
101. Matthys H. Definition and assessment of asthma. Lung 1990; 168:51–56.
102. Mossberg B, Philipson K, Camner P. Tracheobronchial clearance in patients with emphysema associated with alpha$_1$-antitrypsin deficiency. Scand J Respir Dis 1978; 59:1–7.
103. Stahlhofen W, Rudolf G, James AC. Intercomparison of experimental regional aerosol deposition data. J Aerosol Med 1989; 2:285–308.
104. Thomson ML, Pavia D. Particle penetration and clearance in the human lung. Arch Environ Health 1974; 29:214–219.
105. Yeates DB, Gerrity TR, Garrad CS. Particle deposition and clearance in the bronchial tree. Ann Biomed Eng 1981; 9:577–592.
106. Svartengren M, Anderson M, Bylin G, Philipson K, Camner P. Regional deposition of 3.6 μm particles in subjects with mild to moderately severe asthma. J Aerosol Med 1990; 3:197–207.
107. Agnew JE, Pavia D, Clarke SW. Airways penetration of inhaled radioaerosol: an index to small airways function? Eur J Respir Dis 1981; 62:239–255.
108. Ruusa J, Svartengren M, Philipson K, Camner P. Tracheobronchial particle deposition and clearance in immotile cilia syndrome patients. J Aerosol Med 1993; 6: 89–98.
109. Mossberg B, Afzelius BA, Eliasson R, Camner P. On the pathogenesis of obstructive lung disease. A study on the immotile-cilia syndrome. Scand J Respir Dis 1978; 59:55–65.
110. Pavia D, Agnew JE, Sutton PP, Lopez-Vidriero MT, Currie DC, Cole PJ, Clarke SW. Impaired mucus clearance in patients with chronic bronchial sepsis, sinusitis and dextrocardia. Respiration 1988; 53:187–196.
111. Svartengren K, Philipson K, Svartengren M, Nerbrink O, Camner P. Clearance in smaller airways of inhaled 6-μm particles in subjects with immotile-cilia syndrome. Exp Lung Res 1995; 21:667–682.
112. Svartengren M, Anderson M, Bylin G, Philipson K, Camner P. Regional deposition of 3.6 μm particles and lung function in asthmatic subjects. J Appl Physiol 1991; 71:2238–2243.
113. Anderson M, Svartengren M, Bylin G, Philipson K, Camner P. Deposition in asthmatics of particles inhaled in air or helium–oxygen. Am Rev Respir Dis 1993; 147: 524–528.
114. Svartengren K, Philipson K, Svartengren M, Anderson M, Camner P. Tracheobronchial deposition and clearance in small airways in asthmatic subjects. Eur Respir J 1996; 9:1123–1129.
115. Stout SA, Derendorf H. Local treatment of respiratory infections with antibiotics. Drug Intell Clin Pharm 1987; 21:322–329.
116. Odio W, Vanlaer E, Klastersky J. Concentrations of gentamicin in bronchial secretions after intramuscular and endotracheal administration. J Clin Pharmacol 1975; 15:518–524.
117. Ilowite JS, Niederman MS, Fein AM. Delivery of topical antibiotics: pharmacokinetics and clinical problems. Semin Respir Infect 1992; 6:158–167.
118. Ilowite JS, Baskin MI, Sheetz MS, Abd AG. Delivered dose and regional distribu-

tion of aerosolised pentamidine using different delivery systems. Chest 1991; 99: 1139–1144.
119. Slauson DO, Lay JC, Castleman WL, Neilsen NR. Acute inflammatory lung injury retards pulmonary particle clearance. Inflammation 13:185–199, 1989.
120. Englund JA, Piedra PA, Jefferson LS, Wilson SZ, Taber LH, Gilbert BE. High-dose, short-duration ribavirin aerosol therapy in children with suspected respiratory syncytial virus infection. J Pediatr 1990; 117:313–320.
121. Smith DW, Frankel IR, Mathers LH, Tang ATS, Ariagno RL, Prober CG. A controlled trial of aerosolised ribavirin in infants receiving mechanical ventilation for severe respiratory syncytial virus infection. N Engl J Med 1991; 325:24–29.
122. Frank A, Dash CH. Inhaled beclomethasone dipropionate in acute infections of the respiratory tract. Respiration 1985; 48:122–126.
123. Jarstrand C, Camner P, Philipson K. *Mycoplasma pneumoniae* and tracheobronchial clearance. Am Rev Respir Dis 1974; 110:415–419.
124. Camner P, Jarstrand C, Philipson K. Tracheobronchial clearance 5–15 months after infection with *Mycoplasma pneumoniae*. Scand J Infect Dis 1978; 10:33–35.
125. Lidman C, Tynell E, Berglund O, Lindbäck S. Aerosolised pentamidine versus i.v. pentamidine for secondary prophylaxis of *Pneumocystis carinii* pneumonia. Infection 1993; 21:146–149.
126. Lidman C, Berglund O, Tynell E, Lindbäck S, Elvin K. Aerosolised pentamidine as primary prophylaxis for *Pneumocystis carinii* pneumonia: efficacy, mortality and morbidity. AIDS 1994; 8:935–939.
127. Nybo Jensen BN, Nielsen TL, Backer V, Nelsing S, Simonsen L, Flaschs H, Gaub J, Höjlyng N, Nielsen JO, Mathiesen L, Skinhöj P. Aerosolised pentamidine for primary prophylaxis of *Pneumocystis carinii* pneumonia: a controlled, randomised trial. J Acquir Immune Defic Syndr 1993; 6:472–477.
128. Guinet F, Pialoux G, Trotot P, Chauvelle MT, Feuillie V, Sansonetti PH, Dupont B. Prophylaxie de la pneumocystose pulmonaire associée à l'ínfection vih par aérosols de pentamidine. Presse Med 1994; 23:1747–1752.
129. Ng VL, Geaghan SM, Leoung G, Shiboski S, Fahy J, Schnapp LY, Yajko DH, Hopenell PC, Hadley WK. Lack of effect of prophylactic aerosolised pentamidine on detection of *Pneumocystis carinii* in induced sputum or bronchoalveolar lavage specimens. Arch Pathol Lab Med 1993; 117:493–496.
130. Katial R, Honeycutt W, Oswald SG. *Pneumocystis carinii* pneumonia presenting as focal bibasilar uptake on gallium scan during aerosolised pentamidine prophylactics. J Nucl Med 1994; 35:1038–1040.
131. Leoung GS, Feigal DW, Montgomery AB, et al. Aerosolised pentamidine for prophylaxis against *Pneumocystis carinii* pneumonia. N Engl J Med 1990; 323:769–775.
132. Montaner JSG, Lawson LM, Gervais A, Hyland RH, Chan CK, Falutz JM. Aerosol pentamidine for secondary prophylaxis of AIDS related *Pneumocystis carinii* pneumonia. Ann Intern Med 1991; 114:948–953.
133. Milic-Emili J, Henderson J, Dolovich M, Trop D, Kaneko K. Regional distribution of inspired gas in the lung. J Appl Physiol 1966; 21:749–759.
134. Jules-Elysee K, Stover D, Zaman M, Bernard E, White D. Aerosolised pentamidine:

effect on diagnosis and presentation of *Pneumocystis carinii* pneumonia. Ann Intern Med 1990; 112:750–757.

135. O'Riordan TG, Baughman RP, Dohn MN, Smaldone GC. Lobar pentamidine levels and *Pneumocystis carinii* pneumonia following aerosolised pentamidine. Chest 1994; 105:53–56.
136. Smaldone GC, Dickinson GD, Marcial E, Young E, Seymour J. Deposition of aerosolised pentamidine and failure of *Pneumocystis* prophylaxis. Chest 1992; 101:82–87.
137. O'Riordan TG, Smaldone GC. Regional deposition and regional ventilation during inhalation of pentamidine. Chest 1994; 105:395–401.
138. Thomas SHL, O'Doherty MJ, Page CJ, Nunan TO, Bateman NT. Which apparatus for inhaled pentamidine? A comparison of pulmonary deposition via eight nebulisers. Eur Respir J 1991; 4:616–622.
139. O'Doherty MJ, Thomas S, Page C, Barlow D, Bradbeer C, Nunan TO, Bateman NT. Differences in relative efficiency of nebulisers for pentamidine administration. Lancet 1988; 2:1283–1286.
140. Kilburn KH. The innocuousness and possible therapeutic use of aerosol amphotericin B. Am Rev Respir Dis 1959; 80:441–442.
141. Sahni PS. Pulmonary moniliasis. J Pediatr 1957; 50:484–486.
142. Ikemoto H. Treatment of pulmonary aspergilloma with amphotericin B. Arch Intern Med 1965; 115:598–601.
143. Eisenberg RS, Oatway WH. Nebulization of amphotericin B. Am Rev Respir Dis 1971; 193:289–292.
144. Diot P, Rivoire B, Le Pape A, Lemarie E, Dire D, Furet Y, Breteau M, Smaldone GC. Deposition of amphotericin B aerosols in pulmonary aspergilloma. Eur Respir J 1995; 8:1263–1268.
145. Erkkilä S, Fröseth B, Hellström PE, Kaltiokallio K, Taskinen E, Viljanen A, Viljanen B, Selroos O. Inhaled budesonide influences cellular and biochemical abnormalities in pulmonary sarcoidosis. Sarcoidosis 5:106–110, 1988.
146. Spiteri MA, Newman SP, Clarke SW, Poulter LW. Inhaled corticosteroids can modulate the immunopathogenesis of pulmonary sarcoidosis. Eur Respir J 2:218–224, 1989.
147. Spiteri MA, Poulter LW, Clarke SW. Inhaled versus systemic corticosteroids in pulmonary sarcoidosis: a comparison of their immunological and clinical effects. Thorax 1991; 46:322.
148. Alberts C, van der Mark THW, Jansen HM, the Dutch study group on pulmonary sarcoidosis. Inhaled budesonide in pulmonary sarcoidosis: a double-blind, placebo-controlled study. Eur Respir J 1995; 5:682–688.
149. Ueda S, Kawamura K, Ashima K. Lung surfactant—TA in treatments for adult patients suffering from prolonged hypoxemia. Jpn Soc Biol Interface Sci 1988; 19: 60–77.
150. Richman PS, Sprague RG, Robertson B, Merrit TA, Curstedt T. The adult respiratory distress syndrome: first trials with surfactant replacement. Eur Respir J 1989; 2(suppl 3):109S–111S.
151. Nosaka S, Sakai T, Yonekura M, Yoshikawa K. Surfactant for adults with respiratory failure. Lancet 1990; 336:947–948.

152. Van Daal GJ, So KL, Gommes D. Intratracheal surfactant administration restores gas exchange in experimental adult respiratory distress syndrome associated with viral pneumonia. Anesth Analg 1991; 72:589–595.
153. Lachmann B. Animal models and clinical pilot studies of surfactant replacement in adult respiratory distress symptom. Eur Respir J 1989; 2(suppl 3):98S–103S.
154. Kobayshi T, Grossman G, Robertson B, Ueda T. Effects of artificial and natural surfactant supplementation in immature newborn rabbits. Acta Anaesthesiol Scand 1990; 34:216–221.
155. Li WZ, Chen WM, Kobayashi T. Aerosolised surfactant reverses respiratory failure in lung lavaged rats. Acta Anaesthesiol Scand 1994; 38:82–88.
156. Lewis JF, McCaig L. Aerosolised versus instilled exogenous surfactant in a nonuniform pattern of lung injury. Am Rev Respir Dis 1993; 148:1187–1193.
157. Knowles MR, Olivier KN, Hohneker KW, Robinson J, Bennet WD, Boucher RD. Pharmacological treatment of abnormal ion transport in the airway epithelium in cystic fibrosis. Chest 1995; 107(suppl):71S–76S.
158. Turpin SW, Knowles MR, Treatment of pulmonary disease in patients with cystic fibrosis. In: Davis PB, ed. Cystic Fibrosis. New York: Marcel-Dekker, 1993:277–344.
159. Kavanaugh, RE, Unadkat JD, Smith AL. Drug disposition in cystic fibrosis. In: Davis PB, ed. Cystic Fibrosis. New York: Marcel-Dekker, 1993:91–136.
160. Martonen T, Katz I, Cress W. Aerosol deposition as a function of airway disease: cystic fibrosis. Pharm Res 1995; 12:96–102.
161. Hodson M. Antibiotic treatment. Aerosol therapy. Chest 1988; 94(suppl 2):156S–160S.
162. Smith AL, Ramsey B. Aerosol administration of antibiotics. Respiration 1995; 62(suppl 1):19–24.
163. Hodson ME, Penketh ARL, Batten JC. Aerosol carbenicillin and gentamicin treatment, of *Pseudomonas aeroginosa* infection in patients with cystic fibrosis. Lancet 1981; 2:1137–1139.
164. Jensen T, Pedersen SS, Garne S, Heilmann C, Hoiby N, Koch C. Colistin inhalation therapy in cystic fibrosis patients with *Pseudomonas aeruginosa* lung infections. Antimicrob Chemother 1987; 19:831–838.
165. Valerius NH, Koch C, Hoiby N. Prevention of chronic *Pseudomonas aeruginosa* colonisation in cystic fibrosis by early treatment. Lancet 1991; 338:725–726.
166. Wilson FE. Acute respiratory failure secondary to polymyxin inhalation. Chest 1981; 79:237–239.
167. Touw DJ, Brimicombe RW, Hodson ME, Heijerman HGM, Bakker W. Inhalation of antibiotics in cystic fibrosis. Eur Respir J 1995; 8:1594–1604.
168. Zach MS. Discussion. Chest 1988; 94(suppl 2):160S–161S.
169. Steinkamp G, Tümmler B, Gappa M, Albus A, Potel J, Döring G, von der Hardt H. Long-term tobramycin aerosol therapy in cystic fibrosis. Pediatr Pulmonol 1989; 6:91–98.
170. Tomkiewicz RP, App EM, Zayas JG, Ramirez O, Church N. Boucher RC, Knowles MR, King M. Amiloride inhalation therapy in cystic fibrosis. Am Rev Respir Dis 1993; 148:1002–1007.
171. Bennett W, Olivier K, Zemen K, et al. Acute effect of aerosolized uridine 5′-triphos-

phate (UTP) +/− amiloride on mucociliary clearance in cystic fibrosis. Am J Respir Crit Care Med 1994; 149:A670.
172. Köhler D. Aerosols for systemic treatment. Lung 1990; 168(suppl):677–684.
173. Graham JR, Malvea BP, Gramm HF. Aerosol ergotamine tartrate for migraine and Horton's syndrome. N Engl J Med 1960; 263:802–804.
174. Köhler D, Schlüter KJ, Kerp L, Matthys H. Nicht radioaktives Verfahren zur Messung der Lungenpermeabilität: inhalation von Insulin. Atemwegs Lungenkr 1987; 13:230–232.
175. Schlüter KJ, Köhler D, Enzmann F, Kerp L. Pulmonary administration of human insulin in volunteers and type I-diabetes. Diabetes 1984; 33(suppl):298.
176. Wigley M, Londona JH, Scott HW, Shipp JC, Waldmann RH. Insulin across respiratory mucosa by aerosol delivery. Diabetes 1971; 20:552–556.
177. Bick RL, Ross ES. Clinical use of intrapulmonary heparin. Semin Thromb Hemost 1985; 11:213–221.
178. Mahadoo J, Hiebert M, Wright CJ, Jaques LB. Vascular distribution of intratracheally administered heparin. Ann NY Acad Sci 1981; 370:650–655.
179. Neri Serneri GG, Rovelli F, Gensini GF, Pirelli S, Carnovali M, Fortini A. Effectiveness of low-dose heparin in prevention of myocardial reinfarction. Lancet 1987; 1:937–942.
180. Engelberg H. Heparin and the atherosclerosis process. Pharmacol Rev 1984; 36: 91–110.
181. Minti B, Jordan C, Jones JG. Rapid improvement in abnormal pulmonary epithel permeability after stopping cigarettes. Br Med J 1981; 282:1183–1186.
182. Shulman AG. Heparin for prevention of atherosclerosis. N Engl Med 1988; 319: 1154–1155.
183. Huchon GJ. Respiratory clearance of solutes. Bull Eur Physiopathol Respir 1986; 22:495–510.
184. Jacobs MP, Baughman RP, Hughes J, Fernandez-Ulloa M. Radioaerosol lung clearance in patients with active pulmonary sarcoidosis. Am Rev Respir Dis 1985; 131: 687–689.
185. Pavia D, Bateman JRM, Clarke SW. Deposition and clearance of inhaled particles. Bull Eur Physiopathol 1980; 16:335–366.
186. Oberdörster G. Lung clearance of inhaled insoluble and soluble particles. J Aerosol Med 1988; 1:289–305.
187. Schiessle W, Frey D. Bronchoskopische Beobachtungen nach Inhalation von Farbstoffen bei normalen und krankhaften Verhältnissen im Atemtrakt. In: Nückel H, Schattauer FK, eds. Fortschritte der Biologischen Aerosol-Forschung. Stuttgart, 1962.
188. Kelly L, Kolbe J, Mitzner W, Spannhake EW, Bromberger-Barnea B, Menkes H. Bronchial blood flow affects recovery from constriction in dog lung periphery. J Appl Physiol 1986; 60:1954–1959.
189. Brown AR, Pickrell JA. Propellant-driven aerosols for delivery of proteins in the respiratory tract. J Aerosol Med 1995; 8:43–58.
190. Weissman DN, Bice DE, Crowell RE, Schuyler MR. Intrapulmonary antigen deposition in the human lung: local responses. Am J Respir Cell Mol Biol 1994; 11: 607–614.

191. Dahl R, Ringdal N, Ward SM, Stampone P, Donnel D. Equivalence of asthma control with new CFC-free formulation HFA-134a beclomethasone dipropionate and CFC beclomethasone dipropionate. Br J Clin Pract 1997; 51:11–15.
192. Tansey I. The technical transition to CFC-free inhalers. Br J Clin Pract 1997; 89(suppl):22–27.
193. Tobin MJ, Jenouri G, Danta I, Kim C, Watson H, Sackner MA. Response to bronchodilator drug administration by a new reservoir aerosol delivery system and a review of other auxilliary systems. Am Rev Respir Dis 1982; 126:670–675.
194. Pauwels R, Lamont H, Hidinger K, Straeten MVD. Influence of an extension tube on the bronchodilator efficacy of terbutaline delivered from a metered dose inhaler. Respiration 1984; 45:61–66.
195. Pedersen S. Aerosol treatment of bronchoconstriction in children with or without a tube spacer. N Engl J Med 1983; 308:1328–1330.
196. Morris J, Milledge JS, Moszoro H, Higgins A. The efficacy of drug delivery by a pearshaped spacer and metered dose inhaler. Br J Dis Chest 1984; 78:383–389.
197. Kim CS, Eldrige MA, Sackner MA. Oropharyngeal deposition and delivery aspects of metered-dose inhaler aerosols. Am Rev Respir Dis 1987; 135:157–164.
198. Newman SP, Clark AR, Talaee N, Clarke SW. Pressurised aerosol deposition in the human lung with and without an ''open'' spacer device. Thorax 1989; 44:706–710.
199. Vidgren P, Vidgren M, Paronen P, Vainio P, Nuutinen J. Effects of Inspirease holding chamber on the deposition of metered dose inhalation aerosols. Eur J Drug Metab Pharmacokinet 1991; 3:419–425.
200. Barry PW, O'Callaghan C. Poor output of salbutamol from a spacer device: effect of spacer static charge and multiple actuations (abstr). Thorax 1994; 49:402P.
201. Callaghan CO, Lynch J, Cant M, Robertsson C. Improvement in sodium cromoglycate delivery from a spacer device by use of an antistatic lining, immediate inhalation, and avoiding multiple actuations of drug. Thorax 1993; 48:603–606.
202. Everard ML, Clark AR, Milner AD. Drug delivery from holding chambers with attached facemask. Arch Dis Child 1992; 62:580–585.
203. Newman S, Steed K, Hooper G, Källén A, Borgström L. Comparison of gamma scintigraphy and a pharmacokinetic technique for assessing pulmonary deposition of terbutaline sulphate delivered by pressurised metered dose inhaler. Pharmacol Res 1995; 12:231–236.
204. Oldaeus G, Kubista J, Stahl E. Comparison of Bricanyl turbuhaler and Ventolin rotahaler in children with asthma. Ann Allergy Asthma Immunol 1995; 74:34–37.
205. Borgström L, Bondesson E, Morén F, Trofast E, Newman SP. Lung deposition of budesonide inhaled via Turbuhaler: a comparison with terbutaline sulphate in normal subjects. Eur Respir J 1994; 7:69–73.
206. Vidgren M, Paronen P, Vidgren P. In vivo evaluation of the new multiple dose powder inhaler and the Rotahaler using the gamma scintigraphy. Acta Pharm Nord 1990; 1:3–10.
207. Köhler D. Problematik der dosisgenauen. Inhalation, dargestellt am Beispiel des Pari Provocations testgerätest. Pneumologie 1991; 45 (suppl 2):659–669 [in German with English summary].

208. Everard ML, Clark AR, Milner AD. Drug delivery from jet nebulisers. Arch Dis Child 1992; 67:586–591.
209. Clay MM, Clarke SW. Effect of nebulised aerosol size on lung deposition in patients with mild asthma. Thorax 1987; 42:190–194.
210. Dahlström K, Larsson P. Lung deposition and systemic availability of budesonide inhaled as nebulized suspension from different nebulizers (abstr). Am J Respir Crit Care Med 1996; 153:A339.
211. Gonzalez-Rothi RJ, Schreier H. Pulmonary delivery of liposome-encapsulated drugs in asthma therapy. Clin Immunother 1995; 4:331–337.
212. Schreier H, Gonzalez-Rothi RJ, Stecenko A. Pulmonary delivery of liposomes. J Control Release 1993; 24:209–223.
213. Taylor KMG, Farr SJ. Liposomes for drug delivery to the respiratory tract. Drug Dev Ind Pharm 1993; 19:123–142.
214. Taylor KMG, Taylor G, Kellaway IW, Stevens J. The influence of liposomal encapsulation on sodium cromoglycate pharmacokinetics in man. Pharmacol Res 1989; 6:633–636.
215. Thomas DA, Myers MA, Wichert B, Schreier H, Gonzales-Rothi RJ. Acute effects of liposome aerosol inhalation on pulmonary function in healthy human volunteers. Chest 1991; 99:1268–1270.
216. Gilbert BE, Six HR, Wilson SZ, Wyde PR, Knight V. Small particle aerosols of enviroxime-containing liposomes. Antiviral Res 1988; 9:355–365.
217. Myers MA, Niven R, Straub L, Soucy DW, Niven RW, Kaltenbach M, Hoodi CI, Schreier H, Gonzales-Rothi RJ. Pulmonary effects of chronic exposure to liposome aerosols in mice. Exp Lung Res 1993; 19:1–19.
218. Martin F. Development of lipsosomes for aerosol delivery: recent preclinical and clinical results. J Liposome Res 1990; 1:407–429.
219. Vidgren M, Waldrep JC, Arppe J, Black M, Rodarte JA, Cole W, Knight V. A study of ^{99m}technetium-labelled beclomethasone dipropionate dilauroylphosphatidyl-choline liposome aerosol in normal volunteers. Int J Pharm 1995; 115:209–216.
220. Schreier H, Mobley N, Concessio N, et al. Formulation and in vitro performance of liposome powder aerosols. STP Pharm Sci 1994; 4:38–44.
221. Thomas SHL. O'Doherty MJ, Fidler HM, Page CJ, Treacher DF, Nunan T. Pulmonary deposition of a nebulised aerosol during mechanical ventilation. Thorax 1993; 48:154–159.
222. Manthous CA, Hall JB. Administration of therapeutic aerosols to mechanically ventilated patients. Chest 1994; 106:560–571.
223. O'Doherty MJ, Thomas SHL, Page CG, Treacher DF, Nunan TO. Delivery of a nebulized aerosol to a lung model during mechanical ventilation. Am Rev Respir Dis 1992; 146:383–388.
224. O'Riordan TG, Greco MJ, Smaldone PRJ. Nebulizer function during mechanical ventilation. Am Rev Respir Dis 1992; 145:1117–1122.
225. Fuller HD, Dolovich MB, Posmituck G, Wong Pack W, Newhouse MT. Pressurised aerosol versus jet aerosol delivery to mechanically ventilated patients. Am Rev Respir Dis 1990; 141:440–444.
226. Bishop MJ, Larson RP, Buschman DL. Metered dose inhaler aerosol characteristics

are affected by the endotracheal tube actuator/adapter used. Anesthesiology 1990; 73:1263–1265.
227. Rao JL, Harwood RJ, Groff JL. Evaluation of a reservoir device for metered-dose bronchodilator delivery to intubated adults. Chest 1992; 102:924–930.
228. Gold MI. Treatment of bronchospasm during anesthesia. Anesth Analg 1975; 54: 783–786.
229. Sprague DH. Treatment of intraoperative bronchospasm with nebulized isoetharine. Anesthesiology 1977; 46:222–224.
230. MacIntyre NR, Silver RM, Miller CW, Schuler F, Coleman RE. Aerosol delivery in intubated, mechanically ventilated patients. Crit Care Med 1985; 13:81–84.
231. Gay PC, Patel HG, Nelson SB, Gilles B, Huvmayr RD. Metered dose inhalers for bronchodilator delivery in intubated, mechanically ventilated patients. Chest 1991; 99:66–71.
232. Fernandez A, Lazaro A, Garcia A, Aragon C, Cerda E. Bronchodilators in patients with chronic obstructive pulmonary disease on mechanical ventilation: utilisation of metered-dose inhalers. Am Rev Respir Dis 1990; 141:164–168.
233. Farhangfar R, Safirstein B, Khan MA. Comparison of the efficacy of albuterol delivered as metered-dose inhaler (MDI) with that of a nebulizer in mechanically ventilated patients with chronic obstructive pulmonary disease (COPD) (abstr). Am Rev Respir Dis 1992; 145:A60.
234. Gutierrez CJ, Nelson R. Short-term bronchodilation in mechanically ventilated patients receiving metaproterenol via small volume nebulizer (SVN) or metered-dose inhaler (MDI). Respir Care 1988; 33:910–913.
235. Hess D, Fillman D, Daugherty A, Rexrode WO, Smoker JM, Rhoads JE. Use of metered dose inhalers in intubated patients. Respir Care 1989; 34:1027–1033.
236. Bakow ED, Galgon P, Bachman V, Lucke J. beta-Agonist delivery in-line with a ventilator circuit by either metered dose inhaler or updraft nebulizer in a distal or proximal position. Respir Care 1989; 34:1027–1029.
237. Manthous CA, Schmidt GA, Hall JB, Wood LDH. Metered dose inhaler versus nebulized albuterol for the treatment of bronchospasm in mechanically ventilated patients. Am Rev Respir Dis 1993; 148:1567–1571.
238. Dhand R, Jubran A, Tobin MJ. Response to bronchodilator administration by metered dose inhaler in mechanically ventilated patients with COPD (abstr). Am Rev Respir Dis 1993; 147:A895.
239. Everard ML, Stammers J, Hardy JG, Milner AD. New aerosol delivery system for neonatal ventilator circuits. Arch Dis Child 1992; 67:826–830.
240. Grigg J, Arnon S, Jones T, Clarke A, Silverman M. Delivery of therapeutic aerosols to intubated babies. Arch Dis Child 1992; 67:25–30.
241. Rio MG, Gerhardt T, Hehre D, Feller R, Bancalari E. Effect of beta-agonist nebulization on lung function in neonates with increased pulmonary resistance. Pediatr Pulmonol 1986; 2:287–291.
242. Rao S, Wilson B, Brooks RC. Acute effects of nebulization of *N*-acetylcysteine on pulmonary mechanics and gas exchange. Am Rev Respir Dis 1970; 102:17–20.
243. Zandstra DF, Stoutenbeck CP, Miranda DR. Effect of mucolytic and bronchodilator aerosol therapy on airway resistance in mechanically ventilated patients. Intensive Care Med 1985; 11:316–318.

244. Durbin CD. Aerosol therapy in mechanically ventilated patients. Chest 1994; 106: 336–337.
245. Wong BJ, Hargreave FE. Bioequivalence of metered-dose inhaled medications. J Allergy Clin Immunol 1993; 92:373–379.
246. Nelson HS. Adrenergic therapy for bronchial asthma. J Allergy Clin Immunol 1986; 77:771–785.
247. Twentyman, OP, Finnerty JP, Holgate ST. The inhibitory effect of nebulized albuterol on the early and late asthmatic reactions and increase in airway responsiveness provoked by inhaled allergen in asthma. Am Rev Respir Dis 1991; 144:782–787.
248. Britton JR, Hanley SP, Garrett HV, Hadfield JW, Tattersfield AE. Dose related effects of salbutamol and ipratropium bromide on airway calibre and reactivity in subjects with asthma. Thorax 1988; 43:300–305.
249. Cockcroft DW, Murdock KY. Comparative effects of inhaled salbutamol, sodium cromoglycate and beclomethasone dipropionate on allergen-induced early asthmatic responses, late asthmatic responses, and increased bronchial responsiveness to histamine. J Allergy Clin Immunol 1987; 79:734–740.
250. Wong BJO, Dolovich J, Ramsdale EH, et al. Formoterol compared to beclomethasone and placebo on allergen-induced asthmatic responses. Am Rev Respir Dis 1992; 146:1156–1160.
251. Phillips GD, Richards R, Scott VL, Holgate ST. Sodium cromoglycate and nedocromil sodium inhibit bronchoconstriction provoked by adenosine 5-monophosphate in atopic and non-atopic asthma [abstr]. Am Rev Respir Dis 1988; 137(suppl): 29.

Part Three

INHALATION OF PARTICLES

5

Particle Deposition in the Respiratory Tract

HOLGER SCHULZ, PETER BRAND, and JOACHIM HEYDER

Institute for Inhalation Biology
GSF–Research Center for Environment and Health
Neuherberg/Munich, Germany

I. Introduction and Overview

During inhalation, particles are transported with the inspired air through the extrathoracic airways and the bifurcating tracheobronchiolar system to the gas-exchanging region of the lung. A certain number of these particles are caught in the respiratory system by touching the wet airspace surfaces, a phenomenon generally referred to as *particle deposition*. Therefore, with exhalation, not all particles are recovered. Figure 1A shows the fraction of particles deposited in the respiratory system (total deposition) during quiet mouth breathing as a function of the particle diameter. This fraction is small for particles in the size range between 0.1 and 1 μm. But it becomes larger for smaller and larger particles reaching almost 100% for 0.01- or 10-μm particles. However, the particle size determines not only how many particles are deposited, but also in which region of the respiratory tract these particles are deposited (regional deposition, see Fig. 1B–D). Total and regional deposition are modified further by other physical properties of the inhaled particles (particle density and shape), by the breathing pattern (tidal volume, breathing frequency, and flow rate; Fig. 2), and by the lung geometry (airspace dimensions).

The main question addressed in this chapter is: What is the impact of each

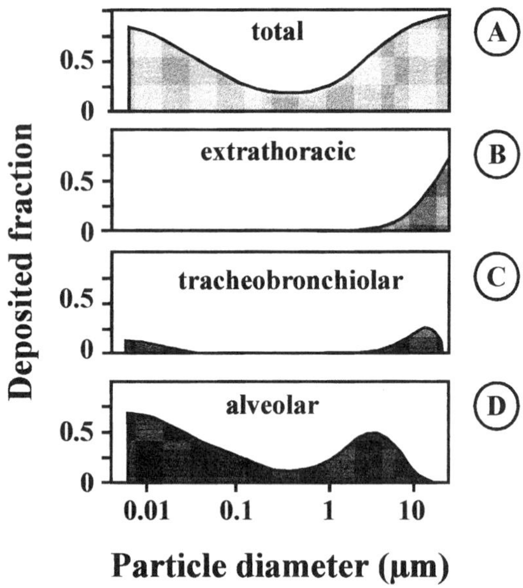

Figure 1 Schematic overview of (A) total deposition fraction and of deposition fraction in (B) the extrathoracic, (C) the tracheobronchial and (D) the alveolar region of the human respiratory system for unit-density spheres during mouth breathing. (From Ref. 163.)

of those factors on particle deposition and deposition pattern and, by knowing the significance of each factor, is it possible to target specific sites within the lung with particles inhaled for therapeutic or diagnostic purposes?

Particle Transport. Particle transport between mouth or nose and the alveoli is governed by convection, resulting from pressure gradients generated along the airways during breathing. Whereas convective bulk flow characterizes the displacement of particles toward the lung periphery or vice versa, convective mixing refers to the amalgam of inhaled with residual air. It occurs as a result of differences in bulk flow pattern during inspiration and expiration and nonuniform intrapulmonary ventilation (1–4).

As the total cross-sectional area of the airways increases rapidly toward the lung periphery (5), flow velocities and, hence, the linear velocity of bulk flow, decrease rapidly within airways from the extrathoracic to the small conducting airways and the alveolated region of the lung (4). Consequently, the residence time of particles is short within the large conducting airways, but increases toward the lung periphery.

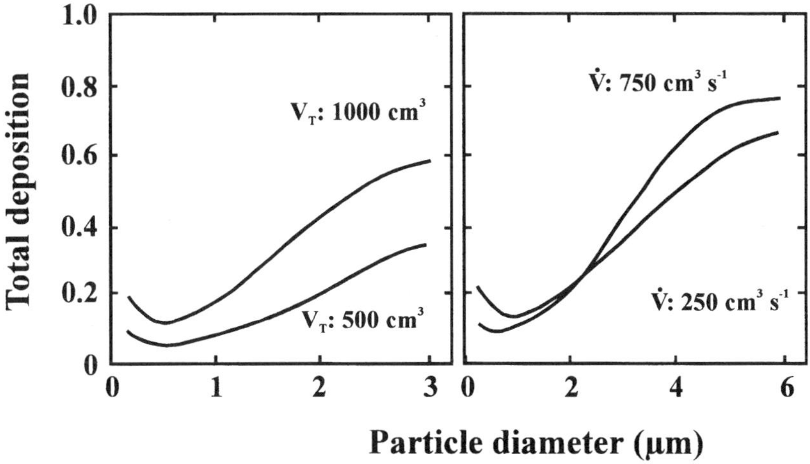

Figure 2 Effect of tidal volume (V_T:500 cm^3 and 1000 cm^3) for a given flow rate of 250 cm^3 s^{-1} (left panel) and of flow rate ($\dot{V}$:250 cm^3 s^{-1} and 750 cm^3 s^{-1}) for a given tidal volume of 1500 cm^3 (right panel) on total deposition fraction of unit density spheres. (From Ref. 10.)

Mechanisms of Mechanical Particle Transport. When particles do not follow, but diverge from, airflow streamlines and thereby come in contact with airspace surfaces, particle deposition occurs. This diverging from airflow streamlines and particle trajectories is mainly due to mechanisms of mechanical particle transport: inertial, gravitational, and diffusional particle transport (Fig. 3). The

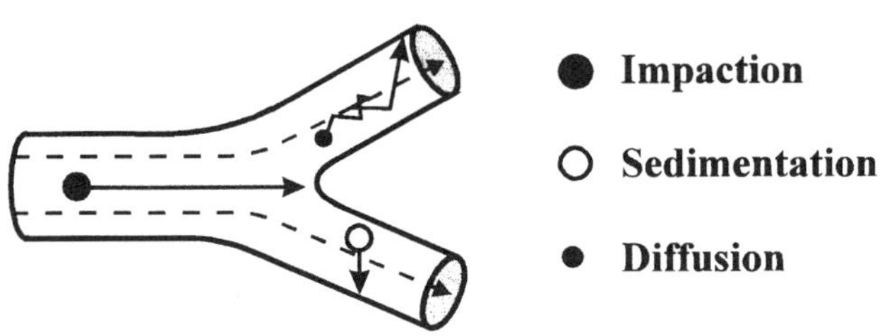

Figure 3 Mechanisms of particle deposition in the respiratory system. Illustrated are the three main deposition mechanisms, impaction, sedimentation, and diffusion, in an airway bifurcation during inhalation.

extent to which each of these mechanisms contributes to the deposition of a specific particle depends on the physical features of that particle.

Diffusion. For particles with a diameter less than 0.5 μm, particle displacement is governed mainly by diffusional transport. Collisions between gas molecules and a particle cause numerous very small random displacements of that particle. The distance a particle will travel by diffusion increases with time and with decreasing particle diameter (Table 1). A 0.1-μm particle can cover a distance of 40 μm in 1 s; a 0.01-μm particle a distance of 350 μm. Hence, the probability of particles to hit airspace surfaces by diffusional transport is larger the smaller the particles are and the longer they remain in the respiratory system. Consequently, the lung periphery with its small airway dimensions favors deposition by diffusion. Residence time is long, and the distance a particle has to travel before it hits an airspace wall is short.

Sedimentation. Particles are continually exposed to gravity and undergo gravitational settling (see Fig. 3). In contrast with diffusional transport, particle displacement by gravitational settling becomes significant for particles larger than 0.5 μm (see Table 1). The distance a particle settles within a given time increases with its mass (i.e., with its density and with its diameter). For instance, a unit-density sphere of 1-μm diameter settles at a distance of 35 μm in 1 s, whereas a unit-density sphere of 10-μm diameter settles at a distance of 3000 μm (see Table 1) within this time. The longer a particle remains in the respiratory system,

Table 1 Mean Displacement of Unit-Density Spheres in 1 s by Gravitational, Inertial, and Diffusional Transport

Diameter (μm)	Settling distance (μm)	Stopping distance (μm)	Diffusional displacement (μm)	Mass (pg)
25.0	18,203.3	1,892.5	1.46	8,181.2
10.0	2,912.9	3,02.8	2.32	523.4
5.0	739.9	75.7	3.30	65.45
2.0	124.0	12.1	5.34	4.19
1.0	33.34	3.02	7.84	0.524
0.5	9.54	0.76	11.85	6.545×10^{-2}
0.2	2.19	0.12	22.31	4.189×10^{-3}
0.1	0.87	0.03	39.19	5.236×10^{-4}
0.05	0.38	0.008	72.96	6.545×10^{-5}
0.02	0.144	0.001	174.53	4.189×10^{-6}
0.01	0.071	0.0003	343.96	5.236×10^{-7}

Temperature: 37°C; atmospheric pressure 1013 hPa, viscosity: 1.9×10^{-5} Pas, stopping distance is given for particles with an initial velocity of 1 m s^{-1}, mass is given per particle.

the larger is the settling distance the particle will cover and, hence, the probability that the particle will touch airspace walls. Therefore, the relative long residence time in the small conducting airways and in the gas-exchanging region of the lung will favor particle deposition by gravitational sedimentation.

Impaction. Inertia is the inherent property of a moving mass to resist accelerations. It may cause particles to continue to move in their original direction and not follow airflow streamlines, such that they deposit on airway walls by impaction (see Fig. 3). The inertia of a particle depends not only on the particle density and the particle diameter, but also, in contrast with gravitational settling and diffusional displacement, on the airflow velocity. A unit-density sphere of 1-μm diameter, traveling with a velocity of 1 or 5 m s^{-1}—which are typical airflow velocities prevailing in the larger conducting airways during quiet breathing and during moderate exercise—stops within a distance of 3 or 15 μm on a sudden cessation of airflow, whereas a unit-density 10-μm sphere continues to travel for 300 or 1500 μm (see Table 1). Inertial impaction will most likely occur in the extrathoracic airways and in the large conducting airways of the lung, where flow velocities are high and rapid changes in airflow direction occur.

In the light of the transport mechanisms causing particle deposition in the respiratory system, the dependency of total deposition on particle diameter, as displayed in Figure 1A, becomes clear. Minimal deposition occurs in the size range between 0.1 and 1 μm, because neither impaction or sedimentation nor diffusion are effective in particle displacement. With decreasing particle diameter, diffusional particle displacement increases so that particle deposition in the respiratory system increases. With increasing particle diameter, the distance covered by sedimentation or impaction increases such that total particle deposition is also enhanced.

In how far do physical particle features determine regional particle deposition? During quiet breathing, inertial impaction appears to be negligible for particles smaller than 2 μm (see Fig. 1B–D), so that those particles escape deposition within the extrathoracic region and the large conducting airways, but they are collected by the time-dependent deposition mechanisms—diffusion and sedimentation—in the small conducting airways and the alveolar region of the lung. Conversely, large particles, with a diameter of about 10 μm, are most likely deposited by impaction in the extrathoracic region, so that only some particles reach the large conducting airways, where they are also deposited by impaction. With decreasing particle diameter, particle displacement by inertia decreases, so that more and more particles escape deposition in the extrathoracic and the large conducting airways. They are caught in the small conducting airways or even in the alveolar region of the lung, either by sedimentation or by diffusion.

Particle Deposition Related to Breathing Patterns. An increase in tidal volume, while keeping the flow rate constant, will transport particles by convection deeper into the lung and increase their mean residence time in the lung.

Hence, more particles reach smaller, peripheral lung structures and more time is available for gravitational and diffusional particle transport. Therefore, an increase in total deposition is found for all particle sizes (see Fig. 2). On the other hand, keeping the tidal volume constant while increasing flow rate enhances total particle deposition for particles larger than 2 μm, but decreases total deposition of smaller particles. This is because the higher flow rate increases the probability for particle losses by impaction in the extrathoracic and large conducting airways, but particle losses by diffusion and sedimentation are decreased because of the shorter available time for deposition.

In summary, deposition occurs solely in alveolated airspaces for particles of minimum deposition. With decreasing and increasing particle size, the site of deposition shifts from distal to proximal airspaces. Consequently, targeting of specific airspaces in the lung with particles is possible if an appropriate particle size is chosen. This targeting can even be improved by making use of appropriate breathing patterns. Details are presented in the following paragraphs.

II. Basics and Definitions

A. Aerosol

An *aerosol* is a suspension of particulate matter in air. It comprises airborne droplets, solid particles, or both; all will be referred to as ‘‘particles’’ in this paper. Because of mechanical particle transport, an aerosol is intrinsically unstable (i.e., particles tend to deposit onto exposed surfaces); also, small aerosol particles at high concentrations tend to aggregate.

Physical Description of an Aerosol

Particle Diameters

Most aerosols are heterodisperse, possibly containing particles of varying sizes, shapes, and densities. The physical description of an heterodisperse aerosol may be misleading if simple geometric terms are used for particle characterization (e.g., the *geometric particle diameter, d*). Hence, equivalent particle diameters related to distinct physical particle properties are often applied. For example, particles may be classified relative to their gravitational settling, and compared by their *aerodynamic diameter* d_{ae}, where d_{ae} is the geometric diameter of a unit-density sphere that has the same gravitational settling velocity as the particle in question. Accordingly, equivalent diameters may be based on particle inertia, or they may be related to diffusional transport (*thermodynamic diameter*, d_{th}). But the light-scattering properties of particles are also applied for classification.

The particle diameters given in this paper refer to the geometric diameter of a unit-density sphere, if not otherwise specified.

Particle Size Distribution

Most frequently, an aerosol is characterized by its particle size distribution. Usually this distribution is reasonably well approximated by a log-normal frequency function (Fig. 4A). If the distribution is based on the logarithm of the particle size, the skewed log-normal distribution is transferred into the bell-shaped, gaussian error curve (see Fig. 4B). Consequently, two parameters are required to describe the particle size distribution of an aerosol: the *median particle diameter* (MD), and an index of dispersion, the *geometric standard deviation* (σ_g). The MD of the log-normal frequency distribution is equivalent to the logarithmic mean and represents the 50% size cut of the distribution. The geometric standard deviation is derived from the cumulative distribution (see Fig. 4C) by

$$\sigma_g = \sqrt{\frac{d_{84}}{d_{16}}} \tag{1}$$

where d_{16} and d_{84} are the particle diameters at the 16 and at the 84% size cut of the distribution. Depending on the biological effect under consideration, the particle size distribution of an aerosol may be related to the number of particles, currently discussed as an important factor for effects of ambient ultrafine particles. Alternatively, it may be related to the mass of particles; for instance, for therapeutic aerosols, for which the mass delivered to the respiratory system is of significance. For particles absorbing toxic constitutes onto their surfaces, the surface area of the particles is the appropriate parameter. Accordingly, the size distribution may be described by the *count median diameter* (CMD), the *mass median diameter* (MMD), or the *surface median diameter* (SMD). The count, the mass, or the surface distribution, all exhibit the same geometric standard deviation, and a clear relation between the means is given, in that CMD is smaller than MMD, whereas SMD is always in-between (see Fig. 4).

Monodisperse–Polydisperse Aerosols

If all particles of an aerosol are of uniform size, an aerosol is termed *monodisperse*. Because in reality perfect monodispersity does not exist, an aerosol is termed monodisperse if the geometric standard deviation of the particle distribution is smaller than 1.2. For deposition analyses, all particles of a monodisperse aerosol are considered to behave as if they had exactly the same diameter as the MD of the size distribution. In *polydisperse* aerosols, particles of widely differing sizes are present, and σ_g is larger than 1.2.

Particle Classes

The upper limit of diameter for respirable particles is approximately 50 μm in humans, but differs among species (6–9). According to their diameter, particles are commonly grouped into different classes: ultrafine, fine, and coarse particles.

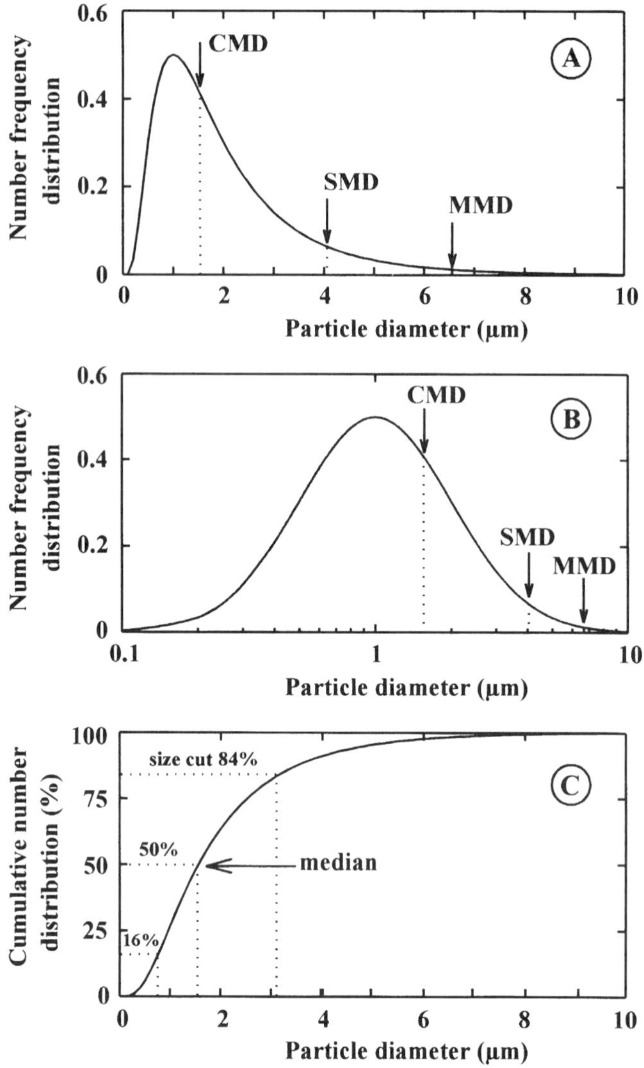

Figure 4 (A, B) Number-frequency distribution and (C) cumulative number distribution of an aerosol of unit-density spheres. Indicated are the count median diameter (CMD), the surface median diameter (SMD), and the mass median diameter (MMD) of the number-frequency distribution. The 16, 50, and 84% size cut of the cumulative number distribution are shown. For further explanation, see text.

Particles smaller than 0.1 μm in diameter are frequently called *ultrafine particles*. The definitions given for fine and coarse particles differ. The Environmental Protection Agency (EPA) convention, originally intended to apply to the two major atmospheric particle distributions, defines particles in the size range between 0.1 and 2.5 μm as *fine particles*, and those larger than 2.5 μm in diameter as *coarse particles*. According to the Health Effects Institute (HEI) convention, particles with diameters between 0.1 and 1 μm are *fine particles*, whereas *coarse particles* are larger than 1 μm in diameter.

In physical terms, particles are classified into different domains relative to their predominant mechanism of mechanical particle transport. Particles smaller than 0.1 μm are related to the *thermodynamic domain* and particles larger than 1 μm to the *aerodynamic domain*. A *transitional domain* is defined for those particles with diameters between 0.1 and 1 μm (10). A detailed overview of the different particle classifications is given in Chapter 1.

B. Deposition

In a mathematical sense, deposition refers to the mean probability for an inspired particle to be caught in the respiratory system. It is derived from particle number or mass balance considerations over a given respired volume, a given number of breaths, or a given time period. Deposition occurs when particles strike the wet airspace surfaces of the respiratory tract, but it also takes place when convective mixing of inhaled with reserve air causes particles not to be recovered on subsequent expirations. The site of initial particle contact with the airspace surface is considered the *site of initial deposition*. Thereafter, particles may rapidly be dislocated by means of mucociliary clearance or by macrophages after phagocytosis (11; see also Chap. 7).

Total, Regional, and Local Particle Deposition

Total deposition fraction or *total deposition* is the fraction of inhaled particles deposited in the entire respiratory system. Total deposition is composed of the sum of regional depositions taking place within distinct regions of the respiratory tract. Two main regions are considered: the extra- and intrathoracic regions. Deposition in the *extrathoracic region* refers to deposition occurring in the nasopharyngeal or oropharyngeal airways and the larynx during nose or mouth breathing. It was previously considered as *laryngeal deposition*, for mouth breathing or *nasopharyngeal deposition*, for nose breathing. *Intrathoracic deposition* is given by the quantity deposited in the *tracheobronchiolar region* (corresponding to the bronchial and bronchiolar region [BB + bb] of the ICRP model; see 138) and in the *alveolar region*.

Particle collection on a subregional level is defined as *local deposition*. For example, local deposition in the nose may refer to deposition occurring in the nasal valve, the nasal mucosa covered with hair, or the turbinated area of the nose. Local deposition also refers to deposition occurring in certain airway generations within the tracheobronchiolar tree.

III. Physical Mechanisms of Particle Deposition in the Respiratory Tract

Particle deposition in the respiratory system is related to distinct physical mechanisms operating on inhaled particles. The most important of these mechanisms are gravitational sedimentation, impaction by inertial forces, and brownian diffusion (see Fig. 3). Electrostatic forces and interception, the latter being significant only for fibers, are generally less important. In this section the physical mechanisms are briefly introduced. Several excellent overviews are available in the literature (12–14).

A. Gravitational Sedimentation

Particles are continuously exposed to gravity and undergo gravitational settling in air. During sedimentation, a particle acquires its terminal settling velocity v when gravitational forces are balanced by viscous resistive forces of the gas. This is described by *Stokes' law*, given here for a spherical particle with geometric diameter d and density ρ

$$\left(\frac{\pi}{6}\right) \rho\, d^3\, g = 3\, \pi\, \eta\, d\, v \tag{2}$$

The force of gravity on the particle is characterized by the left-hand side of the equation, where g is the gravitational constant. The right-hand side represents the resistive forces, where η is the dynamic viscosity of the surrounding medium. For the size region smaller than 1-μm diameter, the *Cunningham slip correction factor* ($C_{s,}$; 15) has to be applied to take the discontinuity of the surrounding medium into consideration. This results in a higher settling velocity than predicted by Stokes' law. The *terminal settling velocity* for spherical particles is then

$$v = \frac{\rho\, d^2\, g\, C_s}{18\, \eta} \tag{3}$$

Settling velocities for particles of different sizes are given in Table 1. Gravitational particle displacement becomes more effective than diffusional displacement for spheres larger than 0.5 μm.

Respirable particles acquire this terminal settling velocity in less than 0.1 ms (13), a fraction of less than 1% of the typical transit time of the airflow in any airway generation of the bronchial tree. For all practical purposes, therefore, particles may be considered to reach their terminal settling velocity instantaneously.

The probability of a particle for depositing on airway walls by gravitational settling is proportional to the distance a particle will cover within the airways; hence, it is proportional to the square of the particle diameter. The *settling distance* in the respiratory system is determined by v times the particle's residence time (t_{rs}). Breath-holding at the end of inspiration increases gravitational deposition, for the residence time and, hence, the settling distance is increased. Considering the respiratory flow rate Q, gravitational deposition is proportional to the parameter d^2/Q.

The efficiency of gravitational deposition is higher in tranquil than in stirred air (16), where particle settling is superimposed on components of convective transport. Convection may move particles back into volume elements previously cleared by gravitational settling. During stirred settling, particle concentration reaches $1/e$ times the original concentration in the same time that is required for complete removal of particles from tranquil air (13).

B. Inertial Impaction

The particle's inertia is related to its momentum (i.e., to the product of the particle's mass and its velocity). A particle's inertia can be assessed by the stopping distance (i.e., by the distance a particle with a given initial velocity will travel in still air in the absence of external forces). Table 1 shows stopping distances of particles traveling with a velocity of 1 m s^{-1}, a typical linear airflow velocity prevailing in the first ten airway generations of the bronchial tree during quiet breathing. It appears that inertial displacement becomes significant during quiet breathing for particles larger than 2 μm.

The likelihood that spheres with the diameter d and density ρ moving in an airstream with linear velocity u will diverge from airflow streamlines is characterized by the dimensionless *Stokes' number* (Stk)

$$\text{Stk} = \frac{\rho\, d^2\, u}{18\, \eta\, G} \tag{4}$$

where G characterizes the geometry of the structure in which particles are traveling (e.g., the diameter of a tube). The higher the Stokes' number, the more readily particles will depart from airflow streamlines, and the more likely they are to be deposited by inertial impaction on airway walls. For respiratory flow rate Q, inertial deposition in a given geometric structure is proportional to the *impaction parameter* d^2Q.

C. Brownian Displacement

Gas molecules are in constant motion because of their thermal energy. The mean free path λ traveled by a molecule in air between successive collisions with other gas molecules is about 0.07 μm under ordinary atmospheric conditions (i.e., about 150 times the molecular diameter). The speed of the gas molecules is about 100 m s^{-1}, leading to a collision frequency of about 5×10^9 s^{-1} (13,17).

For particles with a diameter close to λ, collisions with gas molecules can be considered as discrete events, causing an irregular, wiggling motion of the particle (see Fig. 3). With increasing particle diameter, the number of collisions occurring at one time from different directions increases, such that particle displacement, as the net result of all momentums applied, in effect, is reduced. Mathematically, particle transport by brownian motion is characterized by the *diffusion coefficient* D_P. For a spherical particle with the diameter d, D_P is given by

$$D_P = \frac{\kappa T C_s}{3 \pi \eta d} \tag{5}$$

where η is the viscosity of the surrounding medium, C_s is the slip correction factor, T is the absolute temperature, and κ is the Boltzmann constant. Unlike gravitational displacement or impaction, diffusional transport is independent of particle density, but also depends on particle shape (18,19). The *root mean square diffusional particle displacement* Δ for particulate matter subjected to stochastic transport processes (20)

$$\Delta = \sqrt{2 D_P t} \tag{6}$$

is given for $t = 1$ s in Table 1 for particles of different sizes. Diffusional displacement becomes effective for spheres smaller than 0.5 μm.

The probability for a particle to be deposited by diffusional displacement increases with $(t_{rs}/d)^{1/2}$, where t_{rs} is the residence time in the respiratory system. For the respiratory flow rate, diffusional deposition is a function of the *diffusion parameter* D_P/Q.

D. Interception

Interception takes place when a particle is brought close enough to the airway surface that an edge contacts the surface. Interception is usually important only for fibrous particles, such as asbestos fibers, because deposition by interception requires that the particle size is a significant fraction of the airway diameter. The aerodynamic diameter of fibers is predominantly determined by their geometric diameter and is about three times the fiber diameter, if the length/diameter ratio is larger than 10 (21–23). Hence, a fiber with a diameter of 0.5 μm and a length of 100 μm behaves the same as a 1.5-μm sphere in terms of sedimentation and impaction. Therefore, fibers have a low probability of deposition in the conducting airways by impaction or sedimentation, but interception has to be considered as an important mechanism.

E. Electrostatic Forces

Most ambient particles become neutralized naturally by air ions, but many freshly generated particles are electrically charged. The level of charge may vary widely, depending on the nature of the material, the mode of mechanical generation, and the age of the particles. Charged particles may have an enhanced deposition. For low particle–number concentrations ($< 10^5$ cm^{-3}), deposition increase is assumed to result from the electrostatic image charges generated on the surface of the airways by the charged particles (24). A threshold charge is required to enhance deposition, which Yu (24) found to be about 50 elementary charges for 1-μm particles. For each particle size, deposition increases linearly with the number of elementary charges prevalent on the particles. Electrostatic forces may increase deposition up to a factor of 2, but generally deposition is influenced to a lesser extent, by only about 10% (24–29).

IV. Methods of Assessing Particle Deposition in the Respiratory Tract

A. Experimental Approaches

Noninvasive Techniques

Radioactivity

Radioactive aerosols are frequently used in deposition or medical application studies because they allow noninvasive measurements of high sensitivity and reasonable spatial resolution. The fraction of aerosols deposited in the body is derived from radioactivity balance considerations.

Inhaled particles can be labeled with a variety of radionuclides, emitting β-rays or γ-rays. The β-rays are highly absorbed from tissue, so that they are almost undetectable from outside the body. With β-emitting radionuclides (e.g., ^3H or ^{14}C), particle deposition in the respiratory system or in the mouth can be assessed only from radioactivity recovered on expired-air filters or in lavage fluid from mouth washings.

As body tissues are much more radiolucent for γ-rays, γ-labels can provide information on the amount and the distribution of particles deposited in the respiratory system by using external radioactivity counts. Total deposition is inferred from the activity present in the entire body, whereas regional deposition is assessed from the radioactivity measured over the extrathoracic and the intrathoracic regions. Beside the spatial resolution of γ-count images, time kinetics of particle clearance are commonly used to further separate intrathoracic deposition into tracheobronchiolar and alveolar deposition: Fast-cleared activity is assumed to have been deposited in the tracheobronchiolar region, whereas that cleared slowly is assigned to the alveolated regions of the lung. This functional separation, however, has become a matter of controversial discussion because recent experimental results suggest that a significant fraction of particles deposited in the tracheobronchiolar region is retained much longer than previously assumed (30–32; see also Chap. 7).

Despite continuous technical improvements, deposition measurements based on external γ-counts still suffer some limitations from image nonuniformity, spatial resolution, detection efficiency, and counting linearity (33–35). Gamma rays that originate from different regions of the lungs as well as from the stomach or from the head are attenuated and scattered to variable degrees during their passage through the tissues. Hence, for a reliable interpretation of external γ-counts, it is necessary to apply suitable attenuation factors for different regions of the body. However, these factors can vary by a factor of 5 between subjects, and the use of individual corrections has been recommended for precise deposition measurements (36–43).

For stable γ-labeling of inhaled aerosols, different radioisotopes (e.g., ^{11}C, ^{57}Co, ^{60}Co, ^{67}Ga, ^{111}In, or ^{99m}Tc) are available, providing a wide spectrum of energies, types of radiation, half-lives, and doses. Unfortunately, it is technically difficult to label pharmaceutical agents directly, so that in most medical deposition studies a surrogate of radiolabeled particles or a mixture of drug substance and labeled particles is employed.

Devices Detecting Emitted γ-Rays. The total amount of material deposited in a subject after exposure to a γ-tagged aerosol can be determined in a *whole-body counter*. The energies of γ-quanta are measured by registration of the light pulses they produce in a sodium iodide crystal. Whole-body counters may use only one detector surrounding the subject completely (44), or several smaller detectors (40,45,46). Improved systems employ a *collimator*, which works like a lens and restricts the field of vision of the detector to a certain region of interest (e.g., to the extra- or the intrathoracic regions; 42,47,48). The amount of radioactivity to be detected by a whole-body counter can be small, a typically administered activity is approximately 0.01 MBq.

The *scintillation gamma camera*, developed by Anger in 1953, uses a single, large planar scintillation crystal masked with a honeycomb lead collimator containing as many as 15,000 parallel holes. The scintillations in each element of the crystal are elicited by incoming γ-rays, projected from only a small area of the body. They are sensed by phototubes, and the signals are converted to a two-dimensional radioactivity image reflecting the deposition pattern within the respiratory system. However, only limited information is given about the anatomical location of particles deposited within the lungs. A variety of indices calculated to quantify the deposition pattern in central and peripheral lung structures, among which the ‘‘penetration index’’ is most frequently used, implies that the central regions of the thoracic image represent mostly the large conducting airways (e.g., 33,49–54). However, in three-dimensional space, the presence of small airways and alveoli overlying the central airways within the thorax must be taken into account and precludes a precise separation of materials deposited in these physiologically and anatomically distinct regions (38,50). Radioactivity administered for gamma-camera imaging typically ranges between 2 and 10 MBq.

Three-dimensional images of the distribution of radioactivity in the thorax are obtained by *tomographic emission scanners* (36,37,54,55), using one- or multiple-headed cameras that are rotated along different planes around the source organ. By computational techniques a three-dimensional view of the radionuclide distribution is constructed. Spatial resolution is sufficient to estimate particle deposition in the largest conducting airways, but not in the smaller structures. Tomographic emission scanners are not indicated for total deposition studies, because long patient examination times and large quantities of radioactivity (25 MBq) are needed, and anteroposterior (AP) planar imaging is capable of providing information on total deposition with a similar accuracy (36).

Magnetopneumography

Magnetopneumography was developed by Cohen in 1973 (57) and was used in occupational exposure studies to estimate the quantity of magnetizable mineral dusts in the lungs of welders, coal or asbestos miners, and dental technicians (56–60). The technique consists of applying a magnetic field to the whole thorax or to localized areas and measuring the remanent magnetic field of retained lung particles by sensitive magnetometers. With a calibrated system, the magnitude of the magnetic field gives the amount of accumulated magnetic particles in the respiratory system. In deposition studies on volunteers, magnetide (Fe_3O_4) or hematite (γ-Fe_2O_3) particles have been applied (61,62). Disturbingly, the magnitude of the remanent magnetic field increases in the first days after inhalation. Redistribution of dipole magnetic particles in the lung periphery associated with alveolar macrophage motility is considered to be responsible for this phenomenon (60,63,64). It precludes a reasonable interpretation of magnetometric deposition data to date.

Light-Scattering Photometry (Tyndallometry)

The light-scattering technique enabled Tyndall in 1881 (65), for the first time, to directly observe that inhaled particles are retained in human lungs. Decades later, Altshuler and co-workers (66) were the first to apply this technique for the quantification of total particle deposition in human lungs. Since then, tyndallometry has been used in numerous deposition studies (e.g., 67–75).

Tyndallometry is based on the measurement of the intensity of light scattered by inspired and expired particles while they pass through a light beam close to the entrance of the respiratory system. The scattered light originates from all particles simultaneously present in the beam. Its intensity depends on particle number concentration, but also on diameter and refractive index of the aerosol particles. In applying nonhygroscopic, monodisperse particles, the intensity of the scattered light is solely proportional to particle number concentration. When light-scattering photometry is combined with pneumotachography, a continuous monitoring of particle number concentration in the respired air, as a function of the respired volume, is possible. Total deposition is given by

$$DE_{\mathrm{Tot}} = 1 - \frac{\int_{V_{\mathrm{ex}}} C(V)\, dV}{\int_{V_{\mathrm{in}}} C(V)\, dV} \qquad (7)$$

where V_{in} and V_{ex} are the inspired and expired volumes and $C(V)$ is the corresponding particle number concentration. Currently, this technique is introduced as a ''respiratory aerosol probe'' into clinical studies (76). It can be used to gain not only total deposition, but also particle deposition in so-called volumetric lung compartments (67,77,78). For that purpose, the inspired volume is considered as a succession of many small volume elements. Elements inspired at the onset of inspiration penetrate deeply into the respiratory system, those inspired at the end of inspiration penetrate much less. When a single volume element is labeled with particles, an aerosol bolus is inspired. If particle deposition is determined from a series of boluses inhaled into different volumetric lung regions—''series bolus delivery technique''—a simple algorithm can be used to estimate deposition in these volumetric compartments (67). In that case, the lung region is characterized by the volume of respired air transporting the particle bolus convectively into the respiratory system. Model simulations have to be used in a second step to convert volumetric lung regions to distinct anatomical regions (e.g., to the alveolated region or to the conducting airways).

Invasive Techniques

Postmortem measurements in laboratory animals supply information about regional or local deposition patterns in the lungs at better spatial resolution than noninvasive techniques can provide. Most frequently, radioactively labeled particles are applied, but magnetically labeled particles, microspheres, or fluorescent particles have also been used to quantify deposition throughout the lung on a macroscopic or microscopic level (79). Most of the invasive techniques require special lung fixation procedures before retention analysis to avoid translocation or particle loss during the fixation procedure (11,74). Rapid microwave fixation (80–82), intravascular perfusion techniques (74,83), and cryofixation (84) have been applied (see also Chap. 6).

Measurement Techniques

No single technique can provide all possible information on intrapulmonary particle deposition, so that the choice of the technique clearly depends on the question to be answered.

Lung or lobe dissection provides estimates about regional particle deposition on a macroscopic scale. Lobe-to-lobe, apex-to-base, or ventral-to-dorsal differences can be assessed. *Piece dissection* is used to estimate overall deposition heterogeneity throughout the lung or within a lung region. Regions with a high or a low particle load can be identified (80,85,86). The next level of detail is provided by *autoradiographs* (81,86–89). Thin lung slices are placed in direct contact with x-ray films and a crisp image of the distribution of radioactivity over the surface of the slice is obtained. With an overlay tracing of the lung slice, particle distribution can be mapped in detail. Quantitative information is obtained by computer-assisted correlation of anatomical features with the film density (89).

Unbiased stereological sampling techniques in combination with morphometrical analysis are required to obtain information about how particles are distributed throughout distinct anatomical compartments of the lung (e.g., respiratory bronchioles or alveolar ducts, 90–93; see also Chap. 6). This type of approach can also provide information about the dose of particles per surface area retained in the various compartments of the lung. In combination with confocal microscopy, the anatomical site of particle deposition can be examined in three dimensions (Fig. 5; 83,84).

To localize particles or soluble remanents of particles within cells or on the level of subcellular compartments, electron microscopic techniques are necessary (i.e., *electron spectroscopic imaging* and *electron energy loss spectroscopy*; 95,96).

Deposition in Physical Models

Experimental studies in idealized bronchial structures (e.g., 97–103) or in replicates of casts (e.g., 104–112) allow "inhalation" of substantial amounts of particles into easily accessible structures without having to deal with secondary redistribution phenomena caused by continuous particle clearing or lung preparation processes. They are performed to obtain information on primary deposition patterns with finer spatial resolution than is possible in in vivo experiments. These types of measurements may also be considered as the experimental match, validating theoretical approaches on particle deposition (see later). Mean local deposition rates, but also the heterogeneity of particle deposition within bifurcating zones, were investigated. Many studies (98–103,105,111) specifically focused on localization of so-called hot-spots, which are sites of enhanced deposition within the larynx or the tracheobronchiolar tree and may be most important rela-

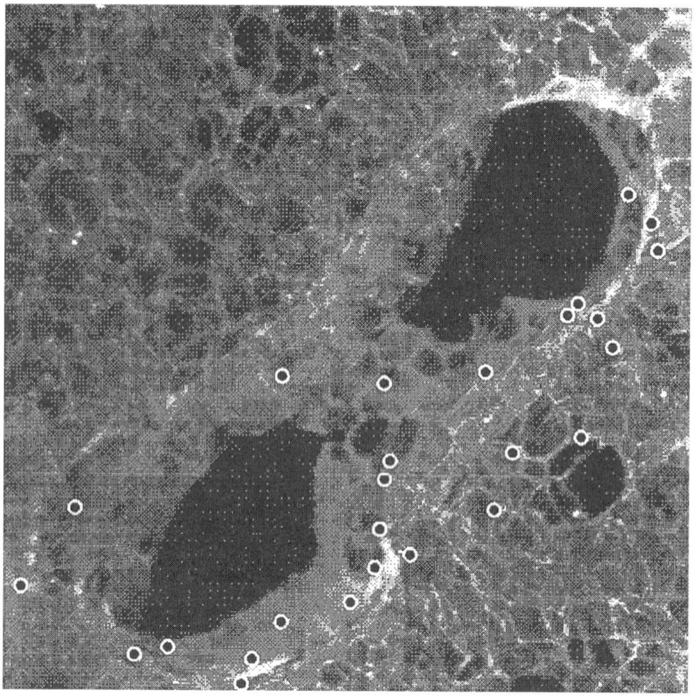

Figure 5 Sites of particle deposition assessed by confocal microscopy. Deposition sites of red and green fluorescent particles with a diameter of 2 μm are shown in a bifurcation of a canine bronchiole surrounded by lung parenchyma. Please note, particles are marked with a thin white circle to improve their appearance in this black and white copy.

tive to human health hazards arising from airborne particles. To a lesser extent, the influence of specific airflow fields on the pattern of intrabronchial deposition has been studied (98,99). In models of single bifurcations or of few successive airway generations, structural parameters of bifurcations (e.g., branching angles or symmetry) were varied systematically to evaluate factors governing the process of deposition within these model bifurcations (98,99,103).

Limitations arise particularly when studies are performed in idealized tubular structures, because geometric features of the conducting airways are simplified to an extent that may result in unrealistic airflow fields and unreasonable particle deposition patterns. Replicates of bronchial casts provide a more realistic flow geometry. Often constant airflows are used, which to some extent can only mimic the effects of in vivo flow variations. Little information is available, however, on whether particle deposition patterns resulting from constant-flow inspirations are the same as those resulting from variable-flow inspirations.

B. Model Simulations

Mathematical Models

In the last decades, various mathematical approaches have been introduced to predict the amount, the anatomical sites, and the underlying mechanisms of particle deposition in the respiratory system. Modeling particle deposition requires idealized assumptions about the structure of the respiratory system (morphometric model), the particle transport through the airways (gas dynamics model) and toward the airway surfaces (mechanical particle transport model), and about the physiological parameters characterizing breathing patterns (physiological model). Having chosen an appropriate set of assumptions, the physical laws of mass, heat, and momentum conservation are employed to quantify the dynamics of interest and to determine their effect on particle deposition. Depending on the method and the degree of idealization, there are many different ways to create deposition models, and there is ample work on this subject available in the literature (113–116). Regardless of the approach chosen, all models published so far were capable of characterizing deposition in the respiratory system reasonably well in comparison with existing experimental data.

The models introduced by Findeisen (117), Altshuler (118), and Taulbee and Yu (119) are considered ''primary deposition models,'' in that each proposed original and independent mathematical formalisms to describe particle transport onto airway surfaces. Incidently, they are also based on different models of the geometric structure of the human lung. Later, the formalisms of the primary models were adopted and modified by many authors, resulting in so-called ''secondary deposition models'' (120–134). Recent models have been proposed by the U.S. National Council on Radiation Protection and Measurements (NCRP; 136–137) and by the Task Group on Human Respiratory Tract Models for Radiological Protection (ICRP; 137,138).

In 1935, the meteorologist Findeisen was the first to introduce a lung deposition model. The geometric structure of the lung is treated as a system of nine regions, arranged in series and characterized according to the functional and anatomical features of different-sized airway structures. The model neglects extrathoracic airways and starts with the trachea, the last region contains the alveolar sacs. Particle transport through airways occurs solely by convective bulk flow, whereas mixing processes are neglected. Particle loss onto airway surfaces is considered as a function of impaction, sedimentation, and diffusion, which are assumed to act independently of each other. Findeisen's estimations of total thoracic particle loss for the size range between 0.03 and 10 μm are shown in Figure

6. Interestingly, despite the relative simplicity of his model, subsequent, more sophisticated models, as well as experimental data, in principle, confirmed his predictions. This holds true for modifications of the Findeisen model by Landahl (121,122), who added a region representing mouth and pharynx, and by Beeckmans (123,124), who further considered convective mixing in particle transport processes. The first international attempt to assess regional particle deposition in the lung was based on the Findeisen–Landahl–Beeckman modeling (126).

In contrast to Findeisen's approach, the model proposed by Altshuler (118) is spatially continuous, in that the entire respiratory tract is considered a continuous filter bed. Altshuler's model was not adopted by other authors, but applied in several studies of his own group (139,140).

Taulbee and Yu (119) developed a formalism to assess particle number concentration in the human lung at any lung depth and any time during the breathing cycle, so that their model is spatially and temporally continuous and allows the simulation of arbitrary breathing conditions. The applied gas dynamics model

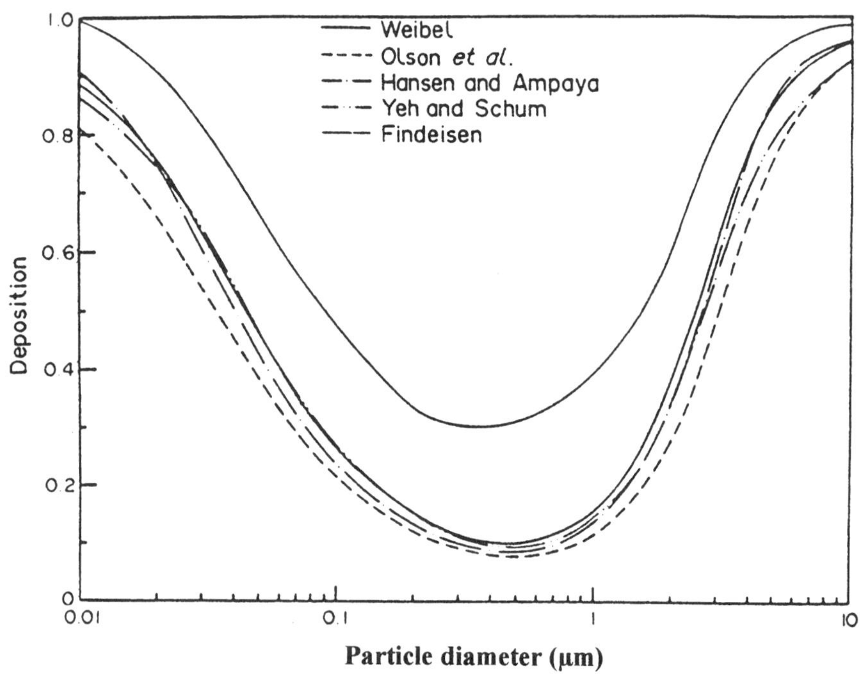

Figure 6 Total deposition fraction of unit-density spheres during mouth breathing: Data were modeled for a tidal volume of 1000 cm^3 and a rate of 15 breaths per minute and for different morphometric models of the human lung. (From Ref. 150.)

considers longitudinal mixing in conducting airways and convective mixing between inhaled and residual air in alveolated airways. The morphometrical model approximates the many generations of the airways by a trumpet-shaped structure, with a variable, continuously increasing cross section along its depth.

This ''trumpet model'' was originally introduced by Scherer et al. (141) for simulations of intrapulmonary gas transport and is based on a morphometric data set proposed by Weibel (5). In Weibel's model, the structural parameters of each airway generation are described by average values, so that all airways of a given generation are identical, as are all pathways leading to a specific airway generation. The model is, therefore, termed ''symmetrical'' or ''deterministic.''

Most of the later proposed secondary deposition models use symmetrical morphometric model structures (e.g., 121,125,127–129,144), whereas some others are based on a system of asymmetrically branching airways (e.g., 130,132–134,145–147). Various simulations neglect the existence of alveoli, whereas others add all the alveoli to the last airway generation or add increasing numbers of alveoli to consecutive airway generations within an acinus. However, the influence of using different morphometric data sets is small, and calculated total or regional deposition does not vary considerably from one model to another (see Fig. 6; 115,148–150).

A so-called stochastic airway model was proposed by Koblinger and Hofmann (146,147). It is based on statistical relations (evaluated on airway casts) between geometrical parameters of a given parent airway and those of the two branching daughter airways. This model shows a significant variability of airway lengths, diameters, and numbers of airway generations along different pathways. The transport of inspired particles occurs by randomly selecting at each bifurcation the sequence of airways an individual particle is passing through. Interestingly, the effect on calculated total or regional deposition again appears to be minor when compared with other lung models. However, within the intrathoracic airways, deposition appears to be partially shifted to more distal airways. Furthermore, this model may provide insight into the deposition variability potentially present in the lung within airways of a given generation (115,133,134,147).

All of the foregoing deposition models are based on the assumption of uniform particle distribution within and among airways. However, local deposition per unit surface area is frequently important for the assessment of possible risks from ambient air pollution, and local accumulations of particles can occur in bifurcating systems. Nowadays, computational techniques and capacities allow theoretical deposition models to focus on local particle deposition in subunits of the respiratory system (e.g., in the oropharyngeal cavity) or in three-dimensional airway bifurcation models. Air velocity fields are computed by numerical modeling techniques solving the Navier–Stokes equation in the respective model geometry (151–158). Particles are then virtually entrained in the airstream, and particle trajectories are simulated by solving the equations for particle motion. Local particle deposition patterns within the three-dimensional model are inferred from the intersection of particle trajectories with the adjacent model surfaces. So far, the effects of asymmetries in airway diameters, branching angles, or flow division, and the influence of the gravitational angle at bifurcations have been studied in idealized airway models. Recently, a new approach was introduced by Perzl et al. (159) to make real-lung geometries available for computational deposition modeling. Two-dimensional images of a canine cast obtained by high-resolution computed tomography were combined to yield a three-dimensional volume data set. After image processing, a three-dimensional polygonial surface representation from the cast was created, showing excellent conformity with the original cast. Based on this surface representation, a finite-element mesh was generated, allowing computational fluid dynamics in realistic conducting airway structures (160). These numerically modeled airflow fields can even be verified in hollow replicates of these computational surface representations by measuring experimentally the flow fields applying the laser-light-sheet imaging method (161,162).

Empirical Models

A different approach to deposition modeling is the empirical one, in which semiempirical functions, derived from experiments or theory, are developed to quantify deposition for a wide range of particle sizes and breathing conditions. The empirical models consider the respiratory system to be a series of filters representing the various anatomical or functional regions of the system. Parameters characterizing particle motion by impaction, sedimentation, and diffusion are developed, and the dependence on the filtration efficiencies of the respective regions is determined. By means of the least-square method, the parameters are optimized to fit experimental data (112,163–168). An advantage of this type of modeling is that it presents relatively clear-cut algebraic approximations that provide qualified estimates of regional particle deposition. It also represents a tool for interpolating and extrapolating missing experimental data on a simple basis.

V. Total Deposition

Numerous studies have investigated total deposition in human lungs for a variety of test particles under different experimental conditions. Schlesinger (8) summarized those studies performed in healthy subjects using monodisperse, charge-neutralized, nonhygroscopic, and nonfibrous aerosols. Corrections for different ventilation conditions were not applied. The data as a function of particle size and the breathing mode are given in Figure 7. For mouth and nose breathing, total deposition in humans exhibits a minimum of about 15% for particles in the 0.1- to 1-μm–size range, for which neither impaction nor sedimentation or diffusion are effective in particle displacement. Sedimentation and/or impaction gov-

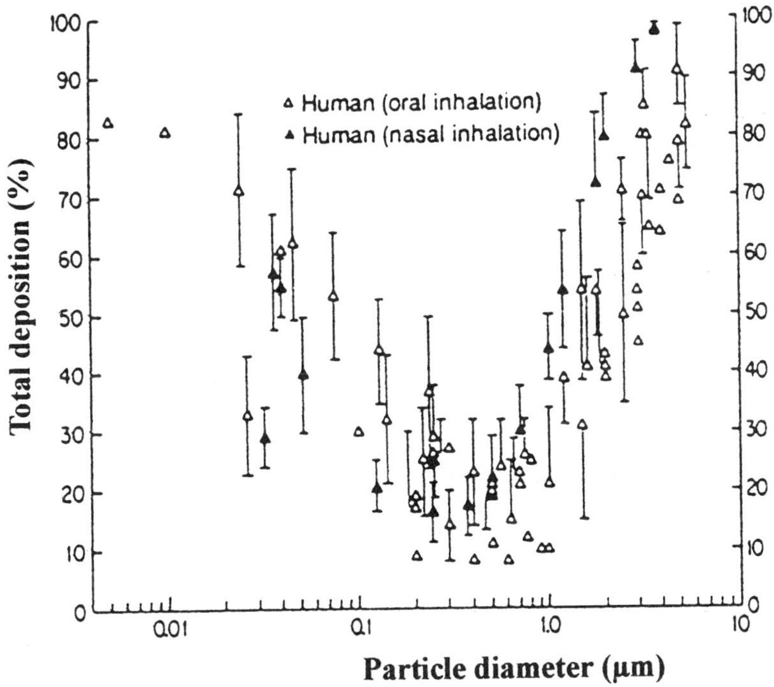

Figure 7 Total deposition data (percentage deposition of amount inhaled) in humans as a function of particle size: Shown are mean values with standard deviations when available. Particle diameters are aerodynamic for those > 0.5 µm and thermodynamic for those < 0.5 µm. (From Ref. 8.)

erns deposition for particles with aerodynamic diameters larger than 1 µm, whereas diffusional displacement determines the deposition of ultrafine particles.

For particles with aerodynamic diameters larger than 1 µm, nasal inhalation generally results in higher total deposition rates than during oral breathing, underlining the greater particle-collecting efficiency of the nasal passage. There is no difference in total deposition between nasal and oral breathing for particles smaller than 1 µm, although little differences for particles in the nanometer range have been reported (169,170).

There is a considerable scatter in the deposition data, although, in general, the same trend can be inferred from the different studies. The heterogeneity may be partly related to the different kinds of test particles and methods applied. But the scatter, in particular, is caused by the intersubject variability in airway morphology and the various breathing patterns used for particle inhalation (71,72,

169–175). Quantifying the biological variability in deposition by the coefficient of variation reveals that, in healthy human subjects, coefficients of 0.38 and 0.19 were observed for 1 and 3-μm–particle deposition under spontaneous-breathing conditions. Under these conditions, coefficients of variation for minute ventilation, tidal volume, and breathing frequency were found to be about 0.2 (176,177). For controlled-breathing conditions, total deposition variability was diminished, and the respective coefficients of variation reduced to 0.27 and 0.13 (71).

Empirical model calculations of total deposition in the human respiratory system are given by Heyder et al. (163) and Rudolf et al. (165–168). From the empirical Eq.(8) for extrathoracic (DE_{ET}), tracheobronchiolar (DE_{TB}), and alveolar deposition (DE_{A}), total deposition (DE_{Tot}) can be assessed by

$$DE_{Tot} = DE_{ET} + DE_{TB} + DE_{A} \tag{8}$$

VI. Regional Deposition

A. Extrathoracic Deposition

Even during quiet breathing, flow velocities in the extrathoracic airways are relatively high. Therefore, residence time of particles within these regions is short and most of the airflow through nasal or oropharyngeal airways is turbulent (178,179). For particles in the aerodynamic domain, deposition is governed mainly by impaction. Particle deposition in the ultrafine-sized range is controlled principally by diffusion, but may be enhanced by the complex interactions of diffusion and turbulent airflow (180–182).

Nose Breathing

The specific anatomical features of the nose, such as nasal hairs or the nasal valves, support the high filtration efficiency of the nose and favor deposition mainly at the entrance of the nasal cavity (183). With nose breathing, laryngeal deposition has been neglected by most authors, for most of those particles that are likely to be retained at the larynx have already been removed by the nasal filter. Hence, because deposition only within the nasopharyngeal airways has been considered, extrathoracic deposition during nose breathing has been previously termed nasopharyngeal deposition.

Aerodynamic Domain

Figure 8 summarizes experimental data (184) obtained on inspiratory collection efficiencies of the human nose as a function of the impaction parameter $d_{ae}^2\,Q$ (d_{ae}, aerodynamic particle diameter; Q, respiratory flow rate). This parameter is applied to account for different flow rates and particle sizes between experimental studies. Despite substantial scatter of the data, the particle collection efficiency

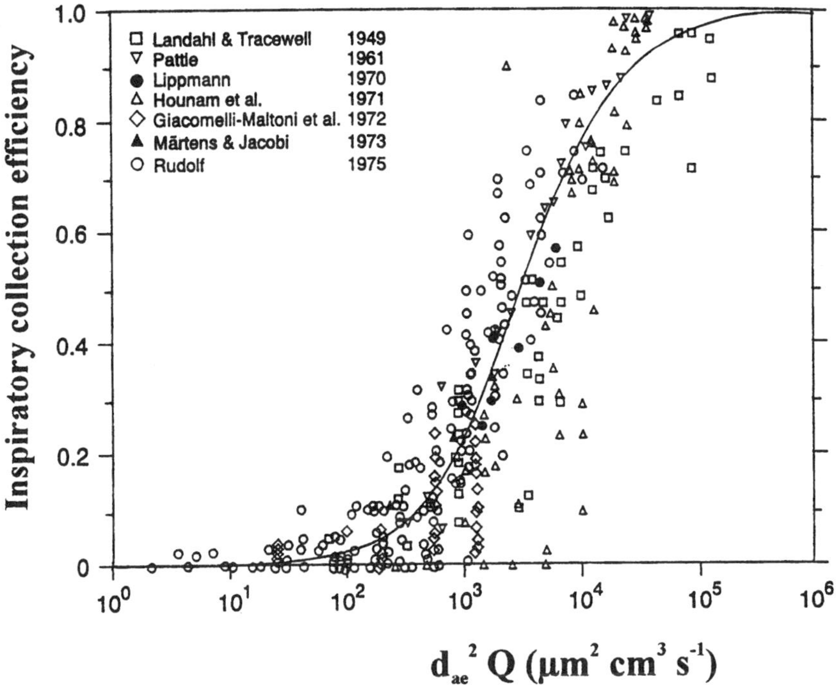

Figure 8 Inspiratory collection efficiency of the human nose as a function of the impaction parameter $d_{ae}^2 Q$: The curve represents a hyperbolic approximation; d_{ae}, aerodynamic particle diameter; Q, inspiratory flow rate. (From Ref. 184.)

of the nose appears to increase in a sigmoidal manner with increasing values of $d_{ae}^2 Q$. The targeting of particles to the nasal region, therefore, requires an aerosol with coarse particles to be inhaled with large flow velocities. For increasing the deposited fraction, it is more effective to increase particle size than flow rate. Mean inspiratory flow rates at rest and exercise are in the order of 250 cm^3 s^{-1} and 1000 cm^3 s^{-1}, so that the respective impaction parameters for 3-μm particles are 2250 μm^2 cm^3 s^{-1} and 9000 μm^2 cm^3 s^{-1}. The latter value also holds for 6-μm particles during quiet breathing. The corresponding experimental data shows nasal deposition efficiencies of 0.05 to 0.6 for 3-μm particles inhaled during quiet breathing. For 3-μm particles inhaled at 1000 cm^3 s^{-1} or for 6-μm particles inhaled at 250 cm^3 s^{-1}, deposition rates are 0.25 to 0.8. The scatter in experimental data is related to mainly the intersubject variability of the anatomical features of the nose (185–187). Cheng and co-workers (185) characterized nasal geometry of ten subjects using magnetic resonance imaging (MRI) and acoustic rhinometry. They found that particle deposition onto nasal airway walls increases with increasing nasal surface area and airway complexity, and with decreasing nasal cross-sectional area. Also, a significant variability in deposition arises within individuals from physiologically occurring periodic variations in the nasal resistance and cross-sectional area that distribute airflow from one side to the other by as much as 20–80%.

There are several approaches to characterize nasal deposition by mathematical (120,122) or by empirical models (163,165–168,173,184,188,189). For particles of 1 μm or larger, Rudolf et al. (168) estimated inspiratory particle collection efficiency of the nose ($E_{ET\text{-}N}$) by

$$E_{ET\text{-}N} = 1 - (2.05 \times 10^{-4}\, d_{ae}^2\, Q + 1)^{-1} \tag{9}$$

This empirical model assumes the inspiratory flow rate Q to be constant.

Empirical models neglect expiratory nasal deposition, for it appears to be insignificant relative to inspiratory collection efficiency. Stahlhofen (184) considers the fraction of the tidal volume flowing through the nose during inspiration to be $1 - V_{ET}/V_T$. The fraction of particles deposited in the extrathoracic region during nasal breathing $DE_{ET\text{-}N}$ is then given by

$$DE_{ET\text{-}N} = \left[1 - \left(\frac{V_{ET}}{V_T}\right)\right] E_{ET\text{-}N} \tag{10}$$

where V_T is the tidal volume and V_{ET} is the extrathoracic volume. V_{ET} is approximated to 50 cm^3 for male adults and to 40 cm^3 for female adults (168). Deposition data predicted by the model for a tidal volume of 1000 cm^3, at flow rates of 250 $cm^3\ s^{-1}$ and 1000 $cm^3\ s^{-1}$ are shown in Figure 9. For all particles in the aerodynamic size range, the higher flow rate clearly enhances nasal collection efficiency. For a given particle size and flow rate, variations in tidal volume have almost no effect on the fraction of deposited particles [see Eqs. (9) and (10)], but the absolute number or mass of particles retained in the nose changes proportionally with the tidal volume.

Thermodynamic Domain

Deposition of particles of the thermodynamic size range has not been studied extensively in humans. Cheng and co-workers (185) measured deposition efficiencies for 4-, 8-, 20-, and 150-nm particles in ten healthy adult, male volunteers. For nose-in mouth-out breathing at flow rates of 333 $cm^3\ s^{-1}$, deposition fractions for these particle sizes were 36.7 ± 10.6 (mean ± SD), 21.2 ± 8.9, 11.1 ± 7.7, and 5.2 ± 3.8%. However, because expiratory deposition in the mouth is not negligible for particles in the thermodynamic domain, these values overestimate nasal deposition. The large SD values indicate that intersubject deposition variability is notable in the thermodynamic domain. Mean nasal deposition, as de-

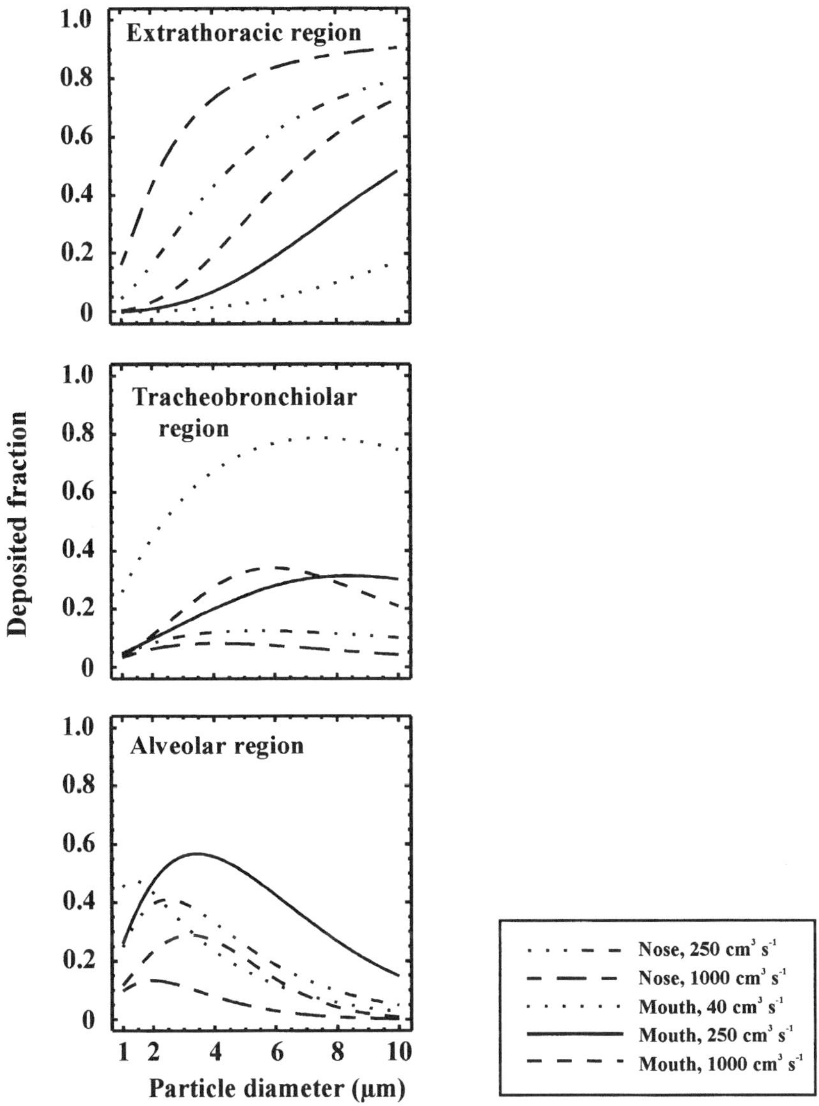

Figure 9 Effect of flow rate on regional deposition: Regional deposition fraction curves are shown for nose and mouth breathing as predicted by the empirical model of Rudolf et al. (167) for male adults. Calculations were performed for a tidal volume of 1000 cm^3 at flow rates of 40, 250, and 1000 $cm^3\ s^{-1}$.

rived from data on total deposition, was estimated to be 15 and 4% for 5- and 10-nm particles at flow rates of 250 $cm^3\ s^{-1}$ (169,170). In the subnanometer-sized range, particle filtration of the nose appears to be almost complete. Inspiratory nasal deposition of 0.53- to 0.62-nm particles ranged between 0.94 and 0.99 in three subjects during quiet-breathing conditions (182).

Complementary to the experiments in human subjects, measurements were performed in hollow replicates of human nasal airway casts (106,108,112,116, 181,190). Particle collection efficiency obtained in nasal airway casts can be approximated by an exponential function of the diffusion parameter (D_p/Q)

$$E_{\text{ET-N}} = 1 - \exp\left(-12.65\, D_p^{1/2}\, Q^{-1/8}\right) \tag{11}$$

(112), which indicates that the dependence on respiratory flow rate Q is weaker than that on particle diffusivity D_p. In the thermodynamic domain, expiratory particle collection efficiency of the nose is approximately 10% higher than inspiratory efficiency (106).

Mouth Breathing

Aerodynamic Domain

Figure 10 summarizes human experimental data (184) on extrathoracic deposition during mouth breathing as a function of the impaction parameter $d_{ae}^2\, Q$. There is substantial scatter in the data, but similar to nasal deposition, the dependence on $d_{ae}^2\, Q$ appears to be sigmoidal. However, it must be emphasized that for $d_{ae}^2\, Q < 10^4$, deposition during mouth breathing is considerably smaller than during nose breathing. During a quiet inspiration, the nose retains about 30% of 3-μm particles, whereas less than 5% of the particles are caught in the extrathoracic region with mouth breathing (see also Fig. 9).

Most of the experimental data of Figure 10 were obtained in human subjects inspiring particles through a tubular mouthpiece held between the teeth. Several studies show that this mode of inhalation causes deposition to occur mainly in the larynx, especially on the upper surface of the vocal cords (48,165,191), whereas almost no particles are lost in the oral cavity or the pharynx. Therefore, extrathoracic deposition during mouth breathing was previously termed laryngeal deposition. During natural mouth breathing, deposition in the oral cavity was higher and quite variable depending much on the degree of mouth opening, flow rate, and breathing frequency (172,192,193).

Empirical models (163,165–168,184) characterize oral collection efficiency ($E_{\text{ET-M}}$) for particles 1 μm or larger, as a function of the impaction parameter $d_{ae}^2\, Q$:

$$E_{\text{ET-M}} = 1 - \left[1.1 \times 10^{-4}\left(d_{ae}^2 \times Q^{0.6} \times V_T^{-0.2}\right)^{1.4} + 1\right]^{-1} \tag{12}$$

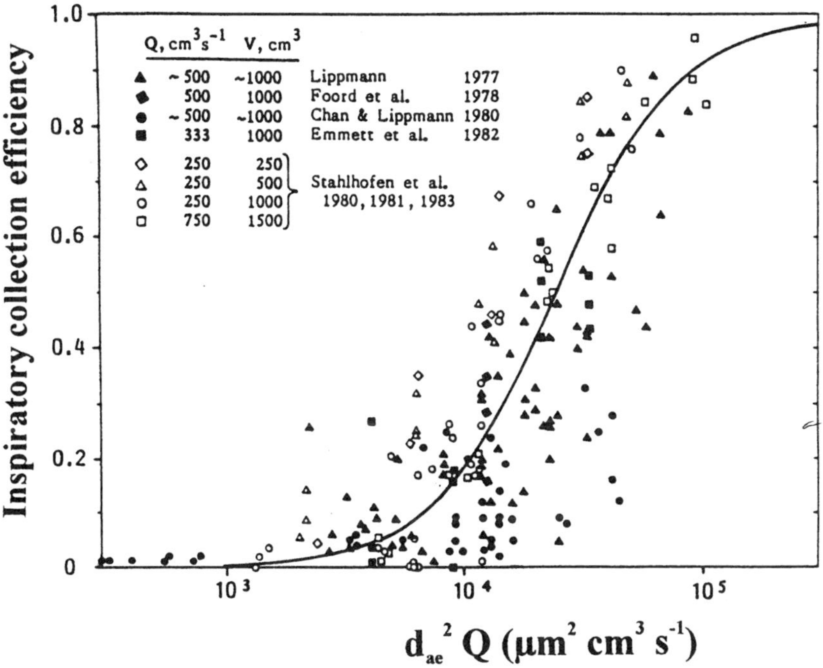

Figure 10 Inspiratory extrathoracic deposition data in humans during mouth breathing as a function of the impaction parameter $d_{ae}^2\,Q$: The curve represents a hyperbolic approximation. d_{ae}, aerodynamic particle diameter; Q, inspiratory flow rate. (From Ref. 184.)

Extrathoracic deposition during mouth breathing ($DE_{ET\text{-}M}$) is derived from the collection efficiency weighted by the fraction of tidal volume $(1 - V_{ET}/V_T)$ flowing through this region

$$DE_{ET\text{-}M} = \left[1 - \left(\frac{V_{ET}}{V_T}\right)\right] E_{ET\text{-}M} \tag{13}$$

Expiratory deposition is again considered to be negligible in comparison with inspiratory deposition (163,184). Figure 9 shows deposition data predicted by the model for breathing conditions during rest and exercise. The model assumes a constant respiratory flow rate Q, but takes into account that the collection efficiency decreases with increasing tidal volume V_T. It shows that oral deposition is less dependent on flow rate than is nasal deposition, as Q is weighted by a power exponent of 0.6. Therefore, the aerodynamic particle diameter is the main determinant of oral collection efficiency and, for targeting particles into this region, coarse particles should be inhaled (see Figs. 9 and 13). Moreover, for increasing the deposited fraction of particles, it is much more efficient to increase particle size than flow rate. Similar to nose breathing, the fraction of particles deposited in the oral region, for a given particle size and flow rate, is generally independent of the tidal volume inhaled [see Eqs. (12), (13); Fig. 11]. But one must consider that the number or the mass of removed particles increases almost linearly with increasing tidal volume.

Thermodynamic Domain

Oral deposition of ultrafine particles determined in physical replicates of oropharyngeal airways was slightly smaller than that measured in nasal casts (109,181,194). However, measurements performed in three healthy adults suggest that there is zero deposition for 0.1-, 0.07-, and 0.05-μm particles inhaled through the mouth under different breathing conditions (163).

B. Intrathoracic Deposition

Experimentally determined deposition efficiencies of the intrathoracic region have usually been inferred from measurements with radioactively labeled particles. The fast-cleared fraction of thoracic activity has been assumed to be deposited in the tracheobronchiolar region, whereas the slow-cleared fraction has been assigned to the alveolar region of the lung (see Chap. 7). Recently, this distinction has become a matter of controversy, for experiments suggest that some of the activity deposited in the conducting airways is cleared much slower than previously assumed (30–32). Some investigators, therefore, prefer to use the term "fast-cleared and slow-cleared thoracic deposition," instead of tracheobronchiolar and alveolar deposition, for the description and analysis of deposition studies using radioactivity.

Tracheobronchiolar Deposition: Fast-Cleared Thoracic Deposition

Aerodynamic Domain

Particles escaping from deposition in the extrathoracic regions enter the lung through the tracheobronchiolar airways. Because flow velocities in the airways decrease rapidly from large to small conducting airways, inertial impaction determines particle deposition only in the most central airways. With decreasing airway diameter, gravitational sedimentation gains more and more importance and dominates deposition within the small bronchial airways. As inertial impaction grows stronger with increasing particle mass, the site of deposition is shifted from the peripheral to the proximal airways with increasing particle size (see Figs. 14 and 15). During expiration, only sedimentation is of importance, because those larger particles that escape inertial deposition during inspiration are subse-

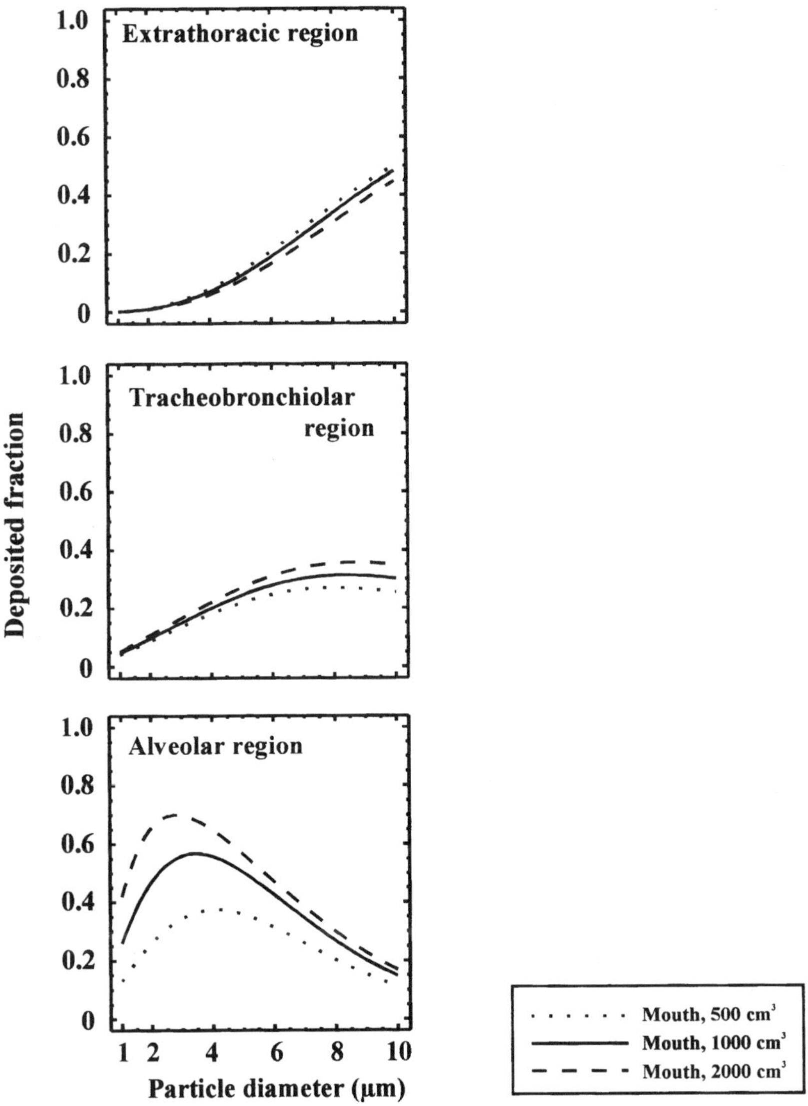

Figure 11 Effect of tidal volume on regional deposition: Regional deposition fraction curves are shown for mouth breathing as predicted by the empirical model of Rudolf et al. (167) for male adults. Estimates were done for tidal volumes of 500, 1000, and 2000 cm^3 at a flow rate of 250 $cm^3\ s^{-1}$.

quently collected in the small conducting airways or in the alveolar region of the lung.

Experimental data, from several investigators who measured intrathoracic particle deposition during mouth breathing, were summarized by Stahlhofen et al. (184). Figure 12 shows these data as a function of the aerodynamic particle diameter. Because large particles are effectively collected by the extrathoracic airways, intrathoracic deposition does not increase or decrease monotonically with particle diameter, but exhibits maximal values for particles with diameters between 4 and 8 μm. It appears to be lowest for particles smaller than 1 μm.

There is a remarkable variability between deposition data collected in different studies. As an example, deposition of 3-μm particles may range between almost zero and a particle loss of close to 50%. Beside those subject-specific factors cited before, technical and experimental confounders are discussed. There were significant differences in measuring procedures and in definitions applied to describe the fast-cleared portion of thoracic particles (184). Moreover, recent investigations suggest hygroscopic growth and leaching of test particles as a possible source of measurement error, resulting in an overestimation of the deposited fraction.

Empirical models (163,165–168) characterize the collection efficiency of the tracheobronchiolar region (E_{TB}) for particles 1 μm or larger as:

$$E_{TB} = 1 - \exp\{-1.24\,[4 \times 10^{-6}\,\mathrm{CF}^{2.8}\,(d_{ae}^2\,Q)^{1.15}] - 1.24\,[(0.009 + 0.165\,t_b^{1.5})\,d_{ae}\,t_b^{-0.25}]\} \tag{14}$$

CF is a correction factor accounting for gender. It is 1 for adult men and 1.075 for adult women. The residence time of particles in small bronchial airways, t_b, is

$$t_b = \frac{V_{b\text{-}FRC}\,(2 + V_T/\mathrm{FRC})}{2\,Q} \tag{15}$$

V_T is the tidal volume and FRC is the functional residual capacity of the lung. FRC is assumed to be 3300 cm^3 for male and 2660 cm^3 for female adults in the coefficients for Eq. (14). $V_{b\text{-}FRC}$ represents the volume of the small bronchial airways at an FRC level, set to 48 and 39 cm^3 in adult men or women (168). Equation (14) characterizes inertial E_{TB} relative to the impaction parameter $d_{ae}^2\,Q$, and sedi-

Figure 12 Tracheobronchial and alveolar deposition data in humans during mouth breathing as a function of aerodynamic particle diameter: The solid curves represent the approximate mean of all experiments, the broken curve gives a "conservative" estimate based on data by Stahlhofen et al. (From Ref. 184.)

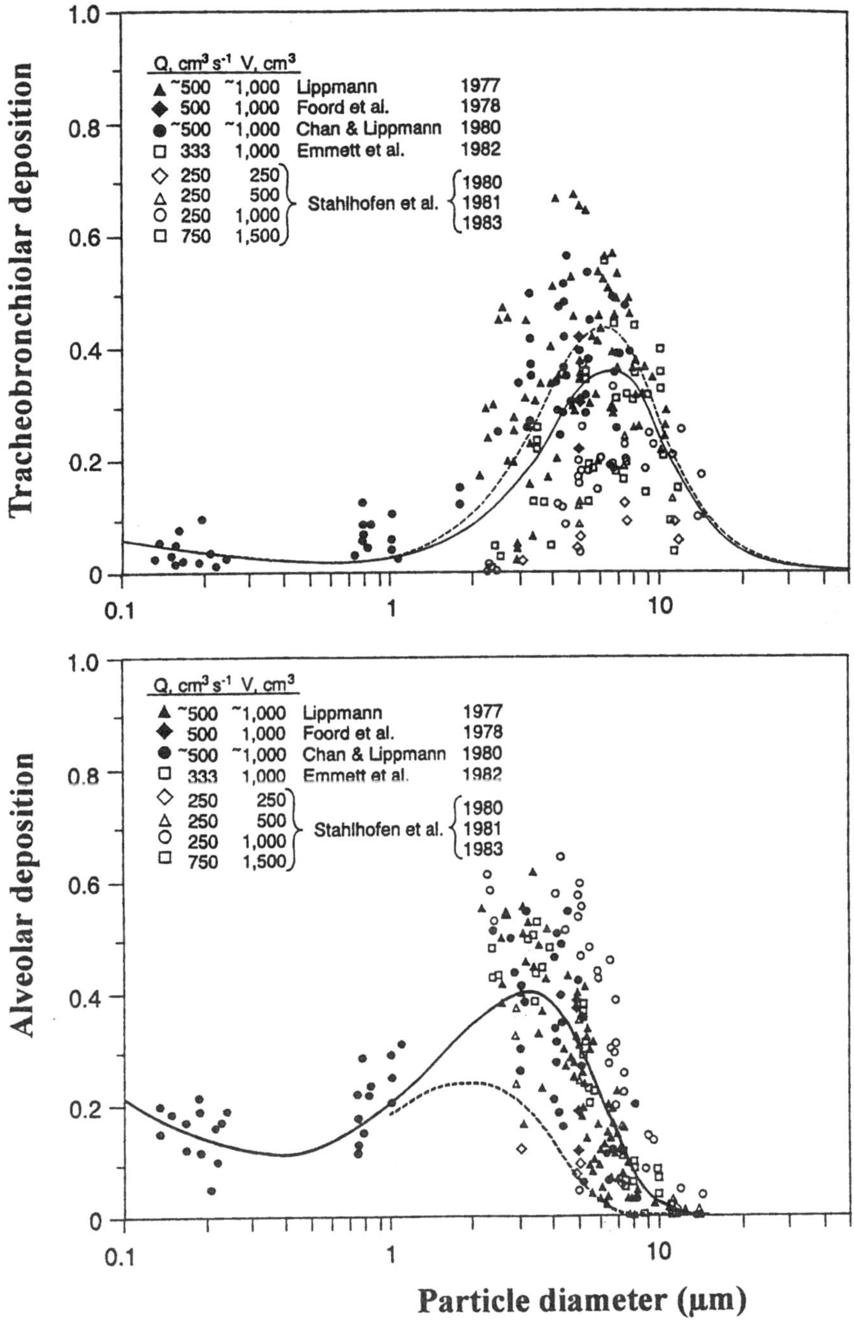
Tracheobronchiolar deposition
Q, cm³ s⁻¹ V, cm³
~500 ~1,000 Lippmann 1977
500 1,000 Foord et al. 1978
~500 ~1,000 Chan & Lippmann 1980
333 1,000 Emmett et al. 1982
250 250
250 500
250 1,000
750 1,500
Stahlhofen et al. 1980 1981 1983
1.0
0.8
0.6
0.4
0.2
0
0.1
1
10
Alveolar deposition
Q, cm³ s⁻¹ V, cm³
~500 ~1,000 Lippmann 1977
500 1,000 Foord et al. 1978
~500 ~1,000 Chan & Lippmann 1980
333 1,000 Emmett et al. 1982
250 250
250 500
250 1,000
750 1,500
Stahlhofen et al. 1980 1981 1983
1.0
0.8
0.6
0.4
0.2
0
0.1
1
10
Particle diameter (μm)

mentational E_{TB} by considering particle diameter and the residence time of particles in small bronchial airways. It further accounts for the expansion of airways during inhalation, but it is based on a constant respiratory flow.

Because the number of particles deposited in the tracheobronchiolar region will be decreased by particle losses during inspiration in the extrathoracic region $(1 - E_{ET})$, the empirical expression for tracheobronchiolar particle deposition (DE_{TB}) is

$$DE_{TB} = \left[1 - \left(\frac{V_{ET}}{V_T}\right)\right](1 - E_{ET})\,E_{TB} \qquad (16)$$

Depending on the mode of breathing, E_{ET} is the deposition efficiency for mouth breathing $(E_{ET\text{-}M})$ or for nose breathing $(E_{ET\text{-}N})$.

Targeting Particles into the Tracheobronchiolar Region

The deposited fractions of particles, as predicted by the foregoing model, are presented in Figures 9 and 11. For targeting particles into the tracheobronchiolar region, the mode of choice is obviously mouth breathing (see Fig. 9). Within the physiological range of flow velocities, inhaling at 1000 $cm^3\,s^{-1}$ leads to somewhat higher deposition of particles between 3 and 7 μm, with a slight peak at 6 μm. However, this high flow rate also causes extrathoracic deposition to double (see Fig. 9), which because of possible side effects often must be avoided in inhalation therapy. In this situation, inhaling particles between 4 and 6 μm at 250-$cm^3\,s^{-1}$ inspiratory flow appears to be appropriate for targeting particles to the tracheobronchiolar region and for keeping extrathoracic deposition low.

However, in inhalation therapy, the mass of the therapeutic substance delivered to the extrathoracic, tracheobronchiolar, or alveolar region by the deposited particles is the primary parameter of interest. This mass, in fact, depends on the deposited fraction, but it is essentially determined by the output of the nebulizer. The output of a nebulizer, in return, depends on the nebulized number of particles per volume element and the produced particle size. The size is of importance because the mass of a particle increases substantially with increasing particle diameter (see Table 1). To illustrate this, based on the deposition fractions given in Figure 9, the amount of substance delivered to the three regions by 1000 inhaled unit-density spheres during mouth breathing was determined for particle sizes between 0.1 and 10 μm. The results in Figure 13 show that the total mass

Figure 13 Amount of substance deposited per 1000 inhaled unit-density spheres in the extrathoracic, the tracheobronchial, and the alveolar region during mouth breathing for a tidal volume of 1000 cm^3 and flow rates of 40, 250, and 1000 $cm^3\,s^{-1}$. Estimates are based on deposition fractions given in Figure 9.

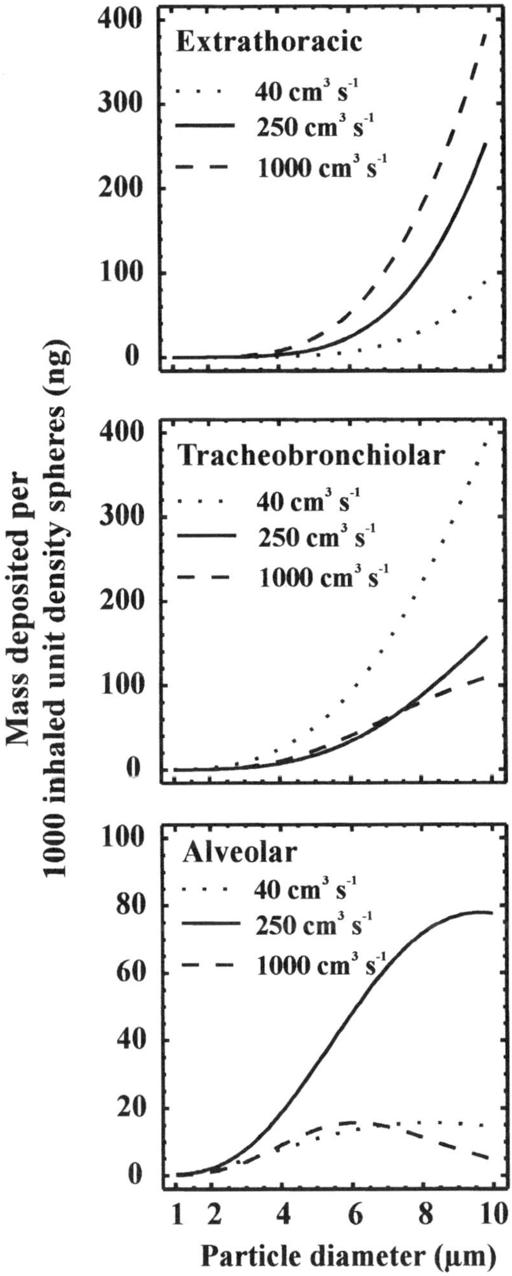
Extrathoracic
40 cm³ s⁻¹
250 cm³ s⁻¹
1000 cm³ s⁻¹
Tracheobronchiolar
40 cm³ s⁻¹
250 cm³ s⁻¹
1000 cm³ s⁻¹
Alveolar
40 cm³ s⁻¹
250 cm³ s⁻¹
1000 cm³ s⁻¹
Mass deposited per 1000 inhaled unit density spheres (ng)
0
100
200
300
400
0
100
200
300
400
0
20
40
60
80
100
1 2 4 6 8 10
Particle diameter (μm)

deposited in the extrathoracic region during mouth breathing increases considerably for particles larger than 4–6 μm during quiet breathing, but even more during exercise. The amount of therapeutic substance deposited in the tracheobronchiolar region is comparable for any particles smaller than 8 μm at 250 or at 1000 $cm^3\ s^{-1}$. For larger particles, despite a decrease in the deposited fraction (see Fig. 9), the mass delivered to the tracheobronchiolar region still increases, slightly more at 250 $cm^3\ s^{-1}$ than at 1000 $cm^3\ s^{-1}$. Therefore, the breathing mode of choice is quiet inhalation of 4- to 6-μm particles if extrathoracic deposition must be avoided. If extrathoracic deposition is noncritical, about five times more therapeutic substance can be deposited per breath in the tracheobronchiolar region when 8- to 10-μm particles are inhaled with quiet mouth breathing. These estimates, however, do not take into account that, with ''real'' nebulizers, the number output usually decreases with increasing particle size. But according to Ferron et al. (195), this is less than a factor of 5 for the particle size range of interest.

The deposited fraction in the conducting airways is almost independent of tidal volume (see Fig. 11), so that the total number of deposited particles changes in proportion to the inhaled aerosol volume. Augmentation of the inhaled volume by an increase in tidal volume also increases alveolar deposition (see Fig. 11 and next paragraph), such that if a low alveolar deposition is required, inhalation of repeated small tidal volumes appears to be more appropriate than that of fewer but larger ones.

Recently, an interesting new approach to target 6-μm particles into the conducting airways was proposed by Anderson (196) and Svartengren (197). They used very slow inspiratory flow rates, of about 40 $cm^3\ s^{-1}$. At this flow rate, the residence time within the conducting airways is long, and deposition is entirely related to sedimentation, which causes the retained fraction in the tracheobronchiolar region to increase substantially. Predicted deposition rates for this type of breathing maneuver are included in Figure 9. The deposited fraction can be expected to be almost constant and larger than 0.6 for particles larger than 4 μm. Owing to the diminished effects of impaction, extrathoracic deposition in the larynx is substantially decreased in comparison with the physiological flow rates discussed in the foregoing (see Fig. 9). Extrathoracic deposition is less than 0.05 for particles smaller than 6 μm and close to 0.1 for 8-μm particles. The corresponding amount of material deposited in the larynx or in the conducting airways can be inferred from Figure 13. If we consider all effects, 6- to 8-μm particles appear to be most suitable for very slow inhalation procedures. The notably enhanced amount of substance delivered to the tracheobronchiolar region makes this technique a very interesting approach for new inhalation therapies. However, specific devices have to be applied for patients to be able to maintain such low flow rates.

Thermodynamic Domain

Experiments performed in three healthy adults who inhaled 0.1-, 0.07-, and 0.05-μm particles, using various breathing maneuvers, showed that these particles are not retained in the tracheobronchiolar airways (163).

Alveolar Deposition: Slow-Cleared Thoracic Deposition

Aerodynamic Domain

Those particles escaping the extrathoracic and the tracheobronchiolar filters reach the alveolated region of the lung. Figure 12 summarizes alveolar deposition during mouth breathing (184), data are taken from the same studies as the foregoing. Discrepancies between studies appear to be less pronounced than for tracheobronchiolar deposition. Alveolar deposition probability peaks at about the same particle size range as does tracheobronchiolar deposition, but a slight advantage for smaller particles to be deposited in the alveoli is detectable. Deposition for particles smaller than 1 μm is twice as likely in the alveoli as in the conducting airways.

The dominant mechanism resulting in alveolar particle deposition is gravitational settling, in addition diffusional displacement becomes more and more significant for particles smaller than 0.5 μm (see Table 1). The efficiency of the alveolar region to collect particles owing to their sedimentation is determined by considering the distance a particle settles while staying in this region. Accordingly, in empirical expressions (163,165–168) the deposition efficiency in the alveolar region (E_A) is assessed as a function of the parameter $d_{ae}^2\, t_A$ for particles 1 μm or larger.

$$E_A = 1 - \exp\left[-0.171\ \mathrm{CF}\ (d_{ae}^2\, t_A)^{2/3}\right] \tag{17}$$

where t_A is the residence time of particles during inspiration in the alveolar region:

$$t_A = \frac{V_T - V_D}{Q} \tag{18}$$

CF is a correction factor applied for gender, V_D is the dead space volume, composed of the extrathoracic and the tracheobronchiolar volumes. It is approximated to 147 and 118 cm^3 for male and female adults (168). The deposited fraction in the alveolar region (DE_A) is

$$DE_A = \left[1 - \left(\frac{V_D}{V_T}\right)\right](1 - E_{ET})\,(1 - E_{TB})\,E_A \tag{19}$$

where E_{ET} is the deposition efficiency for mouth breathing ($E_{ET\text{-}M}$) or for nose breathing ($E_{ET\text{-}N}$).

Targeting Particles into the Alveolar Region

Differences in DE_A between nose and mouth breathing, as predicted by the empirical model, are shown in Figure 9. For each flow rate, differences in alveolar deposition become obvious for particles larger than 1.5 μm, because large particles undergo effective filtration in the nose. Because the collection efficiency of the upper airways is small for small particles, most of the inspired particles smaller than 1.5 μm reach the alveolar region. Given the model data presented in Figure 9, the mode of choice for an inhalation therapy aimed at targeting particles into the alveolar region is quiet inhalation of an aerosol with 2- to 4-μm particles during mouth breathing. This provides about 50% of the inhaled particles to this region and keeps the burden delivered to the extra- and intrathoracic airways low (see Figs. 9 and 13). Increasing tidal volume while maintaining a low flow rate further increases alveolar deposition (see Fig. 11) because particles are convectively transported deeper into the lung and the residence time of particles in the alveolar region is increased. Similarly, a breath-hold, performed at end-inspiration, improves the collection efficiency. According to the empirical model, for instance, a 1000-cm^3 breath, inhaled at 250 $cm^3\ s^{-1}$, results in 55% deposition of 3-μm particles in the alveolar region. A 3-s breath-hold at the end of inspiration enhances deposition to 65%.

Thermodynamic Domain

There are almost no experimental data on alveolar deposition available for this domain. Heyder et al. (163) measured deposition in three healthy adults for 0.1-, 0.07-, and 0.05-μm particles. At a flow rate of 250 $cm^3\ s^{-1}$ and a tidal volume of 500 cm^3, alveolar deposition was 21, 27, and 33%. Increasing tidal volume to 1000 cm^3, while keeping the flow rate constant, raised the removed fraction consistently to values of 34, 43, and 52%. With a flow rate of 750 $cm^3\ s^{-1}$ and a tidal volume of 1500 cm^3, deposition was 25, 36, and 45%. Independent of the breathing maneuver, the fraction of particles collected in the alveolar region increased with decreasing particle size. Both the residence time and the tidal volume appear to be significant determinants of particle deposition in this region.

VII. Factors Modifying Particle Deposition

A. Lung Geometry: Age- and Gender-Specific Differences

During development from infancy to adulthood, the respiratory system undergoes substantial changes in airway structure and lung volume, accompanied by considerable differences in spontaneous-breathing conditions (198–206). Even in adults, distinct sex-related and racial differences are established for structural and conventional lung function parameters (207–211). However, only limited information is available in how far particle deposition in the respiratory system is affected by age, gender, or race.

Deposition in Infants and Children. For this population, deposition data are rare (212–215). Total deposition of particles sized 1–3 μm was measured in 29 healthy children (6.7–14 years) during controlled and spontaneous mouth breathing (214,215), using the respiratory aerosol probe (see Sec. IV.A, under Noninvasive Techniques). Spontaneously breathing children exhibited slightly smaller tidal volumes than adults, but had a higher respiratory rate, so that minute ventilations were almost identical. As in adults, total deposition in children increased with increasing particle size, being approximately 15% for 1-μm particles, 50% for 2.3-μm particles, and 75% for 3-μm particles. The intersubject variability observed in children was comparable with that in adults. For spontaneous, as well as for controlled breathing, deposition decreased slightly with increasing body size, suggesting that smaller lung dimensions favor deposition. This assumption is supported by the fact that deposition values for all particle sizes are higher in children than in adults. In comparison with adults, total deposition in children was increased by an average factor of 1.5, ranging between 1.2 and 1.9 for different particle sizes and breathing patterns. Furthermore, the amount of particles deposited per unit surface area is increased by a factor of 4–5 in children, because the surface area of their respiratory system is only about one third (40 m^2) that of adults (5).

We are unaware of deposition studies in healthy neonates or infants, probably owing to concerns over the use of radiotracers in this population (33). There are some deposition studies, related to therapeutic drug delivery, in spontaneously breathing or ventilated infants with lung diseases (216 218). Also, filter and animal lung models have been used to assess deposition in infants (219–222). One of the limitations of these studies is that deposition is often related to the amount of radioactivity delivered into the nebulizer unit and not to what is actually inhaled. Hence, there is a clear necessity for improved deposition studies to better understand health risks from environmental air pollutions or to improve inhalation therapy in neonates and infants.

Gender Differences in Adults

Lung structure and breathing pattern are considered to be different in adult men and women. The average female thorax is smaller, and the conducting airway size is only about 75% that in men (223). In addition, resting minute ventilation and respiratory flow rates are lower in women than in men. During controlled as well as spontaneous mouth breathing, deposition of particles of the aerodynamic domain was slightly, but consistently, lower in women than in men (213,224,225). Analysis of regional deposition revealed that this was related to a higher extrathoracic and tracheobronchiolar deposition rate (225). Considering that deposition within these regions is largely determined by impaction, deposition was reassessed as a function of the impaction parameter $d^2_{ae}\,Q$. Still there remained an unexplained few percent difference between deposition in women and in men. This difference was most likely attributed to structural differences between men and women (225) in the conducting airways. The empirical model calculations introduced earlier try to account for that by applying a correction factor and by considering gender-specific lung and airway volumes.

B. Exercise

Adults. Ventilation is increased during exercise according to the higher oxygen demand of the body. In adults, this is usually accomplished by an increase in tidal volume and breathing frequency; hence, respiratory flow rates are also high. In addition, breathing is often switched from the nasal to an oronasal or oral route, especially at high levels of exercise (193). In some studies (213,225), total deposition estimated breath-by-breath increased for 1- to 5-μm particles in male and female adults, even during light exercise. Other studies failed to detect clear changes in the deposition rate per breath under various levels of exercise (226,227). Deposition studies under controlled-breathing conditions (70,170) show that increasing tidal volume at a given respiratory rate increases total deposition for all respirable particles. These changes are minimal for particles between 0.1 and 1 μm, for which total deposition is small. Keeping tidal volume constant while increasing respiratory rate decreases total particle deposition for all particle sizes. The most obvious changes here are in the transitional particle-size range. Hence, because of individual breathing patterns, individual features of lung geometry, and different particle sizes studied, physical exercise may result either in an unchanged or an enhanced deposition rate per breath. This is also reflected by a remarkably increased intersubject variability in particle deposition during exercise. Despite these individual differences, the increase in minute ventilation from rest to exercise always enhances deposition per unit of time. This increase is roughly proportional to the increase in minute ventilation.

Children. For particle sizes between 1 and 3 μm, deposition under ventilatory conditions of rest and light exercise was measured in 41 children by Becquemin et al. (212,213). Exercise caused per-breath deposition of 1-μm particles to decrease from about 20 to 15%, whereas the deposition of 2- and 3-μm particles was almost unaffected. Because the higher ventilatory demand under light exercise was accomplished mainly by an increase in breathing frequency, respiratory flows were increased, but the residence time of particles in the respiratory system was shortened. This caused 1-μm particle deposition, which is mainly governed by sedimentation, to decrease. It appears that, for 2- and 3-μm particles, the decreased deposition probability by sedimentation was balanced by an increased effect of impaction, so that total deposition remained unaffected. Therefore, it may be speculated that regional deposition was affected with a partial shift in deposition toward more central airways. Again, it is important to emphasize that the increase in minute ventilation in response to exercise increased deposition per unit of time considerably for all three particle sizes despite a decreased or unchanged deposition rate per breath.

C. Influence of Gas Composition

Replacing ambient air nitrogen (N_2) by carrier gases with differing physical properties is expected to alter flow profiles in the conducting airways, thereby affecting convective particle transport and deposition patterns within the lungs. According to basic fluid dynamics, alteration of kinematic viscosity (η/σ) is presumed to result in more laminar flows in the airways when N_2 is replaced by helium. More turbulent flow occurs when sulfurhexafluoride (SF_6) is used as a carrier gas, which has about five times the molecular weight of N_2 (228).

Svartengren (229) and Anderson and co-workers (230,231) studied 2.5-μm–Teflon particle deposition (ρ, 2.13 kg m^{-3}; d_{ae}, 3.6 μm) in healthy subjects with and without induced bronchoconstriction and in patients with asthma breathing air or a helium–oxygen mixture (He–O_2). More laminar airflow owing to the use of He–O_2 shifted the site of particle deposition to the lung periphery and resulted in higher deposition rates in the alveolar region, but in lower rates in mouth, throat, and in the tracheobronchiolar region. This effect was more marked for constricted airways, both in healthy subjects with a two- to threefold increase in airway resistance and in asthmatics. It was more pronounced at higher, than at moderate, flow rates. Schulz et al. (232) applied the series bolus delivery technique (see Sec. IV.A, under Noninvasive Techniques) in mechanically ventilated dogs to study local deposition of smaller particles in different gas compositions. Deposition of 0.5-, 1-, and 2-μm particles, was unaltered breathing He–O_2. In SF_6–O_2, the deposited fraction of 2-μm particles was enhanced throughout the lung. It was increased for 1-μm particles in deep lung regions, but it was generally not affected for 0.5-μm particles.

These results show that the extent and the preferable site of particle deposition within the lungs can be modified by the physical properties of the atmospheric carrier gas. However, specific combinations of particle properties and flow fields within the airways are required.

VIII. Local Particle Deposition

Numerous studies have been carried out in the last decades to obtain detailed information about collection efficiencies and deposition patterns on a subregional level within the respiratory system. A complete overview is beyond the scope of the present chapter, but the studies introduced in the following discussion should give the reader an idea about approaches and results.

A. Local Deposition Within the Tracheobronchiolar and Alveolar Region

Gerrity and co-workers (129) modeled local deposition in the tracheobronchiolar tree. Estimates were based on the morphometric lung model proposed by Weibel (5) and on Landahl's formalism of particle deposition (121; see Sec. IV.B, under Mathematical Models). Deposition in each of the airway generations was assessed at a tidal volume of 700 cm^3, a flow rate of 500 $cm^3\ s^{-1}$, and a breath-hold of 0.5 s at end-inspiration. Figure 14 shows the results given as percentage of deposition per airway generation for particles with aerodynamic diameters ranging between 1.6 and 15.8 μm. The percentage quoted is the deposited fraction of those aerosol particles that pass through the glottis. The smallest particles exhibited expected deposition rates below 2% in the conducting airways (generation number 0–16) and a clear tendency to deposit in more peripheral lung structures. For 3.2- and 4.8-μm particles, deposition followed principally the same pattern, but was enhanced both in the lung periphery and in the conducting airways. Deposition of 4.8-μm particles appeared to peak at airway generations 3–7. For particles larger than that, the deposition pattern changed, in that the deposited fraction was reduced in the lung periphery and the predominant site of particle deposition was shifted toward central airways. Peak deposition occurred at the fifth airway generation, ranging between 7 and 16% for 8- and 15.8-μm particles. Relative to health effects from inhaled particles, the authors calculated the surface area densities of deposited particles in the various airway generations. Peak density occurred at generation 3 (i.e., within the segmental and subsegmental bronchi), and it was orders of magnitude higher there than in smaller conducting airways or in peripheral lung structures. This observation is interesting in light of studies done on the frequency and location of bronchial carcinomas (111,233). There was a close correspondence between deposition density and frequency of reported cancer at those sites.

Recently, Kim and co-workers (67) applied the series bolus delivery technique (see Sec. IV.A, under Noninvasive Techniques) to assess local deposition in the lungs of 11 healthy young adults. During mouth breathing, 1-, 3-, and 5-μm particles were inhaled at flow rates of 150, 250, and 500 $cm^3\ s^{-1}$ and at a tidal volume of 500 cm^3. Local collection efficiencies and deposited fractions were determined for ten volumetric lung compartments (50–500 cm^3). For all particle sizes and flow rates, local collection efficiency increased with increasing volumetric lung depth of the compartment. For the highest flow rate, collection efficiency was lowest throughout all compartments. The deposited fraction of 1-μm particles varied per volumetric lung compartment between almost zero and 3%, with a tendency for higher deposition rates in larger lung depth if lower flow rates were applied (Fig. 15). With increasing particle size, deposition was enhanced, and the preferential site of deposition was shifted from the distal to the proximal compartments of the lung. Peak deposition occurred in volumetric lung regions between 75 and 200 cm^3; it was approximately 15% for 5-μm particles independent of flow rate. Based on the morphometric lung model of Weibel (5), surface area concentrations were estimated and were greater in the most proximal region of the lung than in distal parts, regardless of particle size and flow rate.

When comparing the experimental data with those modeled by the same group (129), there is reasonable agreement for peak values and general patterns of local deposition within the conducting airways (i.e., within a volumetric lung region of 200 cm^3 or the first 16 airway generations). Absolute estimates of deposition within the tracheobronchiolar region, however, are higher than the corresponding experimental values. For example, Kim and co-workers reported tracheobronchiolar deposition of 3- and 5-μm particles to be 11 and 26% for a flow rate of 250 $cm^3\ s^{-1}$, whereas approximately 30 and 50% are expected from the model (see Fig. 14). This disagreement may be partly explained by the differences in breathing pattern and by other factors already discussed by the authors (67). However, it shows that despite the large body of knowledge gained in the past 50 years, there is still a clear necessity for close cooperation between experimental and theoretical researchers to further improve the understanding of even the most basic processes governing particle deposition in the respiratory tract.

B. Local Deposition Within Airway Bifurcations

Collection efficiencies and deposition patterns of inhaled particles on the level of bifurcating airways have been studied experimentally in idealized y-shaped tube models (98,99). The dimensions of the single bifurcation models were adapted from Weibel's human lung data for airway generations 3–5. Branching patterns of the bifurcation were varied for branching angles, geometric symmetry of daughter tubes, and symmetry of flow division at the bifurcation. To assess local deposition patterns within each of the model tubes, the parent and daughter tubes were divided into several sections. Fluorescent-labeled particles of 3, 5, and 7 μm were applied for laminar and transitional flow and the number of particles deposited in each of the tube sections was inferred from fluorometric measurements. During inhalation, collection efficiency in airway models increased with increasing flow rate and particle size, ranging for 3-μm particles, between almost zero deposition and 15%, and for 7-μm particles, between 20 and 70%. Total deposition appeared to be almost independent of the branching angle of daughter tubes, even for asymmetrical branching models. An even inspiratory airflow division at the bifurcation resulted in balanced deposition rates in the two daughter branches. But even with uneven inspiratory flow divisions of as much as 1 : 3 between daughter branches, deposition efficiencies and patterns deviated only slightly from that of even flow division. The distribution of deposited material

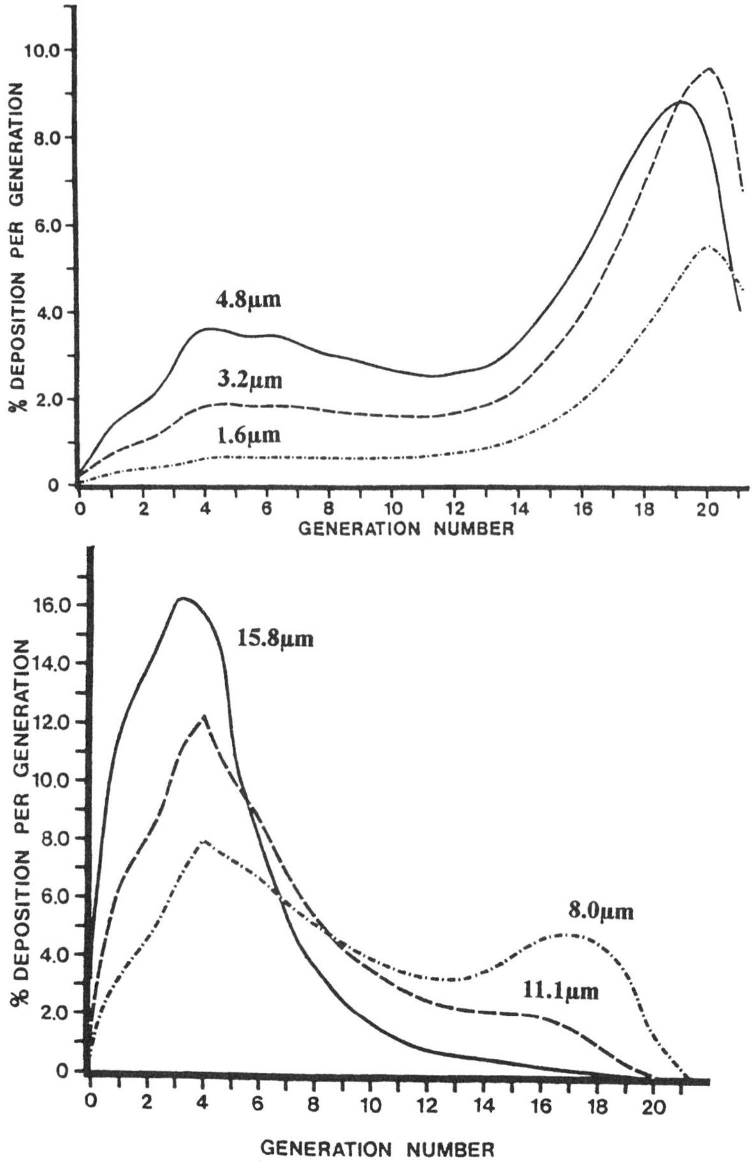

Figure 14 Modeled local deposition in the tracheobronchial and alveolar region: Deposition estimates were carried out for the symmetrical morphometric model of Weibel (5) at a tidal volume of 700 cm^3, an inspiratory flow rate of 500 $cm^3\ s^{-1}$, and an end-inspiratory pause of 0.5 s. The percentage deposition per airway generation is given for particles with aerodynamic diameters ranging between 1.6 and 15.8 μm. The percentage quoted is the fraction of all aerosol particles that pass through the glottis. (From Ref. 129.)

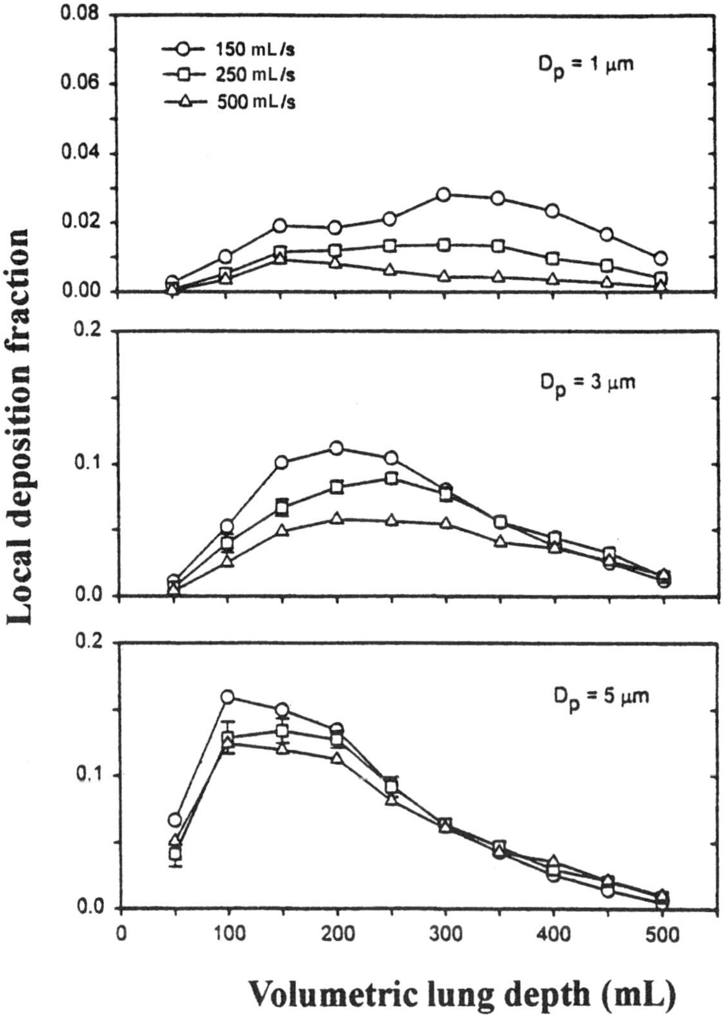

Figure 15 Experimental data on local deposition fraction from 11 young adults: Deposition fractions of 1-, 3-, and 5-µm particles are shown for ten volumetric lung compartments in lung depths between 50 and 500 cm^3. A tidal volume of 500 cm^3 was inhaled from functional residual capacity at flow rates of 150, 250, and 500 $cm^3\ s^{-1}$. Error bars (±SE) are shown for a flow rate of 250 $cm^3\ s^{-1}$. (From Ref. 67.)

was extremely uneven among the tube sections of the models. During inhalation, major deposition occurred in those daughter tube sections adjacent to the bifurcation. With increasing particle size or flow rate, deposition within these daughter sections increased from 70 to 90% of the total amount deposited in the model. During exhalation, peak deposition occurred again in those sections adjacent to the bifurcation, but now mainly in the adjacent parent tube section. This high surface density of particle deposition at bifurcations holds not only for coarse particles with impaction-determined deposition, but was also observed for ultrafine particles (105). For ultrafine particles, however, density differences between bifurcations and along the airway lengths were not so profound.

Spatial deposition patterns within airway bifurcations have been studied numerically (151–153,158; see Sec. IV.B, under Mathematical Models). Corresponding to the airway bifurcation models applied experimentally by Kim and coworkers, airway bifurcation geometries were constructed in a three-dimensional computer mesh and deposition patterns inferred from modeled airflow fields and particle trajectories. In general, there was a good agreement between the experimental results and the theoretical predictions. As an example, Figure 16 shows modeled deposition sites of 2000 randomly selected 5-μm particles ($\rho = 0.891$ g cm^{-3}) inhaled at a flow rate of 133 cm^3 s^{-1}. The parent branch has a diameter of 0.5 cm and the geometry of the bifurcation is symmetrical relative to daughter diameter (0.4 cm) and branching angle (45°), but flow division was changed from symmetrical to asymmetrical, with Q_{dA}/Q_{dB} being the ratio of flows rates in daughter branches A and B. For symmetrical flow division, the deposition pattern also appeared to be symmetrical. Most of the inhaled particles deposited as a hot-spot near the carina, but some particles were also found at the inner airway length of daughter branches. As the flow rate increased in daughter branch A relative to that in daughter branch B, the intensity and extension of the hot-spot in daughter branch A increased. With increasing asymmetry of flow division, the hot-spot in daughter B seemed first to recede to the carina, but then another hot-spot began to develop in the center of that daughter branch (see Fig. 16). These studies show that a homogeneous surface density of deposited particles within the tracheobronchiolar airways appears to be unrealistic. The given example may further illustrate the variability in deposition patterns and the complex mechanisms determining the site of particle deposition within an airway bifurcation.

However, more recent studies suggest (158,160–162,234) that flow regimens and particle trajectories crucially depend on the geometric boundary conditions, so that unrealistic deposition patterns may occur in simplified and idealized airway structures. This has to be disproved or verified in future studies, but it appears reasonable that coming studies must focus their interest on experimentally and numerically determined deposition patterns within realistic airway sys-

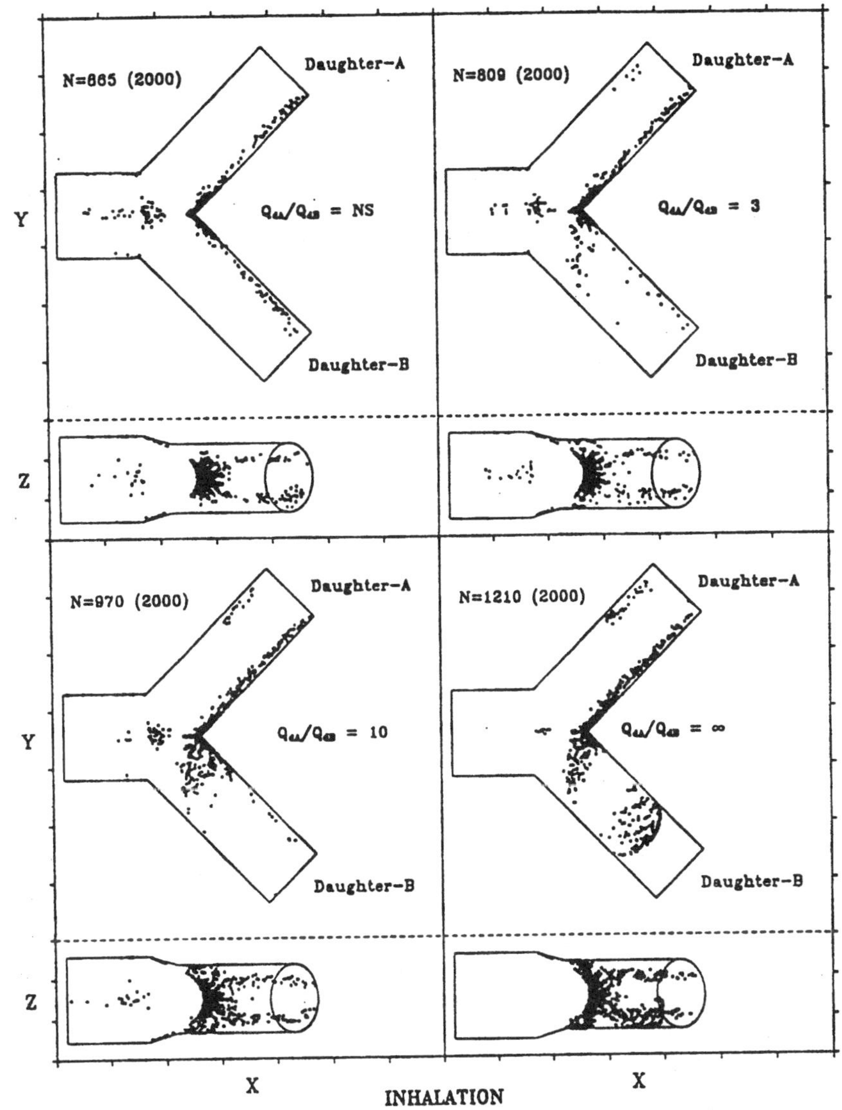

Figure 16 Modeled local deposition patterns in idealized airway structures: The effect of asymmetry in flow division on inspiratory deposition patterns of 5-μm particles (σ = 0.891 g cm^{-3}) is shown for four different flow–rate ratios between daughter branch A and branch B. (From Ref. 153.)

tems, especially because these approaches have now become available with modern computational techniques (159–162).

Nomenclature

CMD	count median diameter of a particle number frequency distribution (μm)
CF	correction factor applied for gender [see Eqs. (14) and (17)]
C_s	Cunningham slip correction factor
C(V)	particle number concentration of the respired volume (cm^{-3})
DE	deposition fraction; particles deposited in a given structure, as a fraction of all particles entering the respiratory system
DE_{Tot}	total deposition
DE_{ET}	extrathoracic deposition
$DE_{ET\text{-}N}$	extrathoracic deposition for nose breathing
$DE_{ET\text{-}M}$	extrathoracic deposition for mouth breathing
DE_{TB}	tracheobronchiolar deposition
DE_A	alveolar deposition
D_P	diffusion coefficient of a particle ($cm^2\ s^{-1}$)
D_p/Q	diffusion parameter (cm^{-1})
d	geometric particle diameter (μm)
d_{ae}	aerodynamic particle diameter (μm)
d_{th}	thermodynamic particle diameter (μm)
d_{16}	particle diameter at the 16% size cut of the cumulative particle size frequency distribution
d_{84}	particle diameter at the 84% size cut of the cumulative particle size frequency distribution
d_{ae}/Q	impaction parameter ($\mu m\ s\ cm^{-3}$)
FRC	functional residual capacity, gas volume in the lung at the end of a normal expiration (cm^3)
G	factor characterizing the geometry of an obstacle (m)
g	gravity constant ($9.81\ m\ s^{-2}$)
MD	median particle diameter of a particle size frequency distribution (μm)
MMD	mass median diameter of a particle mass frequency distribution (μm)
Q	respiratory flow rate ($cm^3\ s^{-1}$)
SMD	surface median diameter of a particle surface frequency distribution (μm)
Stk	Stokes' number
T	absolute temperature (K)
t_a	residence time of particles in the alveolar region (s)
t_b	residence time of particles in the small bronchial airways (s)
t_{rs}	residence time of particles in the respiratory system (s)
u	linear airflow velocity ($m\ s^{-1}$)
$V_{b\text{-}FRC}$	volume of the bronchioles at FRC level (cm^3)
V_{ET}	extrathoracic airway volume (cm^3)
V_{ex}	expired volume (cm^3)
V_{in}	inspired volume (cm^3)

V_T	tidal volume (cm^3)
Δ	root mean square diffusional displacement of particles ($cm\ s^{-1}$)
E	particle collection efficiency; particles deposited in a given structure as a fraction of all particles entering that structure
E_{ET}	particle collection efficiency of the extrathoracic airways
$E_{ET\text{-}N}$	extrathoracic particle collection efficiency for nose breathing
$E_{ET\text{-}M}$	extrathoracic particle collection efficiency for mouth breathing
E_{TB}	particle collection efficiency of the tracheobronchiolar region
E_A	particle collection efficiency of the alveolar region
η	dynamic viscosity of the surrounding medium ($kg\ s^{-1}\ m^{-1}$)
κ	Boltzmann constant (1.38×10^{-23} J K^{-1})
λ	mean free path of gas molecules (μm)
σ	gas density ($kg\ m^{-3}$)
σ_g	geometric standard deviation of a log-normal particle size distribution
v	terminal settling velocity of a particle ($\mu m\ s^{-1}$)
ρ	particle density ($kg\ m^{-3}$)

References

1. Heyder J, Blanchard JD, Feldman HA, Brain JD. Convective mixing in human respiratory tract: estimates with aerosol boli. J Appl Physiol 1988; 64:1273–1278.
2. Paiva M, Engel L. Gas mixing in the lung periphery. In: Chang HK, Paiva M, eds. Respiratory Physiology. An Analytical Approach. New York: Marcel Dekker, 1989:245–276.
3. Schulz H, Heilmann P, Hillebrecht A, Gebhart J, Meyer M, Piiper J, Heyder J. Convective and diffusive gas transport in canine intrapulmonary airways. J Appl Physiol 1992; 72:1557–1562.
4. Ultmann JS. Gas transport in the conducting airways. In: Engel L, Paiva M, eds. Gas Mixing and Distribution in the Lung. New York: Marcel Dekker, 1985:63–136.
5. Weibel ER. Morphometry of the Human Lung. Heidelberg: Springer Verlag, 1963.
6. Breysse P, Swift DL. Inhalability of large particles into the human nasal passage: in vivo studies in still air. Aerosol Sci Technol 1990; 13:459–464.
7. Ménache MG, Miller FJ, Raabe OG. Particle inhalability curves for humans and small laboratory animals. Ann Occup Hyg 1995; 39:317–328.
8. Schlesinger RB. Biological disposition of airborne particles: basic principles and application to vehicular emissions. In: Watson AY, Bates RR, Kennedy D, eds. Air Pollution, the Automobile, and Public Health. Washington, DC: National Academy Press, 1988:239–298.
9. Swift DL. Design of the human respiratory tract to facilitate removal of particles and gases. AICh E Symp Ser 1976; 72(156):137–144.
10. Heyder J. Particle transport onto human airway surfaces. Eur J Respir Dis 1982; 63(suppl 119):29–50.
11. Geiser M, Baumann M, Cruz-Orive LM, Im Hof V, Waber U, Gehr P. The effect of particle inhalation on macrophage number and phagocytic activity in the intrapul-

monary conducting airways of hamsters. Am J Respir Cell Mol Biol 1994; 10:594–603.
12. Fuchs, NA. The Mechanics of Aerosols. New York: Dover Publications, 1989.
13. Hinds WC. Aerosol Technology. New York: John Wiley and Sons, 1982.
14. Willeke K, Baron, PA. Aerosol Measurement. Principles Techniques and Applications. New York: van Nostrand Reinhold, 1992:23–40.
15. Allan MD, Raabe OG. Slip correction measurements of spherical solid aerosol particles in an improved Milikan apparatus. Aerosol Sci Technol 1985; 4:69–86.
16. Gebhart J, Heyder J, Stahlhofen W. Use of aerosols to estimate pulmonary airspace dimensions. J Appl Physiol 1981; 51:465–476.
17. Chang HK. General concepts of molecular diffusion. In: Engel LA, Paiva M, eds. Gas Mixing and Distribution in the Lung. New York: Marcel Dekker, 1985:1–22.
18. Heyder J, Scheuch G. Diffusional transport of nonspherical aerosol particles. Aerosol Sci Technol 1983; 2:41–44.
19. Scheuch G, Heyder J. Dynamic shape factor of nonspherical aerosol particles in the diffusion regime. Aerosol Sci Technol 1990; 12:270–277.
20. Einstein A. On the kinetic molecular theory of thermal movements of particles suspended in a quiescent fluid. Ann Phys 1905; 17:549–560.
21. Asgharian B, Yu CP. Deposition of inhaled fibrous particles in the human lung. J Aerosol Med 1988; 1:37–50.
22. Asgharian B, Yu CP. Deposition of fibers in the rat lung. J Aerosol Sci 1989; 20: 355–366.
23. Timbrell V. An aerosol spectrometer and its applications. In: Mercer TT, Morrow PE, Stöber W, eds. Assessment of Airborne Particles. Springfield IL: CC Thomas, 1972:290–330.
24. Yu CP. Theories of electrostatic lung deposition of inhaled aerosols. Ann Occup Hyg 1985; 29:219–227.
25. Melandri C, Tarroni G, Prodi V, de Zaiacomo T, Formignani M, Lombardi CC. Deposition of charged particles in the human airways. J Aerosol Sci 1983; 14:657–669.
26. Jones AD, Johnston AM, Vincent JH. Static electrification of airborne asbestos dust. In: Marple VA, Liu BYH, eds. Aerosols in the Mining and Work Environment. Ann Arbor, MI: Ann Arbor Science, 1983:613–631.
27. Jones AD, Vincent JH, Johnston AM, McMillin CH. Effects of electrostatic charge on the pulmonary deposition of mineral dust aerosols inhaled by rats. J Aerosol Sci 1988; 19:565–575.
28. Vincent JH, Johnston WB, Jones AD, Johnston AM. Static electrification of airborne asbestos: a study of its causes, assessment and effects on deposition in the lungs of rats. Am Ind Hyg Assoc J 1981; 42:711–721.
29. Cohen BS, Xiong JQ, Li W. The influence of charge on the deposition behaviour of aerosol particles with emphasis on single charged nanometer sized particles. In: Marijnissen JCM, Gradon L, eds. Aerosol Inhalation: Recent Research Frontiers. Dordrecht: Kluwer Academic, 1996:153–164.
30. Stahlhofen W, Gebhart J, Rudolf G, Scheuch G. Measurement of lung clearance with pulses of radioactively labelled particles. J Aerosol Sci 1986; 17:333–336.

31. Stahlhofen W, Scheuch G, Bailey MR. Investigations of retention of inhaled particles in the human bronchial tree. Radiat Prot Dosim 1995; 60:311–319.
32. Scheuch G, Stahlhofen W, Heyder J. An approach to deposition and clearance measurements in human airways. J Aerosol Med 1996; 9:35–41.
33. Everard ML. Studies using radiolabelled aerosols in children. Thorax 1994; 49: 1259–1266.
34. Diot P, Baulieu J-L, Lemarié E. Nuclear medicine and lung diseases. Paris: Springer Verlag, 1993.
35. Rosenthal MS, Cullom J, Hawkins W, Moore SC, Tsui BMW, Yester M. Quantitative SPECT imaging: a review and recommendations by the Focus Committee of the Society of Nuclear Medicine Computer and Instrumentation Council. J Nucl Med 1995; 36:1489–1513.
36. Chan HK. Use of photon emission computed tomography in aerosol studies. J Aerosol Med 1993; 6:23–36.
37. Ferron GA, Erbe F, Fürst G, Haider B, Haller J, Köhl B, Kreyling WG, Schumann G, Stocker M, Heyder J. A scintillation counter for measuring removal of radioactive particles from dog lungs. J Aerosol Sci 1989; 20:1297–1300.
38. Gonda I. Scintigraphic techniques for measuring in vivo deposition. J Aerosol Med 1996; 9:S59–S67.
39. Itoh H, Smaldone GC, Swift DL, Wagner HN. Quantitative measurement of total aerosol deposition: comparison of three different techniques. J Aerosol Sci 1985; 16:367–371.
40. Morsey SM, Eckhardt B, Stahlhofen W, Pohlit W. Optimization studies of a whole-body counter to cope with possible dynamic transfer between neighboring compartments. Health Phys 1978; 35:325–332.
41. Smaldone GC. Factors in measurement of dose by gamma scintigraphy. J Aerosol Med 1996; 9:S69–S76.
42. Stahlhofen W, Gebhart J, Heyder J. Experimental determination of the regional deposition of aerosol particles in the human respiratory tract. Am Ind Hyg Assoc J 1980; 41:385–398.
43. Suzuki S. Detection efficiency of NaI (Tl) crystals and loss of positron resolution caused by photon interactions in the crystals in γ-cameras. Int J Appl Radiat Isot 1982; 33:411–414.
44. Boecker BB, Thomas RG, McClellan RO. Accumulation and retention of 137-Cs fused aluminiosilicate particles by beagle dogs after repeated inhalation exposures. In: Walton WH, ed. Inhaled Particles IV. Oxford: Pergamon, 1977:551–561.
45. Cuddihy RG, Boecker BB. Controlled administration of respiratory tract burdens of inhaled radioactive aerosols in beagle dogs. Toxicol Appl Pharmacol 1973; 25: 597–605.
46. Morrow PE, Gibb FR, Johnson L. Clearance of insoluble dust from the lower respiratory tract. Health Phys 1964; 10:543–555.
47. Heyder J, Gebhart J, Stahlhofen W. Inhalation of aerosols: particle deposition and retention. In: Willeke K, ed. Generation of Aerosols and Facilities for Exposure Experiments. Ann Arbor, MI: Ann Arbor Scientific, 1980:65–103.
48. Stahlhofen W. Human data on deposition. In: Smith H, Gerber G, eds. Lung Model-

ling for Inhalation of Radioactive Materials. Commission of the European Communities. 1984:39–62.
49. Fleming JS, Nassim M, Hashish AH, Bailey AG, Conway J, Holgate S, Halson P, Moore E, Martonen TB. Description of pulmonary deposition of radiolabeled aerosol by airway generation using a conceptual three dimensional model of lung morphology. J Aerosol Med 1995; 8:341–356.
50. Newman SP, Pavia D. Aerosol deposition in man. In: Móren F, Newhouse MT, Dolovich MB, eds. Aerosols in Medicine. Principles, Diagnosis and Therapy. Amsterdam: Elsevier, 1993:193–217.
51. Anderson PJ, Dolovich MB. Aerosols as diagnostic tools. J Aerosol Med 1994; 7: 77–88.
52. Agnew JE. Characterizing lung aerosol penetration. J Aerosol Med 1991; 4:237–249.
53. Dolovich MB, Sanchis J, Rossman C, Newhouse MT. Aerosol penetrance: a sensitive index of peripheral airway obstruction. J Appl Physiol 1976; 40: 468–471.
54. Phipps PR, Gonda I, Bailey D, Borham P, Bautovich G, Anderson SD. Comparison of planar and tomographic gamma scintigraphy to measure the penetration index of inhaled aerosols. Am Rev Respir Dis 1989; 139:1516–1523.
55. Schuster DP. Positron emission tomography: theory and its application to study of lung disease. Am Rev Respir Dis 1989; 139:818–840.
56. Cohen D. Ferrimagnetic contamination in the lungs and other organs of the human body. Science 1973; 180:745–748.
57. Cohen D, Crowther TS, Gibbs GW, Becklake MR. Magnetic lung measurements in relation to occupational exposure in asbestos miners and millers in Quebec. Environ Res 1981; 26:535–550.
58. Freedman AP, Robinson SE. Evaluation of magnetopneumography for assessing thoracic accumulation of welding fume. In: Erné SN, Hahlbohm HD, Lübbig H, eds. Biomagnetism. Berlin: Walter de Gruyter, 1981:489–495.
59. Kalliomäki PL, Karp PK, Katila T, Makipaw P, Jaar P, Tossavainen A. Magnetic measurements of pulmonary contamination. Scand J Work Environ Health 1976; 4:232–239.
60. Stahlhofen W, Möller M. Behaviour of magnetic micro-particles in the human lung. Radiat Environ Biophys 1993; 32:221–238.
61. Valberg PA, Brain JD. Generation and use of three types of iron oxide aerosol. Am Rev Respir Dis 1979; 120:1013–1024.
62. Möller W, Stahlhofen W, Roth C. Improved spinning top aerosol generator for the production of high concentrated ferrimagnetic aerosols. J Aerosol Sci 1990; 21: S435–S438.
63. Brain JD, Bloom SB, Valberg PA, Gehr P. Correlation between the behavior of magnetic iron oxide particles in the lungs of rabbits and phagocytosis. Exp Lung Res 1984; 6:115–131.
64. Freedman AP, Robinson SE, Street MR. Magnetopneumographic study of human alveolar clearance in health and disease. Ann Occup Hyg 1988; 32:809–820.
65. Tyndall J. Essays on the Floating Matter of the Air. London: Longmans Green, 1881.
66. Altshuler B, Yarmus L, Palmes ED, Nelson N. Aerosol deposition in the human

respiratory tract. I. Experimental procedures and total deposition. AMA Arch Ind Health 1957; 15:293–303.

67. Kim CS, Hu SC, DeWitt P, Gerrity TR. Assessment of regional deposition of inhaled particles in human lungs by serial bolus delivery method. J Appl Physiol 1996; 81:2203–2213.
68. Palmes ED, Wang CS. An aerosol inhalation apparatus for human single breath deposition studies. Am Ind Hyg Assoc J 1971; 32:43–46.
69. Giacomelli-Maltoni G, Melandri C, Prodi V, Tarroni G. Deposition efficiency of monodisperse particles in human respiratory tract. Am Ind Hyg Assoc J 1972; 33: 603–610.
70. Heyder J, Armbruster L, Gebhart J, Grein E, Stahlhofen W. Total deposition of aerosol particles in the human respiratory tract for nose and mouth breathing. J Aerosol Sci 1975; 6:311–329.
71. Heyder J, Gebhart J, Stahlhofen W, Stuck B. Biological variability of particle deposition in the human respiratory tract during controlled and spontaneous mouthbreathing. Ann Occup Hyg 1982; 26:137–147.
72. Heyder J, Gebhart J, Scheuch G. Influence of human lung morphology on particle deposition. J Aerosol Sci 1988; 1:81–88.
73. Gebhart J, Heigwer G, Heyder J, Roth C, Stahlhofen W. The use of light scattering photometry in aerosol medicine. J Aerosol Med 1988; 1:89–112.
74. Im Hof V, Scheuch G, Geiser M, Gebhart J, Gehr P, Heyder J. Techniques for the determination of particle deposition in lungs of hamsters. J Aerosol Med 1989; 2: 247–259.
75. Schulz H, Schulz A, Heyder J. Influence of intrinsic particle properties on parameters of aerosol bolus dispersion. Exp Lung Res 1996; 22:393–407.
76. Westenberger S, Gebhart J, Jaser S, Knoch M, Köstler R. A novel device for the generation and recording of aerosol micro-pulses in lung diagnostics. J Aerosol Sci 1992; 23:S449–S452.
77. Heyder J, Blanchard JD, Brain JD. Particle deposition in volumetric regions of the human respiratory tract. Ann Occup Hyg 1988; 32:71–79.
78. Brand P, Scheuch G, Schulz H, Meyer T, Kohlhäufl M, Heyder J, Häussinger K. Ermittlung der Verteilung inhalierter Aerosolteilchen mit der Aerosolbolustechnik. In: Scheuch G, ed. Aerosole in der Inhalationstherapie. München-Deisenhofen: Dustri-Verlag, 1997:27–40.
79. Sweeney TD, Brain JD. Pulmonary deposition: determinants and measurement techniques. Toxicol Pathol 1991; 4:384–397.
80. Sweeney TD, Brain JD, LeMott S. Anesthesia alters the pattern of aerosol retention in hamsters. J Appl Physiol 1983; 54:37–44.
81. Valberg PA, Brain JD, Sneddon SL, LeMott SR. Breathing pattern influences aerosol deposition sites in excised dog lungs. J Appl Physiol 1982; 53:824–837.
82. Logan GR, Schnitt SJ, Dvorak AM. Rapid microwave fixation of human tissue for light microscopic immunoperoxidase identification of diagnostically useful antigens. Lab Invest 1987; 57:585–591.
83. Pinkerton KE, Gallen JT, Mercer RR, Wong VC, Plopper CG, Tarkington BK. Aerosolized fluorescent microspheres detected in the lung using confocal scanning laser microscopy. Microsc Res Technol 1993; 26:437–443.

84. Godleski JJ, Hastings CL, Katler M, Sweeney TD. Preservation of the relationship of airway mucus and epithelium by slam freezing. In: Baily GW, ed. Proceedings of the 49th Annual Meeting of the Electron Microscopy Society of America. San Francisco: San Francisco Press, 1991:72–73.
85. Brain JD, Knudson DE, Sorokin SP, Davis MA. Pulmonary distribution of particles given by intratracheal instillation or by aerosol inhalation. Environ Res 1976; 11: 13–33.
86. Sweeney TD, Brain JD, Tryka AF, Godleski JJ. Retention of inhaled particles in hamsters with pulmonary fibrosis. Am Rev Respir Dis 1983; 128:138–143.
87. Herz RH. The Photographic Action of Ionizing Radiations. New York: Wiley-Interscience, 1969.
88. Rogers AW. Techniques of Autoradiography. New York: Elsevier, 1978.
89. Sweeney TD, Skornik WA, Brain JD, Hatch V, Godleski JJ. Chronic bronchitis alters the pattern of aerosol deposition in the lung. Am J Respir Crit Care Med 1995; 151:482–488.
90. Geiser M, Im Hof V, Gehr P, Cruz-Orive LM. Histological and stereological analysis of particle retention in the conducting airways of hamster lungs. J Aerosol Med 1990; 3:131–145.
91. Geiser M, Cruz-Orive LM, Waber U, Im Hof V, Gehr P. Particle retention in airways estimated by unbiased stereology and photometry. J Aerosol Sci 1995; 8: 149–165.
92. Sweeney TD, Blanchard JD, Carter JE, Brain JD. Delivery of aerosolized drugs to the lungs with a metered dose inhaler: quantitative analysis of regional deposition. J Aerosol Sci 1990; 21:350–351.
93. Zeltner TB, Sweeney TD, Skornik WA, Feldman HA, Brain JD. Retention and clearance of 0.9 μm particles inhaled by hamsters during rest or exercise. J Appl Physiol 1991; 70:1137–1145.
94. Kreyling WG, Blanchard JD, Godleski JJ, Häussermann S, Heyder J, Hutzler P, Schulz H, Sweeney TD, Takenaka S. Shallow aerosol bolus inhalation in beagle dogs: sites of retention and clearance. Eur Respir J 1995; 8:352S.
95. Godleski JJ, Stearns RC, Katler M, Hastings CL. Detection of elements by electron spectroscopic imaging and analysis of electron energy loss spectra in alveolar macrophages prepared by slam-freeze molecular distillation processing. EMSA Proc 1990; 48:776–777.
96. Godleski JJ, Kreyling WG. Localisation of cobalt in the matrix of airway cartilage. Am Rev Respir Dis 1990; 141:A525.
97. Bell KA, Friedländer SK. Aerosol deposition in models of a human lung bifurcation. Staub Reinhalt Luft 1973; 33:178–182.
98. Kim CS, Iglesias AJ. Deposition of inhaled particles in bifurcating airway models: I. Inspiratory deposition. J Aerosol Med 1989; 2:1–14.
99. Kim CS, Iglesias AJ, Garcia L. Deposition of inhaled particles in bifurcating airway models: II. Expiratory deposition. J Aerosol Med 1989; 2:15–27.
100. Kim CS, Fisher DM, Lutz DJ, Gerrity TR. Particle deposition in bifurcating airway models with varying airway geometry. J Aerosol Sci 1994; 25:567–581.
101. Kinsara AA, Loyalka SK, Tompson RV, Miller WH, Holub RF. Deposition patterns

of molecular phase radon progeny (^{218}Po) in lung bifurcations. Health Phys 1995; 68:371–382.
102. Martonen TB, Hofmann W, Lowe JE. Cigarette smoke and lung cancer. Health Phys 1987; 52:213–217.
103. Lee WC, Wang CS. Particle deposition in a system of repeatedly bifurcating tubes. In: Walton WH, ed. Inhaled Particles IV. Oxford: Pergamon Press, 1977:49–59.
104. Guilmette RA, Gagliano TJ. Construction of a model of human nasal airways using in vivo morphometric data. Ann Occup Hyg 1994; 38(suppl 1):69–75.
105. Cohen BS, Sussman RG, Lippmann M. Ultrafine particle deposition in a human tracheobronchial cast. Aerosol Sci Technol 1990; 12:1082–1091.
106. Yamada Y, Cheng YS, Yeh HC, Swift DL. Inspiratory and expiratory deposition of ultrafine particles in a human nasal cast. Inhal Toxicol 1988; 1:1–11.
107. Yamada Y, Koizumi A, Fukuda S, Inaba J, Cheng YS, Yeh HC. Deposition of ultrafine monodisperse particles in a human tracheobronchial cast. Ann Occup Hyg 1994; 38(suppl 1):91–100.
108. Cheng YS, Yamada Y, Yeh HC, Swift DL. Diffusional deposition of ultrafine aerosols in a human nasal cast. J Aerosol Sci 1988; 19:741–751.
109. Cheng YS, Yamada Y, Yeh HC, Swift DL. Deposition of ultrafine aerosols in a human oral cast. Aerosol Sci Technol 1990; 12:1075–1081.
110. Martonen TB, Lowe J. Assessment of aerosol deposition patterns in human respiratory tract casts. In: Marple VA, Lui BYH, eds. Aerosols in the Mining and Industrial Work Environments: Fundamentals and Status. Ann Arbor, MI: Ann Arbor Science, 1983: 151–164.
111. Schlesinger RB, Lippmann M. Selective particle deposition and bronchogenic carcinoma. Environ Res 1978; 15:424–431.
112. Swift DL, Montassier N, Hopke PK, Karpen-Hayes K, Cheng YS, Su YF, Yeh HC, Strong JC. Inspiratory deposition of ultrafine particles in human nasal replicate cast. J Aerosol Sci 1992; 23:65–72.
113. Heyder J, Rudolf G. Mathematical models of particle deposition in the human respiratory tract. J Aerosol Sci 1984; 15:697–707.
114. Morrow PE, Yu CP. Models of aerosol behavior in airways. In: Móren F, Newhouse MT, Dolovich MB, eds. Aerosols in Medicine. Principles, Diagnosis and Therapy. Amsterdam: Elsevier, 1993:157–193.
115. Hofmann W. Lung morphometry and particle transport and deposition: overview of existing models. In: Marijnissen JCM, Gradon L, eds. Aerosol Inhalation: Recent Research Frontiers. Dordrecht: Kluwer Academic, 1996:91–102.
116. Swift DL. Use of mathematical aerosol deposition models in predicting the distribution of inhaled therapeutic aerosols. In: Hickey A, ed. Inhalation Aerosols: Physical and Biological Basis for Therapy. New York: Marcel Dekker, 1996:51–81.
117. Findeisen W. Über das Absetzen kleiner, in der Luft suspendierter Teilchen in der menschlichen Lunge bei der Atmung. Pflügers Arch Physiol 1935; 236:367–379.
118. Altshuler B. Calculation of regional deposition of aerosol in the respiratory tract. Bull Math Biophys 1959; 21:257–270.
119. Taulbee DB, Yu CP. A theory of aerosol deposition in the human respiratory tract. J Appl Physiol 1975; 38:77–85.

120. Scott WR, Taulbee DB, Yu CP. Theoretical study of nasal deposition. Bull Math Biol 1978; 40:581–603.
121. Landahl HD. On the removal of air-borne droplets by the human respiratory tract: I. The lung. Bull Math Biophys 1950; 12:43–56.
122. Landahl HD. Particle removal by the respiratory system: note on the removal of airborne particulates by the human respiratory tract with particular reference to the role of diffusion. Bull Math Biophys 1963; 25:29–37.
123. Beeckmans JM. Correction factor for size-selective sampling, results based on a new computed alveolar deposition curve. Ann Occup Hyg 1965; 8:221–231.
124. Beeckmans JM. The deposition of aerosols in the respiratory tract. I. Mathematical analysis and comparison with experimental data. Can J Physiol Pharmacol 1965; 43:157–172.
125. Beeckmans JM. Deposition of asbestos particles in the human respiratory tract. Int Environ Stud 1970; 1:31–34.
126. ICRP Task Group on Lung Dynamics. Deposition and retention models for internal dosimetry of the human respiratory tract. Health Phys 1966; 10:1163–1174.
127. Mitchel RE. Aerosol retention in the lungs as a function of respiration rate and particle size. Ph.D. dissertation. Ohio State University, 1971.
128. Harris RL, Fraser DA. A model for deposition of fibers in the human respiratory system. Am Ind Hyg Assoc J 1976; 37:73–89.
129. Gerrity TR, Lee PS, Haas FJ, Marinelli A, Werner P, Lourenco RV. Calculated deposition of inhaled particles in the airway generations of normal subjects. J Appl Physiol 1979; 47:867–873.
130. Gerrity TR, Garrard CS, Yeates DB. Theoretic analysis of sites of aerosol deposition in the human lung. Chest 1981; 80:898–901.
131. Yeh HC, Schum GM. Models of human lung airways and their application to inhaled particle deposition. Bull Math Biol 1980; 42:461–480.
132. Hofmann E, Steinhäuser F, Pohl E. Dose calculations for the respiratory tract from inhaled natural radioactive nuclides as a function of age. Health Phys 1979; 37: 517–532.
133. Hofmann W, Koblinger L. Monte Carlo modeling of aerosol deposition in human lungs. Part II: Deposition fractions and their sensitivity to parameter variations. J Aerosol Sci 1990; 21:675–688.
134. Hofmann W, Koblinger L. Monte Carlo modeling of aerosol deposition in human lungs. Part III: Comparison with experimental data. J Aerosol Sci 1992; 23:51–63.
135. Phalen RF, Oldham MJ, Kleinman MT, Crocker TT. Tracheobronchial deposition predictions for infants, children, and adolescents. Ann Occup Hyg 1988; 32:11–21.
136. Phalen RF, Cuddihy RG, Fisher GL, Moss OR, Schlesinger RB, Swift DL, Yeh HC. Main features of the proposed NCRP respiratory tract model. Radiat Prot Dosim 1991; 38:179–184.
137. Yeh HS, Cuddihy RG, Phalen RB, Chang IY. Comparison of calculated respiratory tract deposition of particles based on the proposed NCRP model and the new ICRP66 model. Aerosol Sci Technol 1996; 25:134–140.
138. ICRP Publication 66. Human Respiratory Tract Model for Radiological Protection. New York: Elsevier Science, 1994.

139. Altshuler B, Nelson N, Kuschner M. Estimation of lung tissue dose from the inhalation of radon and daughters. Health Phys 1964; 10:1137–1161.
140. Altshuler B, Palmes ED, Nelson N. Regional aerosol deposition in the human respiratory tract. In: Davies CN, ed. Inhaled Particles and Vapours II. Oxford: Pergamon Press, 1967:323–337.
141. Scherer PW, Shendalman LH, Greene NM. Simultaneous diffusion and convection in single breath lung washout. Bull Math Biophys 1972; 34:393–412.
142. Olson DE, Dart GE, Filley GF. Pressure drop and fluid flow regime of air inspired into the human lung. J Appl Physiol 1970; 28:482–494.
143. Taulbee DB, Yu CP, Heyder J. Aerosol transport in the human lung from analysis of single breaths. J Appl Physiol 1978; 44:803–812.
144. Crawford DJ. Identifying critical human subpopulations by age groups: radioactivity and the lung. Phys Med Biol 1982; 27:539–552.
145. Yeh HC, Hulbert AJ, Phalen RF, Raabe OG. Mathematical considerations for particle deposition in the tracheobronchial tree: equations and lung model. LF-49 Inhalation Toxicology Research Institute Annual Report. Albuquerque, NM; Lovelace Foundation for Medical Education and Research, 1979.
146. Koblinger L, Hofmann W. Analysis of human lung morphometric data for stochastic aerosol deposition calculations. Phys Med Biol 1985; 30:541–556.
147. Koblinger L, Hofmann W. Monte Carlo modeling of aerosol deposition in human lungs. Part I: Simulation of particle transport in a stochastic lung structure. J Aerosol Sci 1990; 21:661–674.
148. Ferron GA, Hornik S, Kreyling WG, Haider B. Comparison of experimental and calculated data for the total and regional deposition in the human lung. J Aerosol Sci 1985; 16:133–143.
149. Hofmann W, Mainelis G. A comparative study of submicron particle deposition in human lungs. J Aerosol Sci 1993; 24:S359–S360.
150. Yu CP, Diu CK. A comparative study of aerosol deposition in different lung models. Am Ind Hyg Assoc J 1982; 43:54–65.
151. Balásházy I, Hofmann W. Particle deposition in airway bifurcations—I. Inspiratory flow. J Aerosol Sci 1993; 24:745–772.
152. Balásházy I, Hofmann W. Particle deposition in airway bifurcations—II. Expiratory flow. J Aerosol Sci 1993; 24:773–786.
153. Balásházy I, Hofmann W. Deposition of aerosols in asymmetric airway bifurcations. J Aerosol Sci. 1995; 26:273–292.
154. Gradon L, Orlicki D. Deposition of inhaled aerosol particles in a generation of the tracheobronchial tree. J Aerosol Sci, 1990; 21:3–19.
155. Li WI, Perzl M, Heyder J, Langer R, Brain JD, Englmeier KH, Niven RW, Edwards DA. Aerodynamics and aerosol particle deaggregation phenomena in model oral–pharyngeal cavities. J Aerosol Sci 1996; 27:1269–1286.
156. Katz IM, Martonen TB. Flow patterns in three-dimensional laryngeal models. J Aerosol Med 1996; 9:501–512.
157. Katz IM, Martonen TB. Three-dimensional fluid particle trajectories in the human larynx and trachea. J Aerosol Med 1996; 9:513–520.
158. Heistracher T, Hofmann W. Physiologically realistic models of bronchial airway bifurcations. J Aerosol Sci 1995; 26:497–509.

159. Perzl MA, Schulz H, Paretzke HG, Englmeier KH, Heyder J. Reconstruction of the lung geometry for the simulation of aerosol transport. J Aerosol Med 1986; 9: 409–418.
160. Perzl MA, Li W, Edwards DA, Tippe A, Lasser R, Schulz H, Heyder J. Three Dimensional Air Flow Simulations in Realistic Airway Geometries. Aerosol Med 1997; 10:254.
161. Tippe A, Häußermann S. In vitro measurements of flow within bronchial bifurcations. Eur J Physiol 1995; 430(suppl):R156.
162. Tippe A, Perzl MA, Li W, Schulz H. Flow in Bifurcation Models: Comparison Between Experiment and Numerical Simulation. Aerosol Med 1997; 10: 254.
163. Heyder J, Gebhart J, Rudolf G, Schiller CF, Stahlhofen W. Deposition of particles in the human respiratory tract in the size range 0.005–15 μm. J Aerosol Sci 1986; 17:811–825.
164. Cohen BS, Asgharian B. Deposition of ultrafine particles in the upper airways: an empirical analysis. J Aerosol Sci 1990; 21:789–797.
165. Rudolf G. A mathematical model for the deposition of aerosol particles in the human respiratory tract. J Aerosol Sci 1984; 15:195–199.
166. Rudolf G, Gebhart J, Heyder J, Scheuch G, Stahlhofen W. Modelling the deposition of aerosol particles in the human respiratory tract. J Aerosol Sci 1983; 14:188–192.
167. Rudolf G, Gebhart J, Heyder J, Schiller CF, Stahlhofen W. An empirical formula describing aerosol deposition in man for any particle size. J Aerosol Sci 1986; 17: 350–355.
168. Rudolf G, Köbrich R, Stahlhofen W. Modelling and algebraic formulation of regional aerosol deposition in man. J Aerosol Sci 1990; 21:S403–S406.
169. Schiller CF, Gebhart J, Heyder J, Rudolf G, Stahlhofen W. Factors influencing total deposition of ultrafine aerosol particles in the human respiratory tract. J Aerosol Sci 1986; 17:328–332.
170. Schiller CF, Gebhart J, Heyder J, Rudolf G, Stahlhofen W. Deposition of monodisperse insoluble aerosol particles in the 0.005 to 0.2 μm size range within the human respiratory tract. Ann Occup Hyg 1988; 32(suppl 1):41–49.
171. Anderson PJ, Hiller FC, Mazumder MK. Deposition of 0.02–0.2 μm particles in the human respiratory tract: effects of variations in respiratory pattern. Ann Occup Hyg 1988; 32(suppl 1):91–100.
172. Bennett WD. Human variation in spontaneous breathing deposition fraction: a review. J Aerosol Med 1988; 1:67–80.
173. Miller FJ, Martonen TB, Ménache MG, Graham RC, Spektor DM, Lippmann M. Influence of breathing mode and activity level on the regional deposition of inhaled particles and implications for regulatory standards. Ann Occup Hyg 1988:32(suppl 1):3–10.
174. Davies CN, Lever M, Rothenberg S. Experimental studies of the deposition of particles in the human lungs. In: Walton HA, ed. Inhaled Particles IV. Oxford: Pergamon 1977:151–162.
175. Bennett WD, Smaldone GC. Human variation in the peripheral air-space deposition of inhaled particles. J Appl Physiol 1987; 62:1603–1610.

176. Tobin MJ, Chadha TS, Jenouri G, Birch SJ, Gazeroglu K, Sackner MA. Breathing patterns 1. Normal subjects. Chest 1983; 84:202–205.
177. Shea SA, Walter J, Murphy K, Guz A. Evidence for individuality of breathing patterns in resting healthy man. Respir Physiol 1987; 68:331–344.
178. Swift DL, Proctor DF. A dosimetric model for particles in the respiratory tract above the trachea. Ann Occup Hyg 1988; 32(suppl 1):1035–1044.
179. Hahn I, Scherer PW, Mozell MM. Velocity profiles for airflow through a large-scale model of the human nose. J Appl Physiol 1993; 75:2273–2287.
180. Schlichting H. Boundary-Layer Theory (Trans. by Kestin J). Stanford: McGraw-Hill, 1968.
181. Cheng YS, Su YF, Yeh HC, Swift DL. Deposition of thoron progeny in human head airways. Aerosol Sci Technol 1993; 18:359–375.
182. Swift DL, Strong JC. Nasal deposition of ultrafine ^{218}Po aerosols in human subjects. J Aerosol Sci 1996; 27:1125–1132.
183. Fry FA, Black A. Regional deposition and clearance of particles in the human nose. Aerosol Sci 1973; 4:113–124.
184. Stahlhofen W, Rudolf G, James AC. Intercomparison of experimental regional aerosol deposition data. J Aerosol Med 1989; 2:285–308.
185. Cheng KH, Cheng YY, Yeh HC, Guilmette RA, Simpson SQ, Yang YH, Swift DL. In vivo measurements of nasal airway dimensions and ultrafine aerosol deposition in the human nasal and oral airways. J Aerosol Sci 1996; 27:785–801.
186. Guilmette RA, Wicks JD, Wolff RK. Morphometry of human nasal airways in vivo using magnetic resonance imaging. J Aerosol Med 1989; 2:365–377.
187. Rasmussen TR, Swift DL, Hilberg O, Pedersen OF. Influence of nasal passage geometry on aerosol particle deposition in the nose. J Aerosol Med 1990; 3:15–25.
188. Rudolf G. Deposition von Aerosolteilchen in der Nase. [Deposition of aerosol particles in the nose]. Dissertation. University Frankfurt/Main, Frankfurt, Germany, 1975.
189. Zhang L, Yuh CP. Empirical equations for nasal deposition of inhaled particles in small laboratory animals and humans. Aerosol Sci Technol 1993; 19:51–56.
190. Gradon L, Yu CP. Diffusional particle deposition in the human nose and mouth. Aerosol Sci Technol 1989; 11:213–220.
191. Emmett PC, Aitken RJ. Measurement of the total and regional deposition of inhaled particles in the human respiratory tract. J Aerosol Sci 1982; 13:549–560.
192. Bowes SM III, Swift DL. Deposition of inhaled particles in the oral airway during oronasal breathing. Aerosol Sci Technol 1989; 11:157–167.
193. Niinimaa V, Cole P, Mintz S, Shephard RJ. Oronasal distribution of respiratory airflow. Respir Physiol 1981; 43:69–75.
194. Swift DL, Cheng YS, Su YF, Yeh HC. Ultrafine aerosol deposition in the human nasal and oral passages. Ann Occup Hyg 1994; 38:77–81.
195. Ferron GA, Busch B, Gebhart J, Roth C. Evaporation of aerosols produced with eleven jet nebulizers. J Aerosol Sci 1996; 27:S381–S382.
196. Anderson M, Philipson K, Svartengren M, Camner P. Human deposition and clearance of 6-µm particles inhaled with an extremely low flow rate. Exp Lung Res 1995; 21:187–195.

197. Svartengren K, Philipson K, Svartengren M, Anderson M, Camner P. Tracheobronchial deposition and clearance in small airways in asthmatic subjects. Eur Respir J 1996; 9:1123–1129.
198. Phalen RF, Oldham MJ, Schum GM. Growth and ageing of the bronchial tree: implications for particle deposition calculations. Radiat Prot Dosim 1991; 38:15–21.
199. Hugonaud C, Gehr P, Weibel EW, Burri PH. Adaptation of the growing lung to increased oxygen consumption II. Morphometric analysis. Respir Physiol 1977; 29: 1–10.
200. Cudmore RE, Emery JL, Mithal A. Postnatal growth of the bronchi and bronchioles. Arch Dis Child 1962; 37:481–484.
201. Stocks J, Quanjar PH. Reference values for residual volume, functional residual capacity and total lung capacity. Eur Respir J 1995; 8:492–506.
202. DeGroodt EG, Quanjer PH, Wise ME, van Zomeren BC. Changing relationships between stature and lung volumes during puberty. Respir Physiol 1986; 65:139–153.
203. Hislop A, Muir DCF, Jacobsen M, Simon G, Reid L. Postnatal growth and function of the preacinar airways. Thorax 1072; 27:265–274.
204. Schrader PC, Quanjer PH, Olievier ICW. Respiratory muscle force and ventilatory function in adolescents. Eur Respir J 1988; 1:368–375.
205. Schrader PC, Quanjer PH, van Zomeren BC, Wise ME. Changes in the FEV_1–height relationship during pubertal growth. Bull Eur Physiopathol Respir 1984; 20: 381–388.
206. Schrader PT, Quanjer PH, Borsboom G, Wise ME. Evaluating lung function and antropometric growth data in a longitudinal study on adolescents. Hum Biol 1984; 56:365–381.
207. Buist AS, Gheo H, Anthonisen NR, Cherniack RM, Ducic S, Macklem PT, Manfreda J, Martin RR, McCarthy D, Ross BB. Relationship between single-breath N_2 test and age, sex, and smoking habit in three north American cities. Am Rev Respir Dis 1979; 120:305–318.
208. Bode FR, Dosman J, Martin RR, Gheo H, Macklem PT. Age and sex differences in lung elasticity and in closing capacity in nonsmokers. J Appl Physiol 1976; 41: 129–135.
209. Becklake M, Crapo RO. Lung function testing: selection of reference values and interpretative strategies. Am Rev Respir Dis 1991; 144:1202–1218.
210. Chiang ST, Wang BC, Chi YL, Hsieh YC. Ventilatory components of lungs in relation to sex and age. Am Rev Respir Dis 1971; 104:175–181.
211. Sherrill DL, Lebowitz MD, Knudson RJ, Burrows B. Continuous longitudinal regression equations for pulmonary function measures. Eur Respir J 1992; 5:452–462.
212. Becquemin MH, Roy M, Bouchikhi A, Teillac A. Deposition of inhaled particles in healthy children. In: Hofmann W, ed. Deposition and Clearance of Aerosols in the Human Respiratory Tract. Vienna: Facultas, 1987:22–27.
213. Becquemin MH, Yu CP, Roy M, Bouchikhi A. Total deposition of inhaled particles related to age: comparison with age-dependent model calculations. Radiat Prot Dosim 1991; 38:23–28.

214. Schiller-Scotland CF, Hlawa R, Gebhart J, Wönne R, Heyder J. Total deposition of aerosol particles in the respiratory tract of children during spontaneous and controlled mouth breathing. J Aerosol Sci 1992; 23:S457–S460.
215. Schiller-Scotland CF, Hlawa R, Gebhart J, Heyder J, Roth C. Wönne R. Particle deposition in the respiratory tract of children during spontaneous and controlled mouth breathing. Ann Occup Hyg 1994; 38(suppl 1):117–125.
216. Fok TF, Monkman S, Dolovich M, Gray S, Coates G, Paes B, Rashid F, Newhouse M, Kirpalani H. Efficiency of aerosol medication delivery from a metered dose inhaler versus jet nebulizer in infants with bronchopulmonary dysplasia. Pediatr Pulmonol 1996; 21:301–309.
217. Grigg J, Amon S, Jones T, Clarke A, Silverman M. Delivery of therapeutic aerosols to intubated babies. Arch Dis Child 1992; 67:25–30.
218. Wattenberg KL, Clark AR, Kelly HW, Murphy S. Delivery of aerosolised medication to intubated babies. Pediatr Pulmonol 1991; 10:136–141.
219. Arnon S, Grigg J, Nikander K, Silverman M. Delivery of micronized budesonide suspension by metered dose inhaler and jet nebulizer into neonatal ventilator circuit. Pediatr Pulmonol 1992; 13:172–175.
220. Cameron D, Arnot R, Clay M, Silverman M. Aerosol delivery in neonatal ventilator circuits: a rabbit lung model. Pediatr Pulmonol 1991; 10:208–212.
221. Flavin M, MacDonald M, Dolovich M, Coates G, O'Brodovich H. Aerosol delivery to the rabbit lung with infant ventilator. Pediatr Pulmonol 1986; 2:35–39.
222. O'Callaghan C, Hardy J, Stammers J, Stephenson TJ, Hull D. Evaluation of techniques for delivery of steroids to lungs of neonates using a rabbit model. Arch Dis Child 1992; 67:20–24.
223. Warwick R, Williams PL. Gray's Anatomy. Philadelphia: WB Saunders, 1973.
224. Brown JS, Gerrity TR, Bennett WD, Kim CS, House DE. Dispersion of aerosol boluses in the human lung: dependence on lung volume, bolus volume, and gender. J Appl Physiol 1995; 79:1787–1795.
225. Pritchard JN, Jefferies SJ, Black A. Sex differences in the regional deposition of inhaled particles in the 2.5–7.5 μm size range. J Aerosol Sci 1986; 17:385–389.
226. Bennett WD, Messina MS, Smaldone G. Effect of exercise on deposition and subsequent retention of inhaled particles. J Appl Physiol 1985; 59:1046–1054.
227. Morgan WKC, Ahmad D, Chamberlain JM, Clague HW, Pearson MG, Vinitski S. The effect of exercise on the deposition of an inhaled aerosol. Respir Physiol 1984; 56:327–338.
228. Schulz H, Schulz A, Eder G, Heyder J. Influence of gas composition on convective and diffusive intrapulmonary gas transport. Exp Lung Res 1995; 21:853–876.
229. Svartengren M, Anderson K, Philipson K, Camner P. Human lung deposition of particles suspended in air or in helium/oxygen mixture. Exp Lung Res 1989; 15: 575–585.
230. Anderson M, Svartengren M, Philipson K, Camner P. Deposition in man of particles inhaled in air or helium–oxygen at different flow rates. J Aerosol Med 1990; 3: 209–216.
231. Anderson M, Svartengren M, Bylin G, Philipson K, Camner P. Deposition in asthmatics of particles inhaled in air or helium–oxygen. Am Rev Respir Dis 1993; 147: 524–528.

232. Schulz H, Schulz A, Heilmann P, Heyder J. Can drug delivery to the lungs be influenced by breathing different gas compositions? J Aerosol Med 1993; 6:42s.
233. Garland LH, Beier RL, Coulson W, Heald JH, Stein RL. The apparent sites of origin of carcinomas of the lung. Radiology 1962; 78:1–11.
234. Ferron GA, Brand P, Schulz A, Tippe A, Heyder J. Improvements in deposition modeling. J Aerosol Med 1993; 6(suppl):24.

6

Structural and Interfacial Aspects of Particle Retention

MARIANNE GEISER, VINZENZ IM HOF, and PETER GEHR

University of Bern
Bern, Switzerland

SAMUEL SCHÜRCH

Health Sciences Center
University of Calgary
Calgary, Alberta, Canada

I. Introduction

Inhaled particles may land on the surface of the lungs' airspaces. Upon making contact with the airway or alveolar wall, the processes of retention and clearance of these particles begin. The retention of particles depends on many factors, among these are (1) particle size, shape, solubility, surface chemistry, and elastic properties of both the particles and the lung surface; (2) the anatomical location of the deposition site (conducting airways, alveoli), which is important for the route and distance of particle clearance; (3) the structures the particle interacts with at the site of deposition, including the surfactant film at the air–liquid interface; the aqueous phase; free cells, such as macrophages, lymphocytes, and granulocytes; the epithelial cells; and dendritic cells that reside at the basal side of the epithelium. All these factors determine the fate of a deposited particle: the length of time it is retained before being cleared or dissolved. Hence, these factors are important for the beneficial or pathogenic potential of the retained particles.

In the present chapter we first describe structural aspects of the conducting airways and alveoli, including the epithelial cells, the extracellular aqueous layer, and the surfactant film at the air–liquid interface.

In the second part, we focus on the biophysical aspects of particle retention, mainly on the interactions of particles with the surfactant film at the air–wall interface in the airways. Not only the surface tensions of the film and the particles are important for particle retention, but also, line tension forces that operate at the three-phase line at the air–particle–substrate interfaces. The effect of these forces largely depends on particle size.

In the third part, we describe the methods of studying particle retention. We thereby focus on techniques that allow quantitative studies concomitant with qualitative ultrastructural analyses, and on new methods to preserve the extracellular lining layer with the surfactant film at the air–liquid interface.

The last part highlights the significance of particle retention, especially because the mucous layer is not an impermeable barrier for particles deposited at the air–wall interface. Even relatively large retained particles appear partially immersed into the aqueous phase, whereas smaller particles are totally submerged. The interaction of particles with surfactant during the immersion process, followed by their exposure to substances of the aqueous layer, and the vicinity of immersed particles to the epithelial cells, macrophages, and to dendritic cells significantly enhance the biological effect of retained particles.

II. Structural Aspects

A. The Conducting Airways

The anatomy of the airway tree—namely, its branching pattern, the length, diameter, and branching angles of the individual airway branches—have been extensively studied in humans and animals (1–6). In addition, the volume of the conducting airways (trachea, bronchi, and bronchioles), which is 5–10% of the total lung volume, is known from quantitative morphological studies of the lung (7,8). Direct measurements of the airway surface area, an important parameter in the study of particle–lung interactions, are scarce, because unbiased stereology for anisotropic (not randomly oriented) structures has only recently become available. Using such methods the airway surface was estimated to be 1–2% of the total inner lung surface area [human (9), mice (10,11)].

The Epithelial Cells of the Conducting Airways

The thickness and the cellular composition of the airway epithelium vary with airway generations and among species. In general, the thickness is greatest (tall columnar pseudostratified) in the trachea, and smallest (simple low cuboidal) in the bronchioles. Nine different cell types have been identified in the epithelium and submucosal glands of the conducting airways in adult mammals: basal, ciliated, mucous (goblet), serous, Clara, small mucous granule, neuroendocrine, brush, and intermediate cells (12,13). In several species, including humans (14), dog (15), ferret (16), and cats (17), basal, mucous, and ciliated cells predominate in the epithelium of the proximal conducting airways (trachea and bronchi) and serous and mucous cells in the submucosal (tracheobronchial) glands. In the same species, the distal airways (i.e., peripheral conducting airways; bronchioles) are lined by mainly ciliated and Clara cells (18). In other species, mucous cells are scarce in the trachea and bronchi, and either Clara [rabbits (19), mice (20), hamsters (17,21)] or serous cells (rats; 22) are the dominant secretory cells of both the proximal and distal airways. In rhesus monkey, however, ciliated, goblet, small mucous granule, and basal cells are found throughout the airway tree, including the respiratory bronchioles, whereas the Clara cell is restricted to the respiratory bronchioles (23). The significant interspecies heterogeneity of the secretory cells in airways suggests differences in the composition and, hence, also in the structure of airway secretions.

In addition to the epithelial cells, the dendritic cells, which reside at the base of the epithelium and reach up to the tight junctions, with numerous intercellular (dendritic) cytoplasmic processes, constitute a principal cell population in the airways. The dendritic cells are extensively described in Chapter 11.

The Aqueous Lining Layer of the Conducting Airways

The aqueous lining layer that covers the surface of the conducting airways consists of water, ions, sugars, proteins, proteoglycans, glycoproteins, and lipids (24). It originates from the airway epithelium and the submucosal glands (25,26). It is not known to what extent the secretions mix. The thickness of the aqueous lining layer is reported to be a few micrometers in the trachea and to diminish to a little more than 1 μm in the distal airways [human and rat (27), guinea pig (28)]. Moreover, the aqueous lining layer of peripheral airways in guinea pigs is not evenly distributed in either the circumferential or longitudinal direction and its thickness varies with airway inflation (28). Therefore, it was suggested that the geometry of the aqueous lining layer is highly dynamic and that movements of liquid across the airway wall and along the airway tree are important factors in establishing the thickness of the lining layer in a healthy state.

The aqueous lining layer has been described (29) as a two-phase system, consisting of a sol phase (hypophase; periciliary fluid) adjacent to the epithelial cells and above a gel phase (epiphase; mucus). The periciliary phase is considered as a continuous aqueous layer of relatively low viscosity, with its depth maintained at a little less than the ciliary length. This allows the ciliary tips to penetrate into the overlaying, more viscous mucous gel phase during the propulsive (effective) strokes (30) and claw the mucus forward to transport all sorts of particles, including cells, cell debris, and dust, contained in it toward the pharynx (31). The existence, thickness, and continuity of the gel phase are debated relative to the different airway compartments and between the differing species. On the one hand, mucus has been reported to be noncontinuous and to be present as streets, flakes, or plaques in large rat airways and human bronchi (27,32,33) or to be focally distributed in rat large airways (34). On the other hand, mucus was described as a superficial continuous layer in bovine, rat, and rabbit tracheae and bronchi (35–38).

The nature of the interface between the sol and gel phase is also unclear. These phases were reported to be separated by osmiophilic ''membranes'' (39–42), and Girod et al. (43) demonstrated osmiophilic vesicles between the sol and gel phase. Morgenroth and Bolz (40) suggested that these osmiophilic structures act as a lubricant to facilitate the sliding of mucus on the sol phase. Recently, a thin mucous layer that extends to the tips of the cilia and into the sol phase was shown in guinea pig and rat tracheae (44). In our laboratory, a structurally distinct gel phase that is separated from a sol phase layer could not be confirmed in the most recent studies, neither in hamster airways (45) nor in horse trachea (46). In addition, a distinct gel phase could not be established in the peripheral airways of guinea pigs (28), rats (47), or rabbits (37).

The existence of osmiophilic material in various forms in the aqueous lining layer has been previously reported (34,35,41,45,47,48). The appearance of osmiophilic material at the air–liquid interface in the form of a film covering the aqueous lining layer is of special interest for the retention of particles and will be discussed later in further detail.

Also, submerged in either the sol or the gel phase are free cells, such as granulocytes, lymphocytes, or macrophages. The latter are most frequent, and they constitute a resident cell population in the conducting airways. We and others have shown that macrophages engulf deposited particles in conducting airways [hamster (49), mouse (50), rat (51)]. Thereby the phagocytes are attracted to the site of particle deposition (49,52,53).

The Air–Liquid Interface of the Conducting Airways

Gil and Weibel (47) demonstrated, for the first time, the existence of an osmiophilic line covering the bronchiolar fluid. In addition, they showed the continuity between bronchiolar and alveolar linings. Recently, such a film was also demonstrated in the trachea and large airways in human, rat, hamster, guinea pig, and horse (27,44–46). This film frequently appeared to be multilaminated. Figure 1 represents a transmission electron micrograph showing an osmiophilic film at the air–liquid interface in a horse trachea after fixation with osmium tetroxide dissolved in perfluorocarbon fluid (45). The existence of a surfactant film at the air–liquid interface in the trachea and large airways is supported by the following additional evidence: The surface tension in large, accessible airways has been measured in vivo by placing oil droplets onto tracheae or bronchi of anesthetized sheep, dog, and horse (54–56). The measured surface tension of approximately

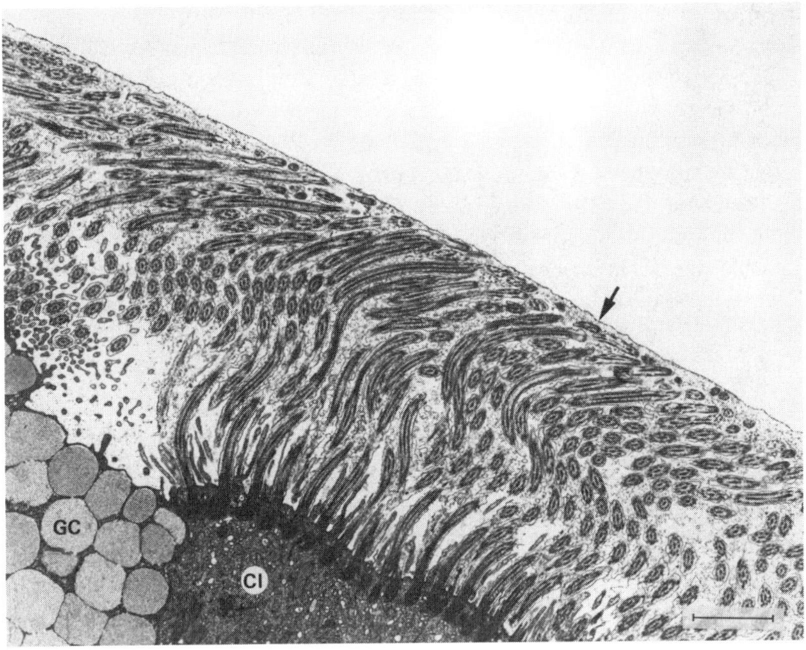

Figure 1 Transmission electron micrograph of normal horse trachea after osmium tetroxide–perfluorocarbon fixation: The air–liquid interface is covered by an osmiophilic film (arrow). The aqueous lining layer surrounds and covers the cilia. GC, goblet cell; CI, ciliated cell; bar = 2 μm.

30 mN/m at the air–liquid interface in horses (54,55) indicates the accumulation of surface-active molecules at this interface. Without an accumulation of such molecules, the surface tension of the aqueous phase would be much higher, between 45 and 60 mN/m, typical for the level of the surface tensions of biopolymers, such as proteins, surface polymers of blood cells, and polysaccharides (57–59).

It appears that a substantial part of the airway surfactant is derived from the alveolar region, but there is also evidence for local production of surfactant. Widdicombe (41) reviewed the possible sources and potential biological role of tracheal surfactants. He concluded that the trachea contains a complex mixture of lipids, including surface-active phospholipids not characteristic of alveolar surfactant. Experiments (60) have shown that nonciliated cells of the bronchioles produce surface-active material and that these cells are involved in ion and water transport. Other studies (43) demonstrated phospholipids in secretory cells of airway submucosal glands, suggesting local production of phospholipids in the airways. Furthermore, nonciliated airway epithelial cells are capable of synthesizing surfactant apoproteins (61–63). There is indirect evidence (64) showing that surface-active material from the alveolar region may reach large airways. Recently, the phospholipids and surfactant proteins (SP) of tracheal aspirates were compared with those of alveolar surfactant (65). Phospholipids of tracheal aspirate surfactant showed the same composition as alveolar surfactant, but SP-A was decreased and SP-B and SP-C were absent in the former. The authors concluded that the substantial amounts of phospholipids and phosphatidylcholine molecular species in tracheal aspirates may have derived from alveolar surfactant. However, adsorption and minimal and maximal surface tension of tracheal aspirate surfactant were impaired compared with those of alveolar surfactant.

B. The Lung Parenchyma

The Transition Zone

The first respiratory structures appear in the respiratory bronchioles. Their airway wall is interrupted by single alveoli. The epithelium of the respiratory bronchioles contains fewer ciliated cells, and at the alveolar rim it appears continuous with the alveolar epithelial cells. Because of the dual function of these airways (conductive and active in gas exchange) this portion of airways is called the transition zone. Respiratory bronchioles may be absent or short and comprise only one to two generations, as seen in small laboratory animals, or the respiratory bronchioles extend over three to five generations, as in humans and other large mammals (66,67).

Beyond the respiratory bronchioles, several generations of alveolar ducts follow. Their wall is completely interspersed with alveoli. This part of the lung is called the gas-exchange zone.

The Gas Exchange Zone

The Epithelial Cells of the Alveoli

The alveolar epithelium consists of two major cell types. It covers a total surface area of approximately 140 m^2 in humans (7). Ninety-three percent of the surface area (human, baboon, and rat; 68), or even more (dog, rabbit, hamster, mouse, and other species; 69) is covered by the squamous type I cells, and 7% or less by the cuboidal type II cells. The structural basis for the gas exchange is the interalveolar septum, which forms the wall between two alveoli. In this location air and blood come into close contact, and they are separated by a tissue barrier with an average thickness of only 2 μm (human; 7). Over large areas in humans and in many other species (69) the thickness is even less than 1 μm.

The Aqueous Lining Layer and the Air–Liquid Interface of the Alveoli

The alveolar epithelium is covered by an ultrathin-lining layer consisting of an aqueous hypophase covered by a film of surfactant (70–73). The aqueous subphase is thicker (on the average 0.89 μm in rats; 70) in the corners of the alveolus where the alveolar walls meet and become thin (0.14 μm), over flat portions of the alveolar wall, and protruding features such as capillaries (0.09 μm). Alveolar surfactant is produced by type II cells (74,75). The surfactant film at the air–liquid interphase has been reported to be thinner than that in airways (47).

Submerged in this lining layer are alveolar macrophages. Their phagocytic and microbiocidal potential is the major reason the alveoli remain sterile and clean. The structure and function of alveolar macrophages are frequently reviewed and studied (76,77), partly because these cells are readily accessible by bronchoalveolar lavage (BAL).

III. Interfacial Aspects: Interaction of Particles with the Air–Liquid Interface (Surfactant)

A. Mechanical Functions of the Surfactant Film

Pulmonary surfactant stabilizes the gas-exchange region of the lung by reducing the surface tension at the air–liquid interface of the alveoli, particularly during expiration. This is the principal and well-known mechanical function of pulmonary surfactant.

In contrast, the mechanical functions of airway surfactant are not well established. One of the functions is particle transport from the alveoli to the ciliated airways by a surface tension gradient (78,79), another is particle translocation toward the epithelium in airways. In the present chapter we will focus on the latter mechanical function of the airway surfactant film.

Particles, after their deposition in the airspaces of the lung, are wetted and displaced toward the epithelium by the surfactant film during the retention process. This translocation of particles by capillary forces is one of the mechanical functions of the surfactant film. In vitro experiments demonstrated that the extent of particle immersion depends on the surface tension of the surfactant film. The lower the surface tension, the greater is the immersion of the particles into the aqueous phase (42,56). Figure 2 illustrates in vitro the effect of a surfactant film, at two different surface tensions, on particle displacement in a modified Langmuir–Wilhelmy balance.

Figure 3 shows polymethylmethacrylate (PMMA) particles retained on a guinea pig trachea. Smaller particles are totally submerged into the subphase below an osmiophilic film. That smaller particles are completely submerged was confirmed by serial sections. On top of these smaller particles there is a thin layer of mucus below the osmiophilic film. This layer appears to be thin and resembles a sheet of Saran wrap covering the particles (Fig. 4). Large PMMA particles show various degrees of displacement into the subphase.

In Figure 5, large PMMA particles of more than 30 μm in diameter appear

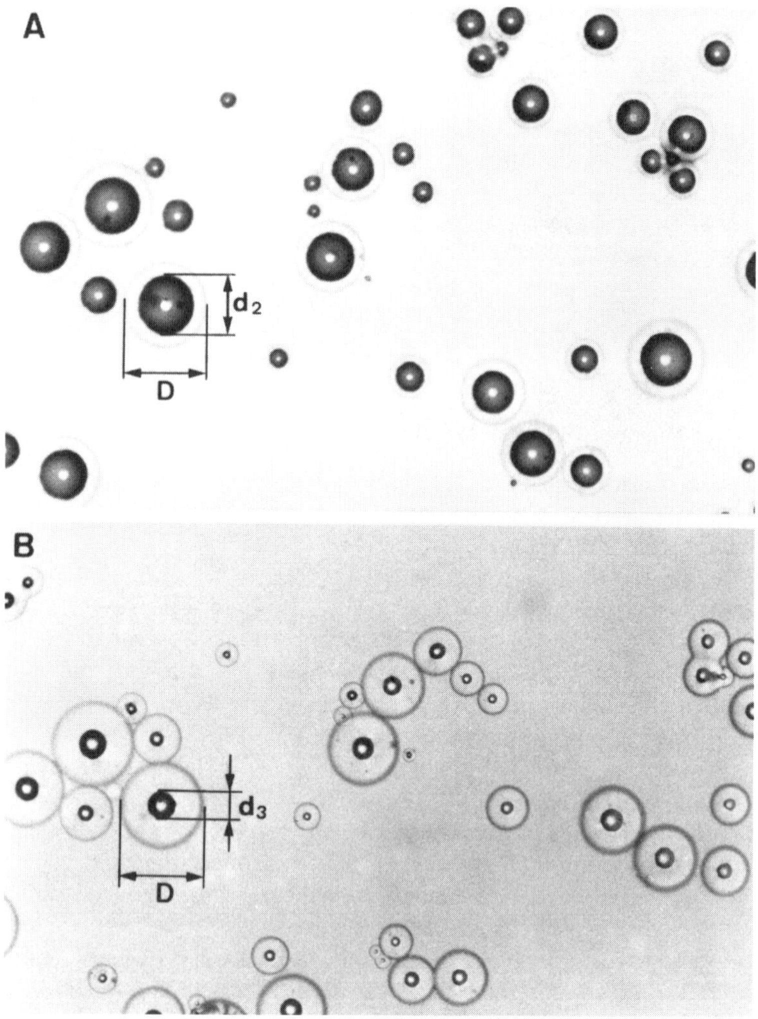

Figure 2 Polymethylmethacrylate (PMMA) microspheres on a dipalmitoylphosphatidylcholine (DPPC) monolayer supported by an aqueous subphase (density 1.26 g/mL) at (A) a surface tension of 40 mN/m, and (B) at 30 mN/m. Note the appearance of the labeled particle at decreasing film surface tensions. D (80 μm) indicates the total diameter, d is the diameter of the segment exposed to air; d is decreasing with the surface tension, indicating increasing particle immersion. (From Ref. 56.)

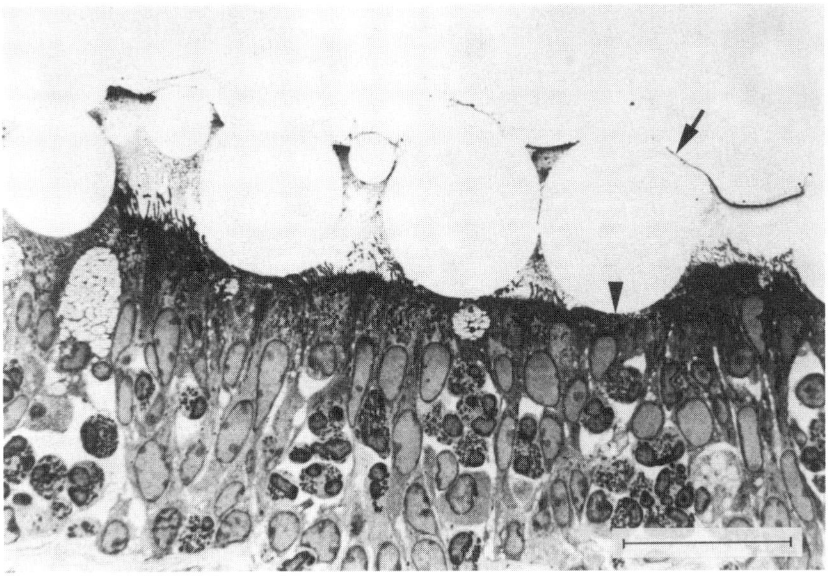

Figure 3 A light micrograph of a guinea pig trachea fixed by immersion in osmium tetroxide–perfluorocarbon 5 min after exposure to a polydispersed aerosol of PMMA (diameter 10–100 μm). The microspheres are submerged beneath an osmiophilic film (arrow) and indent the underlying epithelium (arrowhead). Toluidine blue staining; bar = 30 μm.

only partially covered by mucus. There is a circular three-phase line where the three interfaces (air, liquid, and solid) meet. There is no mucus layer covering the spherical segment above the circular line on the particle.

The mucus layer is not an impermeable barrier for particles deposited at the air–wall interface. Relatively large retained particles appear partially immersed into the aqueous phase, whereas smaller particles are totally submerged (see Figs. 3–5).

B. Properties of the Substrate (Aqueous Lining Layer)

Respiratory mucus is a complex mixture of glycoproteins, proteoglycans, lipids, and smaller quantities of other proteins (82). Glycoproteins appear to be the most important component conferring viscoelastic properties to the mucus (see also Chap. 13).

Mucus is both viscous and elastic and also shows cohesion. The latter two characteristics appear to determine the threadforming ability of mucus or its spi-

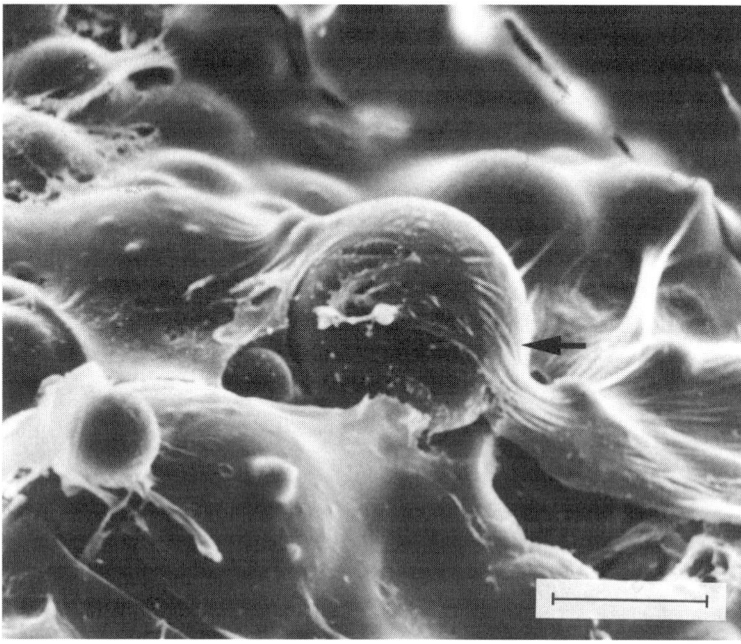

Figure 4 Scanning electron micrograph of a normal guinea pig trachea treated as in Figure 3. Small particles appear totally submerged beneath the mucous layer. Note the Saran-like thin mucous sheet partially covering the large microsphere (arrow); bar = 20 μm. (From Ref. 80.)

nability. Mucus is a nonnewtonian fluid, for its viscosity decreases with increasing rate of shear. The viscosity is important for trapping and retaining particles, whereas elasticity appears to be more important than viscosity in the efficiency of transport. When mucus is stretched and released it may return to near its original dimension. Some of the stored energy is dissipated in overcoming the viscous force. The time taken to use up the stored energy against viscous resistance is a measure of the relaxation time, which relates to the moduli of elasticity and viscosity (81).

In summary, the rheological characteristics of normal mucus are very well matched with the characteristics of the ciliary propulsion system. Mucociliary transport depends on the interplay between three components—the cilia, periciliary fluid, and mucus—with the surfactant film at the mucus–air interface (44,45,81). The glycoproteins are most important in providing the appropriate levels of elasticity, viscosity, and cohesiveness for mucous flakes and sheets to be optimally propelled (82).

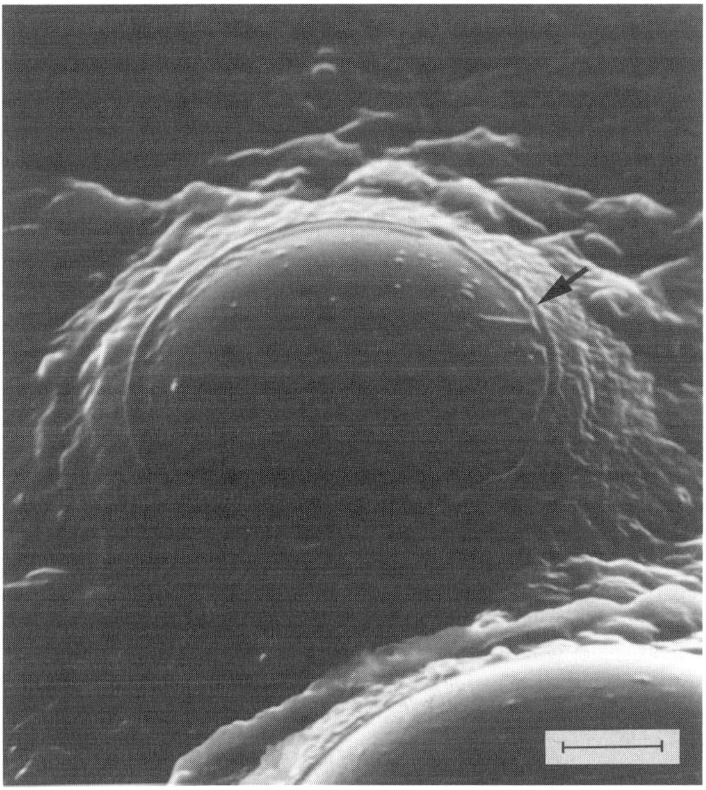

Figure 5 Scanning electron micrograph of a normal guinea pig trachea treated as in Figure 3: Large PMMA particles are partially submerged into the subphase. There is no mucous layer covering the particle above the circular three-phase line (arrow), where the three interfaces, air, liquid, and solid, meet; bar = 10 μm. (From Ref. 44.)

Particles are thought to stick to the viscous and ''sticky'' mucus. However, they do not just stick to the mucus, they appear to be displaced or even engulfed by the mucous layer. The surfactant film at the air–liquid interface is the first structural element of the airway mucosa that particles encounter at their deposition followed by retention.

In our model studies (42,56) we investigated the surface tension properties of the surfactant film at the air–liquid interface. In the studies conducted in vitro, using a modified Langmuir–Wilhelmy balance, we have not considered the structure of the subphase and its viscoelastic properties: the subphase was taken as a newtonian fluid.

Figure 6 shows polystyrene (PS) particles of an average diameter of 11.9 μm retained on a freshly excised piece of sheep trachea and on a surfactant film of dipalmitoylphosphatidylcholine (DPPC) in a modified Langmuir–Wilhelmy balance. The surface tension in both cases is approximately 30 mN/m, measured by a drop-spreading technique on the trachea and by a Wilhelmy plate in the surface balance. The aqueous substrate for the film in the balance was 0.9% NaCl with 55% sucrose. The density of the substrate was 1.26 g/mL, considerably higher than that of the particle (1.05 g/cm^3). Most of the particles retained on the tracheal surface appear to be submerged in the substrate, and only a small segment of the spheres is exposed to air above the three-phase line. This is equivalent to the situation in the surface balance.

Thus, this experiment demonstrates that, for particle immersion, the aqueous substrate on the trachea may be mimicked in vitro by a viscous newtonian fluid the density of which is higher than that of the particle, provided the surface tension of the surfactant film in the balance is the same as that at the tracheal wall–air surface.

In Figure 3, the largest particles, about 40 μm in diameter, seem to be only partially coated with film material, whereas the smaller particles, 10–15 μm in diameter, appear totally submerged. Could this be explained by the enhanced resistance against further displacement of the larger particles once the particles established contact with the underlying epithelium? Are the smaller particles totally submerged because they did not meet the resistance of the epithelium against displacement? Again, in vitro experiments in the Langmuir–Wilhelmy balance might help clarify the question of the displacement of large particles compared with that of small particles.

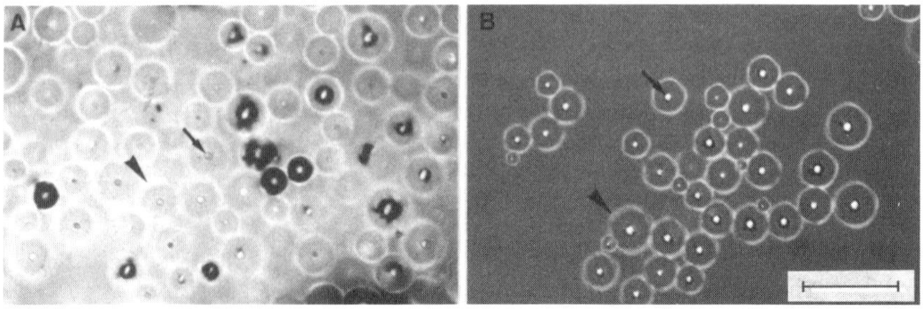

Figure 6 Light micrograph of polystyrene microspheres (11.9 μm in diameter) submerged (A) in the aqueous subphase on the wall of excised sheep trachea and (B) on a DPPC monolayer supported by a subphase of sucrose and NaCl in water, both at a surface tension of 30 mN/m. The arrowheads point to the total particle diameter, the arrows to the segments exposed to air; bar = 30 μm. (From Ref. 42.)

Figure 7 shows PMMA microspheres, in the size range of 10–60 μm, on a DPPC film at approximately 30 mN/m supported by a saline–sucrose substrate; its density of 1.26 g/mL is higher than that of PMMA (1.19 g/cm^3).

The smaller particles are wetted by the substrate to a substantially greater extent than the larger ones. This can be quantified by calculating the height at the spherical segment exposed to air from the diameter of the sphere D and the radius of the segment exposed to air d. In this case, the particles did not establish contact with the underlying solid bottom of the surface balance because the aqueous substrate was at least 1-cm deep.

We, therefore, may conclude from the experiments illustrated by Figures 3, 5, and 7 that small plastic particles (PS or PMMA) smaller than about 20 μm in diameter are substantially more wetted or displaced by a fluid phase covered with a surfactant film than particles larger than 30 μm in diameter and that this effect is not related to the thickness of the subphase. Hence, we have sought

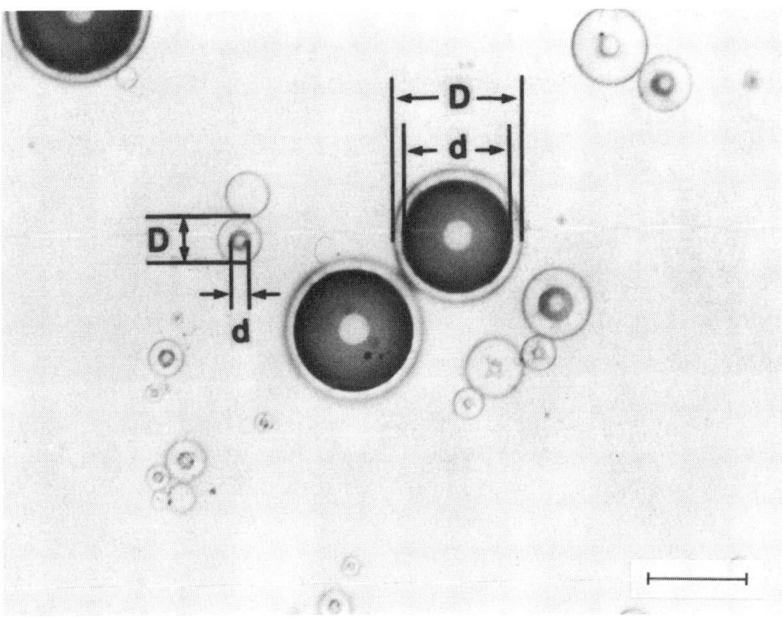

Figure 7 Light micrograph of PMMA microspheres (diameter 10–80 μm) on a DPPC film at 30 mN/m, supported by a saline–sucrose subphase. D indicates the total diameter, d is the diameter of the segment exposed to air. The ratio d/D for the small particles is much smaller than that for the larger particles. This indicates greater immersion into the subphase of the small particles compared with the large particles; bar = 50 μm.

other mechanisms to explain the dependence of particle displacement on particle size. These possible mechanisms are presented in the following section.

IV. Biophysical Aspects of Particle Retention

A. Theoretical Background

Explanations for the difference in displacement according to size are offered from the field of surface thermodynamics, dealing with not just dividing interfaces and the related surface tensions, but also with dividing lines and the related line tensions; whereas the interaction of particles of differing size (e.g., glass, metal, or plastic) with a variety of polymeric (plastic) substrates has been investigated by adhesion science and technology. An understanding of the mechanics of particle adhesion is important in the semiconductor industry, in xerography, and in graphic arts (83).

We will first summarize some of the approaches employed in studying particle adhesion to materials that exhibit elastic properties. Quesnel et al. (84) have discussed the similarity between the tendency of a fluid drop to wet a surface of a solid and the tendency to "wet" when solids are brought together (e.g., a glass particle and a plastic substrate).

For a liquid to wet a solid by spreading means that the free energy of the total system decreases during spreading. In other words, if the free energy needed to form the interface between the liquid and the solid is smaller than the free energy gained by eliminating the free surface, the liquid should spread. This thermodynamic argument does not include kinetic effects and states only what is energetically favorable.

When solids are brought together, the tendency to wet follows the same thermodynamic principles as those for a fluid droplet to spread on a solid surface. However, the finite shear strength of the solid prevents the achievement of a thermodynamic equilibrium. The materials deform elastically or plastically in response to the large stresses generated by the surface forces. Furthermore, the geometry of the interacting surfaces is important for the geometry of the deformations. For example, the adhesive interactions between spherical glass particles and a polyurethane substrate generate a meniscus of cylindrical symmetry (85).

The surface forces between glass spheres (2- to 60-μm radius) with an elastic modulus (Young's modulus) of 7×10^{10} Pa and a polyurethane substrate having a Young's modulus of approximately 5×10^{6} Pa are sufficiently strong to generate a substantial meniscus in the more compliant polyurethane (85). For example, for a glass particle of a radius of approximately 3.0 μm, the height of the meniscus generated in the polyurethane substrate was about 0.5 μm or approximately 20% of the radius of the glass sphere.

When a more compliant substrate of polystyrene, which contained 20%

plasticizer, was employed, with glass spheres of 4.0–11.0 μm in radius, the larger particles appeared to be approximately 40% embedded, whereas the smaller particles, 4.0 μm in radius, were embedded much more, by approximately 90%.

These experimental results suggest that for a given substrate, provided that it is more compliant than the particle material, the particles become more embedded as their size is reduced. These experiments were conducted with substrates having a Young's modulus several orders of magnitude greater than that of mucus. Normally, the shear modulus G of mucus is measured (e.g., by magnetic rheometry, as described by King; 86). The shear modulus is typically between 10 and 100 Pa, measured over the frequency range of 0.2–20 Hz. This shear modulus translates into Young's modulus E of 30–300 Pa. Thus, mucus is much more compliant than the plastic substrates just discussed, and particles deposited on the air–wall interface in the airways are expected to be embedded and submerged into the aqueous airway coating with ease. The likely role of airway surfactant for the adhesive interactions is the modification of the thermodynamic work of adhesion W_A, which is related to the surface free energies of the particle and the substrate. The free energy of the substrate–air interface is reduced to approximately 30 mJ/m^2 by the presence of a surfactant film, as shown by the drop-spreading experiments (54–56). This alteration in the free energy of the substrate implies greater particle wettability in the presence of a surfactant film and, thus, greater particle displacement into the subphase.

The work of adhesion is an important quantity in the semiempirical theories originally developed in 1971 by Johnson, Kendall, and Roberts (JKR theory). We refer to the articles by Rimai et al. (85) and Quesnel et al. (84) for the formulas. In the JKR theory, the contact radius is a function of particle radius, the thermodynamic work of adhesion, and the elastic moduli (Poisson ratio and Young's modulus) of the interacting particle and substrate.

Derjaguin et al. (87,88) proposed an alternative approach from the molecular level, combining van der Waals interactions between a rigid particle and a compliant substrate with empirically determined mechanical properties of the substrate.

Substantial progress has been made in the explanations of the mechanisms related to the adhesion of particles to elastic substrates. Nevertheless, the phenomenon that small particles (e.g., glass) become embedded to a greater extent into a more compliant, elastic substrate than larger particles cannot be explained by employing current models of adhesion (85).

Because, in reality, intermolecular interactions determine both the mechanical properties and the interfacial energies at various interfaces, recent advances have been made to construct adhesion models by assuming that particle and substrates interact through particular potentials (e.g., a Lennard-Jones potential; 84). These models take into account observations that can be made by using atomic force techniques. For example, when a particle comes close to a surface the attractive potential is sufficiently large that it causes the particle to jump into contact with the substrate. Energy loss mechanisms in the presence of elastic deformations, the interfacial energy between surfaces, and the elastic properties of the materials are modeled. We can expect that these new models will bridge the gap between the thermodynamic approach to adhesion and that from the molecular level.

In the following, we assume that the elastic properties of the substrate below the surfactant film can be neglected, so that the substrate can be modeled as a newtonian fluid. We consider this approximation reasonable in view of the in situ observation of particle displacement on a tracheal surface and of the observation of equivalent particle displacement in vitro on a surfactant film formed on a saline–sucrose solution having a density higher than that of the particle. In the latter experiment, the film surface tension was adjusted to approximately 30 mN/m, the surface tension found on the trachea by the drop-spreading approach (54–56).

B. Particle Wettability: Surface Tension and Line Tension

Although the principles of surface thermodynamics, the interfacial free energies, and the work of adhesion play an important role in models of particles' adhesion to polymeric substrates; the thermodynamic quantities associated with dividing lines between differing phases—the edge energy or line tension—have not been considered in these adhesion models.

In the following we focus on the thermodynamics of dividing lines. The thermodynamic theory of capillarity developed by Gibbs in the last century was generalized by Boruvka and Neumann (89) to include the effects of line tension and curvature on the expression for mechanical equilibrium (90–92). Analogous with surface tension, *line tension* may be defined as the free energy per unit length of the three-phase contact line, or alternatively, as tensile force acting in this line (90).

Consider a sessile drop on an ideal solid surface in equilibrium with the liquid's vapor. The mechanical equilibrium condition for any point in the three-phase contact line is given by Boruvka and Neumann (89):

$$\gamma_{lv} \cos \theta = \gamma_{sv} - \gamma_{sl} - \sigma K_{gs} \qquad (1)$$

where γ is the surface or interfacial tension, σ is the line tension, and K_{gs} is the geodesic curvature of the three-phase contact line in the plane of the solid surface; *l*, *v*, *s* refer to liquid, vapor, and the solid phases, respectively. Equation (1) is called the modified Young equation, which considers the contribution of the line tension to the equilibrium of the three-phase line (89). If the solid surface is planar, smooth, homogeneous, and rigid, and the effects of gravity can be neglected, then the drop is axisymmetrical and the three-phase line is a perfect circle. The geodesic curvature is then given simply by $K_{gs} = r^{-1}$, where r is the radius of the three-phase contact circle in the plane of the solid surface (90,93).

Under these conditions and with $r \to \infty$, Eq. (1) is replaced by the classic Young equation:

$$\gamma_{lv} \cos \theta_\infty = \gamma_{sv} - \gamma_{sl} \quad (2)$$

combining Eqs. (2) and (1) yields

$$\cos \theta = \cos \theta_\infty - \sigma (\gamma_{lv} \times r)^{-1} \quad (3)$$

Figure 8 represents a sessile drop resting on a solid substrate, without line tension and with positive line tension increasing the contact angle θ. Equation (3) shows that the contact angle θ varies with the radius of the three-phase contact circle, suggesting that the value of line tensions can be determined by measuring the dependence of the contact angle on drop size, provided that both line tension and the interfacial tensions are constant.

The measurements of line tension have generated a controversy over its magnitude and whether it is positive or negative (for a review see, 90,91,93). For example, Exerowa et al. (91) found that the line tension of the contact line at the Newton black film–bulk solution can be either positive or negative, depending on the composition of the solution. Duncan et al. (90) found from contact angle measurements on sessile drops of a variety of fluids in the surface tension range from about 23 mJ/m² (decane) to 63 mJ/m² (glycerol) that the line tension was positive and increased from about 1.9 to ~5.4 μJ/m monotonically with the solid–liquid interfacial tension. Wallace and Schürch (94,95) also found positive line tensions from measurements of the contact angles oil droplets made in water on a DPPC film formed at the interface between water and a perfluorocarbon

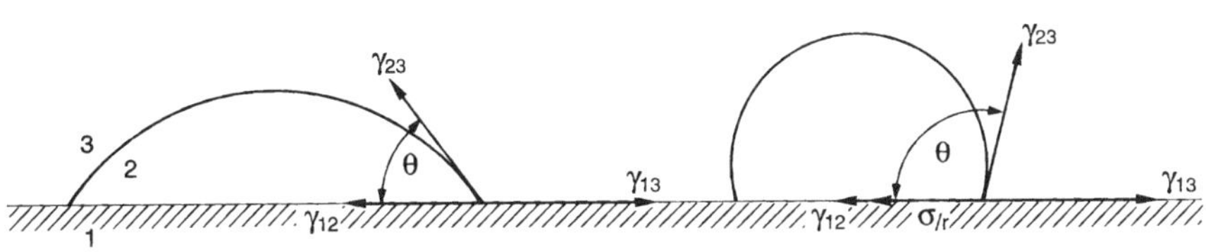

Figure 8 Schematic drawing of a sessile drop resting on a solid substrate: Phases 1, 2, and 3 represent the solid, fluid, and vapor phases, respectively: (Left) the Young equation $\gamma_{13} = \gamma_{23} \cos \theta + \gamma_{12}$ represents mechanical equilibrium without the line tension contribution. (Right) the modified Young equation (see text) $\gamma_{13} - \gamma_{12} - \sigma/r = \gamma_{23} \cos \theta$ represents mechanical equilibrium for any point at the three-phase contact line, where σ is the line tension and r^{-1} is the curvature of the circular three-phase line. Note: The positive line tension contribution modifies (increases) the contact angle.

fluid. In that system, line tension was also positive, but about three orders of magnitude smaller than the values found by Duncan et al. (90).

The magnitude of line tension obtained by different experimental approaches appears to vary over several orders of magnitude, from 10^{-11}–10^{-10} J/m (74) to about 10^{-6} J/m (90,96,97), and line tension can also assume negative values (91). Negative line tension means that the free energy of a particular system is reduced by the extension of the three-phase line.

In summary, different investigators have obtained different results for the magnitude and sign of line tension by using different experimental approaches and materials. Unless the same materials and experimental setups are used, the comparison of the results are not sensible (98).

C. Analysis and Discussion

The complete analysis of particles subjected to forces caused by dividing surfaces (surface tension forces) and dividing lines (line tension forces) would be beyond the scope of the present chapter, thus a brief summary of the analysis is given. We follow the study of Chen and co-workers (98), who generalized the classic Neumann triangle relation, suggested over a century ago (99), to include line tension. The position of a spherical particle resting in a planar liquid interface subjected to surface and line tension forces is then discussed by employing the approach by Aveyard and Clint (100).

Figure 9 represents an equilibrium position of a large and a smaller microsphere. The interfacial tensions γ and the line tension term, $\sigma\kappa$, are shown in vector notation (A), κ is the curvature vector, the value of κ is equal to r^{-1} for a sphere (B), $\mathbf{m}_1$, $\mathbf{m}_2$, and $\mathbf{m}_3$ are the unit vectors in the direction of γ_{12}, γ_{23}, and γ_{13}, respectively. The mechanical equilibrium condition (force balance equation) for the circular contact line (98) is:

$$\gamma_{12}\mathbf{m}_1 + \gamma_{23}\mathbf{m}_2 + \gamma_{13}\mathbf{m}_3 + \sigma\kappa = 0 \quad (4)$$

It can be seen from Eq. (4) that the line tension term σ/r can have a dominant effect if the local curvature r^{-1} is large.

Forces related to gravity (weight and buoyancy) are neglected because, for particles of a radius equal to or smaller than 100 μm, these forces related to gravity are several orders of magnitude smaller than surface tension forces (56).

The line tension contribution σ/r does not directly contribute to the displacement of the particle in the direction vertical to the fluid surface. Line tension contributes indirectly to the force balance by modifying the contact angle. If the three-phase contact line is above the equatorial plane of the sphere, $\theta_2 < \theta_1$ for $r_2 < r_1$ (see Fig. 9). For the three-phase line below the equator, line tension would increase the contact angle.

Aveyard and Clint (100) have simplified the analysis for a spherical particle

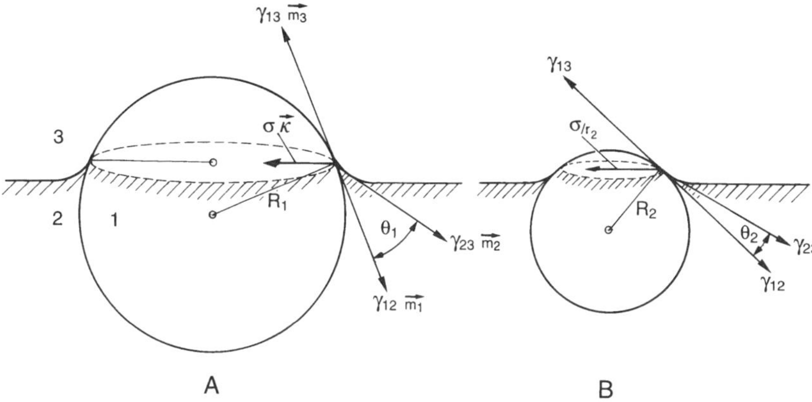

Figure 9 Schematic drawing of two spherical particles of different size at the liquid–vapor interface: The particles are partially wetted by the fluid, which forms a meniscus at the particle (1) fluid, (2) vapor, (3) three-phase line. Note: in addition to the interfacial tensions γ, the positive line tension σ, acts in the three-phase line, and tends to minimize its length. The line tension contribution $\sigma\kappa$, being proportional to the curvature κ (or to r^{-1} for a circle) contributes indirectly to the mechanical equilibrium of any point in the three-phase line by modifying the contact angle θ. Because $r_2 < r_1$, $\sigma/r_2 > \sigma/r_1$, and $\theta_2 < \theta_1$, the three-phase line is above the equatorial plane of the sphere.

with uniform wetting properties over its surface, which means that the contact angle θ is independent of position in the absence of line tension. In addition, they assumed that the particle is sufficiently small so that the liquid–vapor interface is effectively planar (i.e., the height of the meniscus owing to capillary rise can be neglected. According to Figure 10, the force-balance equation along the tangent to the solid surface at the contact line is

$$\gamma_{13} + \sigma \cos \theta \, (R \sin \theta)^{-1} - \gamma_{12} - \gamma_{23} \cos \theta = 0 \tag{5}$$

Aveyard and Clint (100) have used Eq. (5) to obtain curves of θ against dimensionless line tension $\sigma = \sigma/\gamma_{23}R$.

We have used the approach by Aveyard and Clint (100) to estimate the minimum radius of a PMMA microsphere for which a position in the interface would be possible. Smaller microspheres would be totally submerged.

With a line tension of 4×10^{-8} J/m (94) and a contact angle θ_0 approximately 50° (101) at $\sigma = 0$, the smallest PMMA (surface free energy ~ 38 mJ/m^2) microsphere with a possible position in the interface would have a radius of

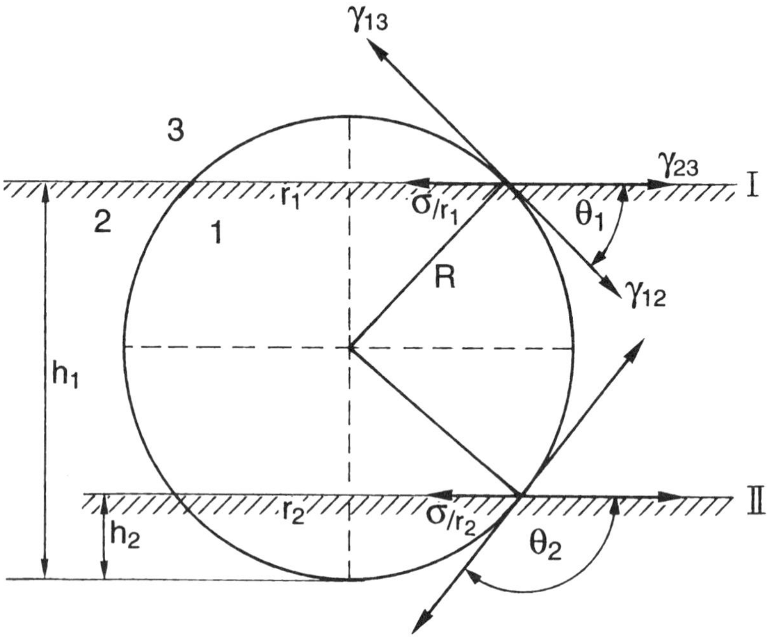

Figure 10 Schematic drawing of spherical particle small enough that the liquid–vapor interface is effectively planar. Phases 1, 2, and 3 indicate the solid sphere (1), liquid (2), and vapor (3), respectively. (I) The particle in its equilibrium position immersed to a height h_1 in the liquid–vapor interface. If an increasing positive line tension σ, is assumed, the three-phase line, radius r_1, tends to contract (i.e., the contact angle θ_1 decreases), promoting particle immersion into the liquid. (II) The particle in its equilibrium position immersed to a height h_2 in the liquid–vapor interface. An increasing positive line tension σ, again tends to contract the three-phase line, and tends to prevent further particle immersion into the liquid phase (see text). A negative line tension, on the other hand, would promote further immersion.

R_m approximately 13 μm, or a diameter of 26 μm. Microspheres smaller than about 26 μm in diameter would be totally submerged.

However, the model calculations were conducted for an ideal microsphere with uniform wetting properties (100). Real surfaces such as those of PMMA particles, although macroscopically smooth, might be rough and heterogeneous. Roughness and heterogeneity substantially influence the wetting behaviors of solid surfaces by fluids.

Because of the uncertainty about the magnitude of both contact angle and line tension, there is not yet a definitive answer for the magnitude of the effect of line tension on the displacement of small particles at the surface of airways. However, the consistently observed greater immersion of small particles than that of larger particles in vitro, as well as in situ, in airways, supports the concept that line tension plays a significant role in particle displacement.

So far we have discussed only the wetting of particles for contact angles less than 90° (see Fig. 9); that is, we considered only particles that had initially been immersed into the liquid phase by at least 50% before further immersion by a positive line tension was considered. Yet particles do land on the surface from the air phase; that is, for the expansion of the contact, a new interface with the corresponding contact line has to be formed. This formation of the new contact is hindered by a force barrier owing to the positive line tension (92). At the onset of the contact, when r is very small, σ/r is large.

Gravity might play a role in the initial-wetting process, when the surface tension forces caused by the geometry at the bottom of the sphere are very small (56). Some other activation energy might play a role in the further wetting process during immersion up to the equator of the spherical particle. Aveyard and Clint (100) mentioned that thermal energy may contribute to the position of very small particles at interfaces, whereas capillary waves on a liquid surface would affect the position of larger particles, such as those considered in the present discussion.

Further experiments should clarify how the molecular spacing or composition of the airway surfactant film might change after the initial contact of the particle with the film molecules. Because the magnitude and the sign of the line tension depend on the composition of the three-phase linear region, we cannot exclude that line tension might initially be very small, such that there would be no appreciable barrier for the initial particle wetting, or this wetting could even be initially promoted by a negative line tension.

In summary, experimental results demonstrate consistently greater immersion of smaller particles into a liquid substrate covered with a surfactant film than that for larger particles. The exact mechanism, especially the initial-wetting process is not yet understood and requires further experiments. Line tension remains a possible explanation for the dependence of particle displacement on particle size.

V. Methods of Studying Particle Retention

A. Particle Retention Studies

To study particle retention, noninvasive and invasive techniques are available (102). Noninvasive methods use radioactive, fluorescent, or magnetic particles. So far they are the only feasible techniques in humans, and they allow repeated measurements in the same individual. These techniques are extensively discussed in Chapter 5. However, even single-photon emission computed tomography

(SPECT; 103,104), which provides three-dimensional information on the distribution of radionuclides in the body, cannot give detailed information on the location of particles relative to the airway wall and the structures the particles are associated with. Morphometric, although invasive, techniques which require the fixation of the lungs, tissue sampling, embedding, and cutting into histological sections, allow a more precise analysis of the localization of the particles. With these techniques, the distribution and number of particles retained in airways and alveoli can be determined (105–107). Unbiased stereological methods for total-number estimation are available (the fractionator; 108,109). In addition to unbiased estimates of total number, every particle can be allocated to the lung compartment, and the structures it is associated with can be identified. The only requirement is that each particle can be identified, there is no restriction on the shape or size of particles. We have adapted these techniques to study particle retention and clearance in airways and alveoli of hamsters (110–113).

B. Preservation of the Extracellular Lining Layer

The preservation of the extracellular lining layer is difficult, owing to its location at the surface of epithelial cells adjacent to air, and its high-water and low-protein content. Various chemical fixation methods have been developed, such as intravascular perfusion of fixatives, to preserve the surface of small airways and alveoli (47,114), or the application of fixative vapors either alone or together with intravascular perfusion (rat; 34 and guinea pig; 48). Recently, the use of fixatives dissolved in a nonpolar (hydrophobic) perfluorocarbon fluid has been described and the authors report better conservation of osmiophilic components of the extracellular lining layer (35,44,45,115). Furthermore, cryofixation techniques have been developed that can be used for ultrastructural analysis and also for immunohistochemical analysis or the investigation of the distribution of elements in the aqueous lining layer (116,117). With the development of the low-temperature, (cryo-)scanning electron microscopy, it has become possible to preserve lung water in the frozen hydrated state during prolonged examination (118). The rapid freezing followed by low-temperature scanning electron microscopy was used to measure the thickness and continuity of the alveolar lining layer (70). Currently, the freezing techniques are successfully applied only to extrapulmonary airways and subpleural alveoli.

VI. Significance of Particle Retention

Most lung diseases are caused by inhaled particulate compounds, such as cigarette smoke, viruses, bacteria, pollen, and occupational or environmental pollutants (i.e., toxic or radioactive aerosols). An increasing number of diagnostic and especially therapeutic aerosols (bronchodilators, anti-inflammatory drugs, antibiotics, antiproteases, surfactant, insulin, and others) are also delivered to the respiratory tract. The fate of these inhaled soluble or insoluble particles, regardless of whether their effect is considered to be useful or noxious, critically depends on the site of deposition and, above all, their retention and clearance.

At deposition, the solubility, shape, size, and surface properties of the particle largely determine its fate and, hence, also its resident time in the respiratory tract, with consequences for the generation of lung disease. As shown by the model studies outlined in the foregoing, wetting and displacement of spherical particles at the air–aqueous substrate interface depend on the surface forces and likely, also, on line tension effects. These forces also determine whether or not the particle is brought into close contact with the epithelium. The line tension effect on particle displacement is significant for relatively small spherical particles (i.e., diameter <17 μm). Furthermore, surface and line tension forces depend on the interfacial properties of the interacting systems, including the particles themselves and the surrounding aqueous medium, with the interfacial film between medium and particle. For example, particles having a low surface free energy, such as Teflon, will generally be immersed less than high-energy particles, such as glass. Hydrated particles, such as bacteria, with a surface free energy of about 70 mJ/m^2, would be substantially more wetted and displaced than hydrophobic plastic particles.

Forces caused by the free energy in interfaces and dividing lines might also contribute substantially to particle–cell interaction. These interactions are considered nonspecific, in contrast with specific receptor–ligand interactions. Thus, nonspecific interactions may contribute to the uptake of particles by cells that are not professional phagocytes, such as epithelial cells of the airways. These findings have implications for particle pathogenicity and persistence of small particles in the submicron range (119; see also Chap. 9).

In addition to particle size and interfacial chemistry, shape also plays a role in particle wetting: the sharper the edges of a particle, the less likely the particle will be wetted and displaced. Oliver et al. (120) have shown theoretically and experimentally, using a circular sapphire disk with a 90° edge, that sharp edges inhibit the spreading of liquids.

Whether a particle is deposited in the conducting airways or in the alveoli will also influence its resident time, for different clearance mechanisms and routes are effective, and the distance a particle must be transported to be removed from the respiratory tract is variable. In addition to the location of particle deposition, the structures of the extracellular lining layer, and free cells, such as macrophages and the epithelial cells, are important for the retention and clearance of particles (41,42,56,121–123). Macrophages phagocytose particles in the airways, as well as in the gas-exchange region (50,51,76,111,124). They accumulate at the sites where particles have been deposited (49,52,53). However, for the retention of ultrafine particles, macrophages do not seem to be important; because ultrafine particles are seldom found phagocytosed by macrophages (125). The uptake of ultrafine particles by epithelial cells has been studied by Ferin and co-workers (125,126). These authors showed a prolonged retention time and a special clearance across the epithelium.

The location of particles relative to the epithelial cells might determine their pathogenic or beneficial potential. The proximity of, for example, radioactive particles to sensitive structures, such as mitotic or stem cells, might influence the progeny of the airway lining and, by their location near the vasculature, systemic effects might be achieved (127).

Knowledge of these structures and their functions is important for the assessment of occupational and daily risks of exposure to increasing amounts of air pollutants, as well as for further treatment of airway and other diseases by inhalation of therapeutic aerosols (122,128–131).

References

1. Weibel ER. Morphometry of the Human Lung. New York: Academic Press, 1963.
2. Raabe OG, Yeh HC, Schum GM, Phalen RF. Tracheobronchial Geometry: Human, Dog, Rat, Hamster. Albuquerque, NM: Lovelace Foundation, 1976.
3. Horsfield K, Dart G, Olson DE, Filley GF, Cumming G. Models of the human bronchial tree. J Appl Physiol 1971; 31:207–217.
4. Phalen RF, Yeh HC, Schum GM, Raabe OG. Application of an idealized model to morphometry of the mammalian tracheobronchial tree. Anat Rec 1978; 190:167–176.
5. Yeh HC, Schum GM, Duggan T. Anatomic models of the tracheobronchial and pulmonary regions of the rat. Anat Rec 1979; 195:483–492.
6. Yeh HC, Schum GM. Models of human lung airways and their application to inhaled particle deposition. Bull Math Biol 1980; 42:461–480.
7. Gehr P, Bachofen M, Weibel ER. The normal human lung: ultrastructure and morphometric estimation of diffusion capacity. Respir Physiol 1978; 32:121–140.
8. Gehr P, Mwangi DK, Ammann A, Maloiy GMO, Taylor CR, Weibel ER. Design of the mammalian respiratory system. V. Scaling morphometric pulmonary diffusing capacity to body mass: wild and domestic animals. Respir Physiol 1981; 44:61–86.
9. Pache JC, Roberts N, Vock P, Zimmermann A, Cruz-Orive LM. Vertical LM sectioning and parallel CT scanning designs for stereology: application to human lung. J Microsc 1993; 170:9–24.
10. Gaeng D, Geiser M, Cruz-Orive LM, Larsen SE, Schaffner T, Laissue JA, Altermatt HJ. Paradoxical effects of bleomycin and heavy water in mice. Int J Cancer 1995; 62:784–790.
11. Geiser M, Baumann M, Dorin JR, Porteous DJ, Gehr P, Kraemer R. Is the lung morphology altered in cystic fibrosis mutant mice? Am J Respir Crit Care Med 1995; 151:A737.

12. Breeze RG, Wheeldon EB. The cells of the pulmonary airways. Am Rev Respir Dis 1977; 116:705–777.
13. Jeffrey PK. Morphologic features of airway surface epithelial cells and glands. Am Rev Respir Dis 1983; 128:S14–S20.
14. Van Hayak H. The Human Lung. New York: Hafner Publishing, 1960.
15. Frasca JM, Auerbach O, Parks VR, Jamieson JD. Electron microscopic observations of the bronchial epithelium of dogs: I. Control dogs. Exp Mol Pathol 1968; 9:363–379.
16. Hyde DM, Samuelson DA, Blakeney WH, Kosch PC. A correlative light microscopy, transmission and scanning electron microscopy study of the ferret lung. Scanning Electron Microsc 1979; 3:891–898.
17. Plopper CG, Mariassy AT, Wilson DW, Alley JL, Nishio SJ, Nettesheim P. Comparison of nonciliated tracheal epithelial cells in six mammalian species: ultrastructure and population densities. Exp Lung Res 1983; 5:281–294.
18. Plopper CG. Comparative morphologic features of bronchiolar epithelial cells. The Clara cell. Am Rev Respir Dis 1983; 128:S37–S41.
19. Plopper CG, Halsebo JE, Sonstegard KS, Nettesheim P. Distribution of nonciliated bronchiolar epithelial (Clara) cells in intra- and extrapulmonary airways of the rabbit. Exp Lung Res 1983; 5:79–98.
20. Pack RJ, Al-Ugaily LH, Morris G. The cells of the tracheobronchial epithelium of the mouse: a quantitative light and electron microscope study. J Anat 1981; 132: 71–84.
21. Becci PJ, McDowell EM, Trump BF. The respiratory epithelium. II. Hamster trachea, bronchus, and bronchioles. J Natl Cancer Inst 1978; 61:551–561.
22. Jeffrey PK, Reid L. New observations of the rat airway epithelium: a quantitative and electron microscopic study. J Anat 1975; 120:295–320.
23. Plopper CG, Heidsieck JG, Weir AJ, St George JA, Hyde DM. Tracheobronchial epithelium in the adult rhesus monkey: a quantitative histochemical and ultrastructural study. Am J Anat 1989; 184:31–40.
24. Robinson NP, Kyle H, Webber SE, Widdicombe JG. Electrolyte and other chemical concentrations in the tracheal airway and mucus. J Appl Physiol 1989; 66:2129–2135.
25. Jacquot J, Hayem A, Galabert C. Functions of proteins and lipids in airway secretions. Eur Respir J 1992; 5:343–358.
26. Widdicombe JG. Airway mucus. Eur Respir J 1989; 2:107–115.
27. Mercer RR, Russel ML, Crapo JD. Mucous lining layers in human and rat airways (abstr). Am Rev Respir Dis 1992; 145:A355.
28. Yager D, Cloutier T, Feldman H, Bastacky J, Drazen JM, Kamm RD. Airway surface liquid thickness as a function of lung volume in small airways of guinea pig. J Appl Physiol 1994; 77:2333–2340.
29. Lucas AM, Douglas LC. Principles underlying ciliary activity in the respiratory tract. II: A comparison of nasal clearance in man, monkey and other mammals. Arch Otolaryngol 1934; 20:518–541.
30. Sleigh MA. Ciliary function in mucus transport. Chest 1981; 80(suppl):791–795.
31. Kilburn KH. A hypothesis for pulmonary clearance and its implications. Am Rev Respir Dis 1968; 98:449–463.

32. Van As A, Webster I. The morphology of mucus in mammalian pulmonary airways. Environ Res 1974; 7:1–12.
33. Van As A. Pulmonary airway defence mechanisms: an appreciation of integrated mucociliary activity. Eur J Respir Dis 1980; 61(suppl 111):21–24.
34. Yoneda K. Mucous blanket of rat bronchus. Am Rev Respir Dis 1976; 114:837–842.
35. Sims DE, Westfall JA, Kiorpes AL, Horne MM. Preservation of tracheal mucus by nonaqueous fixative. Biotech Histochem 1991; 66:173–180.
36. Luchtel DL. The mucous layer of the trachea and major bronchi in the rat. Scanning Electron Microsc 1978; 2:1089–1098.
37. Luchtel DL. Mucociliary interactions in rabbit intrapulmonary airways. Cell Motil 1982; 1(suppl 1):77–81.
38. Sturgess JM. The mucous lining of major bronchi in the rabbit lung. Am Rev Respir Dis 1977; 115:819–827.
39. Allegra L, Bossi R, Braga P. Influence of surfactant on mucociliary transport. Eur J Respir Dis 1985; 67(suppl 142):71–76.
40. Morgenroth K, Bolz J. Morphological features of the interaction between mucus and surfactant on the bronchial mucosa. Respiration 1985; 47:225–231.
41. Widdicombe JG. Introduction. Endobronchial surface active phospholipids: morphology, biochemistry, function and therapeutic aspects. Eur J Respir Dis 1985; 67(suppl 142):1–5.
42. Gehr P, Schürch S, Berthiaume Y, Im Hof V, Geiser M. Particle retention in airways by surfactant. J Aerosol Med 1990; 3:27–43.
43. Girod S, Fuchey C, Galabert C, Lebonvallet S, Bonnet N, Ploton D, Puchelle E. Identification of phospholipids on secretory granules of human submucosal gland respiratory cell. J Histochem Cytochem 1991; 39:193–198.
44. Lee MM, Schürch S, Roth SH, Jiang X, Cheng S, Bjarnason S, Green FHY. Effect of acid aerosol exposure on the surface properties of airway mucus. Exp Lung Res 1995; 21:835–851.
45. Geiser M, Im Hof V, Siegenthaler W, Grunder R, Gehr P. Ultrastructure of the extracellular lining layer in hamster airways: is there a two-phase system? Microsc Res Technol 1997; 36:428–437.
46. Gerber V, Geiser M, Gehr P, Schürch S, Im Hof V. Ultrastructure of the extracellular lining layer in horse tracheae (abstr). Am J Respir Crit Care Med 1997; 155: A436.
47. Gil J, Weibel ER. Extracellular lining of bronchioles after perfusion–fixation of rat lungs for electron microscopy. Anat Rec 1971; 169:185–200.
48. Hulbert WC, Forster BB, Laird W, Pihl CE, Walker DC. An improved method for fixation of the respiratory epithelial surface with the mucous and surfactant layers. Lab Invest 1982; 47:354–363.
49. Geiser M, Baumann M, Cruz-Orive LM, Im Hof V, Waber U, Gehr P. The effect of particle inhalation on macrophage number and phagocytic activity in the intrapulmonary conducting airways of hamsters. Am J Respir Cell Mol Biol 1994; 10:594–603.
50. Sorokin SP, Brain JD. Pathways of clearance in mouse lungs exposed to iron oxide aerosols. Anat Rec 1975; 181:581–626.

51. Stirling C, Patrick G. The localization of particles retained in the trachea of the rat. J Pathol 1980; 131:309–320.
52. Warheit DB, Chang LY, Hill LH, Hook GER, Crapo JD, Brody AR. Pulmonary macrophage accumulation and asbestos-induced lesions at sites of fiber deposition. Am Rev Respir Dis 1984; 129:301–310.
53. Warheit DB, Overby LH, George G, Brody AR. Pulmonary macrophages are attracted to inhaled particles through complement activation. Exp Lung Res 1988; 14:51–66.
54. Im Hof V, Schürch S, Straub R, Gehr P. Surfactant in the trachea of the horse (abstr). Eur Respir J 1990; 3(suppl 10):257S.
55. Im Hof V, Gehr P, Gerber V, Lee MM, Schürch S. In vivo determination of surface tension in the horse and in vitro model studies. Respir Physiol 1997; 109:81–93.
56. Schürch S, Gehr P, Im Hof V, Geiser M, Green F. Surfactant displaces particles toward the epithelium in airways and alveoli. Respir Physiol 1990; 80:17–32.
57. Holm BA. Surfactant in activation in adult respiratory distress syndrome. In: Robertson B, van Golde LMG, Batenburg JJ, eds. Pulmonary Surfactant: From Molecular Biology to Clinical Practice. Amsterdam: Elsevier, 1992:667–684.
58. Ikada Y, Suzuki M, Tamada Y. Polymer surfaces possessing minimal interaction with blood components. In: Shalaby SW, Hoffmann AS, Rattner BD, Horbett TA, eds. Polymers as Biomaterials. New York: Plenum Press, 1984:135–147.
59. Neumann AW, Absolom DR, Francis DW, Omenyi SN, Spelt JK, Policova Z, Thomson C, Zingg W, van Oss CJ. Measurement of surface tension of blood cells and proteins. Ann NY Acad Sci 1983; 416:276–298.
60. Auten RL, Watkin RM, Shapiro DL, Horowitz S. Surfactant apoprotein A (SP-A) is synthetized in airway cells. Am J Respir Cell Mol Biol 1990; 3:491–496.
61. Khoor A, Gray ME, Hull WM, Whitsett JA, Stahlman MT. Developmental expression of SP-A and SP-A mRNA in the proximal and distal respiratory epithelium in the human fetus and newborn. J Histochem Cytochem 1993; 41:1311–1319.
62. Khoor A, Stahlman MT, Gray ME, Whitsett JA. Temporal–spatial distribution of SP-B and SP-C proteins and mRNAs in developing respiratory epithelium of human lung. J Histochem Cytochem 1994; 42:1187–1199.
63. Voorhout WF, Veenendaal T, Kuroki Y, Ogasawara Y, van Golde LMG, Geuze HJ. Immunocytochemical localization of surfactant protein D (SP-D) in type II cells, Clara cells, and alveolar macrophages of rat lung. J Histochem Cytochem 1992; 40:1589–1597.
64. Clements JA, Oyarzún MJ, Baritussio A. Secretion and clearance of lung surfactant: a brief review. Prog Respir Res 1981; 15:20–26.
65. Bernhard W, Haagsman HP, Tschering T, Poets CF, Postle AD, van Eijk ME, von der Hardt H. Conductive airway surfactant: surface-tension function, biochemical composition, and possible alveolar origin. Am J Respir Cell Mol Biol 1997; 17:41–50.
66. Phalen RF, Oldham MJ. Tracheobronchial airway structure as revealed by casting techniques. Am Rev Respir Dis 1983; 128:S1–S4.
67. Tyler WS. Small airways and terminal units. Am Rev Respir Dis 1983; 128:S32–S36.

68. Crapo JD, Barry BE, Gehr P, Bachofen M, Weibel ER. Cell number and cell characteristics of the normal human lung. Am Rev Respir Dis 1982; 125:740–745.
69. Stone KC, Mercer RR, Gehr P, Stockstill B, Crapo JD. Allometric relationships of cell numbers and size in the mammalian lung. Am J Respir Cell Mol Biol 1992; 6:235–243.
70. Bastacky J, Lee CYC, Goerke J, Koushafar H, Yager D, Kenaga L, Speed TP, Chen Y, Clements JA. Alveolar lining layer is thin and continuous: low-temperature scanning electron microscopy of rat lung. J Appl Physiol 1995; 79:1615–1628.
71. Gil J. Histological preservation and ultrastructure of alveolar surfactant. Annu Rev Physiol 1985; 47:753–763.
72. Gil J, Weibel ER. Improvements in demonstration of lining layer of lung alveoli by electron microscopy. Respir Physiol 1969; 8:13–36.
73. Weibel ER, Gil J. Electron microscopic demonstration of an extracellular duplex lining layer of alveoli. Respir Physiol 1968; 4:42–57.
74. Askin FB, Kuhn C. The cellular origin of pulmonary surfactant. Lab Invest 1971; 25:260–268.
75. Chevalier G, Collet AJ. In vivo incorporation of choline-^{3}H, leucine-^{3}H and galactose-^{3}H in alveolar type II pneumocytes in relation to surfactant synthesis. A quantitative radioautographic study in mouse by electron microscopy. Anat Rec 1972; 174:289–310.
76. Brain JD. Macrophages in the respiratory tract. In: Fishman AP, Fisher AB, eds. Handbook of Physiology. Vol 1. Circulation and Nonrespiratory Functions. Bethesda: American Physiological Society, 1985:447–471.
77. Valberg PA, Blanchard JD. Pulmonary macrophage physiology: origin, motility, endocytosis. In: Parent RA, ed. Comparative Biology of the Normal Lung. Boca Raton FL: CRC Press, 1992:681–724.
78. Horn LW, Davis SH. Apparent surface tension hysteresis in dynamical systems. J Colloid Interface Sci 1975; 51:459–478.
79. Podgórski A, Gradon L. An improved mathematical model of hydrodynamical self-cleansing of pulmonary alveoli. Ann Occup Hyg 1993; 37:347–365.
80. Lee MM, Green FHY, Bjarnasson S, Zhang Y, Schürch S. Surface properties of airway mucus exposed to acid aerosol. In: Liepsch D, ed. Biofluid Mechanics. Düsseldorf: VDI Verlag, 1994:133–144.
81. Sleigh MA, Blake JR, Liron N. The propulsion of mucus by cilia. Am Rev Respir Dis 1988; 137:726–741.
82. Silberberg A. Biorheological matching: mucociliary interaction and epithelial clearance. Biorheology 1983; 20:215–222.
83. Rimai DS, De Mejo LP, Bowen RC. Mechanics of particle adhesion. In: Rimai DS, De Mejo LP, Mittal KL, eds. Fundamentals of Adhesion and Interfaces. Utrecht: VSP, 1995:1–23.
84. Quesnel DJ, Rimai DS, De Mejo LP. Molecular dynamic modeling of particle adhesion. J Adhesion 1995; 51:49–69.
85. Rimai DS, De Mejo LP Bowden RC. Mechanics of particle adhesion. J Adhesion Sci Technol 1994; 8/11:1333–1355.
86. King M. Interrelation between mechanical properties of mucus and mucociliary transport: effect of pharmacologic interventions. Biorheology 1979; 16:57–68.

87. Derjaguin BV, Muller VM, Toporov YUP. Effect of contact deformation on the adhesion of particles. J Colloid Interface Sci 1975; 53:314–326.
88. Derjaguin BV, Muller VM, Toporov YUP. On the role of molecular forces in contact deformations [Critical remarks concerning Dr. Tabor's report]. J Colloid Interface Sci 1978; 67:314.
89. Boruvka L, Neumann AW. Generation of the classical theory of capillarity. J Chem Phys 1977; 66:5464–5476.
90. Duncan D, Li D, Gaydos J, Neumann AW. Correlation of line tension and solid–liquid interfacial tensions from the measurement of drop size dependence of contact angles. J Colloid Interface Sci 1995; 169:256–261.
91. Exerowa D, Kashchiev D, Platikanov D, Toshev BV. Linear energy with positive and negative signs. Adv Colloid Interface Sci 1994; 49:303–339.
92. Toshev BV, Platikanov D, Scheludko A. Line tension in three-phase equilibrium systems. Langmuir 1988; 4:489–499.
93. Li D. Drop size dependence of contact angles and line tensions of solid–liquid systems. Colloids Surfaces 1996; 116:1–23.
94. Wallace JA, Schürch S. Line tension of a sessile drop on a fluid–fluid interface modified by a phospholipid monolayer. J Colloid Interface Sci 1988; 124:452–461.
95. Wallace JA, Schürch S. Line tension of sessile drops placed on a phospholipid monolayer at the water–fluorocarbon interface. Colloids Surfaces 1990; 43:207–221.
96. Gaydos J, Neumann AW. The dependence of contact angles on drop size and line tension. J Colloid Interface Sci 1987; 120:76–86.
97. Li D, Neumann AW. Determination of line tension from drop size dependence of contact angles. Colloids Surfaces 1990; 43:195–206.
98. Chen P, Gaydos J, Neumann AW. The contact line quadrilateral relation: a generalization of the Neumann triangle relation to include line tension. Langmuir 1996; 12:5956–5962.
99. Adamson AW. Physical Chemistry of Surfaces. 5th ed. New York: John Wiley & Sons, 1990:1–777.
100. Aveyard R, Clint JH. Particle wettability and line tension. J Chem Soc Faraday Trans 1996; 92:85–89.
101. Neumann AW, Good AJ, Hope CJ, Sejpal M. Equation of state approach to determine surface tensions of low energy solids from contact angles. J Colloid Interface Sci 1974; 49:291–304.
102. Brain JD, Valberg PA. Deposition of aerosol in the respiratory tract. Am Rev Respir Dis 1979; 120:1325–1373.
103. Chan HK. Use of single photon emission computed tomography in aerosol studies. J Aerosol Med 1993; 6:23–36.
104. Mortonen TB, Yang Y, Hwang D, Fleming JS. Computer model of human lung morphology to complement SPECT analysis. Int J Biomed Comput 1995; 40:5–16.
105. Sweeney TD, Blanchard JD, Carter JE, Brain JD. Delivery of aerosolized drugs to the lungs with a metered-dose inhaler: quantitative analysis of regional deposition. J Aerosol Sci 1990; 21:350–354.
106. Zeltner TB, Sweeney TD, Skornik WA, Feldman HA, Brain JD. Retention and

clearance of 0.9 μm particles inhaled by hamsters during rest or exercise. J Appl Physiol 1991; 70:1137–1145.

107. Pinkerton KE, Gallen JT, Mercer RR, Wong VC, Plopper CG, Tarkington BK. Aerosolized fluorescent microspheres detected in the lung using confocal scanning laser microscopy. Microsc Res Technol 1993; 26:437–443.
108. Gundersen HJG. Stereology of arbitrary particles. A review of unbiased number and size estimators and the presentation of some new ones, in memory of William R. Thompson. J Microsc 1986; 143:3–45.
109. Pakkenberg B, Gundersen, HJG. Total number of neurons and glial cells in human brain nuclei estimated by the disector and the fractionator. J Microsc 1988; 150: 1–20.
110. Cruz-Orive LM. On the empirical variance of a fractionator estimate. J Microsc 1990; 160:89–95.
111. Geiser M, Cruz-Orive LM, Im Hof V, Gehr P. Assessment of particle retention and clearance in the intrapulmonary conducting airways of hamster lungs with the fractionator. J Microsc 1990; 160:75–88.
112. Geiser M, Cruz-Orive LM, Waber U, Im Hof V, Gehr P. Particle retention in airways estimated by unbiased stereology and photometry. J Aerosol Med 1995; 8: 149–165.
113. Geiser M, Leupin N, Maye I, Im Hof V, Gehr P. Retention of puff ball (*Calvatia excipuliformis*) spores in the intrapulmonary conducting airways of hamsters (abstr). Am J Respir Crit Care Med 1997; 155:A955.
114. Im Hof V, Scheuch G, Geiser M, Gebhart J, Gehr P, Heyder J. Techniques for the determination of particle deposition in lungs of hamsters. J Aerosol Med 1989; 2: 247–259.
115. Thurston RJ, Hess RA, Kilburn KH, McKenzie WN. Ultrastructure of lungs fixed in inflation using a new osmium–fluorocarbon technique. J Ultrastruct Res 1976; 56:39–47.
116. Godleski JJ, Hastings CL, Katler M, Sweeney TD. Preservation of the relationship of airway mucus and epithelium by slam freezing. In: Bailey GW, ed. Proceedings 49th Annual Meeting of the Electron Microscopy Society of America. San Francisco: San Francisco Press, 1991:72–73.
117. Puchelle E, Beorchia A, Ménager M, Zahm JM, Ploton D. Three-dimensional imaging of the mucus secretory process in the cryofixed frog respiratory epithelium. Biol Cell 1991; 72:159–166.
118. Bastacky J, Hook GR, Finch GL, Goerke J, Hayes TL. Low-temperature scanning electron microscopy of frozen hydrated mouse lung. Scanning 1987; 9:57–70.
119. Oberdörster G, Ferin J, Lehnert BE. Correlation between particle size, in vivo particle persistence, and lung injury. Environ Health Perspect 1994; 102(suppl. 5):173–179.
120. Oliver JF, Huh C, Mason SG. Resistance to spreading of liquids by sharp edges. J Colloid Interface Sci 1977; 59:568–581.
121. Rensch H, von Seefeld H, Gebhardt KF, Renzow D, Sell PJ. Stop and go particle transport in the peripheral airways? A model study. Respiration 1983; 44:346–350.
122. Im Hof V, Patrick G. Particle retention and clearance. J Aerosol Med 1994; 7:39–47.

123. Geiser M, Im Hof V, Cruz-Orive LM, Gehr P. Histological and stereological analysis of particle retention in the conducting airways of hamster lungs. J Aerosol Med 1990; 3:131–145.
124. Brain JD. Lung macrophages: how many kinds are there? What do they do? Am Rev Respir Dis 1988; 137:507–509.
125. Ferin J, Oberdörster G. Translocation of particles from pulmonary alveoli into the interstitium. J Aerosol Med 1992; 5:179–187.
126. Ferin J, Oberdörster G, Penney DP. Pulmonary retention of ultrafine and fine particles in rats. Am J Respir Cell Mol Biol 1992; 6:535–542.
127. Derom E, Joos G, Kips J. Peleman R, Pauwels R. Factors influencing pulmonary absorption of inhaled drugs. Eur Respir Rev 1994; 4:71–74.
128. Sanchis J. New trends in aerosol therapy: the clinicians view. Eur Respir Rev 1994; 4:106–107.
129. Laube B, Georgopoulos A, Adams G III. Preliminary study of the efficacy of insulin aerosol delivered by oral inhalation in diabetic patients. JAMA 1993; 16:2106–2109.
130. Piazza FM, Johnson SA, Ottolini MG, Schmidt HJ, Damell MRR, Hemming VG, Prince GA. Immunotherapy of respiratory syncytial virus infection in cotton rats (*Sigmodon fulviventer*) using IgG in a small-particle aerosol. J Infect Dis 1992; 166:1422–1424.
131. Patton JS, Platz RM. Pulmonary delivery of peptides and proteins for systemic action. Adv Drug Deliv Rev 1992; 8:179–196.

7

Clearance of Particles Deposited in the Lungs

WOLFGANG G. KREYLING

GSF–Research Center for Environment and Health
Neuherberg/Munich, Germany

GERHARD SCHEUCH

GSF–Research Center for Environment and Health, Gauting/Munich, and
Institute for Aerosol Medicine InAMed GmbH
Gemuenden, Germany

I. Introduction

During respiration, a fraction of inhaled aerosol particles deposits on the epithelium of the respiratory tract. While being retained, particles are subject to various interactions with the fluids, cells, and tissues of the respiratory tract. With use of a parameter to characterize the amount of particulate matter, such as mass m, number N, and such, a time-dependent function $R_{(t)}$ describes the kinetics of particle retention.

$$R(t) = f\ (t, R(0), m(t), N(t)\ .\ .\ .\ .) \tag{1}$$

where $R(0)$ is the amount of particulate matter deposited expressed by the chosen parameter. *Particle clearance* is usually defined as the fraction of particles eliminated from the respiratory tract in a given time interval. Hence, it can be described by the fractional rate of change CL(t) of particle retention as a function of time t:

$$\mathrm{CL}(t) = \left(\frac{1}{R(t)}\right)\left(\frac{dR(t)}{dt}\right) \tag{2}$$

Note that particle clearance is commonly distinguished between different anatomical sites, such as the alveolar region (peripheral lung), conducting airways of the lungs, and extrathoracic airways. From a microscopic view, however, particle clearance implies movement from the initial deposition location of each individual particle. Particle displacement is caused by numerous reactions between the fluids, cells, and tissues of the respiratory tract and the deposited particulate matter to keep the large epithelial surface area clean and sterile, and to protect its primary function: gas exchange of oxygen and carbon dioxide. These reactions are maintained by the immune system of the respiratory tract as a part of the immune system of the entire body. Their common feature is that they usually include recognition of the foreign body, followed by its relocation, elimination, digestion, decomposition, and inactivation. The immune reactions themselves are complex interactions with the foreign body, acting in parallel or sequentially. They involve various cell types and also extracellular matrix and fluids containing interactive molecules and components. To address the complexity of such reactions, they will be termed ''mechanisms involved in the clearance of foreign bodies from the respiratory tract,'' or in short, *clearance mechanisms*. As a result, particles may be eliminated from the respiratory tract following distinct clearance pathways.

Clearance mechanisms are different at different locations in the respiratory tract and also depend on the nature of the deposited foreign body (i.e., the physical, chemical, and biological properties of the particulate matter).

This chapter does not attempt to review the entire range of clearance mechanisms provided by the respiratory tract for all kinds of deposited particles. It does not address the clearance of particles that are readily soluble in the epithelial lining fluid, nor specific immune reactions triggered by viable particles. It reviews clearance mechanisms of particles deposited in the lung, with emphasis on slow-clearance mechanisms.

II. Particle Clearance in the Intrathoracic Airways

Inhaled particles deposited in the intrathoracic airways are cleared by several mechanisms, resulting in two major clearance pathways: particle transport and absorption of dissolved material. Particle transport is directed either toward the larynx, from which they are swallowed into the gastrointestinal tract (GIT) or toward the lymphatic system. Material cleared by absorption is eliminated mainly by the blood.

The rates and amounts of material cleared by each mechanism depend primarily on the site of particle deposition and the physicochemical properties of the material (1,2). The following discussion addresses the clearance of particles that do not dissolve readily.

Particles that are deposited in thoracic airways are cleared mostly by mucociliary transport, which results from the concerted action of cilia on the airway epithelial surface, forming metachronous waves and propelling the mucous blanket toward the larynx. Mucociliary clearance may be assisted by coughing, but mainly in diseased lungs. However, there is evidence that not all particles located on the airway walls are cleared rapidly by mucociliary action. A fraction of particles, taken up by airway macrophages, remain in the airways for a long time, eventually being cleared by mucociliary transport (3,4). Furthermore, a small fraction of particles may be found in the airways outside macrophages many weeks after inhalation (5,6).

Particle transport by mucociliary clearance is a much faster process than those in which macrophages are involved. Mucociliary clearance, therefore, can be easily distinguished from slow-particle transport processes in the airways and the peripheral lungs by sequential measurements of the retained material. In humans the most commonly used technique is based on the inhalation of aerosol particles labeled with gamma-emitting radionuclides and their detection in the lungs using external gamma-ray detectors (7–9).

A. Mucociliary Clearance

The conducting airways of the tracheobronchiolar tree are characterized by branching generations, beginning with the trachea and ending with the terminal bronchioli. Airway walls are covered with a layer of epithelial cells comprising ciliated cells, goblet cells, and a variety of other secretory cells. The proportions of these cells differ in different airway generations within and between different species (10). The epithelium is covered with a layer of mucus. This layer is composed of a sol phase of low viscosity (hypophase), in which the cilia beat, and an overlaying gel phase of higher viscosity (epiphase) that can be moved by the ciliary motion. It is still controversial whether a viscosity gradient exists between sol and gel phase or whether there are two distinct phases. The thickness of this layer of mucus decreases from the trachea down to the bronchioli (11).

The cilia are essential to move the layer of mucus. They have a diameter of about 0.25 μm and variable lengths between 5 and 50 μm, depending on their function and location. Cilia length is greatest in the central airways (trachea and main bronchi) and decreases toward the terminal bronchioli (12). The density of ciliated and secretory cells per unit surface area also decreases toward the peripheral airways.

Mucus behaves as a nonnewtonian fluid; that is, the viscosity decreases with increased applied force. The measurement of mucus's viscosity and elasticity, therefore, depends on the given shear rate and stress. The viscoelastic properties of mucus in normal humans showed no great differences from those observed in normal dogs, but high variability within individuals (13). Yeates (14) measured mucus' viscosity in healthy dogs. At low rates of strain it varied between 200 and 2000 poise (P), and at high rates between 1 and 10 P. For comparison the viscosity of water is 0.01 P.

There is controversy in the literature over whether or not the mucous blanket on the epithelium of airways is continuous (15–18). Most observations have been made in laboratory animals, such as rabbits, hamsters, and rats. Many observations indicate that the mucous layer is not uniform around the circumference of each airway (2). Some investigators found that the mucus in the small airways consists of discrete particles or islands with diameters of about 4–10 μm (17). The size of these islands of mucus increases with increasing airway size. In the lobar bronchi diameters of about 100 μm were found and, in the main bronchi and the trachea, the mucus became a uniform layer. Other authors did not support these observations of discontinuous mucus. In rabbits they found uniform mucous layers, which distally became thinner, from the trachea down to the bronchioli (19).

Hence, mucociliary transport is a complex interaction of ciliary beat and elastoviscous properties of the overlaying mucus and its (dis)continuity in the various airway generations. Mucociliary action is an important function of the airway walls, and the determination of this function is essential to assess the functional and structural integrity of the conducting airways. To study this function, suitably labeled particles are deposited in the airways and mucus' transport is determined by external measurement of the label.

Transport Velocity of Mucus in the Trachea

Measurements of linear mucus' velocities in the human trachea were conducted mainly with two methods: inhalation or instillation.

Inhalation. Rapid inhalation (fast inspiration and exhalation) of radiolabeled 5- to 8-μm–diameter particles leads to inhomogeneous particle deposition, resulting in accumulated particle deposits (boluses) in the vicinity of bifurcations owing to particle impaction. The linear velocity is measured by following boluses of radioactivity moving on the wall of the trachea toward the larynx with a gamma-camera.

Instillation. Particles are instilled by bronchoscopy directly onto the tracheal epithelium. Radiolabeled particles can be measured by a gamma-camera (20–23) or by scintillation detectors (8,24–28). The motion of large particles has been measured directly using cinephotography (29) or radiography (30,31).

The mean linear velocity of mucus, obtained from ten studies using instillation, was 14 ± 5.5 mm/min, whereas that obtained from 13 studies using inhalation was 5.3 ± 1.3 mm/min (2). The velocities measured after bronchoscopic instillation were higher and more variable than those measured after inhalation. This could be due to stimulation of the mucociliary transport system, either by reflex or local irritation caused by the local anesthetic or by passing the bronchoscope down the trachea and hitting its epithelium. The observed differences in tracheal mucous velocities indicate that instillation is a more invasive and less physiological method than inhalation.

Foster et al. (32) also measured mucociliary clearance in the main bronchi after inhalation of radiolabeled particles, using a gamma-camera. For healthy nonsmokers, a linear velocity of 2.4 ± 0.5 mm/min was measured in the bronchi, compared with 5.5 ± 0.4 mm/min in the trachea. Furthermore, they (32) found a correlation between tracheal and bronchial mucous velocities. There is no direct information available about mucous velocities in more distal airways. From the foregoing observation, it can be assumed that linear mucous velocity will decrease in more peripheral airways. By making assumptions about the properties of mucus during its transport from distal airways towards the trachea, mucous velocity has been modeled by several authors (33–36). From these calculations the mucus-transport velocity in terminal bronchioli could be more than three orders of magnitude lower than in the trachea.

Transport of Mucus in Airways

Measurements of mucociliary clearance in lungs of healthy human subjects were performed by inhaling radiolabeled aerosol particles. Retention of these particles was measured either with a gamma-camera or other gamma-ray detectors from outside the lungs. The fast-cleared fraction of the retention function was used as an indicator of mucociliary clearance. The half-time of the mucociliary clearance in healthy humans was t_h(fast) = 2–4 hr, and this fast phase of clearance was finished after about 6–12 hr. Thus, many authors have used 24-hr clearance as a measure of "airway deposition" or "deposition in the tracheobronchial tree." However, this is true only if all particles are cleared from intrathoracic airways by mucociliary clearance within 24 hr. If particles are retained in airways after 24 hr, they cannot be distinguished from those deposited in the peripheral lungs from where particle transport is well known to be slow (see Sec. III).

The aerosol bolus inhalation technique provides a tool to deposit particles preferentially in the airways. A small volume of aerosol is inserted into a breath of clean air at a preselected volume of inhalation. Hence, the aerosol is a label of a fraction of the inhaled air volume. Inhaling a small aerosol bolus (20–50 mL) of particles at the end of a breath (a *shallow bolus*), the particles penetrate only into the lumen of the proximal airways and eventually deposit there. Particle deposition can be enhanced by a postinhalation breath-hold.

Almost complete clearance was observed within the first 6 hr after inhaling monodisperse, gamma-emitting particles with geometric diameters (d_{geom}) larger than 6.5 μm. Particle retention was less than 5% of the initial deposit after 24 hr (37). This 24-hr retention increased only slightly for boluses inhaled into volumes of the respiratory tract between 30 and 110 cm^3 as measured from the entrance of the mouth (volumetric lung depth; VL). This corresponds to about 20–70% of the volume of the conducting airways. These results demonstrate that particles inhaled by shallow aerosol boluses were deposited mainly in the tracheobronchiolar airways and cleared from there.

As a negative control, an aerosol bolus of monodisperse, radiolabeled particles (aerodynamic diameter d_{ae}, 3 μm) was injected at the beginning of an inhalation. Then, the particles were transported deep into the lungs and were deposited in the alveolar region. The measurements showed that less than 5% of the particles were cleared within 24 hr and the retention decreased with a half-time of about 100 days. This was also shown by other investigators, who found that particles were deposited mainly in the alveolar region (2,38,39).

B. Slow Clearance from Intrathoracic Airways

With 3-μm d_{ae} particles in shallow bolus experiments, only about 50% were cleared rapidly (40–42; Fig. 1). The particles remaining in the lungs after 24 hr were cleared with half-times between 5 and 30 days (38,41) and in most investiga-

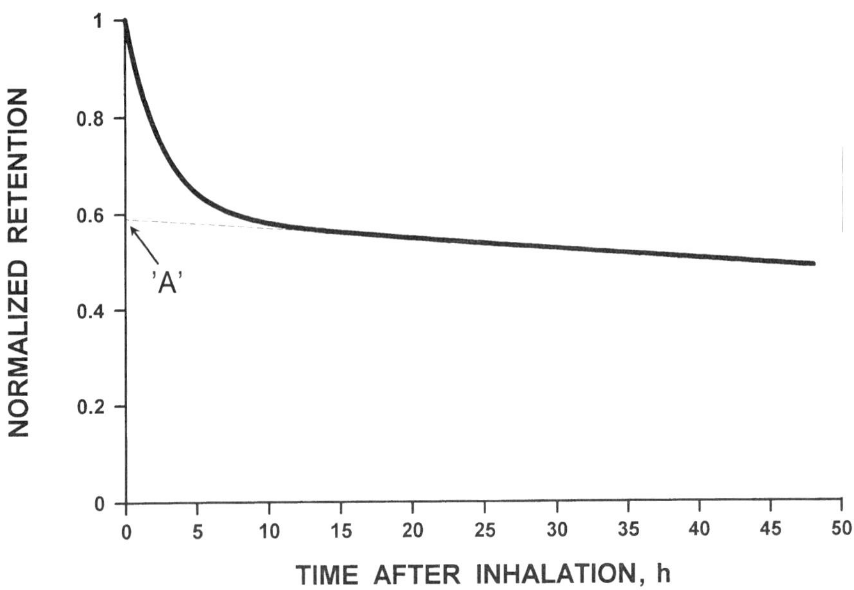

Figure 1 Particle retention in the lungs after a bolus inhalation of iron oxide particles of 3.5-μm–aerodynamic diameter: Inhalation started from functional residual capacity, tidal volume 600 cm^3, volumetric lung depth of the aerosol bolus, VL = 50 mL.

tions significant clearance was found between 24 and 72 hr. For example, clearance between 24 and 48 hr after inhalation was 10–25% of the amount in the lungs at 24 hr. In contrast, in control experiments in which the same particles were inhaled into the whole lung, the fraction cleared between 24 and 48 hr was less than 5%. These clearance patterns imply that a significant fraction of the particles cleared slowly after shallow bolus inhalation were not cleared from the alveolar region.

Increasing the breath-holding time t_p, and the volumetric lung depth of the bolus VL, between 30 and 110 mL led to an increase in total particle deposition, but the fraction of slowly cleared particles, A (see Fig. 1), did not change significantly. If the slowly cleared fraction A had been associated with particle deposition in the nonciliated peripheral lungs, A should increase with increasing VL, because more particles should deposit in the periphery. On the other hand, with increasing t_p more particles should deposit in the central airways, because any particles in the nonciliated airspaces would have been already deposited completely after about 2 sec. (The sizes of nonciliated airspaces are smaller than 0.5 mm, and the settling velocity of 3-μm particles is 0.29 mm/sec; hence, alveolar deposition would have been complete after 2 sec). Only airway deposition, therefore, could increase deposition during increasing t_p. This increased central deposition should have led to an increase in the fraction of fast-cleared particles and, thus, to a smaller *A* value. Neither of these considerations was confirmed by these experiments, indicating that particle deposition was predominant in the airways.

Inhaling shallow aerosol boluses (VL = 52 cm^3) of 3.8-μm–d_{ae} particles at a high flow rate (660–800 cm^3/sec) increased the total particle deposition by impaction. However, the value of A (0.52 ± 0.11) was unchanged from that (0.55 ± 0.07) at the commonly used flow rate of 250 cm^3/sec. This again indicated predominant particle deposition in the airways.

To study the behavior of aerosol particles in the airways, experiments were conducted with hollow human and canine casts, which were complete from the trachea to 1-mm airways. These casts were connected to the inhalation device for aerosol bolus measurements and were ventilated by a piston pump. Aerosol boluses ventilated to a VL of less than 80 mL did not leave the cast out of the 1-mm open-ended airways, but were deposited exclusively in the airways of the cast (43,44).

All these experiments led to the conclusion that the fraction of particles cleared slowly were not deposited in the alveolar region, but were deposited in the airways and were cleared from there more slowly than expected, and as a function of d_g.

Shallow aerosol bolus studies were also performed on dogs ventilated with a servoventilator using red and green fluorescent and ^{99m}Tc-labeled 2-μm–polystyrene particles (45,46). Also, in these dogs, a fraction A was slowly cleared;

except in humans the value of A was not constant for VL, ranging from 50–75% of the series dead space of the canine airways, but increased proportional to VL. About 40% of the particles retained for either 24 or 96 hr after inhalation were found in the small airways with diameters less than 1 mm, confirming slow clearance in airways. However, 60% of the retained particles were observed in alveolar structures. Note, the more monopodial branching pattern of the canine airways results in a larger distribution of path lengths from the beginning of the trachea to alveolated acini than that for the more dichotomously branching human airways (e.g., in an ideally dichotomous-branching system the path lengths to all tubes of a given size are identical). This means, at a VL of 50% of the airway dead space, it is more likely that particles reach alveolar structures in the canine lungs than in the human lungs. This is consistent with the observation that the A value increases linearly with VL in the canine lungs, but is constant in the human lungs. Therefore, the considerably large alveolar particle fraction found in the dog lungs may not be representative of the human lungs. However, that the same fraction of retained particles were observed in small airways 24 and 96 hr after inhalation proves that there is a fraction of slowly clearing particles from small airways in this animal model.

In further experiments, the effect of particle size on the value of A was studied. The clearance of polystyrene particles (labeled with ^{111}In) with diameters above 6.5 μm ($d_{ae} = d_{geom}$, because density $= 1$ g/cm^3) was complete within 24 hr ($A < 0.05$).

In the same subjects who had inhaled the 3.8-μm–d_{ae} particles at a high flow rate, aerosol boluses (VL $= 63$ cm^3) of particles of $d_{ae} = 5.8$ μm were inhaled slowly (200–250 cm^3/sec). This resulted in a similar impaction parameter ($=$ flow rate $\times\ d_{ae}^2$). In this way the site of deposition was adjusted to that of the 3.8-μm particles inhaled rapidly. A was 0.26 ± 0.02 for the 5.8-μm–d_{ae} particles, and was 0.52 ± 0.11 for the 3.8-μm–d_{ae} particles. The large particles had a geometric diameter d_{geom} of 3 μm and the small particles had a d_{geom} of 2 μm. These results suggested that the determining factor for the ratio between slow- and fast-cleared particle fractions is not the site of aerosol deposition in the airways and, therefore, not the aerodynamic diameter, but the geometric diameter of the physical size of the deposited particles.

In Figure 2, the slowly cleared fraction A after inhalation of shallow boluses (VL < 60 mL) is shown as a function of d_{geom} for particles of different materials (37,38,47). The value of A increases with decreasing d_g. These investigations indicate that the physical size of the particle, not the particle material, determines the slowly cleared fraction A. Although larger particles were cleared efficiently by fast mucociliary particle transport within 1 day, the slowly cleared fraction increased with decreasing d_g (i.e., particles of decreasing diameter deposited in the airways are decreasingly accessible to mucociliary transport). As a result, the

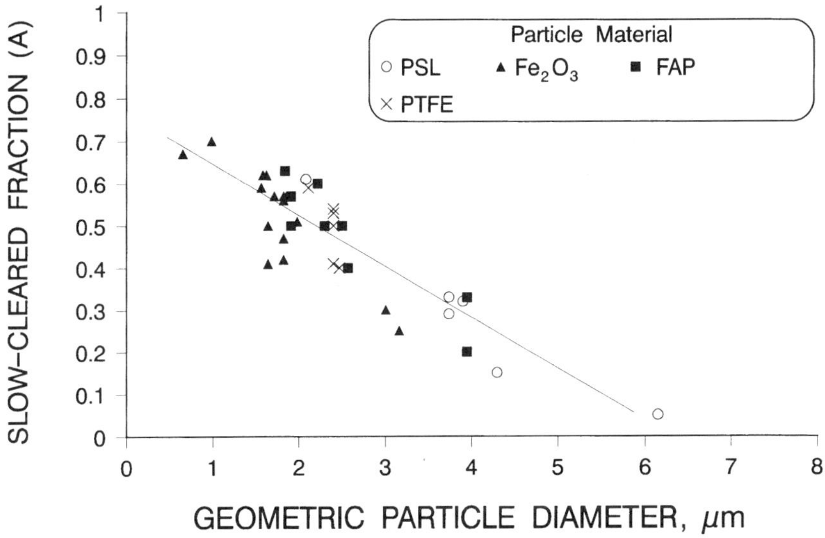

Figure 2 Fraction of slowly cleared particles as function of the geometric particle size: All experiments were done in five healthy subjects with bolus inhalation maneuvers ($V_L < 55$ mL). PSL, polystyrene; FAP, fused aluminum oxide particles; PTFE, Teflon.

slowly cleared fraction was inversely proportional to the geometric particle size (37).

Anderson et al. (48), Svartengren et al. (49), Falk et al. (50) and Camner et al. (51) also observed slow particle clearance from the conducting airways of healthy humans using a different method of aerosol inhalation. They conducted inhalation experiments with d_{ae} = 6-μm particles at two different flow rates (0.5 and 0.05 L/sec). Deposition at the higher (normal) flow rate occurred mainly in central airways by impaction and in the alveolar region by sedimentation. Deposition, at the low-flow rate was enhanced in the last five to six generations of the tracheobronchial tree (i.e., small conducting airways). Deposition in the central airways was reduced because of less impaction at the low-flow rate. Deposition in the alveoli should be negligible because particles are already deposited in the small airways, owing to the large settling velocity (1 mm/sec). Retention of slowly inhaled ^{111}In-labeled Teflon particles was 52% of the initial deposit after 24 hr and 39% after 72 hr (i.e., about 13% was cleared between day 1 and day 3; 49–51). This amount of clearance between day 1 and day 3 was not found when particles were inhaled at the higher-flow rate and cleared from the alveolar region: retention was 51 and 49% after 24 and 72 hr, respectively. Hence, another method of predominant particle deposition in the small conducting airways—aerosol inhalation at a very slow flow rate—also demonstrated the existence of mechanisms leading to a much slower clearance of a fraction of particles deposited in the conducting airways than by mucociliary clearance.

There are two possible explanations for the phenomenon of an intermediate-phase particle clearance from airways:

1. Particles penetrate through the mucous layer onto the epithelial surface and are no longer subject to transport in the overlying mucus. This may happen in all airway generations and phagocytosis by airway macrophages may play a role.
2. Particles that are deposited in small airways with incomplete mucous layer deposit on the epithelium and are retained there. Phagocytosis by airway macrophages may again play a role.

Some investigators have found a significant number of airway macrophages in different species of animals (3,4,52–54), which indicated the involvement of macrophages in the process of a slow-clearance phase from the airways. The possible protective function of these airway macrophages was discussed (55). In rats (5,6) and in hamsters (3,4), most of the particles had already been phagocytosed by macrophages in the airways within 1–2 hr after inhalation or instillation.

Other investigators found many particles located under the mucous layer close to the epithelium. As a result, Schürch and his colleagues (56–58) suggested that the surface tension of the surfactant layers on top and underneath the mucous gel phase may play a role in drawing particles beneath the mucus. Some investigators have found particles retained in the airway walls of rats. However, the fraction of particles located in airway walls was small, about 1% (5). These particles were cleared from the airway walls with half-times of about 100 days.

Some investigators suggest that an impaired mucociliary clearance and the increased retention of particles in the airways might correlate with the occurrence of lung cancer. Churg and Stevens (59) found an association between particles retained in certain airway walls and the occurrence of lung cancer in these lobes. The bronchial mucosa from the lobe with the cancer contained about three times more mineral particles than the lobe without the cancer.

C. Cough Clearance

Particle clearance by cough supports mucociliary clearance, especially under pathophysiological conditions of diseased lungs (60), such as chronic obstructive pulmonary disease (COPD), immotile cilia syndrome (ICS), and cystic fibrosis (CF). An increased secretion in the airways seems to be necessary. During cough, mucus is propelled toward the larynx by the very fast exhalation, with linear air velocities of about 5 m/sec. Cough receptors are found in the trachea and larger bronchi, probably down to the sixth to eighth airway generation (2). Because of the much lower linear velocities in the smaller airways it is likely that cough is not particularly effective distal to the eighth airway generation. Nevertheless, in subjects with strongly impaired mucociliary clearance (e.g., COPD, ICS, or CF) the clearance of particles from the airways by coughing is very efficient. The clearance rates from the entire tracheobronchiolar system are noncontinuous, depending on the frequency and force of coughing and may be slower than mucociliary clearance, but probably these patients can clear almost all material out of the airways by coughing.

Bennett and co-workers (61) investigated the cough-enhanced clearance of mucus in normal healthy subjects. They found a significant increase in the clearance rate during the first 2 hr, but no effect on the amount of clearance in the first 24 hr. They believe that clearance by cough in healthy human subjects may be due to stimulation of the mucociliary apparatus and not to the induced movement of mucus caused by the high velocity of the exhaled air during cough. This supports the assumption that, for an effective cough clearance, an increased secretion is necessary (22).

In conclusion, particles inhaled at the end of a breath are deposited in the conducting airways according to their aerodynamic behavior. Mucociliary clearance is complete for large particles beyond 6-μm d_{geom} deposited in central airways, but may be retarded in small airways. Furthermore, with decreasing physical size of the particles the fraction of slowly cleared particles increases to more than 60% for particles smaller than 1 μm (see Fig. 2). Although there is evidence that airway macrophages play a role in slow particle clearance from the airways, quantitative aspects of the various mechanisms leading to slow clearance in the airways remain to be solved. This issue gains increasing importance, because slow particle clearance from the airways may play a role in the development of airway diseases, including COPD, carcinogenicity in small airways, and others.

III. Clearance from the Peripheral Lung

Historically, long-term particle retention in the lungs was described in coal workers (62) and was associated with lung disease. The term pneumoconiosis was introduced to describe fibrotic lesions found in lung tissue. In this century, it became clear that radioactive particles deposited in the lungs can induce lung cancer as well as acute radiation effects (63). Consequently, the question of the fate of particles deposited in the lungs was raised, acknowledging not only the importance of the administered dose, but also particle retention in the lungs and, hence, particle clearance from the lungs. As a result, both radioactive particles of occupational interest and also particles labeled with gamma-emitting radionuclides were used to study the kinetics of particle retention in various animal species, as well as in humans. A Task Group on Lung Dynamics of the International Commission for Radiological Protection (ICRP) published a summary and gave guidelines for radiation protection in 1966 (64).

However, many of those studies suggested that there are different mechanisms in the lungs and their various regions that interact specifically with deposited particles, leading to different clearance kinetics. Therefore, the ICRP Task Group on Lung Dynamics made several attempts to distinguish between particles of different chemical composition and physical structure, particle clearance pathways, such as particle dissolution versus particle transport, and such. Since then, intensive research has continued mainly to study effects caused by inhaled particles to the peripheral lungs, which was reviewed more recently by a new task group of the ICRP, Human Respiratory Tract Model for Radiological Protection (HRTM) of ICRP-66 (2). Particularly, the concept of particle clearance was adopted by the US Environmental Protection Agency (EPA) in their document, *Air Quality Criteria for Particulate Matter* (65).

A. Long-Term Particle Clearance Pathways and Their Underlying Mechanisms

Several clearance pathways were recognized to play a potential role in the elimination of slowly dissolving, nonviable particles from the epithelium of the peripheral lungs:

1. Particle transport toward the ciliated airways
2. Particle transport to the hilar lymph nodes
3. Particle transport to interstitial sites
4. Particle transport to subpleural spaces
5. Particle retention and relocation on the alveolar epithelium
6. Extracellular particle dissolution in the epithelial lining fluid
7. Intracellular particle dissolution by alveolar macrophages (AM) and other phagocytic cells

The underlying mechanisms maintaining particle clearance (i.e., interactions between lung cells, fluids, and tissues and slowly dissolving, nonviable particles) are multiple and not yet fully understood. The following list is not exhaustive but gives an overall impression of the wide range:

1. Free particle transport on the epithelium by movement of the epithelial lining fluid caused by breathing, heartbeat, secretion processes, or other.

   Toward ciliated airways.

   Toward distal alveolar spaces (sequestration).

2. Free particle transport through the epithelium
   - Into interstitial spaces
   - Toward lymphatic vessels
   - Toward pleural spaces
   - Eventual phagocytosis by interstitial macrophages
3. Recognition and phagocytosis or pinocytosis by phagocytes (AM; polymorphoneutrophilic leukocytes; PMN) on the alveolar epithelium
4. Transport by migration of phagocytes on the alveolar epithelium either by random or chemokinetic movement or directed by chemotactic forces
   - Toward ciliated airways
   - Toward distal alveolar spaces (sequestration)
5. Transport by migration of phagocytes through the epithelium, possibly directed by chemotactic forces
   - Into interstitial spaces
   - Toward lymphatic vessels
   - Toward pleural spaces
6. Phagocytosis or pinocytosis by type I and II epithelial cells
   - Subsequent translocation into interstitial spaces
   - Toward lymphatic vessels
   - Toward pleural spaces
   - Including eventual phagocytosis by interstitial macrophages
7. Reappearance on the alveolar epithelium as free particles or by interstitial macrophages
8. Dissolution in extracellular lung fluids, such as epithelial lining fluid, interstitial fluids, or other
   - Interaction and binding of dissolved particle material to constituents of extracellular fluids and tissues
   - Uptake of dissolved material by cells and subsequent interaction and binding
   - Diffusional transport of dissolved particle material and absorption by blood
9. Intracellular dissolution in phagocytes
   - Interaction and binding of dissolved particle material to cytosolic and membraneous constituents of the phagocyte
   - Transport of dissolved and metabolized particle material out of the cell into epithelial lining fluid, see topic 8.

This list indicates the important role of phagocytes and, in particular, the role of AM. However, recognition and interaction of phagocytes with deposited particles depends not only on contact, adherence, and binding by cell membrane receptors and energy-consuming activation and internalization, but also on the physicochemical properties of the particles. These factors have been excellently reviewed (66). Moreover, there is growing evidence that phagocytosis decreases for both particles larger than 2 and smaller than 0.5 μm, with an optimal particle size at about 1 μm. Similarly, the surface charge of the particles is an important factor, such that hydrophobic particles with either cationic or anionic surfaces are more readily phagocytosed than hydrophilic particles, with diminishing surface charge or zeta potential (67–72). As a consequence, ultrafine particles may be less effectively recognized and phagocytosed by AM, so that they are endocytosed by epithelial cells, resulting in an increasing access of ultrafine particles to interstitial spaces (73–77).

Some of these clearance mechanisms compete with others, such as particle uptake by phagocytes versus epithelial cells and phagocyte migrational parameters. Others run parallel, for instance, particle dissolution parameters are independent of transport parameters no matter whether the latter are associated with free particle transport or mediated by phagocytes. The latter has an important consequence: the clearance pathway of particle dissolution and subsequent uptake of dissolved material by blood (absorption) is independent of particle transport pathways inside and out of the peripheral lungs. This concept was challenged by ICRP-66 (2) and was supported by several studies. Given this assumption, the fractional clearance rate $CL(t)$ of Eq. (2) is the sum of the dissolution and uptake rate $S(t)$ and particle transport rate $M(t)$:

$$CL(t) = S(t) + M[t, g(t), ln(t), p_i(t)] \quad i = 3,4,5 \tag{3}$$

The particle transport rate $M(t)$ is a function of the transport rate toward ciliated airways $g(t)$, the transport rate toward lymphatic drainage $ln(t)$ and intrapulmonary transport rates $p_i(t)$ according to the list of intrapulmonary pathways given in the foregoing.

B. Methods of Studying Distinct Clearance Pathways

There are several established approaches to study clearance pathways and their underlying mechanisms which usually provide information on only a subset of those pathways. Common to all is the use of specific test particles that are uniform in terms of their chemical composition and their physical characteristics, such as structure, density, size, shape, surface, and such. Because in any given region of the peripheral lungs the various clearance mechanisms act in parallel and are competitive, selection of the physicochemical properties of the test particles provides an important tool to allow for only limited interactions between these test particles and lung fluids, tissues, and cells. As a result, specific mechanisms and, hence, distinct pathways can be studied selectively. Requirements to use uniform particles, however, depend on not only the clearance mechanisms to be studied, but also on the application and deposition in the peripheral lungs, which is the subject of another chapter in this book. To study the fate of those test particles they are usually labeled by one or more of the following:

Radioactive isotopes
Fluorescent molecules
Atomic or molecule structures visible by light or electron microscopy
Magnetic crystalline structures

Depending on the type of analysis, the label or a combination of labels is chosen. Note that these studies on clearance pathways and their underlying mechanisms differ distinctly from investigations of the clearance of potentially toxic materials of occupational or environmental interest. The former seek basic understanding of each of the interactions between a well-defined particle material and the fluids, cells, or tissues of the lungs, contributing to a distinct pattern of pathways for particle clearance. The primary interest of the latter is the toxicological risk assessment associated with the exposure of a particle material found under certain occupational or environmental conditions.

Application of Test Particles

After the selection of the physicochemical parameters of test particles, including their aerodynamic properties, the ultimate aim of test particle application is a deposition pattern corresponding to the breathing conditions desired. Hence, the *inhalation of test particles* should have highest priority, particularly, when such studies are anticipated on adult human subjects who can be trained to perform certain breathing patterns. Limitations arise rather quickly with children, patients, or handicapped subpopulations of humans.

In studies on experimental animals, measures need to be taken to achieve a reasonable test inhalation, which usually include restraints or sedation–anesthesia of the spontaneously breathing animal. Because these studies concentrate on clearance pathways from the peripheral lungs, no particle deposition is required, or desired, in the airways, particularly, not in the extrathoracic airways of nose or mouth and larynx. Many of the experimental animal species used are obligatory nose breathers, and their extrathoracic airways are usually very efficient in particle filtration and, therefore, in the reduction of test particle delivery to the alveolar region. The use of an endotracheal tube in the anaesthetized, spontaneously breathing animal enables the extrathoracic airways to be bypassed. This intervention is easily achieved in large animal species, but it has also been applicable in rats (56–58,78). Limitations are breathing at rest, including its variability from breath to breath, which results not only in uncertainties of a factor of 2–10 in dose delivery, but also in a more variable deposition pattern including increased airway deposition, particularly in small ciliated airways. This uncertainty can be reduced by ventilation of the animal and by controlling the accumulating lung deposit when making use of external gamma-ray detection of radiolabeled test particles.

Instillation of test particles provides a precise dosage at a well-defined time point. However, the distribution pattern on the epithelium remains a major concern. The flow of the test particle suspension down the tracheobronchial tree into the alveolar region cannot entirely be predicted, resulting in inhomogeneous deposition patterns and an increased particle deposition in small airways. Also, the liquid phase of the suspension—usually saline—still provides a stimulus and causes a mild inflammatory reaction with increased influx of phagocytes, proteins, and such. In addition, the particle number administered needs to be limited to avoid an additional systemic reaction. As a rule of thumb, the dose should not exceed an inhaled dose deposited during a given time interval unless a high dosage was intended. The time interval considered might be determined by the possible interactions between the test particles and lung fluids, cells, or molecules, or some combination thereof. As a result, the instilled dose should relate to an inhaled dose deposited during 15–60 min.

Another issue, which can be easily controlled before the instillation process, is the degree of agglomeration of test particles forming irregularly shaped multiplets of particles being attached to each other. Because this agglomeration will also affect particle distribution in the peripheral lung as well as the systemic reactions (e.g., phagocytosis and transport by AM), it is desirable to determine the fraction of multiplets in the suspension used for instillation.

Particle Retention in the Lungs

The decreasing amount of particles retained in the lungs describes the overall clearance of particles from the lungs. However, measurement of retention in the lungs is not sufficient to distinguish between distinct particle clearance pathways, unless it is shown that the test particles used interact so specifically that they are cleared prominently by one clearance pathway. Strictly speaking, there is not a single test particle that is subject to only one clearance pathway, but all test particles are subject to a variety of clearance pathways. For example, even though in vivo dissolution can be reduced to the extent that it plays only a minor role in particle clearance, particle transport involves more than one pathway. It is directed not only toward ciliated airways and hence to the larynx, resulting in particle removal from the thorax, but also to other sites of the peripheral lungs and thoracic lymph nodes, resulting in a redistribution of particles within the thorax.

On the other hand, measurement of the kinetics of particle retention in the lungs is necessarily required as a quantitative approach to estimate the fractional contribution of each clearance pathway investigated. Experimentally, there are two approaches to measure the kinetics of particle retention after identical exposures to the test particles:

1. In human subjects, test particles need to contain a label that can be determined by sequential external measurements of the individual subjects. It is required that the label of the test particle is representative of a given parameter of the particle matrix, such as particle mass, surface, or other. The most prominent class of labels used in recent studies are gamma-emitting radionuclides, which allow the radiation dose to be limited to an extent that is considered to be nonhazardous to the subject. External counting and body scans are performed using either high-sensitive scintillation and semiconductor gamma-detectors, or image-providing detectors such as gamma-cameras, single photon emission computer tomography (SPECT), or positron emission tomography (PET).

2. In experimental animals similar noninvasive approaches may be chosen. Additionally or alternatively, invasive techniques may be applied by single-time-point measurements of the respiratory tract and other organs and tissues of each animal after being killed. Retention kinetics are obtained from measurements on animals analyzed at different time points, and by pooling the retention data of all individual animals. The benefit of this invasive procedure is

   a. Precise organ and tissue analysis based on gross or microscopic measurements
   b. Use of any test particles providing an appropriate label, such as those mentioned in the forgoing

A disadvantage, however, is the use of large numbers of animals needed to provide the statistical power of determining the retention kinetics representative for this group of animals (e.g., for a 6-month study, using four animals at each of eight time points selected according to a geometric series (days 0, 1–2, 4, 8, 16, 32, 64, 128–180) results in a total of 32 animals. Generally, the large numbers of animals restricts these studies to rodents and other small animal species.

Sequential Bronchoalveolar Lavages and Morphological Approaches to Particle Localization in the Lung Tissue

Because of the relatively easy access to experimental rodent species, studies were performed in which test particles were administered to groups of rodents either by inhalation or instillation and, subsequently, bronchoalveolar lavages (BAL) were carried out on subgroups of animals at sequential time points (79–84). Because the animals were killed during the process of BAL, exhaustive lavage techniques were developed, with the emphasis on recovering all particles from the epithelium, and on determining the phagocytosed particle fraction in AM recovered in the BAL fluid. In addition, morphometric approaches to localize remaining particles in the lung tissue and lung digestion techniques, allow determination of the ratio of particles retained on the epithelium versus elsewhere in the lungs, including interstitial sites and lymph nodes (77,85–88).

Recovered particle fractions were analyzed according to the particle material and its label, using fluorescent light microscopy and flow cytometry, electron microscopy, chemical analysis, gamma-spectroscopy, or autoradiography. The combination of flow cytometry and monodisperse latex spheres of bright fluorescence of various colors with appropriate surface charges in the diameter range of 0.5–10 μm, provided a particularly effective tool. The fluorescent particles were phagocytosed by AM, but did not significantly initiate other systemic reactions not involved in the process of recognition and phagocytosis of a nonviable foreign body.

Such studies were not usually performed in large animal species because of excessive experimental expenses, ethical objections and such, and the need for large groups of animals (see the estimate in the previous Sec. III.B). One way to estimate the kinetics of particle transport from the alveolar epithelium itself makes use of a combined analysis of radiolabeled uniform particle retention in the lungs and of particle recovery in the lavage fluid of sequential BAL on individual animals over a period of several months. Application of this method prohibits the rigorous lavage techniques used in terminal studies, and it allows only partial lavage of the epithelium to ensure the recovery of the animal from the procedure. The saline solution for BAL washes only a restricted part of the lungs, such as a lung lobe, a segment of a lobe, or at most one lung. Because the lungs or part of the lungs to be lavaged have not been collapsed, the lavage solution does not inflate and float across the entire epithelium, but only part of it. Therefore, it does not dilute the epithelial lining fluid (ELF) of the entire epithelial surface and, in addition, only part of the ELF-diluted lavage fluid is recovered during aspiration. Hence, the limitation of this method is the unknown fraction of ELF in the BAL fluid. However, a standardized procedure and a sufficient number of animals allows averaging over some of the uncertainties. In addition, if only the kinetic change of particle recovery with time is anticipated, sequential, partial BAL provide a tool to estimate the kinetics of particle disappearance from the alveolar epithelium.

Lung Retention and Excretion Analysis by Gamma-Spectroscopy Using Radiolabeled Test Particles

Another approach makes use of uniform test particles labeled with gamma-emitting radionuclides of suitable gamma-energies and half-time. Simultaneous external gamma-spectroscopy over the chest, or whole-body scans, and gamma-spectroscopy of excretion samples, allow estimates of the kinetics of particle retention in the lungs as well as the kinetics of long-term particle transport toward ciliated airways and larynx and subsequently into the gastrointestinal tract (GIT). However, the radiolabel must be shown to stay with the particle matrix in the biological system over the long period of observation, which may be months or years. Because of the large specific surface area of test particles (surface area per unit particle mass) in the micron (0.01–1 m^2/g) and submicron range (1–100 m^2/g), dissolution of the test particles must be controlled very carefully. To test for, and allow for, absorption (the dissolution and uptake to blood of dissolved material) occurring simultaneously with particle transport, serial sacrifice studies with laboratory animals have been established involving gamma-spectroscopy of organs and tissues. Accumulation of the radiolabel in organs and tissues, for which particles deposited in the respiratory tract would not normally clear, is a clear indication that the radiolabel has leached out of the particle matrix. This results in a set of biokinetic pathways inside and out of the body completely different from that of the test particles themselves. The biokinetic behavior will depend on the chemical nature of the nonparticulate (dissolved) material and its interaction with biomolecules of body fluids, cells, and tissues. If particle dissolution occurs in the lungs, it is the variety of initial interactions with biomolecules present in the lungs (i.e., in AM, epithelial cells, lung fluids, or lung tissues) that determine the biokinetic fate. In fact, such reactions might lead to nonparticulate radiolabel retention in the lungs superimposed on test particle retention. This requires careful distinction and greater efforts to analyze the lung tissue.

A suitable approach to assess the coincident effects of particle dissolution and radiolabel leaching from the particles is to conduct supplementary studies in which the radiolabel is administered in an appropriate soluble chemical form and dose to the lungs or systemic circulation. Similarly, supplementary studies are required to allow for the biokinetic fate of particles during GIT passage or maybe even after their entrance into the systemic circulation.

Because particle dissolution during long periods in the lungs is important for many nonviable particles found in the environment or workplace, it is also important to study this clearance pathway and its underlying mechanisms. However, this imposes additional requirements on the physicochemical properties of the test particle and its radiolabel, especially on the particle surface parameters, for this is the interface of material exchange between the particle matrix and the surrounding medium. Generally, the radiolabel should be an isotope of the predominant element in the particle matrix. This implicitly restricts studies on dissolution kinetics to test particles containing metallic compounds. Because differences between the biokinetic fate of the test particle and that of the nonparticulate radiolabel are anticipated, the various interactions between the radiolabel and constituents of the solvent need to be considered. For example, if the particle was phagocytosed by an AM, the concentration of protons, chelating biomolecules, proteolytic and lysosomal enzymes, and such in the membrane-bound phagolysosomal vacuole will be different from conditions in the cytosol or in extracellular lung fluid. As a result, the reaction products in the vacuole will determine the further stages of reactions and translocation inside the cell and, subsequently, outside the cell through the epithelial barrier (either by extracellular or intracellular passage) into lung interstitial tissues, until the radioisotope eventually enters the systemic circulation.

Depending on the chemical nature of the radiolabel and the previous series of metabolic reactions, systemic circulation of the biomolecularly bound radiolabel may lead to rapid and complete excretion, or it may lead to further reactions and accumulation in other organs. If the former occurs, it is straightforward to analyze the expected clearance. The latter event might result in a misleading analysis of the anticipated clearance pathway if the study is based only on gamma-spectroscopic analyses of the chest/whole body, excreta samples, and gross organs. However, with attempts to determine the biomolecular reaction partners in the lungs, in the circulation, and in organs with accumulating radiolabel, this type of analysis provides information on the entire series of metabolic reactions and the potential toxicological aspects of the inhaled material. Thus, such analyses may eventually show that the intake of a given material by inhalation might lead to very different clearance pathways, depending on its physicochemical properties, such as moderate solubility versus insolubility in the lungs.

As many of these investigations cannot be carried out on human subjects because of their invasive character, interspecies comparisons including human subjects and a variety of experimental animal species provide a powerful tool to obtain the maximum information about the behavior of an inhaled material. The concept of interspecies comparison allows mechanistic studies in the animals and, at the same time, allows judgment on whether those mechanisms can be extrapolated and applied to humans. A schematic graph of the various analytical approaches is provided in Figure 3.

Lymph Node Accumulation

Although it is frequently stated (2,89) that particles are accumulated in the tracheobronchial lymph nodes (TBLN) located mainly around the bifurcation of the trachea into the main bronchi, there are no data available on the kinetics of particle transport to TBLN in humans. In small animals, the common approach involves serial sacrifices of groups of animals after appropriate administration of the test particles.

In large experimental animals, with only small numbers available, the kinetics of this clearance pathway can be analyzed using insoluble particles with an appropriate radiolabel and imaging gamma-spectroscopy (gamma-camera). A series of lung scans will provide activity accumulation at the sites of the TBLN as an indicator of particle transport to the TBLN, but this must finally be proved by lymph node tissue analyses at the time of sacrifice. Although careful radiation dose estimates would be required, this approach may also be applicable to human subjects.

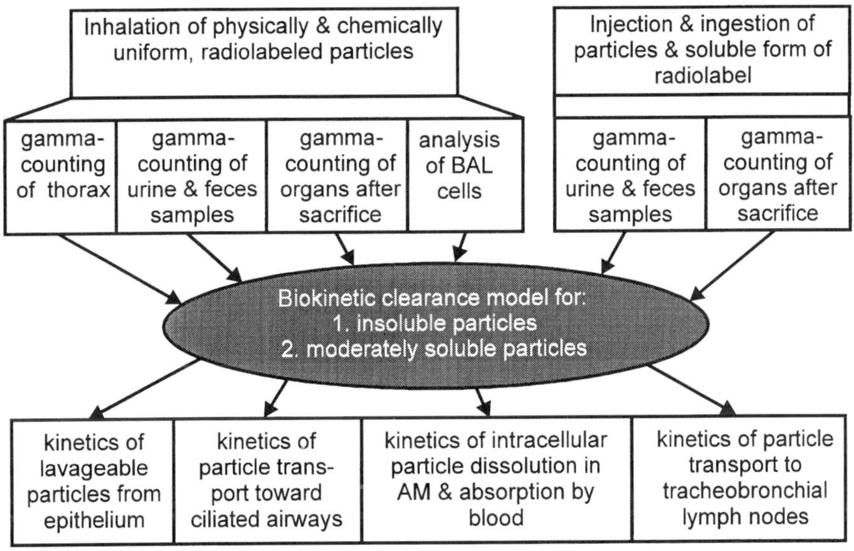

Figure 3 Schematic graph of the various analytical approaches to estimate the kinetics of clearance pathways of uniform test particles with specific physical and chemical properties.

C. Determination of the Kinetics of Particle Clearance Pathways

Kinetics of Particle Transport Toward the Ciliated Airways

The rate-determining step for particle transport from the peripheral lungs to the larynx and thence to the gastrointestinal tract is the time required to transport the particle from an alveolus to the most distal ciliated airways—the terminal bronchioli. Subsequent transport by mucociliary action up the ciliated airways to the larynx is considered to be comparatively rapid. Particle transport toward the ciliated airways and larynx has been determined in various animal species, including humans. A summary of studies, in different animal species and humans, that used different particle materials in which efforts were made to distinguish this particle clearance pathway, particularly, from particle dissolution, is given in Annexe E of the HRTM of ICRP-66 (2). Figure 4 shows the kinetics of the fractional transport rate $g(t)$, which is the daily fraction of particles transported to the larynx, relative to the particles retained in the lungs, according to the following equation:

$$g(t) = \left(\frac{1}{R_t(t)}\right)\left(\frac{dR_t(t)}{dt}\right) - S(t) \qquad (4)$$

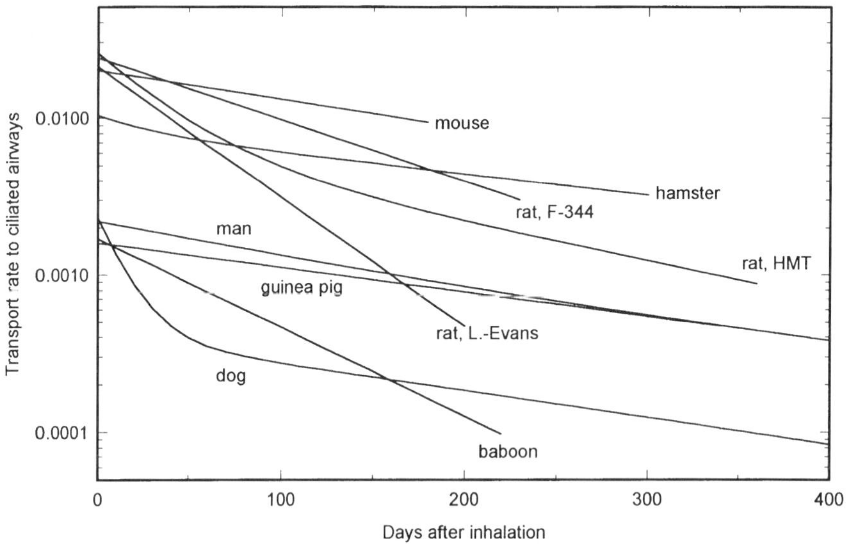

Figure 4 Kinetics of the fractional transport rate $g(t)$ of $^{57}Co_3O_4$ particles from the peripheral lungs toward ciliated airways and, subsequently, to larynx in humans and various experimental animal species: monkeys, dogs, guinea pigs, three strains of rats (HMT, Fischer-344, Long–Evans), hamsters, and mice.

This modification of Eqs. (2) and (3) is valid, since all transport rates $ln(t)$, $p_i(t)$ determining the overall transport rate $M(t)$ besides $g(t)$ lead to only particle redistribution in the thorax and do not change thoracic retention $R_t(t)$.

Data obtained from various animal species and humans were summarized recently (90). All particle transport rates were obtained after inhalation of uniform, moderately soluble cobalt oxide particles labeled with ^{57}Co ($^{57}Co_3O_4$) in a European collaborative study on the interspecies comparison of particle clearance from the lungs (91). Although the particles were moderately soluble in the lungs, it was possible to distinguish the kinetics of particle transport toward ciliated airways from the other clearance pathway out of the lungs, particle dissolution, and absorption. With one exception, in all dogs studied, the particle transport rate was so small compared with particle dissolution, that only the initial phase, during the first month, could be determined. When less soluble $^{57}Co_3O_4$ particles were used, the particle transport rate could be followed for more than 2 years (92). The latter is shown in Figure 4. In all species the dissolved ^{57}Co was rapidly and predominantly excreted in urine.

Although the kinetics of particle transport varied widely between species strain, there was little intersubject variability within each species. Generally, in all species the fractional transport rate was not constant, but decreased monotonically from its initial value immediately after particle inhalation. The transport rates could be described by either one or two exponential terms (90), values of which are given in Table 1.

$$g(t) = G_1 \exp[-(\ln(2)/\tau_{g1})\ t] + G_2 \exp[-(\ln(2)/\tau_{g2})t] \quad (5)$$

where $G_i(i = 1,2)$ are the initial transport rates of each term and $\tau_{gi1}(i = 1,2)$ are the half-times of decline for each term.

The transport kinetics did not significantly differ between various particle materials studied—metal oxides, polystyrene, Teflon, glass (fused aluminosilicate)—or over the particle size range 0.5–5 μm, as shown in Annexe E of ICRP-66 (2). Intersubject variability was small within a given animal species, but was somewhat larger for human subjects. A very recent human study (93), which measured lung retention in ten healthy subjects over 900 days using very slowly dissolving ^{195}Au-labeled Teflon particles, confirmed transport rates of initially 0.0009 decreasing to 0.0004 per day after 1 year of retention.

However, cytotoxic particles, such as Am/PuO_2 showed a dose-dependent retardation of particle transport rates in rats (94). In addition, the transport rates of ultrafine particles, smaller than 0.1 μm in rats (75,76), and of particles larger than 5 μm in rats and dogs were less than those of particles in the size range 0.5–5 μm (95,96). From those observations it was concluded in the HRTM of ICRP-66 (2) that particle transport toward ciliated airways is independent of the particle material, as long as the material is not cytotoxic and as long as the particles are in the range 0.5- to 5-μm diameter.

As shown in Figure 4 the initial rates differed clearly between the species.

Table 1 Parameters of Co_3O_4 Particle Transport Rates According to Eq. (5) for Humans and Various Experimental Animals

Species	$g(t = 0)$ (d^{-1})	G_1 (d^{-1})	τ_{g1} (*d*)	G_2 (d^{-1})	τ_{g2} (*d*)
Man	0.0022	0.0018	120	0.0004	430
Baboon	0.0017			0.0017	53
Beagle dog	0.0023	0.0019	10	0.0004	180
Guinea pig	0.0036			0.0036	430
HMT rat	0.020	0.019	36	0.0066	120
F-344 rat	0.024			0.024	77
Long–Evans rat	0.021			0.021	33
Syrian golden hamster	0.030	0.0022	21	0.0082	220
CBA/H mouse	0.018			0.018	170

Source: Ref. 87.

Although the initial rates for rodents (rats, hamsters, and mice) were about 0.01–0.03/day, the initial rate in guinea pigs was 0.005/day. Initial rates in humans, monkeys, and beagle dogs were similar at 0.001–0.004/day, which were about an order of magnitude lower than those of rodents. The decrease of the transport rate was described by a half-time in the range of 50–500 days, as shown in Table 1. Furthermore, Langenback et al. (97,98) studied lung clearance in sheep using slowly dissolving ^{57}Co-labeled polystyrene particles, and evaluated an initial transport rate of 0.02/day, which is similar to those found in rodents. This remarkable difference between rodents and sheep versus humans, monkeys, dogs, and guinea pigs has an important consequence when integrating the cleared particle fraction over a time period. In rodents and sheep about 90% of the particles deposited in the lung periphery are cleared by this pathway within 6 months. In humans, monkeys, dogs, and guinea pigs, however, less than 30% of particles are cleared during the entire life span because of the decrease in the transport rate, resulting in negligible rates after 6–12 months. There is no conclusive explanation yet for this species difference. The decrease in particle transport rate indicates that the pool of particles on the alveolar epithelial surface empties faster than the total of the retained particles in the lungs. This is discussed together with particle transport through the alveolar epithelial membrane in the following section.

To better understand particle transport toward the ciliated airways, a closer look to possible mechanisms is required. When BAL was performed at times well after the particles were deposited in the lungs, most of lavaged particles were phagocytosed by AM. However, most of the lavaged particles came from particles retained on that part of the alveolar epithelial surface that was lavaged and only a small fraction was recruited from the particles on airway epithelial surfaces and those on their way to the ciliated airways. In rodents, for example, this fraction must be less than 0.01–0.03% of the retained fraction, according to the declining transport rate (see Table 1). In humans, monkeys, and dogs it must be an order of magnitude less. The fraction of nonphagocytosed particles in BAL fluid is in the range of 1–5% of lavaged particles. The origin of this small fraction remains uncertain. It may represent the free particle fraction on the epithelium, or it may be an artifact, because the particles might have been released from AM during the process of BAL and analysis. Hence, from this type of investigation, it is still possible that not only phagocytosed particles, but also free particles, are transported to the ciliated airways. Valberg and Blanchard (66) have reviewed models of free-particle transport caused, for instance, by the intermittent flow of the epithelial lining fluid in alveoli according to the expansion and contraction during breathing, heart beat, ELF secretion, and such. However, all these models lack experimental evidence in the lungs.

Alveolar macrophage-mediated particle transport was inferred from observations of particle-containing macrophages on the luminal surfaces of airways at times well after the particles were deposited in the lungs (80,99). In addition, morphometric studies showed that most of the particles retained in the lungs of rats were associated with AM at similar retention times (79,80). However, the possibility cannot be excluded that free particles that were loosely retained on airway or alveolar epithelial surfaces were lost during tissue processing for microscopical analysis. These observations show that particle transport toward the ciliated airways is predominantly AM-mediated, but it still does not exclude transport of free particles.

Further evidence that particle transport is AM-mediated came from a study by Collier et al. (94), who compared lung retention in HMT rats using either monodisperse ^{57}Co-labeled glass particles (fused aluminosilicate; FAP) or mixed Am–Pu oxide particles both of 1.2-μm d_{ae}. For both particles, in vivo dissolution was so small that it did not significantly contribute to particle clearance from the lungs of rats, which was predominantly maintained by particle transport toward the ciliated airways (100). At an initial lung deposit (ILD) of 0.1 kBq of Am–Pu oxide particles, lung retention was similar for both particles. However, at 2- and 9-kBq ILD, lung retention was increased (i.e., particle transport was retarded). The decreased particle transport was associated with cytotoxic effects of alpha-irradiation of the Am–Pu oxide particles acting either directly on AM motility or by alterations of mediators necessary for AM migration. It seemed unlikely that transport of free particles (i.e., nonphagocytosed particles) would have been affected by the inhaled dose.

Another hypothesis suggested that AM may be passively transported by alveolar fluid currents, but this again lacks experimental evidence. In contrast, Brain et al. (101,102) showed that AMs appear to be in close apposition with, and adherent to the alveolar epithelial surface.

Other evidence on AM-mediated particle transport came from studies of Muhle et al. (103) and Bellmann et al. (104). In these, particle transport toward the ciliated airways of the rat lung was not only retarded during continuous exposure to high concentrations of carbonaceous aerosols, but also during recovery, when the epithelium and AM were loaded much less. This observation was considered to be consistent with the hypothesis that AM were diverted from their route to the ciliated airways. Altered concentration gradients of chemoattractants were discussed as possible underlying mechanisms for the deviation of AM (105,106), based on previous observations: It is well known that AM follow chemotactic concentration gradients. These findings came not only from cell culture studies but also from observations of increased AM concentrations at locations that also showed enhanced concentrations of complement factors—well-known chemoattractants (107–110). From these observations, it was concluded that AM-mediated particle transport toward the ciliated airways was associated with chemotactic concentration gradients on the alveolar epithelium directing AM toward the distal entrance of alveolar acini. Following this hypothesis the chemotactic gradient should be weaker on the epithelium of humans, monkeys, and dogs than of rodents and sheep to account for this lower particle transport rate.

Another hypothesis considers anatomical differences in the acini of rodents and sheep versus humans, monkeys, dogs, and guinea pigs. If, for instance, the path length from an alveolus to the most distal ciliated airways—terminal bronchioli—were shorter in rodents and sheep than in humans, monkeys, dogs, and guinea pigs, then particle transport might be faster, regardless of the mechanism by which the particles are transported. Indeed, according to Tyler and Julian (111), there are ''several'' generations of respiratory bronchioli before the branching into alveolar ducts and sacs in the lungs of humans, monkeys, and dogs, whereas respiratory bronchioli are ''either absent or there is only one short generation'' in the lungs of sheep, rats, hamsters, mice, and guinea pigs. This means that the path length from alveoli to ciliated terminal bronchioli is longer in humans, monkeys, and dogs, than in sheep, rats, hamsters, and mice, which may result in a longer transport time for the former species than for the latter. Hence, this hypothesis fits with all species in this comparison, with the exception of guinea pigs, which show a short path length and yet the particle transport is almost as slow as in humans, monkeys, and dogs. Nevertheless, with the sheep having a short path length and particle transport as fast as rodents, there is a nonrodent large animal species confirming the hypothesis, which otherwise would have had support only from small rodent species versus large animal species.

In summary, there is evidence that (1) particle transport from the peripheral lung toward ciliated airways is mediated by AM, whereas particle transport of free (nonphagocytosed) particles may play a minor role. (2) From interspecies comparisons, the path length from alveoli to ciliated terminal bronchioli may determine the particle transport rate. In addition, it is hard to believe that AM migration on the alveolar epithelium results from random movement, whereas AM recruitment onto the epithelium, and the migration toward, and phagocytosis of particles on the alveolar epithelium are controlled by chemotactic and biomolecular mediators (66,112). The concept of a nonstochastic migration of AM on the alveolar epithelium toward ciliated airways, actively directed by chemotactic attractants, is more consistent with what is known about AM migration.

Kinetics of Particle Transport Through the Alveolar Epithelial Membrane

Studies on rodents have applied exhaustive BAL and lung tissue digestion techniques to balance lavageable versus nonlavageable particles in the peripheral lung over time spans from a few days up to half a year after administration of monodisperse iron oxide or fluorescent latex particles (79,84,113,114). At any of the time points investigated, about 90% of the particles retained in the lungs could be recovered in the BAL fluid, indicating that at least 90% of the retained particles were found on the alveolar epithelium. The particle transport rate toward ciliated airways was estimated to decrease from 0.02/day initially, to 0.007/day, which corresponds well with those discussed in the foregoing section. From these observations it was concluded that in rodents particle transport toward ciliated airways was the dominant clearance pathway for insoluble particles from the epithelium. The small fraction of about 10% of nonlavageable particles at any of the time points was associated with retention on the distal alveolar epithelium or, more likely, in interstitial sites. This was consistent with earlier findings on particle uptake by type I epithelial cells and particle retention at interstitial sites (99,115,116). As a result, particle transport through the alveolar epithelial membrane was considered to be a minor clearance pathway.

In another study (83) on Syrian golden hamsters, using monodisperse, ^{57}Co-labeled FAP, less exhaustive BAL was performed at three different times after inhalation, but the animals were maintained alive, and lung retention measurements by external gamma-spectroscopy continued. Particle retention after BAL continued to decrease with the same exponential slope as before. This indicated the same type of particle clearance took place before and after BAL of these slowly dissolving FAP particles, which was relatively rapid transport towards the ciliated airways and larynx (see foregoing section). When the particle fractions recovered in the lavage fluid were normalized to the particle mass retained in the lungs at the time of lavage, these fractions remained constant at about 0.65 during all three lavages performed throughout a year after particle inhalation. These results showed the particle fraction accessible for lavage remained constant in hamsters, indicating that particles were retained predominantly on the alveolar epithelium and that no major particle redistribution from the alveolar epithelium had taken place.

In two studies on beagle dogs using either monodisperse FAP or polystyrene particles (PSL) both labeled with ^{60}Co (117,118) a series of four partial BALs (see Sec. III.B) were performed at the same three subsegmental locations during 1 year after particle inhalation. When the particle fractions recovered in the lavage fluid were normalized to the particle mass retained in the lungs at the time of lavage and corrected for previous particle removals by BAL, they declined exponentially as shown in Figure 5 for PSL. The decreasing lavageable particle fraction showed that the particles retained in the lungs were continuously less accessible for lavage, indicating that they had been transported from the epithelium to other locations. Possible locations not accessible for lavage were in and beyond the epithelial membrane in interstitial spaces; also, it could not be excluded that some particles were relocated on the epithelium at more distal surfaces not accessible to the lavage fluid.

According to the exponential decrease of recovered particles in the lavage fluid a half-time of decline of about 150 days was observed that described the rate of particle disappearance of 0.005/day from the alveolar epithelium. Interest-

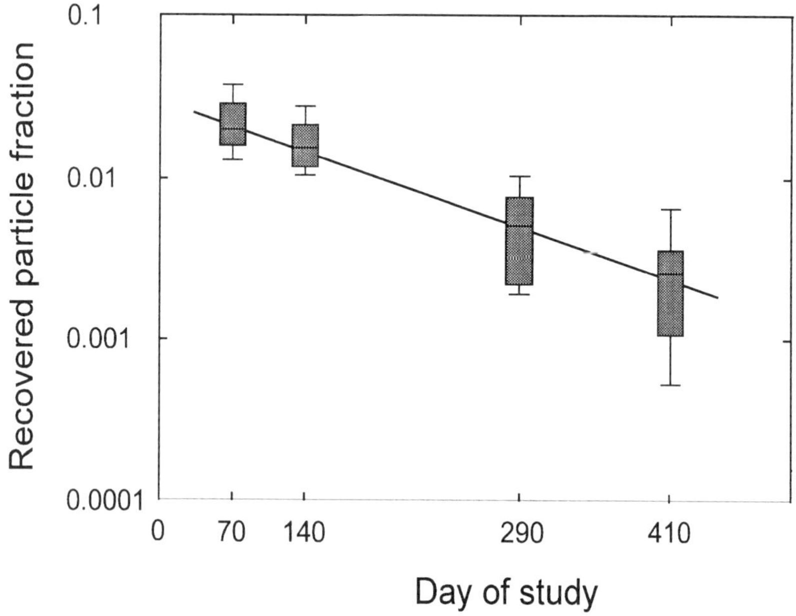

Figure 5 Kinetics of the PSL particle fractions recovered in the lavage fluid of sequential bronchoalveolar lavage during 1 year after inhalation. Fractions were normalized to the particle mass retained in the lungs at the time of lavage and corrected for estimates of previous particle removals by bronchoalveolar lavage.

ingly, this half-time of decline is very similar to the half-time at which the particle transport rate toward ciliated airways declined (see Table 1). In that case, it was postulated that the pool of particles on the alveolar epithelial surface reduced faster than the total of the retained particles in the lungs. Furthermore, the two half-times of decline correlated significantly ($r^2 = 0.82$) between the 16 dogs. This strongly suggested that the reason for the decreasing fraction of particles accessible to transport toward ciliated airways was particle transport into and through the alveolar epithelial membrane toward interstitial sites. If we take the low transport rate toward ciliated airways into account, the dominant fraction of the retained particles was translocated from the alveolar epithelial surface to interstitial sites and perhaps partly to distal alveolar epithelium. Hence, although there was predominant particle transport from the epithelium of the dog's lungs into the interstitium, this transport phenomenon was only minor in the lungs of rats and hamsters. In rodents, particle transport toward ciliated airways dominated. The different efficiencies of clearance pathways from the epithelial surface of HMT rats versus dogs are shown cumulatively in Figure 6. Because the transport rate toward ciliated airways in rodents also declined (with a half-life given in Table 1), this observation indicated some particle relocation from the alveolar epithelium toward interstitial spaces and toward more distal alveolar epithelial surfaces. However, some investigators concluded from their studies on rodents that once AM appeared on the alveolar epithelium they do not migrate across the epithelial membrane back into interstitial sites (102,115). Therefore, the two findings in rodents—declining transport rate toward ciliated airways, but constant normalized lavageable particle fractions—remained contradictory. However, the fraction of particles translocated to interstitial sites was rather small in rodents. Hence, BAL does not provide the appropriate method to confirm this relocated fraction, because it does not determine the small relocated fraction, but rather, the large particle fraction retained on the alveolar epithelium.

The AM may well be able to penetrate the alveolar epithelium, migrating to hilar lymph nodes (87,119,120). BAL in dogs at times long after particle inhalation (121–124) showed that more than 90% of the retained particles on the alveolar epithelium were phagocytosed by AM. Because this fraction dominated the pool from which particles were translocated through the alveolar epithelial

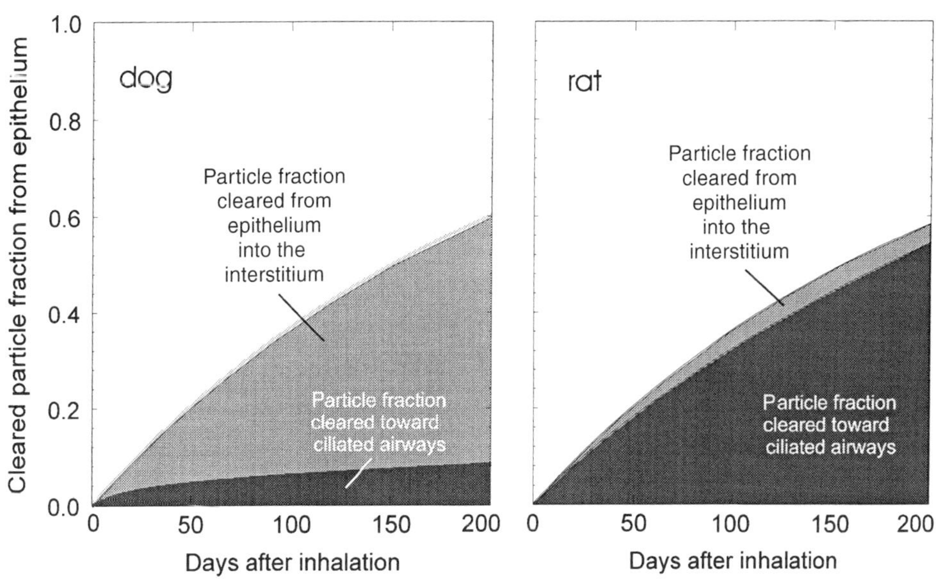

Figure 6 Cumulative efficiencies of clearance pathways of HMT rats versus dogs from the epithelial surface either toward ciliated airways or into and through the alveolar epithelial membrane.

membrane (with a rate of 0.005/day), this strongly suggested that this clearance pathway through the epithelial membrane was AM-mediated. However, free-particle transport by endocytosis of epithelial type I and perhaps type II cells, and subsequent exocytosis into interstitial spaces still cannot be excluded (99,125–127). The latter is particularly important for particles in the ultrafine-particle–size range that are recognized and phygocytosed by AM to a lesser extent than larger particles (see Sec. III.A).

The concept of particle transport through the alveolar epithelium and retention in macrophages at interstitial sites was supported by morphometric analyses of the lungs of monkeys that had been exposed to coal dust or diesel exhaust (128). Particle retention was observed not only at interstitial sites in monkeys, but also in humans (89,129). In addition, the particle clearance studies discussed in the previous section, showed that transport rates toward ciliated airways and half-times of decline of these rates were low and similar in dogs, monkeys, and humans. The decline of these rates was associated in dogs with particle transport through the alveolar epithelial membrane, as described in the foregoing. Because of these similarities, it is plausible to presume kinetics of particle transport through the alveolar epithelial membrane in monkeys and humans similar to those found in dogs. Because of the similarities observed between humans, monkeys, and dogs we postulate that particle transport through the alveolar epithelial membrane is also AM-mediated in humans.

The reason why AM of humans, monkeys, and dogs are predominantly directed toward interstitial sites, whereas AM of rodents are predominantly directed toward ciliated airways, remains an open question that needs further research. Intuitively, this species difference is also considered to be indicative of differences in directed migration of AM, possibly resulting from chemotactic stimuli or the distance from alveoli to terminal bronchioli according to the anatomical differences in respiratory bronchioli, as described in the previous section.

Note that these considerations were based on studies using noncytotoxic particles in the size range 0.5- to 5-μm diameter at exposure levels well below what is considered to result in "overload." Recognition and phagocytosis by AM seem to be optimal for particles in the size range 0.5–2 μm, with a maximum at 1 μm (68,101), which also corresponds to the highest deposition probability in the alveolar region relative to particle size. When numbers of deposited particles are increased to exceed a certain ratio relative to the existing AM population, transport through the alveolar epithelial membrane increased in rodents, as discussed in recent reviews (114,130). Consistent with the diminishing capability of AM for recognition and phagocytosis of ultrafine particles, these particles were reported to be found in epithelial cells and interstitial sites (73–76; see Sec. III.A).

Note also that the fraction of particles recovered in BAL fluid may not necessarily have resided on the epithilium for the entire time before the BAL. It may be representative only of what was currently located on the epithelium during lavage, and may perhaps include particles that were initially transported into the interstitium, but reappeared on the epithilium later (126).

In summary, although there was predominant particle transport from the epithelium of the dog lung into the interstitium, this transport phenomenon was only minor in the lungs of rats and hamsters. Conversely, particle transport toward ciliated airways dominated in rodents, and was low in dogs. Because of similarities in long-term lung retention and the kinetics of AM-mediated particle transport toward the ciliated airways, it is plausible to presume that the kinetics of particle transport through the alveolar epithelial membrane in monkeys and humans is similar to that found in dogs.

Kinetics of Particle Transport to the Hilar Lymph Nodes

ICRP-66 (2) reviewed the available data on particle uptake by TBLN in humans. These data do not provide any direct information on the kinetics of particle accumulation in TBLN; they originate from autopsy measurements. They were presented as ratios of particle concentrations in TBLN versus particle concentrations in lungs, which range from 1 to 20. Note, even at the high concentrations observed in TBLN, the total of retained particles is still a factor of 3 higher in the lungs than in TBLN, because the mass ratio of TBLN and lungs is about a factor of 0.015. However, these data do not consider particles that were retained in the lymphatic vessels not distinguished from the lungs, as described by Cottier et al. (131) in lymphatic vessels of elderly persons. The rather large range of concentration ratios may have resulted from many factors, such as those depending on particle materials, but it also may have reflected human intersubject variability.

Thomas (132) used data obtained mostly from dogs, but also from monkeys killed at various times after inhalation of radioaerosols. He proposed a particle concentration ratio between TBLN and lungs [LN]/[L] as a function of time t:

$$[\mathrm{LN}]/[\mathrm{L}] = 0.0107t^{1.08} \text{ for } 1 < t(d) < 3000 \text{ days} \quad (6)$$

which predicted a value of [LN]/[L] of about 20 at 1000 days after inhalation. It was suggested that dog and monkey provided a good model for particle accumulation in TBLN of humans. Yet, data from dogs and monkeys also indicated a large intersubject variability (133,134).

In contrast, there is much less particle accumulation in TBLN of rodents than in those of dogs (96,130). Comparing this observation with the differences in particle removal from the alveolar epithelial surface of these species (see previous section), this provides another indication for less particle transport through the alveolar epithelium of rodents.

With use of a gamma-camera, the kinetics of uptake of ^{57}Co-labeled FAP and $^{57}Co_3O_4$ particles in TBLN of individual dogs was observed and is shown

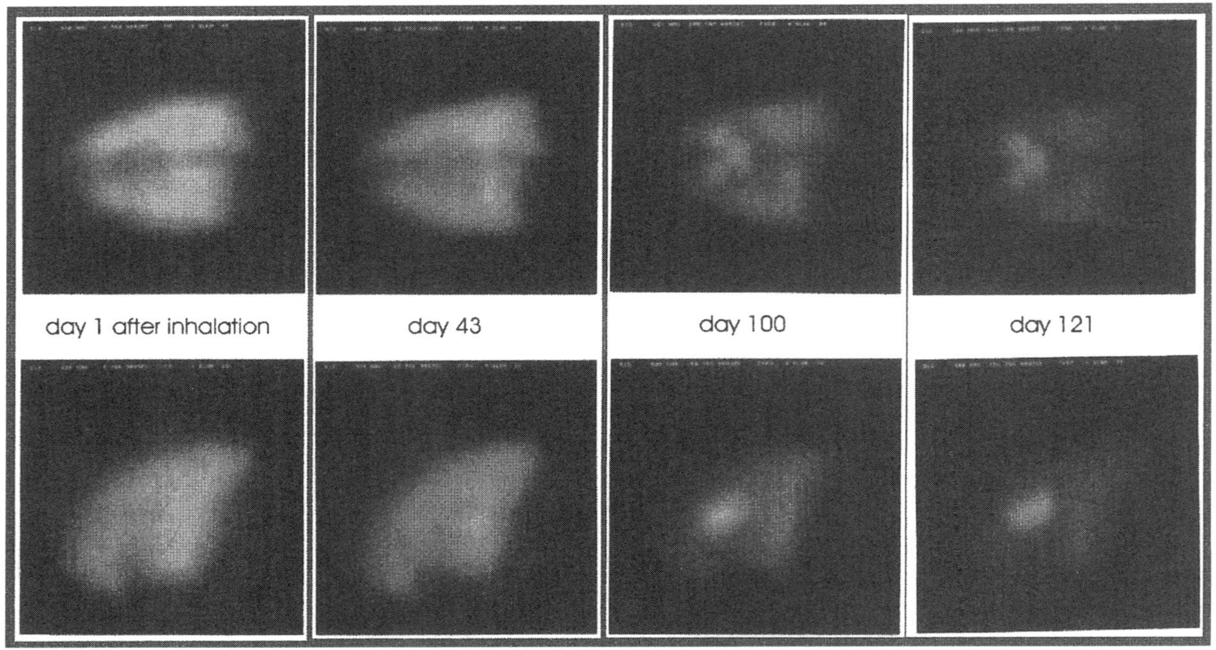

Figure 7 Series of gamma-camera scintigrams of particle retention in the lungs obtained from an individual dog taken at different days after inhalation of $^{57}Co_3O_4$ particles by (upper) a dorsal and a (lower) right lateral view. At sacrifice, particle accumulation observed in the scintigrams was confirmed to be taken up in tracheobronchial lymph nodes.

by a series of sequential gamma-camera scintigrams in Figure 7 (135). The kinetics of particle accumulation in TBLN calculated from these scintigrams are compared with lung retention for both ^{57}Co-labeled FAP and $^{57}Co_3O_4$ in Figure 8 (92,121,136). Whereas ^{57}Co-FAP accumulation continued to increase over the time period of 600 days, $^{57}Co_3O_4$ particles accumulated during the first 100 days after inhalation and decreased subsequently, following the same slope as lung retention. Because the latter resulted from AM-mediated particle dissolution (discussed in the following section), we concluded that macrophage-mediated particle dissolution also took place in the TBLN.

The kinetics of accumulation in TBLN were described by a rate of 0.0015/day (half-life 470 days) for ^{57}Co-labeled FAP and 0.018/day (half-life 40 days) for $^{57}Co_3O_4$ particles. Accumulation rates varying between 0.01 and 0.0015/day were observed in different dogs, indicating a large intersubject variability. Moreover, the accumulated fractions differed between different dogs to the extent that in some dogs it was never possible to analyze the particle accumulation in TBLN from scintigrams because of the limited resolution of the detector. Similarly, intersubject variation between dogs had any correlation between particle size or composition and TBLN accumulation for the various $^{57}Co_3O_4$ particles differing

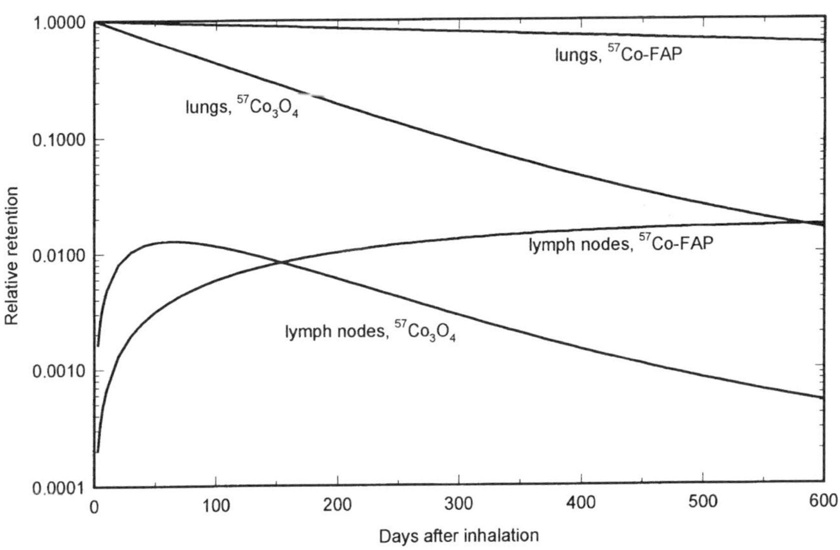

Figure 8 Calculated particle uptake in tracheobronchial lymph nodes of individual dogs after inhalation of moderately soluble $^{57}Co_3O_4$ particles and rather insoluble ^{57}Co-labeled glass (FAP) particles: Particle accumulation in tracheobronchial lymph nodes is compared with lung retention by these dogs.

in size and density, ^{57}Co-labeled FAP, and ^{57}Co-labeled PSL. On the other hand, the same pattern of $^{57}Co_3O_4$ particle accumulation in TBLN of the dog shown in Figure 8 was observed again when $^{57}Co_3O_4$ particles of similar physicochemical parameters were inhaled a second time 3 years after the first inhalation.

Particle transport toward and accumulation in TBLN originates from the pool of particles that has penetrated the alveolar epithelium. This pool contributes to the predominant fraction of particles deposited and retained in the alveolar region of the dog lung that is translocated into the interstitium. However, the large range of rates and fractions of particle accumulation in TBLN is in contrast with particle transport from the epithelium into the interstitium, which shows low intersubject variability and a rather uniform rate of 0.05/day (150-day half-life). These observations indicate that once the particles have arrived in interstitial spaces, particle transport toward lymphatic vessels and TBLN seemed to be maintained by individual factors, leading to a large intersubject variability. The possible mechanisms involved include free-particle transport in the interstitium toward lymphatic vessels under the influence of flow of tissue fluids (125,126,137) versus macrophage-mediated transport, including interstitial as well as alveolar macrophages, directed possibly by chemotaxis (87,119,120).

From reviewing the current literature, ICRP-66 (2) concluded that under physiological conditions, excluding exposure to highly concentrated aerosols, there will be little penetration of particles without specific cytotoxicity through TBLN into systemic circulation.

Concluding, particle accumulation in TBLN observed in individual dogs indicated large intersubject variability, as shown by the wide range of the accumulation rate and the accumulated fraction. Yet, particle accumulation in TBLN of dogs was more pronounced than in TBLN of rodents. In the absence of the kinetics of particle accumulation in human TBLN, the linear kinetics observed in individual dogs, including intersubject variability, may provide a suitable model of assessment of particle accumulation kinetics in human TBLN.

Kinetics of Intracellular Particle Dissolution by Alveolar Macrophages

In addition to particle transport, deposited material is cleared from the respiratory tract by biochemical processes dissociating the particles. Because this is an important clearance pathway for metal-containing particles, such as radionuclide-containing aerosol particles, the HRTM of ICRP-66 (2) discusses this pathway in great detail. Here we will limit considerations to particles that are not readily soluble in the alveolar epithelial-lining fluid. For the more rapid processes, we refer to a recent review (138) that distinguishes the clearance kinetics of hydrophilic versus lipophilic molecules dissolving from soluble particles. Limiting this review to particles that are relatively insoluble in the alveolar epithelial lining fluid means that the initiation of particle dissociation occurs in AM. In general, a relatively insoluble particle is phagocytosed by AM within hours after deposition on the alveolar epithelium (54) and remains there until it is eventually released by autolysis or other processes of the phagocyte (126) for a short time before it is phagoytosed by another AM. Basically, absorption into blood is a two-stage process:

1. Dissolution of particles assuming that the particles are in contact with the cytosolic or vacuolar liquid
2. Transport of the dissolved material to the vasculature and uptake by blood

In the first step, ions or molecules dissociated from the surface of the particle mix freely in the liquid. As the surrounding liquid within a cell or cellular vacuole is continuously exchanged, there will be no equilibrium concentration of ions or molecules leaving the particle surface and precipitating onto it. Furthermore, chemical reactions that result in dissociation will not generally be reversible. Therefore, particle dissolution in the peripheral lungs does not reach equilibrium, but continues until the particle is either dissolved or transformed into another chemical form with another dissolution kinetics.

The dissolution rate is proportional to the particle surface area and specific constants and factors of the particle material and the liquid solvent (139). If m, A_s, d are the particle mass, surface area, and diameter at time t, and ρ is the particle density, $\alpha_s = A_s/d^2$ the surface shape factor, $\alpha_v = m/\rho\, d^3$ the volume shape factor, and k the dissolution rate constant (dissolved mass per unit surface area per unit time) of the given particle material in the solvent, then:

$$\frac{dm}{dt} = -kA_s = -k\alpha_s d^2 = -\frac{k\alpha_s\, m^{2/3}}{(\rho\ \alpha_v)^{2/3}} \tag{7}$$

Hence, the fractional dissolution rate $S(t)$ is:

$$S(t) = -\frac{dm/dt}{m} = \frac{k\alpha_s}{\rho\alpha_v\ d} \tag{8}$$

The model thus predicts that the dissolution rate is inversely proportional to particle diameter and that, if the shape does not change, the fractional dissolution rate will increase with time as the particles become smaller.

Dissolution rates are potentially sensitive to conditions in the medium inside the phagolysosomal vacuole of the AM, making it difficult to simulate intracellular particle dissolution in AM. In fact, dissolution rates in the respiratory tract could well differ according to whether the particles are in the epithelial lining fluid, or phagocytosed by AM. Lundborg et al. (140,141) were the first to

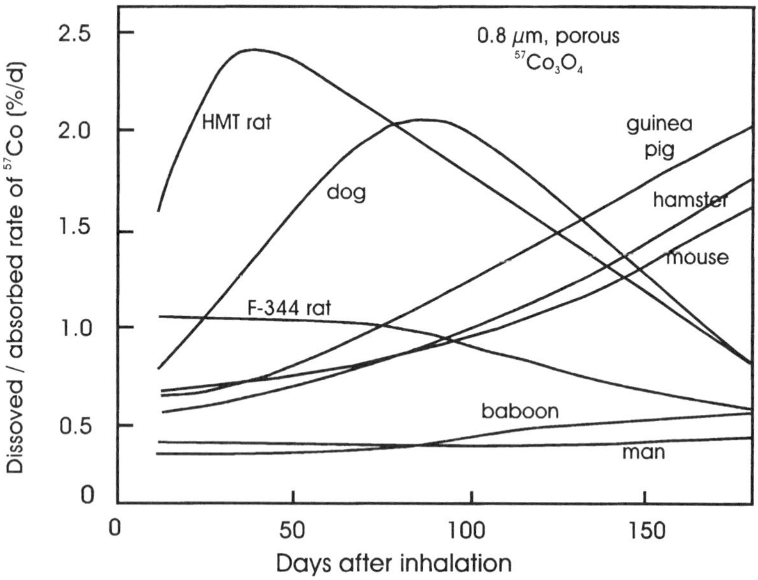
0.8 μm, porous
$^{57}Co_3O_4$
HMT rat
dog
guinea pig
hamster
mouse
F-344 rat
baboon
man
Dissoved / absorbed rate of ^{57}Co (%/d)
Days after inhalation
0
0.5
1.0
1.5
2.0
2.5
0
50
100
150

(a)

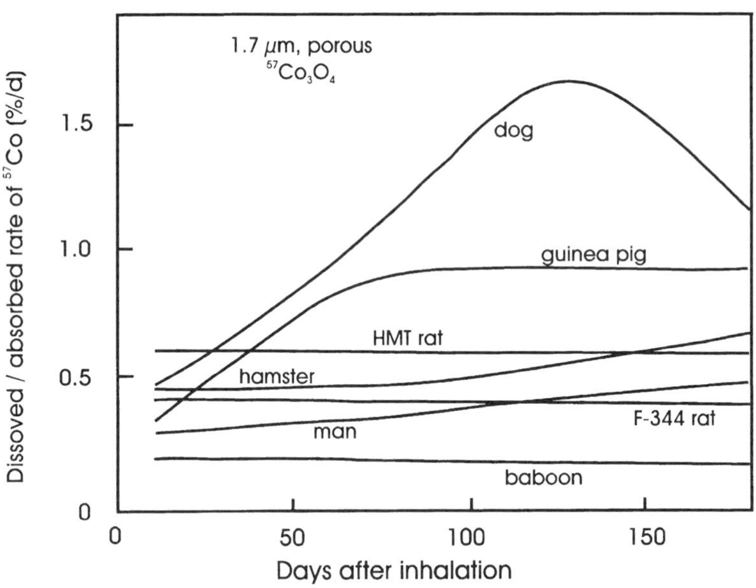
1.7 μm, porous
$^{57}Co_3O_4$
dog
guinea pig
HMT rat
hamster
man
F-344 rat
baboon
Dissoved / absorbed rate of ^{57}Co (%/d)
Days after inhalation
0
0.5
1.0
1.5
0
50
100
150

(b)

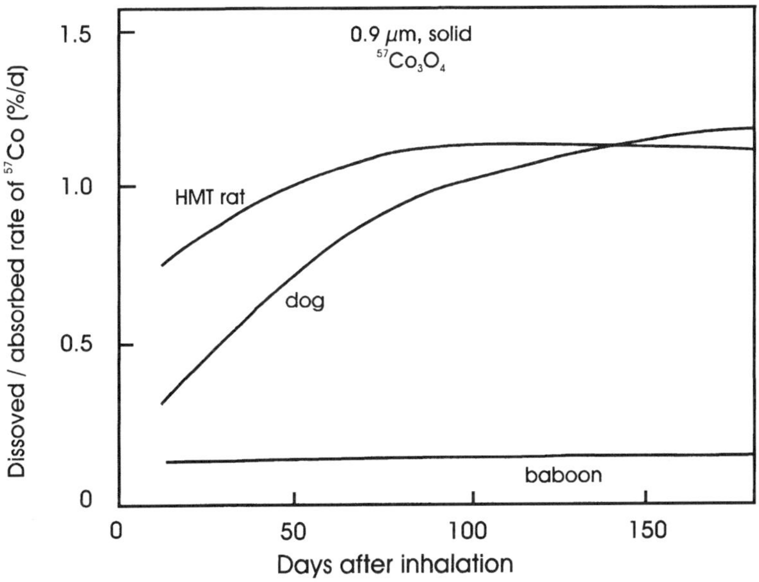

(c)

Figure 9 Kinetics of the fractional dissolution and absorption rates $S(t)$ of dissolved ^{57}Co by blood from moderately soluble $^{57}Co_3O_4$ particles of different specific surface areas in humans and various experimental animal species: monkeys, dogs, guinea pigs, two strains of rats (HMT, Fischer-344), hamsters, and mice: (a) Porous 0.8-μm; (b) porous 1.7-μm; (c) solid 0.9-μm particles.

show that manganese dioxide particles were dissolved faster in rabbit and human AM cultures than in a lung fluid simulant, such as the culture medium.

For the second step of absorption in blood—uptake of the dissolved material by blood—dissolved material must cross several membranous barriers as well as various fluids before it reaches the bloodstream:

1. The vacuolar membrane inside the AM to reach the cytosol
2. The cellular membrane of the AM to reach the alveolar epithelial lining fluid
3. The alveolar epithelium to reach interstitial space
4. The vascular endothelium to finally reach the blood

As each fluid may contain components different from the other fluids, there may be binding partners of the dissolved material that modulate its transport or its retention. Therefore, dissolution in an aqueous medium may not even be a qualitative guide to absorption in vivo. For example, Oberdörster (127) compared the observed lung clearance in rats of the oxides of nickel, zinc, and cadmium, which are all slowly dissolving in water. Nickel oxide was cleared mainly by AM-mediated particle transport toward ciliated airways, with a retention half-time of about 2 months, which corresponds to the transport rates in Figure 4. Zinc oxide dissolved rapidly and was retained with a half-time of about 6 hr. Cadmium oxide also dissolved rapidly in the lungs, but cadmium was retained with a half-time of more than 1 month as a result of chemical binding in the tissues of the lungs.

Generally, the rate-determining step in absorption of material from moderately soluble particles to blood is the intracellular dissolution in AM. This is particularly true if the dissolved material remains in a hydrophilic form and transport is diffusion determined. The latter is inversely related to the molecular weight according to Fick's law (142). For example, water and small molecules cross the epithelium readily, as illustrated by the high resorption of NaCl isotonic solutions used for BAL; the volume absorbed by each lung may reach several hundred milliliters. Observed clearance rates of low molecular weight solutes suggest that there are 0.6- to 1.5-nm pores in the region of the intercellular tight junctions of epithelial cells, including opening up of tight junctions (127). Transcellular transport by pinocytosis (i.e., nonspecific uptake of small droplets of extracellular fluid to form pinocytic vesicles in the epithelial cells) may also occur and may be important for hydrophilic solute molecules too large to diffuse through intercellular pores (127). In contrast, lipophilic molecules are passively transported across the cellular membranes, which provide a much larger surface area for absorption than do the extracellular pathways, generally resulting in much higher absorption rates (142). Transport of dissolved material from the interstitium across the vascular endothelium is usually 10–100 times higher than through the alveolar epithelium because of the higher permeability of the endothelial wall (127). However, these considerations will be modified or may not even apply to dissolved materials that undergo chemical transformation with binding partners present in any of the fluids and membranes to be crossed for absorption by blood.

Therefore, material-specific absorption rates need to be based on in vivo measurements of lung clearance, preferably in humans or in a large animal species, such as primates or dogs. Numerous lung clearance studies in the past on various animal species and on human subjects after accidental exposure to occupational aerosols suggested that absorption from particles was an important clearance pathway. This was unexpected for those materials showing minimal solubility in water, but were slowly dissolving or even moderately soluble in the lungs. These observations became particularly manifest in species such as primates and dogs, which, similar to humans, showed low particle transport rates toward ciliated airways. Most of these studies related to particles containing metal radionuclides produced during the nuclear fuel cycle (2).

In an attempt to compare the kinetics of absorption rates in various animal species and humans, two studies have been performed using three uniform particles of the same chemical compound, but different physical parameters: monodisperse ^{57}Co-labeled cobaltosic oxide (Co_3O_4) of different sizes and densities (i.e., different particle-specific surface areas; 91,123). In the first study (91,143), two moderately porous $^{57}Co_3O_4$ particles (Table 2) were inhaled by human subjects, baboons, beagle dogs, guinea pigs, three strains of rats (HMT, Fischer-344, Long-Evans rats), Syrian golden hamsters, and CBA/H mice. In the second study baboons, beagle dogs, and HMT rats inhaled $^{57}Co_3O_4$ particles of higher density (see Table 2).

Evaluation of absorption rates was followed for at least 6 months by sequential lung retention measurements, excretion analyses, and terminal organ–tissue analyses. Measurements were also made of the biokinetic behavior of the dissolved ^{57}Co following systemic uptake and the fractional absorption of material in the gastrointestinal tract. Because there was little intersubject variation within a given species strain, the mean absorption rates are shown in Figure 9 for each species. Patterns between species differed considerably. For each species, the rates increased with increasing specific surface area of the particles, according to Eq. (7). In those species showing high initial absorption rates, these rates increased with time. In those species, such as baboon and human, however, showing low initial absorption rates the rate remained constant over the 6-month period. This is in good agreement with Eq. (8), which predicts either an increasing absorption rate when there is substantial particle mass loss by a high dissolution rate and, hence, significant reduction of particle diameter; or an almost constant absorption rate when there is a slow dissolution rate resulting in little reduction of the particle diameter. The final decrease of the absorption rate in those species with an initial rapidly increasing rate is because more than 90% of the particle mass was either dissolved or eliminated from the lungs by particle transport. Hence, the pool of particles that was subject to dissolution and absorption simply emptied. Further confirmation of this predicted behavior was found in guinea pigs and hamsters, which showed a maximal absorption rate at a later time point—

Table 2 Parameters of $^{57}Co_3O_4$ Particles Used in Two Collaborative European Interspecies Comparisons of Lung Clearance

Study	I	I	II
Geometric mean diameter; d_{geom}(μm)	0.8	1.7	0.9
Density; ρ(g/cm^3)	2.8	2.8	4.6
Specific surface area; A_s(m^2/g)	15	6	2–3

Source: Refs. 91 and 123.

measurements on these animal species were made for about 300 days (144). Reproducibility of the kinetics of absorption rates was tested in HMT rats using moderately porous $^{57}Co_3O_4$ particles of both sizes (0.8 and 1.7 μm) 1 year later. The absorption rates resulted in the same patterns as observed a year before.

In addition to these interspecies comparisons, more clearance studies performed on dogs were carried out also using $^{57}Co_3O_4$ particles of different physical parameters (92,121,136). In all these studies the initial absorption rate was proportional to the specific surface area of the $^{57}Co_3O_4$ particles and varied more than 1 order of magnitude (145). Note: These studies emphasize that the in vivo absorption rate is not a constant value for a given compound, but this rate clearly depends on physical particle parameters: specific surface area, size, density, porosity, and such. This issue is only qualitatively addressed in HRTM of ICRP-66 (2) by the three compound categories, which classify compounds to be absorbed as fast, moderate, or slow. The dependence of absorption on particle parameters needs more quantitative evaluation in the future. In fact, from the linear relation between the in vivo absorption rate and the specific particle surface area, a dissolution rate constant for cobaltosic oxide in the milieu of the dogs' lungs was derived to be $k_{\text{lung}} = 4.4 \pm 0.3\ 10^{-7}$ g/cm^2 per day. This wholely material-dependent rate constant was in the same range as those found for various other metal oxides (Am, Ba, La, Co, Nb, Ce, Cm) determined in the lungs of dogs (146–152).

To better understand the underlying mechanisms of particle dissolution, several investigators studied particle dissolution in cultures of AM (140,141,153,154). It was confirmed by electron microscopy that particles were contained in membrane-bound vacuoles (phagosomes) onto which primary lysosomes fused, forming phagolysosomes. To quantify the kinetics of intracellular particle dissolution, we developed a 2-week cell culture assay in which uniform, moderately soluble $^{57}Co_3O_4$ particles were quantitatively phagocytosed and continuously dissolved by AM. From the increase with time of the dissolved ^{57}Co fractions a dissolution rate was evaluated (122,136,155–157).

Generally, particles showing increasing dissolution with increasing acidity in aqueous solvents dissolved more rapidly in AM than in simulants of extracellular lung fluids. This indicated that the proton concentration in the phagolysosomal vacuole played an important role in intracellular particle dissolution. Indeed, the phagolysosomal pH value was between 4.3 and 5.3 for human, monkey, dog, rabbit, guinea pig, and rat AM (158–162). When the phagolysosomal pH value was compared with intracellular $^{57}Co_3O_4$ particle dissolution in AM obtained from cattle, dogs, and rats, the particle dissolution rate increased with increasing phagolysosomal proton concentration (156,163). Furthermore, when the phagolysosomal proton concentration was decreased (increased pH value from 4.3 to 5.4) by treating cultured dog AM with chloroquine, the intracellular particle dissolution rate decreased by a factor of 2 (164).

In contrast, uranium oxide particles seemed to be less soluble in AM than in simulants of extracellular lung fluids (165,166). However, on looking more closely at the ultrastructure of the AM these particles had dissolved intracellularly, but the dissolved uranium precipitated as phosphate owing to the high acid phosphatase activity in lysosomes (167). Similar phosphate precipitation was found for chromium, aluminium, gallium, indium, lanthanum, cerium, and thorium, clearly indicating that the dissolved particle material may undergo chemical reactions within AM. For intracellular $^{57}Co_3O_4$ particle dissolution in dog AM, metallothionein—a metal-chelating protein—was induced by dissolved ^{57}Co and was associated with this protein inside the AM (165,168). From this we hypothesize that other chelating molecules present in the cytosol may also play a role in particle dissolution and transport of the dissolved material inside and out of AM.

Intracellular particle dissolution rates obtained from cultured dog AM increased with increasing specific surface area of different $^{57}Co_3O_4$ particles, such that the dissolution rate constant for $^{57}Co_3O_4$ was calculated to be $k_{am} = 4.1 \pm 0.5\ 10^{-7}$ g/cm^2 per day (145). The very close agreement of the two dissolution rate constants—k_{lung} given earlier and k_{am}—showed that the dissolving medium is the same and, hence, that the rate-determining step of $^{57}Co_3O_4$ particle dissolution and subsequent absorption by blood is intracellular dissolution in AM in vivo in the lungs.

In summary, dissolution of particles that are not readily soluble is maintained intracellularly in AM. For those particles, such as many metal oxides, that are more soluble in more acidic aqueous solvents, particle dissolution is faster than in extracellular lung fluids owing to the phagolysosomal pH value of 4.3–5.3. For these particles, intracellular dissolution is an important clearance mechanism. It eventually turns into an essential clearance pathway out of the lungs if the dissolved particle material is not bound to a molecular partner that remains retained in some sites of the lungs, but is transported to blood vessels.

IV. Summary and Conclusion

Particles inhaled at the end of a breath are deposited in the conducting airways, according to their aerodynamic behavior. Mucociliary clearance is complete for particles larger than 6-μm–geometric diameter deposited in central airways, but may be incomplete in small airways. Furthermore, with decreasing physical size of the particles, the fraction of slowly cleared particles increases to more than 60% for particles smaller than 1 μm. Although there is evidence that airway macrophages play a role in slow particle clearance from the airways, the quantitative aspects of the various mechanisms leading to slow clearance in the airways remains to be solved. This issue is of considerable importance, because slow particle clearance from the airways may play a role in the development of airway diseases, including COPD, carcinogenicity in small airways, and others.

Although particle transport from the peripheral lung toward ciliated airways is a predominant pathway of particle clearance in rodents and sheep, it plays only a minor role in the lungs of humans, monkeys, and dogs. In each experimental animal species maintained under controlled conditions, intersubject variability is low. There is evidence (1) that particle transport from the peripheral lung toward ciliated airways is mediated by AM, and particle transport of free (nonphagocytosed) particles may play a role which, however, is considered to be minor. (2) From interspecies comparisons, there is evidence that the path length from alveoli to ciliated terminal bronchioli may determine the particle transport rate. The concept of a nonstochastic, actively directed migration of AM on the alveolar epithelium toward ciliated airways, guided by chemoattractants is more consistent with what is known about AM migration, than that of random movement of AM onto ciliated airways. More experimental studies are needed to confirm, in particular, the underlying mechanisms.

Even though there is predominant particle transport from the epithelium of the dog lung into the interstitium, this transport pathway is minor in the lungs of rats and hamsters. Conversely, particle transport toward ciliated airways dominates in rodents and is a minor pathway in dogs. Because of similarities in long-term lung retention and the kinetics of AM-mediated particle transport toward the ciliated airways, it is plausible to presume kinetics of particle transport through the alveolar epithelium in monkeys and humans similar to those found in dogs. The reasons for the very clear interspecies differences remains to be solved. Also, the nature of transport and its destination in the tissue requires further investigations.

Particle accumulation in tracheobronchial lymph nodes (TBLN) observed in individual dogs indicates large intersubject variability. Yet, particle accumulation in TBLN of dogs is more prominent than in rodents. In the absence of direct information on the kinetics of particle uptake in human TBLN the linear kinetics observed in individual dogs, including intersubject variability, may provide a suitable model for assessment of the kinetics of particle accumulation.

Dissolution of particles that are not readily soluble is maintained intracellularly in alveolar macrophages (AM). For those particles, such as many metal oxides, which are more soluble in more acidic aqueous solvents, particle dissolution is faster than in extracellular lung fluids, owing to the phagolysosomal pH value of 4.3–5.3 and the presence of chelating biomolecules in the AM. For these particles, intracellular dissolution becomes an important clearance mechanism that depends not only on the chemical compound, but also on physical particle parameters, such as the specific surface area. It eventually turns into an essential clearance pathway from the lungs if the dissolved material is not bound to a molecular partner that stays retained in some unit of the lungs, but is transported to blood vessels. In each species strain intersubject variability in dissolution is low. Questions to be solved relate to the role of the various chelating biomolecules in the transport of the dissolved material out of the cell through cells and tissues toward blood vessels.

All phenomena of particle transport or disintegration leading to particle clearance from the lungs or particle relocation within the lungs are concerted systemic reactions involving various cell types and extracellular matrix and fluids containing interactive molecules, mediators, and other components. These responses to foreign material deposited in the respiratory tract are maintained by and also feed back to the immune system. Many of these multiple interactions are not yet fully understood and need further investigations. Furthermore, although the immune response is delicately balanced in good health under ''normal'' conditions, it may become out-of-balance in disease and during exposure to airborne noxae. It remains a considerable challenge to explore the role of particles deposited on the respiratory epithelium in the various steps of initiation and pathogenesis of disease.

Acknowledgments

The authors are very grateful to Dr. Michael R. Bailey, National Radiological Protection Board of the United Kingdom, Chilton UK, for his thorough review and his editorial help to finish this manuscript.

Nomenclature

A	fraction of slowly cleared particles from airways
A_s	surface area of a particle
α_s	surface shape factor of a particle
α_v	volume shape factor of a particle
AM	alveolar macrophage
BAL	bronchoalveolar lavage
CF	cystic fibrosis
CL(t)	particle clearance from the lungs at time t
COPD	chronic obstructive pulmonary disease
d	particle diameter
d_{ae}	aerodynamic particle diameter
d_{geom}	geometric particle diameter, diameter of the physical size of a particle
ELF	epithelial-lining fluid
FAP	fused aluminosilicate particles
$g(t)$	rate of AM-mediated particle transport from the lung periphery towards the larynx
GIT	gastrointestinal tract
ICS	immotile cilia syndrome

ICRP	International Commission for Radiological Protection
ILD	initial particle deposit in the lungs
HRTM	Human Respiratory Tract Model for Radiological Protection of ICRP-66
k	dissolution rate constant (dissolved mass per unit surface area per unit time)
$\ln(t)$	particle transport rate toward lymphatic drainage vessels
[LN]/[L]	particle concentration ratio between TBLN and lungs
$m(t)$	particle mass at time t
$M(t)$	rate of particle transport in the lungs
$p_i(t)$	intrapulmonary transport particle rates
PET	positron emission tomography
PMN	polymorphoneutrophilic leukocytes
PSL	polystyrene–latex particles
$R(t)$	particle retention in the lungs at time t
$R_t(t)$	thoracic particle retention at time t
ρ	density of a particle
$S(t)$	rate of particle dissolution and uptake of the dissolved particle material by blood
SPECT	single-photon emission computer tomography
t_h(fast)	half life of fast-particle clearance from airways by mucociliary action
t_p	time (sec) of breath-hold during an inhalation maneuver
TBLN	tracheobronchial lymph nodes
USEPA	U.S. Environmental Protection Agency
VL	volumetric lung depth

References

1. Morrow PE. Clearance kinetics of inhaled particles. In: Brain JD, Proctor DF, Reid LM, eds. Respiratory Defense Mechanisms Part II. New York: Marcel Dekker, 1977:491–543.
2. Bair WJ, Bailey MR, Cross FT, Cuddihy RG, Gehr P, James AC, Johnson JR, Masse R, Roy M, Sathlhofen W. Human respiratory tract model for radiological protection. ICRP Publication 66. Ann ICRP 1994; 24 (1–3).
3. Geiser M, Im Hof V, Gehr P, Cruz-Orive LM. Histological and stereological analysis of particle retention in the conducting airways of hamster lungs. J Aerosol Med 1990; 3:131–145.
4. Geiser M, Cruz-Orive LM, Im Hof V, Gehr P. Assessment of particle retention and clearance in the intrapulmonary conducting airways of hamster lungs with the fractionator. J Microsc 1990; 160:75–88.
5. Stirling C, Patrick G. The localisation of particles retained in the trachea of the rat. Pathology 1980; 131:309–320.
6. Patrick G, Stirling C. The retention of particles in large airways of the respiratory tract. Proc R Soc Lond B 1977; 198:455–462.
7. Schlesinger RB. Clearance from the respiratory tract. Fundam Appl Toxicol 1985; 5:435–450.

8. Stahlhofen W, Gebhart J, Heyder J. Experimental determination of the regional deposition on aerosol particles in the human respiratory tract. Am Ind Hyg Assoc J 1980; 41:385–399.
9. Morrow PE, Gibb FR, Gazioglu KM. A study of particulate clearance from the human lungs. Am Rev Respir Dis 1968; 96:1209–1221.
10. Deitmer T. Physiology and pathology of the mucociliary system. In: Pfaltz CR, ed. Advances in Oto-Rhino-Laryngology. Basel: Karger, 1989:1–136.
11. Hilding AC. Ciliary streaming in the lower respiratory tract. Am J Physiol 1957; 191:404–410.
12. Pavia D. Lung mucociliary clearance. In: Clarke SW, Pavia D, eds. Aerosols and the Lung. London: Butterworths, 1984:127–155.
13. Wolff RK. Mucociliary function. In: Parent RP, ed. Comparative Biology of the Normal Lung. Boca Raton, FL: CRC Press, 1992:659–680.
14. Yeates DB. Mucus rheology. In: Crystal RG, West JB, eds. The Lung, Scientific Foundations. New York: Raven Press, 1991:197–203.
15. Iravani J, van As A. Mucus transport in the tracheobronchial tree of normal and bronchitis rats. J Pathol 1972; 106:81–93.
16. Sturgess JM. Mucociliary clearance and mucus secretion in the lung. In: Witschi HP, Brain JD, eds. Toxicology of Inhaled Materials. Berlin: Springer Verlag, 1985: 319–367.
17. Van As A. Pulmonary airway clearance mechanisms. Am Rev Respir Dis 1977; 115:721–727.
18. Gil J, Weibel ER. Extracellular lining of bronchioles after perfusion–fixation of rat lungs from electron microscopy. Anat Rec 1971; 169:185–200.
19. Luchtel DL. Mucociliary interactions in rabbit intrapulmonary airways. Cell Motil 1982; 1:77–81.
20. Foster WM, Langenback EG, Bergofsky EH. Lung mucociliary function in man: interdependence of bronchial and tracheal mucus transport velocities with lung clearance in bronchial asthma and healthy subjects. Ann Occup Hyg (Inhaled Particles V) 1982; 26:227–244.
21. Smaldone GC, Perry RJ, Bennet WD, Messina MS, Zwang J, Ilowite J. Interpretation of ''24 hour lung retention'' in studies of mucociliary clearance. J Aerosol Med 1988; 1:11–20.
22. Bennett WD, Chapman WF, Lay JC, Gerrity TR. Pulmonary clearance of inhaled particles 24 to 48 hours post deposition: effect of beta-adrenergic stimulation. J Aerosol Med 1993; 6:53–62.
23. Isawa T, Teshima T, Hirano T, Ebina A, Konno K. Mucociliary clearance mechanism in smoking and nonsmoking normal subjects. J Nucl Med 1984; 25:352–359.
24. Yeates DB, Gerrity TR, Garrard CS. Particle deposition and clearance in the bronchial tree. Ann Biomed Eng 1981; 9:577–592.
25. Albert RE, Lippmann M, Peterson HT, Berger J, Sanborn K, Bohning D. Bronchial deposition and clearance of aerosols. Arch Intern Med 1973; 131:115–127.
26. Albert RE, Lippmann M, Peterson HT. The effects of cigarette smoking on the kinetics of bronchial clearance in humans and donkeys. In: Walton WH, ed. Inhaled Particles III. Oxford: Pergamon Press, 1971:165–180.
27. Albert RE, Lippmann M, Spiegelman J, Strehlow C, Briscoe W, Wolfson P, Nelson

N. The clearance of radioactive particles from the human lung. In: Davies CN, ed. Inhaled Particles and Vapours II. Oxford: Pergamon Press, 1967:361–377.
28. Lippmann M, Albert RE, Yeates DB, Berger JM, Foster WM, Bohning DE. Factors affecting tracheobronchial mucociliary transport. In: Walton WH, ed. Inhaled Particles IV. Oxford: Pergamon Press, 1977: 305–319.
29. Toomes H, Vogt-Moykopf I, Heller WD, Ostertag H. Measurements of mucociliary clearance in smokers and nonsmokers using a bronchoscopic video-technical method. Lung 1981; 159:27–34.
30. Gamsu G, Weintraub RM, Nadel JA. Clearance of tantalum from airway of different caliber in man evaluated by a roentgenographic method. Am Rev Respir Dis 1973; 107:214–224.
31. Friedman M, Scott FD, Poole DO, Dougherty R, Chapman GA, Watson H, Sackner MA. A new roentgenographic method for estimating mucous velocity in airways. Am Rev Respir Dis 1977; 115:67–72.
32. Foster WM. Is 24 hour lung retention an index of alveolar clearance? J Aerosol Med 1988; 1:1–10.
33. Morrow PE, Yu CP. Models of aerosol behavior in airways. In: Moren F, Newhouse MT, Dolovich MB, eds. Aerosols in Medicine, Principles Diagnosis and Therapy. Amsterdam: Elsevier Science, 1985:149–191.
34. Yu CP, Hu JP, Yen BM, Spektor D, Lippmann M. Models for mucociliary particle clearance in lung airways. In: Lee SD, Schneider T, Grant LD, Verkerk PJ, eds. Aerosols: Research, Risk, Assessment and Control Strategies. Chelsea, MI: Lewis, 1986:569–578.
35. Yeates DB, Gerrity TR, Garrard CS. Characteristics of tracheobronchial deposition and clearance in man. Ann Occup Hyg (Inhaled Particles V) 1982; 26:245–257.
36. Cuddihy RG, Yeh HC. Respiratory tract clearance of particles and substances dissociated from particles. In: Mohr U, ed. Inhalation Toxicology: The Design and Interpretation of Inhalation Studies and Their Use in Risk Assessment. New York: Springer-Verlag, 1988:169–193.
37. Scheuch G, Stahlhofen W, Heyder J. An approach to deposition and clearance measurements in human airways. J Aerosol Med 1996; 9:35–41.
38. Stahlhofen W, Scheuch G, Bailey MR. Investigations of retention of inhaled particles in the human bronchial tree. Radiat Prot Dosim 1995; 60:311–319.
39. Stahlhofen W, Gebhart J, Heyder J, Philipson K, Camner P. Intercomparison of regional deposition of aerosol particles in the human respiratory tract and their long-term elimination. Exp Lung Res 1981; 2:131–139.
40. Stahlhofen W, Gebhart J, Rudolf G, Scheuch G. Measurement of lung clearance with pulses of radioactively-labelled aerosols. J Aerosol Sci 1986; 17:333–336.
41. Stahlhofen W. Human lung clearance following bolus inhalation of radioaerosols. In: Crapo JD, Smolko ED, Miller FJ, Graham JA, Hayes AW, eds. Extrapolation of Dosimetric Relationships for Inhaled Particles and Gases. San Diego, CA: Academic Press, 1987:153–166.
42. Stahlhofen W, Gebhart J, Heyder J, Scheuch G. Deposition pattern of droplets from medical nebulizers in the human respiratory tract. Bull Eur Physiopathol Res 1983; 19:459–463.

43. Scheuch G, Stahlhofen W, Fang CP, Lippmann M. Aerosol recovery after bolus inhalations into an airway cast. J Aerosol Sci 1993; 24:S355–S356.
44. Fang CP, Lippmann M, Scheuch G, Stahlhofen W. Effect of flow rate on aerosol bolus penetration in a hollow canine lung airway cast. Exp Lung Res 1995; 21: 547–558.
45. Kreyling WG, Blanchard JD, Godleski JJ, Häußermann S, Heyder J, Hutzler P, Schulz H, Sweeney TD, Takenaka S. Shallow aerosol bolus inhalation in beagle dogs: sites of retention and clearance. Eur Respir J 1995; 8:352s.
46. Schulz H, Blanchard JD, Godleski JJ, Heyder J, Kreyling WG, Mellert U, Sweeney TD, Ziesenis A. Shallow aerosol bolus inhalation in dogs: respiratory physiology and intrapulmonary deposition. Eur Respir J 1995; 8:439s.
47. Stahlhofen W, Scheuch G, Bailey MR. Measurements of the tracheobronchial clearance of particles after aerosol bolus inhalation. Ann Occup Hyg (Inhaled Particles VII) 1994; 38:189–196.
48. Anderson M, Philipson K, Svartengren M, Camner P. Human deposition and clearance of 6 mm particles inhaled with an extremely low flow rate. Exp Lung Res 1995; 21:187–195.
49. Svartengren K, Philipson K, Svartengren M, Anderson M, Camner P. Tracheobronchial deposition and clearance in small airways in asthmatic subjects. Eur Respir J 1996; 9:1123–1129.
50. Falk R, Philipson K, Svartengren M, Jarvis N, Bailey M, Camner P. Clearance of particles from small ciliated airways. Exp Lung Res 1997; 23:495–515.
51. Camner P, Anderson M, Philipson K, Bailey A, Hashish A, Jarvis N, Bailey M, Svartengren M. Human bronchiolar deposition and retention of 6, 8 and 10 μm particles. Exp Lung Res 1997; 23:517–534.
52. Brain JD, Godleski JJ, Sorokin SP. Quantification, origin, and fate of pulmonary macrophages. In: Brain JD, Proctor DF, Reid LM, eds. Respiratory Defense Mechanisms. New York: Marcel Dekker, 1977:849–892.
53. Sorokin SP, Brain JD. Pathways of clearance in mouse lungs exposed to iron oxyde aerosols. Anat Rec 1975; 181:581–626.
54. Brain JD. Macrophages in the respiratory tract. In: Fishman AP, Fisher AB, eds. Handbook of Physiology. Bethesda, MD: American Physiology Society, 1985:447–471.
55. Brain JD. Lung magrophages: how many kinds are there? what do they do? Am Rev Respir Dis 1988; 137:507–509.
56. Schürch S, Gehr P, Im Hof V, Geiser M, Green FHY. Surfactant displaces particles toward the epithelium in airways and alveoli. Respir Physiol 1990; 80:17–32.
57. Gehr P, Schürch S, Berthiaume Y, Im Hof V, Geiser M. Particle retention in airways by surfactant. J Aerosol Med 1990; 3:27–43.
58. Gehr P, Im Hof V. The fate of particles deposited in the airways. J Aerosol Med 1991; 4:6.
59. Churg A, Stevens B. Association of lung cancer and airway particle concentration. Environ Res 1988; 45:58–63.
60. Leith DE. Cough. In: Brain JD, Proctor DF, Reid LM, eds. Respiratory Defense Mechanisms. New York: Marcel Dekker, 1977:545–592.

61. Bennett WD, Foster WM, Chapman WF. Cough-enhanced mucus clearance in the normal lung. J Appl Physiol 1990; 69:1670–1675.
62. Zenker FA. Von Staubinhalationskrankeiten in der Lunge. Dtsch Arch Klin Med 1867; 2:116–117.
63. Lorenz E. Radioactivity and lung cancer, a critical review of lung cancer in the mines of Schneeberg and Joachimsthal. J Natl Cancer Inst 1944; 5:1–15.
64. Morrow PE, Bates DV, Fish BR, Hatch TF, Mercer TT. ICRP Taskgroup on Lung Dynamics 1966 deposition and retention models for internal dosimetry of the human respiratory tract. Health Phys 1966; 12:173–207.
65. USEPA United States Environmental Protection Agency Office of Research and Development. Air Quality Criteria for Particulate Matter. Washington DC: EPA/600//P-95/001cF, 1996.
66. Valberg PA, Blanchard JD. Pulmonary macrophage physiology: origin; motility; endocytosis. In: Parent RC, ed. Treatise on Pulmonary Toxicology: Comparative Biology of the Normal Lung. New York: CRC Press, 1992:681–724.
67. Hahn FF, Newton GJ, Bryant PL. In vitro phagocytosis of respirable-sized monodisperse particles by alveolar macrophages. In: Sanders CL, Schneider RP, Dagle GE, Ragan HA, eds. Springfield, VA: National Technical Information Service, Proceedings of the 16th Annual Hanford Biology Symposium 1977: 424–435.
68. Tabata Y, Ikada Y. Effect of size and surface charge of polymer microspheres on their phagocytosis by macrophage. Biomaterials 1988; 9:356–362.
69. Seymour L, Schacht E, Duncan R. The effect of size of polystyrene particles on their retention within the rat peritoneal compartment, and on their interaction with rat peritoneal macrophages in vitro. Cell Biol Int Rep 1991; 15:277–286.
70. Ishikawa Y, Muramatsu N, Ohshima H, Kondo T. Effect of particle size on phagocytosis of latex particles by guinea pig polymorphonuclear leucocytes. J Biomater Sci Polym Ed 1991; 2:53–60.
71. Ayhan H, Tuncel A, Bor N, Piskin E. Phagocytosis of monosize polystyrene-based microspheres having different size and surface properties. J Biomater Sci Polym Ed 1995; 7:329–342.
72. Gonzalez O, Smith PL, Goodman SB. Effect of size, concentration, surface area, and volume of polymethacrylate particles on human macrophages in vitro. J Biomed Mater Res 1996; 30:463–473.
73. Takenaka S, Dornhöfer-Takenaka H, Muhle H. Alveolar distribution of fly ash and of titanium dioxide after long-term inhalation by Wistar rats. J Aerosol Sci 1986; 17:361–364.
74. Takenaka S, Muhle H. Clearance of inhaled insoluble particles from the alveolar regions via the extraalveolar perivascular sheath. In: Schikarski W, Fissan HJ, Friedlander SK, eds. Aerosols: Formation and Reactivity. Oxford: Pergamon Press, 1986:318–321.
75. Ferin J, Oberdörster G, Penney DP, Soderholm SC, Gelein R, Piper HC. Increased pulmonary toxicity of ultrafine particles. I. Particle clearance, translocation, mophology. J Aerosol Sci 1990; 21:381–384.
76. Ferin J, Oberdörster G, Soderholm SC, Gelein R. Pulmonary tissue access of ultrafine particles. J Aerosol Med 1991; 4:57–68.

77. Ferin J, Oberdörster G, Penney DP. Pulmonary retention of ultrafine and fine particles in rats. Am J Respir Cell Mol Biol 1992; 6:535–542.
78. Oberdörster G, Cox C, Gelein R. Intratracheal instillation versus intratracheal inhalation of tracer particles for measuring lung clearance function. Exp Lung Res 1997; 23:17–34.
79. Lehnert BE, Morrow PE. Association of 59-iron oxide with alveolar macrophages during alveolar clearance. Exp Lung Res 1985;9:1–16.
80. Lehnert BE, Valdez YE, Lehnert NM, Saunders GC, Steinkamp JA. Airway intraluminal macrophages: evidence of origin and comparisons to alveolar macrophages. Am J Respir Cell Mol Biol 1990; 3:377–391.
81. Lehnert BE, Ortiz JB, Valdez YE, Steinkamp JA. Influence of particulate load on macrophage proliferation. Toxicologist 1990; 10:399.
82. Lehnert BE, Ortiz JB, London JE, Valdez YE, Cline AJ, Sebring RJ, Tietjen GL. Migratory behaviors of alveolar macrophages during alveolar clearance of light and heavy burdens of particles. Exp Lung Res 1990; 16:451–479.
83. Ellender M, Hodgson A, Wood KL, Moody JC. Effect of bronchopulmonary lavage on lung retention and clearance of particulate material in hamsters. Environ Health Perspect 1992; 97:209–213.
84. Morgan A, Kellington JP, Collier CG, Hodgson A. Labelling rat alveolar macrophages with fluorescent microspheres. Inhal Toxicol 1995; 7:255–267.
85. Ferin J, Feldstein ML. Pulmonary clearance and hilar lymph node content in rats after particle exposure. Environ Res 1978; 16:342–352.
86. Harmsen AG, Mason MJ, Muggenburg BA, Gillett NA, Jarpe MA, Bice DE. Migration of neutrophils from the lung to tracheobronchial lymph node. J Leukoc Biol 1980; 41:95–103.
87. Harmsen AG, Muggenburg BA, Snipes MB, Bice DE. The role of macrophages in particle translocation from lungs to lymph nodes. Science 1985; 230:1277–1280.
88. Zeltner GM, Sweeney TD, Skornik WA, Feldman HA, Brain JD. Retention and clearance of 0.9 μm particles inhaled by hamsters during rest and exercise. J Appl Physiol 1991; 70:1137–1145.
89. Roggli VL, Shelburne JD. Mineral pneumoconiosis. In: Dail DH, Hammar SP, eds. Pulmonary Pathology. New York: Springer Verlag, 1988:589–617.
90. Kreyling WG. Interspecies comparison of lung clearance of ''insoluble'' particles. J Aerosol Med 1990; 3:S93–S110.
91. Bailey MR, Kreyling WG, André S, Batchelor A, Black A, Collier CG, Drosselmeyer E, Ferron GA, Foster P, Haider B, Hodgson A, Métivier H, Moores SR, Morgan A, Müller HL, Patrick G, Pearman I, Pickering S, Ramsden D, Stirling C, Talbot RJ. An interspecies comparison of the lung clearance of inhaled monodisperse cobalt oxide particles—part I: objectives and summary of results. J Aerosol Sci 1989; 20:169–188.
92. Kreyling WG, Schumann G, Ortmaier A, Ferron GA, Karg E. Particle transport from the lower respiratory tract. J Aerosol Med 1988; 1:351–369.
93. Philipson K, Falk R, Gustafsson J, Camner P. Long-term lung clearance of 195 Au-labeled Teflon particles in humans. Exp Lung Res 1996; 22:65–83.
94. Collier CG, James AC, Ellender M. The effect of alpha-irradiation on retention of particles in the rat lung. Ann Occup Hyg 1988; 32:1007–1015.

95. Snipes MB, Clem M. Retention of microspheres in the rat lung after intratracheal installation. Environ Res 1981; 24:33–41.
96. Snipes MB, Boecker BB, McClellan RO. Retention of monodisperse or polydisperse aluminosilicate particles inhaled by dogs, rats and mice. Toxicol Appl Pharmacol 1983; 69:345–362.
97. Langenback EG, Bergofsky EH, Halpern JG, Foster WM. Determining deposition sites of inhaled lung particles and their effect on clearance. J Appl Physiol 1990; 68:1427–1434.
98. Langenback EG, Bergofsky EH, Halpern JG, Foster WM. Supramicron-sized particle clearance from alveoli: route and kinetics. J Appl Physiol 1990; 69:1302–1308.
99. Sorokin SP, Brain JD. Pathways of clearance in mouse lungs exposed to iron oxide aerosols. Anat Rec 1975; 181:581–626.
100. Bailey MR, Hodgson A, Smith H. Respiratory retention of relatively insoluble particles in rodents. J Aerosol Sci 1985; 16:279–293.
101. Brain JD, Frank NR. Alveolar macrophage adhesion: wash electrolyte composition and free cell yield. J Appl Physiol 1973; 34:75–80.
102. Brain JD, Godleski JJ, Sorokin SP. Quantification, origin and fate of pulmonary macrophages. In: Brain JD, Proctor DF, Reid LM, eds. Respiratory Defense Mechanisms Part 2. New York: Marcel Dekker, 1977:849–892.
103. Muhle H, Bellmann B, Heinrich U. Overloading of lung clearance during chronic exposure of experimental animals to particles. Ann Occup Hyg (Inhaled Particles VI) 1988; 32:141–147.
104. Bellmann B, Muhle H, Creutzenberg O, Kilpper R, Morrow PE, Mermelstein R. Reversibility of clearance impairment after subchronic test toner inhalation. Exp Pathol 1989; 37:234–238.
105. Morrow PE. Possible mechanisms to explain dust overloading of the lungs. Appl Toxicol 1988; 10:369–384.
106. Yu CP, Chen YK, Morrow PE. An analysis of alveolar macrophage mobility kinetics at dust overloading of the lungs. Fundam Appl Toxicol 1989; 13:452–459.
107. Warheit DB, Chang LY, Hill LH, Hook GER, Crapo JD, Brody AR. Pulmonary macrophage accumulation and asbestos-induced lesions at sites of fiber deposition. Am Rev Respir Dis 1984; 129:301–310.
108. Warheit DB, George G, Hill LH, Snyderman R, Brody AR. Inhaled asbestos activates a complement-dependent chemoattractant for macrophages. Lab Invest 1984; 52:505–514.
109. Warheit DB, Hill LH, George G, Brody AR. Time course of chemotactic factor generation and the corresponding macrophage response to asbestos inhalation. Am Rev Respir Dis 1986; 134:128–133.
110. Warheit DB, Overby LH, George G, Brody AR. Pulmonary macrophages are attracted to inhaled particles through complement activation. Exp Lung Res 1988; 14:51–66.
111. Tyler WS, Julian MD. Gross and subgross anatomy of lungs, pleura, connective tissue septa, distal airways, and structural units. In: Parent RC, ed. Treatise on Pulmonary Toxicology: Pulmonary Toxicology: Comparative Biology of the Normal Lung. New York: CRC Press, 1992.
112. Crystal RG, West JB. The Lung. New York: Raven Press, 1991.

113. Lehnert BE, Valdez YE, Tietjen GL. Alveolar macrophages–particle relationships during lung clearance. Am J Respir Cell Mol Biol 1989; 1:145–154.
114. Lehnert BE, Ortiz JB, Steinkamp JA, Tietjen GL, Sebring RJ, Oberdörster G. Mechanisms underlying the particle redistribution phenomenon. J Aerosol Med 1992; 5: 261–279.
115. Adamson IYR, Bowden DH. Adaptive responses of the pulmonary macrophagic system to carbon. II. Morphologic studies. Lab Invest 1978; 38:430–438.
116. Brody AR, Hill LH, Adkins B Jr, O'Connor RW. Chrysotile asbestos inhalation in rats: deposition pattern and reaction of alveolar epithelium and pulmonary macrophages. Rev Respir Dis 1981; 123:670–679.
117. Kreyling WG, Ferron GA, Fürst G, Heilmann P, Neuner M, Ruprecht L, Schumann G, Takenaka S, Heyder J. Long-term exposure of dogs to a sulfite aerosol: III. Macrophage mediated long-term particle clearance. Inhalation Toxicology 1992; 4:197–233.
118. Kreyling WG, Dirscherl P, Ferron GA, Heilmann P, Josten M, Miaskowski U, Neuner M, Reitmeir P, Ruprecht L, Schumann G, Takenaka S, Ziesenis A, Heyder J. Health effects of sulfur-related environmental air pollution: III. Nonspecific respiratory defense capacities. Inhalation Tox 1999; 11: In press.
119. Corry D, Kulkarni P, Lipsomb MF. The migration of broncho-alveolar macrophages into hilar lymph nodes. Alveolar macrophage. J Pathol 1984; 115:321–328.
120. Gillet AM, Harmsen AB, Stegelmeier B. Translocation by macrophages from lung to lymph nodes. J Aerosol Med 1989; 2:29–39.
121. Kreyling WG, Ferron GA, Haider, B. An interspecies comparison of the lung clearance of inhaled monodisperse cobalt oxide particles—part IV: lung clearance of inhaled cobalt oxide particles in beagle dogs. J Aerosol Sci 1989; 20:219–232.
122. Kreyling WG, Godleski JJ, Kariya ST, Rose RM, Brain JD. In vitro dissolution of uniform cobalt oxide particles by human and canine alveolar macrophages. Am J Respir Cell Mol Biol 1990; 2:413–422.
123. Kreyling WG, André S, Collier CG, Ferron GA, Métivier H, Schumann G. Interspecies comparison of lung clearance after inhalation of monodisperse, solid cobalt oxide aerosol particles. J Aerosol Sci 1991; 22:509–535.
124. André S, Métivier H, Masse R. An interspecies comparison of the lung clearance of inhaled monodisperse cobalt oxide particles—part III: lung clearance of inhaled cobalt oxide particles in beagle dogs. J Aerosol Sci 1989; 20:205–218.
125. Lauweryns JM, Baert JH. Alveolar clearance and the role of the pulmonary lymphatics. Am Rev Respir Dis 1977; 115:625–683.
126. Lehnert BE, Valdez YE, Stewart CC. Translocation of particles to the tracheobronchial lymph nodes after lung deposition: kinetics and particle–cell relationships. Exp Lung Res 1986; 10:245–266.
127. Oberdörster G. Lung clearance of inhaled insoluble and soluble particles. J Aerosol Med 1988; 1:289–330.
128. Nikula KJ, Avila KJ, Griffith WC, Mauderly JL. Sites of particle retention and lung tissue responses to chronically inhaled diesel exhaust and coal dust in rats and cynomolgus monkeys. Environ Hlth Perspectives 1997; 105:1231–1234.
129. Stöber W, Einbrodt HJ, Klosterkötter W. Quantitative studies of dust retention in

animal and human lungs after chronic inhalation. In: Davis CN, ed. Inhaled Particles and Vapours II. Oxford: Pergamon Press, 1966:409–418.
130. Snipes MB. Long-term retention and clearance of particles inhaled by mammalian species. Toxicology 1989; 20:175–211.
131. Cottier H, Meister F, Zimmermann A, Kraft R, Burkhardt A, Gehr P, Poretti G. Accumulation of anthracotic particles along lymphatics of the human lungs: relevance to "hot spot" formation after inhalation of poorly soluble radionuclides. Radiat Environ Biophys 1987; 26:275–286.
132. Thomas RG. Transport of relatively insoluble materials from the lung to lymph nodes. Health Phys 1968; 14:111–117.
133. Bair W, Métivier H, Park, JF. Comparison of early mortality in baboons and dogs after inhalation of $^{239}PuO_2$. Radiat Res 1980; 82:588–610.
134. Park JF, Apley GA, Buschbom RL, Dagle GE, Fisher DR, Gideon KM, Kashmitter JD, Powers GJ, Ragan HA, Weller RE, Wierman EL. Inhaled plutonium oxide in dogs. Pacific Northwest Laboratory Annual Report for 1985 to the DOE Office of Energy Research. Part 1: Biomedical Sciences. Springfield: National Technical Information Service, 1986:3–17.
135. Kobzik L, Godleski JJ, Brain JD. Selective down-regulation of alveolar macrophage oxidative response to opsonin-independent phagocytosis. J Immunol 1990; 144(11): 4312–4319.
136. Kreyling WG, Ferron GA, Haider B. Metabolic fate of inhaled Co aerosols in beagle dogs. Health Phys 1986; 51:773–795.
137. Leak LV. Lymphatic removal of fluids and particles in the mammalian lung. Environ Health Perspect 1980; 35:55–76.
138. Oberdörster G. Lung dosimetry: pulmonary clearance of inhaled particles. Aerosol Sci Technol 1993; 18:279–289.
139. Mercer TT. On the role of particle size in the dissolution of lung burdens. Health Phys 1967; 13:1211–1224.
140. Lundborg M, Lind B, Camner P. Ability of rabbit alveolar macrophages to dissolve metals. Exp Lung Res 1984; 7:11–22.
141. Lundborg M, Eklund A, Lind B, Camner P. Dissolution of metals by human and rabbit alveolar macrophages. Br J Ind Med 1985; 42:642–655.
142. Effros RM, Mason GR. Measurements of pulmonary epithelial permeability in vivo. Am Rev Respir Dis 1983; 127:S59–S65.
143. Kreyling WG, Cox C, Ferron GA, Oberdörster G. Lung clearance in Long–Evans rats after inhalation of porous, monodisperse cobalt oxide particles. Exp Lung Res 1993; 19:445–467.
144. Collier CG, Bailey MR, Hodgson A. An interspecies comparison of the lung clearance of inhaled monodisperse cobalt oxide particles—part V: lung clearance of inhaled cobalt oxide particles in beagle dogs. J Aerosol Sci 1989; 20:233–248.
145. Kreyling WG. Aerosol particle parameters maintaining lung clearance by intracellular dissolution and translocation. J Aerosol Sci 1990; 21:371–374.
146. Barnes JE, Kanapilly GM, Newton GJ. Cobalt-60 oxide aerosols: methods of production and short-term retention and distribution kinetics in the beagle dog. Health Phys 1976; 30:391–398.
147. Cuddihy RG, Griffith WC. A biological model describing tissue distribution and

whole body retention of barium and lanthanum in beagle dogs after inhalation and gavage. Health Phys 1972; 23:621–633.

148. Cuddihy RG, Gomez SR, Pfleger RC. Inhalation exposures of beagle dogs to cerium aerosols: physical, chemical and mathematical analysis. Health Phys 1975; 29:257–265.
149. Cuddihy RG, Boecker BB, Griffith WC. Modelling deposition and clearance of inhaled radionuclides. In: Biological Implications of Radionuclides Released from Nuclear Industries. Vol 2. Vienna: IAEA, 1979:175–188.
150. McClellan RO, Boyd HA, Gallegos AF, Thomas RG. Retention and distribution of ^{244}Cm following inhalation of $^{244}CmCl_3$ and ^{244}CmO 1.73 by dogs. Health Phys 1972; 22:877–885.
151. Mewhinney JA, Griffith WC, Muggenburg BA. The influence of aerosol size on retention and translocation of ^{241}Am following inhalation of $^{241}AmO_2$ by beagles. Health Phys 1982; 42:611–628.
152. Mewhinney JA, Griffith WC. Models of Am metabolism in beagles and humans. Health Phys 1982; 42:629–644.
153. Marafante E, Lundborg M, Vahter M, Camner P. Dissolution of two arsenic compounds by rabbit alveolar macrophages in vitro. Fundam Appl Toxicol 1987; 8: 382–388.
154. André S, Métivier H, Lantenois G, Boyer M, Nolibé D, Masse R. Beryllium metal solubility in the lung, comparison of metal and hot-pressed forms by in vivo and in vitro dissolution assays. Hum Toxicol 1987; 6:2330–2340.
155. Kreyling WG, Ferron GA, Godleski JJ, Haider B, Kariya ST. The dissolution of monodisperse, porous cobaltosic oxide particles in the dog's lungs and in its alveolar macrophages. In: Schikarski W, Fissan HJ, Friedlander SK, eds. Aerosols: Formation and Reactivity. Oxford: Pergamon Press, 1986:232–236.
156. Kreyling WG, Beisker W, Miaskowski U, Neuner M, Heilmann P. Intraphagolysosomal pH and intracellular particle dissolution in canine and rat alveolar macrophages. In: Seemayer NH, Hadnagy N, eds. Environmental Hygiene III. Heidelberg: Springer Verlag, 1992:19–23.
157. Harper RA, Stirling C, Townsend KMS, Kreyling WG, Patrick G. Intracellular particle dissolution in macrophages isolated from the lungs of the Fischer (F-344) rat. Exp Lung Res 1994; 20:143–156.
158. Nyberg K, Johansson A, Camner P. Intraphagosomal pH in alveolar macrophages studied with fluorescein-labeled amorphous silica particles. Exp Lung Res 1989; 15:49–62.
159. Nyberg K, Johansson A, Rundquist J, Camner P. Estimation of pH in individual alveolar macrophage phagolysosomes. Exp Lung Res 1989; 15:499–510.
160. Nyberg K, Johansson U, Johannsson A, Camner P. Phagolysosomal pH in alveolar macrophages. Environ Health Perspect 1992; 97:149–152.
161. Kreyling WG, Nyberg K, Nolibé D, Collier CG, Camner P, Heilmann P, Lirsac P, Lundborg M, Matejkova E. Interspecies comparison of phagolysosomal pH in alveolar macrophages. Inhal Toxicol 1991; 3:91–100.
162. Heilmann P, Beisker W, Miaskowski U, Camner P, Kreyling WG. Intraphagolysosomal pH in canine and rat alveolar macrophages: flow cytometric measurements. Environ Health Perspect 1992; 97:115–120.

163. Kreyling WG, Beisker W, Berg I, Gercken G, Miaskowski U, Neuner M, Schlüter T, Heilmann P. Particle clearance functions of alveolar macrophages of different species: intracellular particle dissolution and phagolysosomal pH. Eur Respir J 1992; 4:70.
164. Luedtke K-U. Mechanismen der Lösung anorganischer Partikel in kultivierten Alveolarmakrophagen. PhD dissertation, Technical University of Munich, Munich, Germany, 1996.
165. Poncy J-L, Metivier H, Dhilly M, Verry M, Masse R. In vitro dissolution of uranium oxide by baboon alveolar macrophages. Environ Health Perspect 1992; 97:127–130.
166. Ansoborlo E, Chalabreysee J, Hengé-Napoli M-H. In vitro chemical and cellular applied to uranium trioxide with different hydration states. Environ Health Perspect 1992; 97:139–145.
167. Galle P, Berry JP, Galle C. Role of alveolar macrophages in precipitation of mineral elements inhaled as soluble aerosols. Environ Health Perspect 1992; 97:145–147.
168. Lüdtke K-U, Forderkunz S, Neuner M,Summer K-H, Kreyling WG. Mechanisms of intracellular dissolution of cobalt oxide particles by canine alveolar macrophages. Eur Respir J 1994; 7:70.

Part Four

MOLECULAR AND CELLULAR RESPONSES OF THE LUNG TO INHALED PARTICLES

8

Alterations in Gene Expression in Pulmonary Cells Following Particle Interactions

JACOB N. FINKELSTEIN and EDWARD G. BARRETT

University of Rochester School of Medicine and Dentistry
Rochester, New York

I. Introduction

When one considers the cellular heterogeneity of the normal lung, it is reasonable to recognize that the response of the lung to toxicant-induced injury and the subsequent repair processes be equally complex. The cellular dynamics of the lung injury process has been the subject of intense investigation by many investigators using multiple model systems. As the use of new and powerful tools in cellular and molecular biology has been extended to these systems, their true complexity has begun to be appreciated. Particularly relevant to the current discussion are the studies that have provided additional insights into the cellular origins of the lungs' response to injury and the role that individual cell types may play in directing the tissue responses. From such studies, the prominent role of polypeptide growth factors and cytokines, and the effects of injury on cell-specific expression of several genes have become apparent.

Nowhere have these tools had a more profound effect on the development of new paradigms than in the area of the pulmonary response to inhaled particles and fibers. The pulmonary response to inhaled particulates has been the subject of comprehensive investigation for many years. Studies of the deposition and clearance of such inhaled materials have provided a useful framework for a more in-depth study of the cellular and molecular events that are involved in the acute and chronic manifestations of particle-induced lung injury (1–4). Much of the initial phase of such studies has described physiological aspects of the pulmonary response to particles including investigations of phagocytosis (5–7), development of markers of acute injury (5–10), and quantitation of inflammatory cell recruitment (11).

An important aspect of the early studies of particle-induced inflammation was the attempt to identify the key mediators of the inflammatory response and the subsequent tissue injury. Numerous chemotactic factors and activities were identified from studies of in vivo and in vitro dust exposures including such potent agents as complement fragments (e.g., C5a; 12,13), prostaglandins (14,15), leukotrienes, and other lipid mediators (16–19). The role of these substances in the recruitment and activation of macrophages and neutrophils has been clearly demonstrated. More distal to the initial inflammatory events has been the study of the relation between these acute inflammatory processes and the chronic diseases related to particle inhalation. The role of altered expression of polypeptide growth factors and mediators in the process of pulmonary fibrosis has long been appreciated (20–29) a paradigm that has been extended to the question of particle (or fiber)-induced tumorogenesis (30,31).

As with the acute inflammatory events, the alveolar macrophage has been seen as a central figure in this process. Macrophage activation has been postulated to be the key event in the vast array of pulmonary response to inhaled substances. Our understanding of this process has also matured as the tools available to examine detailed intracellular events have become more available. Work by several authors (25,29,32–40) has suggested that production of both inflammatory and fibrotic mediators is not limited to classic inflammatory cells, that pulmonary parenchymal elements, including epithelial cells (type II; Clara cells), and fibroblasts may also contribute to the milieu. In the subsequent discussion, we will attempt to review aspects of the pulmonary response to particles from the perspective of particle-induced cell-specific alterations in gene expression and the possible signaling mechanisms that may be involved.

II. Inflammatory Cytokine Gene Expression

A. Alveolar Macrophages

Most studies of particle-induced pulmonary gene expression have addressed the initial phase of injury, the inflammatory response, and have focused on the expression of inflammatory cytokine genes and their temporal relation to the recruitment of inflammatory cells by the lung (14,41–45). The overwhelming majority of these studies have investigated the production of cytokines and other aspects of altered gene expression by the alveolar macrophage (5,46,47). Such studies have shown the remarkable ability of the resident alveolar macrophage to upregulate its expression of a wide variety of proinflammatory (45,47–50) and profibrotic (21,22) cytokines.

One interesting aspect of the study of cytokine production by macrophages has been the nature of the particle used to initiate the response. As a potent inducer of pulmonary inflammation, fibrosis, and even pulmonary tumors in rats, silica or quartz has been used as the prototypical particle. The molecular and cellular response to crystalline silica is clearly the best characterized of all inhaled particles. Although its relevance to other inorganic or organic dusts has not been rigorously proved, it does provide an effective framework for understanding many of the changes in gene expression that are believed to occur during the pulmonary response to particulates.

A variety of hypotheses relating particle properties to biological effects have been proposed to explain the pulmonary response to various forms of particles. Particle size, surface area, surface composition, and crystal structure have been proposed as key properties influencing particle–tissue interactions. Clearance, and impairment of clearance have also been implicated as mechanistic factors determining the outcome of particulate exposure. Although these are important issues that must be recognized, they are outside the scope of the current chapter.

As described previously, the alveolar macrophage is thought to play a critical role in initiation and potentiation of the inflammatory and repair process following particle exposure (Fig. 1). On interaction with a particle, the alveolar macrophage is stimulated to produce a host of cytokines, chemokines, growth factors, eicosanoids, enzymes, and reactive oxygen or nitrogen species (Table 1; 51,52). Among the various cytokines, interleukin 1 (IL-1) and tumor necrosis factor-alpha (TNF-α) appear to play a prominent role in the particle-induced inflammatory response (53,54), for they are involved in recruitment and stimulation of neutrophils, lymphocytes, and macrophages; they stimulate fibroblast proliferation; they induce the release of other acute-phase proteins; and they contribute to granuloma formation (55,56). Moreover, direct evidence for their role in the pathogenesis of silicosis was obtained by using specific antagonists that inhibited the development of fibrosis (57–59). In addition to IL-1 and TNF-α, the growth factors transforming growth factor-beta (TGF-β) and platelet-derived growth factor (PDGF) may mediate alveolar macrophage-induced proliferation of fibroblasts (60).

The chemokines—macrophage inflammatory protein 2 (MIP-2) and cytokine-induced neutrophil chemoattractant (CINC)—play a role in neutrophil recruitment to the lung following particle exposure, and their expression is partly mediated by the production of TNF-α (55,61). Release of reactive oxygen and nitrogen species (62–66) and neutral proteases and other enzymes (52) during silica exposure are thought to be responsible for the damage to lung tissues that

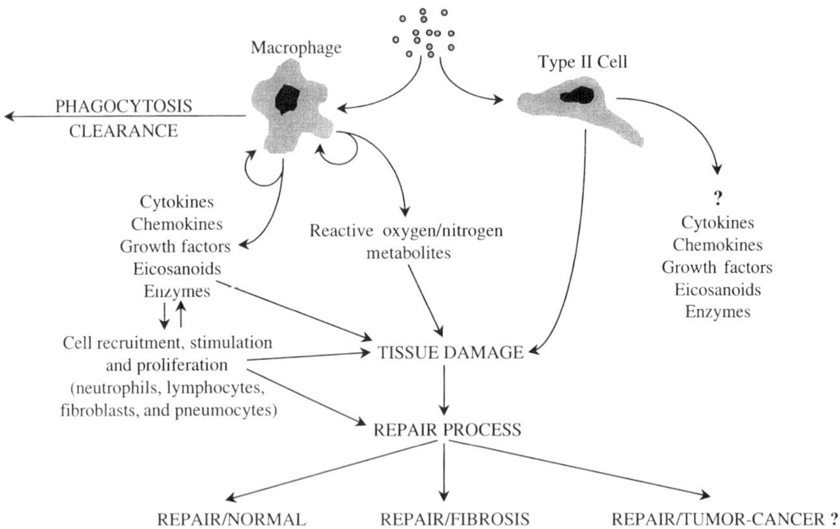

Figure 1 Suggested role of the macrophage and type II cell in particle-induced inflammation.

Table 1 Cytokines, Growth Factors, and Chemokines Expressed by Alveolar Macrophages Following Exposure to Crystalline Silica

Factors	Mouse	Rat	Human	Ref.
TNFα	+	+	+	11, 42, 53, 54
IL-1α	+, +/−	?	?	54, 155
IL-1β	+, +/−	+	+/−	11, 42, 57, 155
IL-6	+/−	?	+/−	57, 155
TGF-α	?	+	?	156
TGF-β	+/−	+	?	57, 157
PDGF	?	+	?	60
MIP-1α	?	+	?	158
MIP-2	?	+	?	49, 158
CINC	?	+	?	49
iNOS	?	+	?	63

+, increased expression; − decreased expression; +/−, no change; ?, not known.

has been found associated with the acute phase of the response to silica and other inflammatory particles.

Increased production of nitric oxide (NO) is dependent on the expression of the appropriate biosynthetic activities. Increased expression of inducible nitric oxide synthase has been observed in macrophages following particle exposure (67), further implicating the role of this molecule in the pathogenesis of particle-induced tissue damage. Beyond their ability to directly injure tissues, reactive oxygen and nitrogen metabolites may also be involved in the regulation of pro-inflammatory cytokine expression.

B. Epithelial Cells

Studies examining the early inflammatory response in the lung following silica exposure have typically focused on the contribution of macrophages, neutrophils, and their products (61,68). However, an additional or alternative means by which silica may initiate an inflammatory response is through direct interaction with the lung epithelium. Alveolar type II epithelial (type II) cells are uniquely situated at the interface between the alveolar airspace of the lung and the capillary circulation, allowing them to respond to airborne stimuli and interact with various cell types, such as endothelial, mesenchymal, alveolar macrophages, and other inflammatory cells. Type II cells play an important role in lung injury through the synthesis and secretion of pulmonary surfactant and by acting as the stem cell for the replacement of damaged type I epithelial cells (29,69–75).

In rats instilled with silica, alterations in type II cell morphology and surfactant metabolism were evident. These changes were partly due to alterations in surfactant protein gene expression and alterations in cell cycle kinetics of a hypertrophic type II cell population that developed in the silica-exposed lung (76–81). These responses could arise from direct interactions between silica particles and type II cells, or from particle-induced alterations in the interaction of the alveolar macrophage and the type II cell, mediated by changes in macrophage-derived growth factors (29,44,71,82–85).

The importance of the inflammatory reaction to the pulmonary response to particles, and the knowledge that epithelial cells are capable of synthesis and secretion of potent inflammatory mediators, have led to the investigation of cytokine expression by epithelial cells following dust exposure. In primary isolated and immortalized cell lines in an in vitro silica exposure model (35), type II cells respond directly to silica (α-quartz) by increasing expression of MIP-2 and CINC mRNA.

Other stimuli also stimulate type II cells to produce inflammatory mediators, such as interferon (IFN), MIP-2, CINC, IL-8, and monocyte chemotactic protein (MCP-1; 29,33,40,86–88). Although evidence is accumulating supporting a more important role for the type II cell in the development of silica-induced pulmonary inflammation, the exact molecular and cellular events leading to the type II cell response remain unclear.

Pulmonary epithelial cells have been extensively characterized as the producers of pulmonary surfactant lipid and protein species and in their role in the repair of epithelial damage through increased cell proliferation and subsequent differentiation. It is also clear that a subpopulation of the respiratory epithelium is capable of uptake, accumulation, and metabolism of inhaled and systemic lipophilic substances (89).

It had long been suspected that the pulmonary epithelium may also play a role in defining the inflammatory environment within the lung. Several investigators have shown that pulmonary epithelial cells can produce a variety of inflammatory cytokines (for review see 90). Of particular relevance to particle-induced pulmonary inflammation has been the demonstration of expression of granulocyte–macrophage colony-stimulating factor (GM-CSF), TGF-β (91), and TGF-α (92) in type II cells. More directly related to the question of inflammatory cell recruitment is the demonstration of the production of the specific chemoattractants IL-8, (40,93) and RANTES (94) by alveolar epithelial cells and cell lines in vivo and in vitro. In addition, more studies have shown increased expression of MIP-1α, MIP-2, and TNF-α following mineral dust exposure (61,95).

As with macrophages, epithelial cells are capable of production of reactive oxygen and nitrogen species. Interestingly, nitric oxide synthase is inducible in pulmonary epithelial cells and cell lines (96–98), in addition to macrophages discussed earlier. This emphasizes the similarity in gene expression of these two pulmonary cell types and makes more compelling the possibility that each makes a unique contribution to the development and progression of particle-induced inflammation, as well as fibrosis. It also suggests a common particle-induced–signaling mechanism may be responsible for the upregulation of the expression of these gene products.

The lung epithelium, in particular the type II cell, may interact with silica through both direct and indirect pathways. Direct particle–cell interactions can lead to increased alveolar–capillary permeability, proliferation, and cytotoxic effects, which are dose-dependent (84,99,100). Such interactions may be mechanistically similar to those that occur with macrophages. Indirect effects, may be mediated through cell–cell-mediator interactions primarily associated with macrophages. Macrophages release several cytokines and growth factors (IL-1, TNF-α, PDGF, and TGF-β_1) that can have effects on type II cell activation and proliferation (28,55,71,83,100–102). Increased MIP-2 mRNA expression has occurred in a rat epithelial cell line following exposure to TNF-α (35,55). The contribution of the type II cell to the pathogenesis of silicosis, or any particle-induced disease, especially the early inflammatory component, however, is still largely unknown.

Surprisingly little information is available about the specific nature or the mechanism of cellular communication between the type II cell and the other lung cells. Type II cells appear to be able to synthesize other growth factors, such as PDGF (102,103), TGF-β (60,104,105), and EGF (92,106), as well as various inflammatory cytokines, including TNF-α (107,108) and GM–CSF (109,110), during fibrotic events in the lung. Evidence from other models of fibrosis suggest that type II cells may interact directly (cell–cell contact or soluble mediator) with fibroblasts, lymphocytes, and macrophages (6,111). A better understanding of the role of cellular interactions in the pulmonary inflammatory response to particles may permit the identification of disease markers that predispose the lung to development of fibrosis.

III. Intracellular Signaling Following Particle Cell Interactions

Although there are many clues to how the development of particle-induced fibrosis progresses, the precise biochemical and molecular mechanisms that mediate the disease remain undefined. Understanding the particle–cell interactions that lead to the activation of specific signal transduction pathways and subsequent gene activation are critical in determining the initiating and propagating events of silicosis. Studies with opsonized and unopsonized latex beads show that alveolar macrophages have differing responses, based on which receptor system is engaged during phagocytosis. Fc-receptor activation during phagocytosis of opsonized beads results in a respiratory burst, release of TNF, and expression of chemokine mRNA (5,6). In contrast, the response to opsonin-independent phagocytosis resulted in no macrophage activation. Quartz–silica and the ''nuisance'' dusts, iron oxide and titanium dioxide (TiO_2), have shown interactions with macrophage opsonin-independent acetyl-low-density lipoprotein (LDL) scavenger receptors where receptor antagonists blocked about 50% of the particle uptake (5). Unlike the interaction of iron oxide, TiO_2, and latex particles with the scavenger receptor, silica interaction did lead to the activation of macrophages. The basis for these conflicting results is unclear, but may be due the ability of silica to interact with other receptor systems. Also, additional components carried by particulates may contribute to cellular activation independent of receptor systems.

Freshly fractured quartz–silica contains free radicals on the surface that have the ability to regulate cytokine gene expression (112,113).

The second-messenger systems involved in signaling and gene activation following silica–cell interactions remain unknown. Studies with fibers have shown that asbestos stimulates superoxide anion production in alveolar macrophages through the phospholipase C–protein kinase C pathway, and opening of verapamil-sensitive calcium channels (114). In contrast, although both asbestos and silica stimulate cytokine release (e.g., TNF and IL-1), silica does not appear to activate this pathway, nor to stimulate superoxide anion production (114). In in vitro studies, in the absence of serum, crystalline silica and, to a lesser extent, amorphous silica cause a dose-dependent increase in intracellular calcium coming from the extracellular space (115,116).

One approach to understanding the mechanism by which particles activate cellular gene expression would be by comparison with other better-characterized agents that lead to the expression of similar gene products. Among the most thoroughly studied agents that mediate macrophage gene expression and cytokine release are endotoxin (lipopolysaccharide; LPS) and interferon gamma (IFN-γ; 117,118). The cellular effects of LPS (119,120), TNF-α (121), and IL-1β (122) are partly mediated by protein tyrosine phosphorylation, and these signaling events are blocked by protein tyrosine kinase (PTK) inhibitors, such as tyrphostins (119,123), herbimycin A (124,125) and genistein (125,126). LPS-induced toxicity and TNF-α release, in particular, have been inhibited with tyrphostins (123). IFN-γ and other cytokines that use the cytokine receptor family of receptors, also act, at least partly, by a PTK pathway known as the Janus family of protein tyrosine kinases (JAKs) and the signal transducer and activator of transcription (STAT) family (127–129). Interestingly, many of the genes that are responsive to LPS and IFN-γ also appear to be induced by silica.

Of the proteins tyrosine phosphorylated on LPS stimulation, several have molecular masses similar to mitogen-activated protein (MAP) kinases (p42 and p44; 130–132). The ability of LPS to activate these MAP kinases could be blocked by the tyrosine kinase inhibitor herbimycin A (130). There are currently two known mechanisms by which different receptors may activate MAP kinases (Fig. 2), which subsequently target different factors, such as phospholipase A_2 and the transcription factors p62TCF/ELK-1 and nuclear factor (NF)–IL-6 in macrophages (130,133,134). The Ras/Raf/MAP kinase pathway however fails to induce NF-κB and stimulates only a modest induction of TNF-α mRNA and protein secretion, which are seen in large amounts following both LPS and silica exposure (135). The identity of the pathway controlling NF-κB is unknown, but the protein tyrosine kinase inhibitor herbimycin A blocks activation of NF-κB in response to LPS (136). Thus, it appears that LPS and possibly silica trigger more than one tyrosine kinase-mediated signaling pathway.

Another tyrosine kinase-mediated pathway is the JAK/STAT pathway, which is involved in signaling through the cytokine receptor superfamily. Various cytokines and growth factors operate through this pathway. Currently, there are six known STAT proteins that on tyrosine phosphorylation differentially bind to more than ten related IFN-γ activation site (GAS) sequences [TT(C/A)CNN-NAA] (128,137). Contribution of STATs toward LPS signaling remains unclear. Studies have reported no STAT-binding activity following LPS exposure to RAW 264.7 macrophages (137); however, another study reported that a new STAT-like factor was involved in LPS, IL-1, and IL-6 signaling, and it recognized a GAS-like element in the IL-1β gene (157). Evidence is also accumulating suggesting that sometimes the JAK pathway may activate MAP-kinase, when the

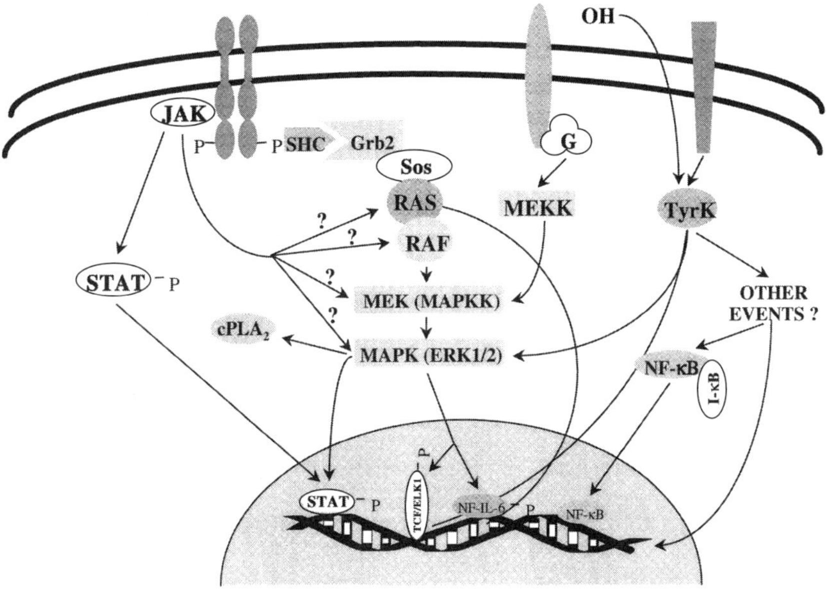

Figure 2 Potential tyrosine kinase-mediated signaling pathways for silica.

MAP-kinase subsequently turns up STAT activity (138). Thus, current evidence suggests that a complex mixture of signaling pathways are involved in macrophage activation following silica–cell interaction (see Fig. 2).

IV. Mechanism of Silica-Induced Changes in Gene Expression

Increasing evidence supports the role of reactive oxygen intermediates (ROI) as mediators of pulmonary inflammation and damage following silica exposure (139). ROI can form on the surface of silica, especially following its fracture (112) or through the generation of a respiratory burst caused by the phagocytosis of silica (66,140). Inducible nitric oxide synthase mRNA expression and nitric oxide production in alveolar macrophages and neutrophils can be induced by silica (62,63). The combination of nitric oxide with superoxide forms a highly reactive toxic species, peroxynitrite, which may play a role in silica-induced lung damage (62,63,141). Also, silica can induce changes in lung antioxidant enzymes (142). In addition, treatment with antioxidants decreases silica-induced expression of TNF in alveolar macrophages and attenuates overall lung injury (113).

Little information is available in the scientific literature on the contribution of ROIs in regulating the type II cell response to direct interactions with silica particles. Increases in manganese superoxide dismutase (Mn-SOD) protein can be localized to type II cells following in vivo silica exposure in rats (143). Type II cells respond to an oxidant stress, such as hyperoxia, by increasing antioxidant enzymes (144) and chemokines (145,146). Thus, it is reasonable to hypothesize that the type II cell response to silica involves an oxidant-mediated component.

The signaling pathways through which silica–type II cell interactions lead to alterations in gene expression remain unclear. Increasing evidence points to ROI or changes in cellular redox status as important mediators in signal transduction and gene regulation. ROI, generated by TNF-α, H_2O_2, and other stimuli, activate the nuclear transcription factor NF-kB (147–151). Also, tyrosine phosphorylation of specific proteins is an important and mandatory initial step in the oxidant-induced activation of NF-kB (152,153). We hypothesize that oxidant-stimulated tyrosine kinase-mediated signaling pathways are an integral part of the type II cell response following silica exposure.

In studies from our laboratory (154), the murine-derived pulmonary epithelial cell line MLE15 responds to both direct interactions with silica particles and to macrophage-derived cytokines by increasing specific chemokine mRNA species. With free radical scavengers and various modifiers of cellular antioxidant status, we have shown that the increase in MLE15 chemokine mRNA following silica exposure is dependent on ROI. We also demonstrated, using a tyrosine kinase inhibitor, that the silica-induced chemokine response in MLE15 cells requires tyrosine kinase activity. Furthermore, specific proteins are tyrosine phosphorylated in the MLE15 cells following silica exposure, and this phosphorylation can be reduced or eliminated using free radical scavengers or modifiers of cellular antioxidant status. Our findings support a pivotal role for the type II cell in mediating the inflammatory response in the lung following exposure to silica.

V. Conclusions

Over the last several years the role of cytokines and chemokines in the pathogenesis of particle-induced lung disease has become widely recognized. Nevertheless, several key mechanistic questions remain unanswered. Despite tremendous advances in our understanding of signaling events and the control of cytokine gene expression, the specific events that occur downstream from the interaction between a particle and a lung cell remain largely unknown and speculative. Furthermore, the relative contributions of individual pulmonary cell types to both the acute and chronic aspects of lung disease induced by particles is still in question. Increasing evidence implicates the type II cell as a potential mediator of pulmonary recruitment and activation of inflammatory cells through the release of a variety of chemokines. How significant this epithelial response is in the overall process will require more precise approaches to measuring changes in gene expression and a better understanding of the mechanisms involved.

Acknowledgments

The authors wish to thank Carl Johnston and Christina Reed for their technical assistance. This work was supported in part by HL 36543, ES 04872, CA 27791, CA 11051, ES 01247, and NASA-NSCORT grant NAGW-2356 and contracts from The Center for Indoor Air Research and the Health Effects Institute.

References

1. Morrow PE. Dust overloading of the lungs—update and appraisal. Toxicol Appl Pharmacol 1992; 113:1–12.
2. Oberdorster G. Lung particle overload: implications for occupational exposures to particles. Regul Toxicol Pharmacol 1995; 21:123–135.
3. Oberdorster G, Ferin J, Lehnert BE. Correlation between particle size, in vivo particle persistence, and lung injury. Environ Health Perspect 1994; 102:173–179.
4. Oberdorster G, Ferin J, Gelein R, Soderholm SC, Finkelstein J. Role of the alveolar macrophage in lung injury: studies with ultrafine particles. Environ Health Perspect 1992; 97:193–199.
5. Kobzik L. Lung macrophage uptake of unopsonized environmental particulates—role of scavenger-type receptors. J Immunol 1995; 155:367–376.
6. Kobzik L, Huang S, Paulauskis JD, Godleski JJ. Particle opsonization and lung macrophage cytokine response. In vitro and in vivo analysis. J Immunol 1993; 151:2753–2759.
7. Brain JD, Knudson DE, Sorokin SP, Davis MA. Pulmonary distribution of particles given by intratracheal instillation or by aerosol inhalation. Environ Res 1976; 11:13–33.
8. Henderson RF, Barr EB, Cheng YS, Griffith WC, Hahn FF. The effect of exposure pattern on the accumulation of particles and the response of the lung to inhaled particles. Fundam Appl Toxicol 1992; 19:367–374.
9. Warheit DB. Interspecies comparisons of lung responses to inhaled particles and gases. Crit Rev Toxicol 1989; 20:1–29.
10. Warheit DB, Carakostas MC, Hartsky MA, Hansen JF. Development of a short-term inhalation bioassay to assess pulmonary toxicity of inhaled particles—comparisons of pulmonary responses to carbonyl iron and silica. Toxicol Appl Pharmacol 1991; 107:350–368.
11. Driscoll KE, Maurer JK, Lindenschmidt RC, Romberger D, Rennard SI, Crosby LP. Respiratory tract responses to dust—relationships between dust burden, lung injury, alveolar macrophage fibronectin release, and the development of pulmonary fibrosis. Toxicol Appl Pharmacol 1990; 106:88–101.

12. Warheit DB, Carakostas MC, Bamberger JR, Hartsky MA. Complement facilitates macrophage phagocytosis of inhaled iron particles but has little effect in mediating silica-induced lung inflammatory and clearance responses. Environ Res 1991; 56: 186–203.
13. Warheit DB, Overby LH, George G, Brody AR. Pulmonary macrophages are attracted to inhaled particles through complement activation. Exp Lung Res 1988; 14:51–66.
14. Kuhn DC, Demers LMP. Influence of mineral dust surface chemistry on eicosanoid production by the alveolar macrophage. J Toxicol Environ Health 1992; 35:39–50.
15. Demers LM, Kuhn DC. Influence of mineral dusts on metabolism of arachidonic acid by alveolar macrophage. Environ Health Perspect 1994; 102:97–100.
16. Shamsuddin M, Hsueh W, Smith LJ. Production of leukotrienes and thromboxane by resident and activated rat alveolar macrophages—a possible role of protein kinase-C. J Lab Clin Med 1992; 120:434–443.
17. Carmankrzan M, Wise BC. Arachidonic acid lipoxygenation may mediate interleukin-1 stimulation of nerve growth factor secretion in astroglial cultures. J Neurosci Res 1993; 34:225–232.
18. Henderson WR. The role of leukotrienes in inflammation. Ann Intern Med 1994; 121:684–697.
19. Shamsuddin M, Anderson J, Smith LJ. Differential regulation of leukotriene and platelet-activating factor synthesis in rat alveolar macrophages. Am J Respir Cell Mol Biol 1995; 12:697–704.
20. Bonner JC. Regulation of platelet-derived growth factor (PDGF) and alveolar macrophage-derived PDGF by alpha 2-macroglobulin. Ann NY Acad Sci 1994; 737:324–338.
21. Brody AR, Bonner JC. Platelet-derived growth factor produced by pulmonary cells. Chest 1991; 99:S50–S52.
22. Brody AR, Bonner JC, Overby LH, et al. Interstitial pulmonary macrophages produce platelet-derived growth factor that stimulates rat lung fibroblast proliferation in vitro. J Leukoc Biol 1992; 51:640–648.
23. Lasky JA, Bonner JC, Tonthat B, Brody AR. Chrysotile asbestos induces PDGF-a chain-dependent proliferation in human and rat lung fibroblasts in vitro. Chest 1996; 109:S26–S28.
24. Liu JY, Morris GF, Lei WH, Corti M, Brody ARP. Up-regulated expression of transforming growth factor-alpha in the bronchiolar–alveolar duct regions of asbestos-exposed rats. Am J Pathol 1996; 149:205–217.
25. Maniscalco WM, Watkins RH, Finkelstein JN, Campbell MH. Vascular endothelial growth factor mRNA increases in alveolar epithelial cells during recovery from oxygen injury. Am J Respir Cell Mol Biol 1995; 13:377–386.
26. Oreilly MA, Staversky RJ, Flanders KC, Johnston CJ, Finkelstein JN. Temporal changes in expression of TGF-beta isoforms in mouse lung exposed to oxygen. Am J Physiol 1997; 16:L60–L67.
27. Maniscalco WM, Watkins RH, Finkelstein JN, Campbell MH. Vascular endothelial growth factor mRNA increases in alveolar epithelial cells during recovery from oxygen injury. Am J Respir Cell Mol Biol 1995; 13:377–386.

28. Brandes ME, Finkelstein JN. The production of alveolar macrophage-derived growth-regulating proteins in response to lung injury. Toxicol Lett 1990; 54:3–22; discussion 1–2.
29. Finkelstein JN. Physiologic and toxicologic responses of alveolar type II cells. Toxicology 1990; 60:41–52.
30. Mossman BT. Carcinogenesis and related cell and tissue responses to asbestos: a review. Ann Occup Hyg 1994; 38:617–624.
31. Saffiotti U, Daniel LN, Mao Y, Shi X, Williams AO, Kaighn ME. Mechanisms of carcinogenesis by crystalline silica in relation to oxygen radicals. Environ Health Perspect 1994; 102:159–163.
32. Breen E, Shull S, Burne S, et al. Bleomycin regulation of transforming growth factor-beta mRNA in rat lung fibroblasts. Am J Respir Cell Mol Biol 1992; 6:146–152.
33. Crestani B, Cornillet P, Dehoux M, Rolland C, Guenounou M, Aubier M. Alveolar type II epithelial cells produce interleukin-6 in vitro and in vivo. Regulation by alveolar macrophage secretory products. J Clin Invest 1994; 94:731–740.
34. Crippen TL, Klasing KC, Hyde DM. Cytokine-induced neutrophil chemoattractant production by primary rat alveolar type II cells. Inflammation 1995; 19:575–586.
35. Driscoll KE, Howard BW, Carter JM, et al. alpha-Quartz-induced chemokine expression by rat lung epithelial cells: effects of in vivo and in vitro particle exposure [see comments]. Am J Pathol 1996; 149:1627–1637.
36. Dunsmore SE, Lee YC, Martinezwilliams C, Rannels DE. Synthesis of fibronectin and laminin by type II pulmonary epithelial cells. Am J Physiol 1996; 14:L215–L223.
37. Hastings RH, Hua XY. Expression of calcitonin gene-related peptide by cultured rat alveolar type II cells. Am J Respir Cell Mol Biol 1995; 13:563–569.
38. Khalil N, O'Conner RN, Flanders KC, Shing W, Whitman CI. Regulation of type II alveolar epithelial cell proliferation by TGF-beta during bleomycin-induced lung injury in rats. Am J Physiol 1994; 267:L498–L507.
39. Klein JM, Fritz BL, McCarthy TA, Wohlfordlenane CL, Snyder JM. Localization of epidermal growth factor receptor in alveolar epithelium during human fetal lung development in vitro. Exp Lung Res 1995; 21:917–939.
40. Paine RD, Rolfe MW, Standiford TJ, Burdick MD, Rollins BJ, Strieter RM. MCP-1 expression by rat type II alveolar epithelial cells in primary culture. J Immunol 1993; 150:4561–4570.
41. Brown GM, Brown DM, Donaldson K. Inflammatory response to particles in the rat lung—secretion of acid and neutral proteinases by bronchoalveolar leucocytes. Ann Occup Hyg 1991; 35:389–396.
42. Gosset P, Lassalle P, Vanhee D, et al. Production of tumor necrosis factor-alpha and interleukin-6 by human alveolar macrophages exposed in vitro to coal mine dust. Am J Resp Cell Mol Biol 1991; 5:431–436.
43. Lenz AG, Krombach F, Maier KLP. Oxidative stress in vivo and in vitro—modulation by quartz dust and hyperbaric atmosphere. Free Radical Biol Med 1992; 12: 1–10.
44. Lesur O, Cantin AM, Tanswell AK, Melloni B, Beaulieu JF, Begin R. Silica expo-

sure induces cytotoxicity and proliferative activity of type-II pneumocytes. Exp Lung Res 1992; 18:173–190.
45. Driscoll KE, Maurer JKP. Cytokine and growth factor release by alveolar macrophages—potential biomarkers of pulmonary toxicity. Toxicol Pathol 1991; 19: 398–405.
46. Kobzik L, Huang SL, Paulauskis JD, Godleski JJ. Particle opsonization and lung macrophage cytokine response—in vitro and in vivo analysis. J Immunol 1993; 151:2753–2759.
47. Savici D, He B, Geist LJ, Monick MM, Hunninghake GW. Silica increases tumor necrosis factor (TNF) production, in part, by upregulating the TNF promoter. Exp Lung Res 1994; 20:613–625.
48. Driscoll KE, Higgins JM, Leytart MJ, Crosby LLP. Differential effects of mineral dusts on the in vitro activation of alveolar macrophage eicosanoid and cytokine release. Toxicol In Vitro 1990; 4:284–288.
49. Driscoll KE, Maurer JK, Higgins J, Poynter J. Alveolar macrophage cytokine and growth factor production in a rat model of crocidolite-induced pulmonary inflammation and fibrosis. J Toxicol Environ Health 1995; 46:155–169.
50. Driscoll KE, Hassenbein DG, Carter J, et al. Macrophage inflammatory protein-1 and protein-2 expression by rat alveolar macrophages, fibroblasts, and epithelial cells and in rat lung after mineral dust exposure. Am J Respir Cell Mol Biol 1993; 8:311–318.
51. Kelley J. Cytokines of the lung. Am Rev Respirat Dis 1990; 141:765–788.
52. Davis GS, Pfeiffer LM, Leslie KE, Hemenway DR. Macrophage–lymphocyte cytokine interactions in silicosis. Chest 1996; 109:S49–S50.
53. Bissonnette F, Cook C, Geoghegan T, et al. Transforming growth factor-alpha and epidermal growth factor messenger ribonucleic acid and protein levels in human placentas from early, mid, and late gestation. Am J Obstet Gynecol 1992; 166:192–199.
54. Ohtsuka Y, Munakata M, Ukita H, et al. Increased susceptibility to silicosis and TNF-alpha production in C57bl/6j mice. Am J Respir Crit Care Med 1995; 152: 2144–2149.
55. Driscoll KE, Hassenbein DG, Carter JM, Kunkel SL, Quinlan TR, Mossman BT. TNFa and increased chemokine expression in the rat lung after particle exposure. Toxicol Lett 1995; 82/83:483–489.
56. Mohr C, Gemsa D, Graebner C, et al. Systemic macrophage stimulation in rats with silicosis—enhanced release of tumor necrosis factor-alpha from alveolar and peritoneal macrophages. Am J Respir Cell Mol Biol 1991; 5:395–402.
57. Piguet PF, Collart MA, Grau GE, Sappino AP, Vassalli P. Requirement of tumour necrosis factor for development of silica-induced pulmonary fibrosis. Nature. 1990; 344:245–247.
58. Piguet PF, Vesin C, Grau GE, Thompson RC. Interleukin-1 receptor antagonist (IL-1ra) prevents or cures pulmonary fibrosis elicited in mice by bleomycin or silica. Cytokine 1993; 5:57–61.
59. Piguet PF, Tacchinicottier F, Vesin C. Administration of anti-TNF-alpha or anti-CD11a antibodies to normal adult mice decreases lung and bone collagen content—

evidence for an effect on platelet consumption. Am J Respir Cell Mol Biol 1995; 12:227–231.
60. Bauman MD, Jetten AM, Bonner JC, Kumar RK, Bennett RA, Brody AR. Secretion of a platelet-derived growth factor homologue by rat alveolar macrophages exposed to particulates in vitro. Eur J Cell Biol 1990; 51:327–334.
61. Driscoll KE, Hassenbein DG, Carter J, et al. Macrophage inflammatory proteins 1 and 2: expression by rat alveolar macrophages, fibroblasts, and epithelial cells and in rat lung after mineral dust exposure. Am J Respir Cell Mol Biol 1993; 8:311–318.
62. Blackford JA Jr, Jones W, Dey RD, Castranova V. Comparison of inducible nitric oxide synthase gene expression and lung inflammation following intratracheal instillation of silica, coal, carbonyl iron, or titanium dioxide in rats. J Toxicol Environ Health 1997; 51:203–218.
63. Blackford JA, Antonini JM, Castranova V, Dey RD. Intratracheal instillation of silica up-regulates inducible nitric oxide synthase gene expression and increases nitric oxide production in alveolar macrophages and neutrophils. Am J Respir Cell Mol Biol 1994; 11:426–431.
64. Nyberg P, Klockars MP. Quartz-induced production of reactive oxygen metabolites by activated human monocyte-derived macrophages. APMIS 1990; 98:823–827.
65. Nyberg PW, Nordman SA, Klockars MLP. Increased mineral dust-induced production of reactive oxygen species by blood monocytes from patients with malignant diseases. APMIS 1994; 102:765–770.
66. Vallyathan V, Mega JF, Shi XL, Dalal NSP. Enhanced generation of free radicals from phagocytes induced by mineral dusts. Am J Respir Cell Mol Biol 1992; 6: 404–413.
67. Pendino KJ, Laskin JD, Shuler RL, Punjabi CJ, Laskin DL. Enhanced production of nitric oxide by rat alveolar macrophages after inhalation of a pulmonary irritant is associated with increased expression of nitric oxide synthase. J Immunol 1993; 151:7196–7205.
68. Rakesh WL, Kumar RK, O'Grady R, Velan GM. Role of lymphocytes in silicosis: regulation of secretion of macrophage-derived mitogenic activity for fibroblasts. Int J Exp Pathol 1992; 73:793–800.
69. Bassett DJ, Bowen-Kelly E, Elbon CL, Reichenbaugh SS. Rat lung recovery from 3 days of continuous exposure to 0.75 ppm ozone. J Toxicol Environ Health 1988; 25:329–347.
70. Belinsky SA, Devereux TR, Foley JF, Maronpot RR, Anderson MW. Role of the alveolar type-II cell in the development and progression of pulmonary tumors induced by 4-(methylnitrosamino)-1-(3-pyridyl)-1-butanone in the A/J mouse. Cancer Res 1992; 52:3164–3173.
71. Brandes ME, Finkelstein JN. Stimulated rabbit alveolar macrophages secrete a growth factor for type II pneumocytes. Am J Respir Cell Mol Biol 1989; 1:101–109.
72. Brandes ME, Finkelstein JN. Induction of the stress response by isolation of rabbit type II pneumocytes. Exp Lung Res 1989; 15:93–111.

73. Dormans JAMA, Vanbree L. Function and response of type II cells to inhaled toxicants. Inhal Toxicol 1995; 7:319–342.
74. Witschi H. Responses of the lung to toxic injury. Environ Health Perspect 1990; 85:5–13.
75. Uhal BD. Cell cycle kinetics in the alveolar epithelium [Review]. Am J Physiol 1997; 16:L1031–L1045.
76. Miles PR, Bowman L, Ma JKH, Ma JYC. Alterations in alveolar type-II cell metabolism induced by tetrandrine and other alkaloids. Toxicol Appl Pharmacol 1993; 119:142–149.
77. Uhal BD, Etter MD. Type-II pneumocyte hypertrophy without activation of surfactant biosynthesis after partial pneumonectomy. Am J Physiol 1993; 264:L153–L159.
78. Viviano CJ, Rooney SA. Early increase in expression of surfactant protein a gene in type II cells from silica-treated rats. Am J Physiol 1997; 17:L395–L400.
79. Hook GER. Alveolar proteinosis and phospholipidoses of the lungs. Toxicol Pathol 1991; 19:482–513.
80. Miller BE, Bakewell WE, Katyal SL, Singh G, Hook GE. Induction of surfactant protein (SP-A) biosynthesis and SP-A mRNA in activated type II cells during acute silicosis in rats. Am J Respir Cell Mol Biol 1990; 3:217–226.
81. Lesur O, Bouhadiba T, Melloni B, Cantin A, Whitsett JA, Begin R. Alterations of surfactant lipid turnover in silicosis: evidence of a role for surfactant-associated protein A(SP-A). Int J Exp Pathol 1995; 76:287–298.
82. Fischer R, Rehn B, Bruch J. Dust specific effects on the macrophage pneumocyte type II cell system—comparing in vitro and in vivo data. Exp Toxicol Pathol 1996; 48:520–522.
83. Melloni B, Lesur O, Cantin A, Begin R. Silica-exposed macrophages release a growth-promoting activity for type-II pneumocytes. J Leukoc Biol 1993; 53:327–335.
84. Lesur O, Melloni B, Cantin AM, Begin R. Silica-exposed lung fluids have a proliferative activity for type-II epithelial cells—a study on human and sheep alveolar fluids. Exp Lung Res 1992; 18:633–654.
85. Melloni B, Lesur O, Bouhadiba T, Cantin A, Martel M, Begin R. Effect of exposure to silica on human alveolar macrophages in supporting growth activity in type II epithelial cells. Thorax 1996; 51:781–786.
86. Williams AO, Knapton AD, Ifon ET, Saffiotti U. Transforming growth factor beta expression and transformation of rat lung epithelial cells by crystalline silica (quartz). Int J Cancer 1996; 65:639–649.
87. Smart SJ, Casale TB. Pulmonary epithelial cells facilitate TNF-alpha-induced neutrophil chemotaxis. A role for cytokine networking. J Immunol 1994; 152:4087–4094.
88. Paine R, Chavis A, Gaposchkin D, et al. A factor secreted by a human pulmonary alveolar epithelial-like cell line blocks T-cell proliferation between G_1 and S-phase. Am J Respir Cell Mol Biol 1992; 6:658–666.
89. Stripp BR, Maxson K, Mera R, Singh G. Plasticity of airway cell proliferation and gene expression after acute naphthalene injury. Am J Physiol 1995; 13:L791–L799.

90. Simon RH, Paine R. Participation of pulmonary alveolar epithelial cells in lung inflammation. J Lab Clin Med 1995; 126:108–118.
91. Khalil N, O'Conner RN, Flanders KC, Unruh H. TGF-beta 1, but not TGF-beta 2 or TGF-beta 3, is differentially present in epithelial cells of advanced pulmonary fibrosis: an immunohistochemical study. Am J Respir Cell Mol Biol 1996; 14:131–138.
92. Madtes DK, Busby HK, Strandjord TP, Clark JG. Expression of transforming growth factor-alpha and epidermal growth factor receptor is increased following bleomycin-induced lung injury in rats. Am J Respir Cell Mol Biol 1994; 11:540–551.
93. Standiford TJ, Kunkel SL, Basha MA, et al. Interleukin-8 gene expression by a pulmonary epithelial cell line—a model for cytokine networks in the lung. J Clin Invest 1990; 86:1945–1953.
94. Vanotteren GM, Standiford TJ, Kunkel SL, et al. Expression and regulation of macrophage inflammatory protein-1 alpha by murine alveolar and peritoneal macrophages. Am J Respir Cell Mol Biol 1994; 10:8–15.
95. Driscoll KE, Carter JM, Howard BW, et al. Pulmonary inflammatory, chemokine, and mutagenic responses in rats after subchronic inhalation of carbon black. Toxicol Appl Pharmacol 1996; 136:372–380.
96. Punjabi CJ, Laskin JD, Pendino KJ, Goller NL, Durham SK, Laskin DL. Production of nitric oxide by rat type II pneumocytes: increased expression of inducible nitric oxide synthase following inhalation of a pulmonary irritant. Am J Respir Cell Mol Biol 1994; 11:165–172.
97. Adcock IM, Brown CR, Kwon O, Barnes PJ. Oxidative stress induces NF kappa B DNA binding and inducible NOS messenger RNA in human epithelial cells. Biochem Biophys Res Commun 1994; 199:1518–1524.
98. Robbins RA, Barnes PJ, Springall DR, et al. Expression of inducible nitric oxide in human lung epithelial cells. Biochem Biophys Res Commun 1994; 203:209–218.
99. Kawanami O, Jiang HX, Mochimaru H, et al. Alveolar fibrosis and capillary alteration in experimental pulmonary silicosis in rats. Am J Respir Crit Care Med 1995; 151:1946–1955.
100. Lesur O, Cantin AM, Tanswell AK, Melloni B, Beaulieu JF, Begin R. Silica exposure induces cytotoxicity and proliferative activity of type II pneumocytes. Exp Lung Res 1992; 18:173–190.
101. Wagner CL, Ryan RM, Forsythe DE, Keenan A, Finkelstein JN. Secretion of transforming growth factor-alpha (TGF alpha) by postnatal rabbit alveolar macrophages. Pediatr Res 1995; 38:49–54.
102. Antoniades HN, Bravo MA, Avila RE, et al. Platelet-derived growth factor in idiopathic pulmonary fibrosis. J Clin Invest 1990; 86:1055–1064.
103. Antoniades HN. Linking cellular injury to gene expression and human proliferative disorders—examples with the PDGF genes. Mol Carcinogen 1992; 6:175–181.
104. Khalil N, O'Connor RN, Unruh HW, et al. Increased production and immunohistochemical localization of transforming growth factor-beta in idiopathic pulmonary fibrosis. Am J Respir Cell Mol Biol 1991; 5:155–162.

105. Khalil N, O'Connor RN, Flanders KC, Unruh H. TGF-beta(1), but not TGF-beta(2) or TGF-beta(3), is differentially present in epithelial cells of advanced pulmonary fibrosis—an immunohistochemical study. Am J Respir Cell Mol Biol 1996; 14: 131–138.
106. Raaberg L, Nexo E, Buckley S, Luo W, Snead ML, Warburton D. Epidermal growth factor transcription, translation, and signal transduction by rat type-II pneumocytes in culture. Am J Respir Cell Mol Biol 1992; 6:44–49.
107. Piguet PF, Ribaux C, Karpuz V, Grau GE, Kapanci Y. Expression and localization of tumor necrosis factor-alpha and its messenger RNA in idiopathic pulmonary fibrosis. A J Pathol 1993; 143:651–655.
108. Nash JRG, McLaughlin PJ, Hoyle C, Roberts D. Immunolocalization of tumour necrosis factor-alpha in lung tissue from patients dying with adult respiratory distress syndrome. Histopathology 1991; 19:395–402.
109. Paine RD, Chavis A, Gaposchkin D, et al. A factor secreted by a human pulmonary alveolar epithelial-like cell line blocks T-cell proliferation between G_1 and S phase. Am J Respir Cell Mol Biol 1992; 6:658–666.
110. Blau H, Riklis S, Kravtsov V, Kalina M. Secretion of cytokines by rat alveolar epithelial cells: possible regulatory role for SP-A. Am J Physiol 1994; 266:L148–L155.
111. Antoniades HN, Nevillegolden J, Galanopoulos T, Kradin RL, Valente AJ, Graves DT. Expression of monocyte chemoattractant protein-1 messenger RNA in human idiopathic pulmonary fibrosis. Proc Natl Acad Sci USA 1992; 89:5371–5375.
112. Vallyathan V, Shi XL, Dalal NS, Irr W, Castranova VP. Generation of free radicals from freshly fractured silica dust. Potential role in acute silica-induced lung injury. Am Rev Respir Dis 1988; 138:1213–1219.
113. Gossart S, Cambon C, Orfila C, et al. Reactive oxygen intermediates as regulators of TNF-alpha production in rat lung inflammation induced by silica. J Immunol 1996; 156:1540–1548.
114. Perkins RC, Scheule RK, Holian AP. In vitro bioactivity of asbestos for the human alveolar macrophage and its modification by IgG. Am J Respir Cell Mol Biol 1991; 4:532–537.
115. Chen J, Armstrong LC, Liu SJ, Gerriets JE, Last JA. Silica increases cytosolic free calcium ion concentration of alveolar macrophages in vitro. Toxicol Appl Pharmacol 1991; 111:211–220.
116. Rojanasakul Y, Wang LY, Malanga CJ, Ma JYC, Banks DE, Ma JKH. Altered calcium homeostasis and cell injury in silica-exposed alveolar macrophages. J Cell Physiol 1993; 154:310–316.
117. Ohmori Y, Hamilton TA. Regulation of macrophage gene expression by T-cell-derived lymphokines. Pharmacol Ther 1994; 63:235–264.
118. Doran JE. Biological effects of endotoxin. Curr Stud Hematol Blood Trans 1992: 66–99.
119. Weinstein SL, Sanghera JS, Lemke K, Defranco AL, Pelech SL. Bacterial lipopolysaccharide induces tyrosine phosphorylation and activation of mitogen-activated protein kinases in macrophages. J Biol Chem 1992; 267:14955–14962.
120. Manthey CL, Brandes ME, Perera PY, Vogel SN. Taxol increases steady-state lev-

els of lipopolysaccharide-inducible genes and protein-tyrosine phosphorylation in murine macrophages. J Immunol 1992; 149:2459–2465.

121. Kohno M, Nishizawa N, Tsujimoto M, Nomoto H. Mitogenic signalling pathway of tumour necrosis factor involves the rapid tyrosine phosphorylation of 41,000-M_r and 43,000-M_r cytosol proteins. Biochem J 1990; 267:91–98.
122. Ahlers A, Belka C, Gaestel M, et al. Interleukin-1-induced intracellular signaling pathways converge in the activation of mitogen-activated protein kinase and mitogen-activated protein kinase-activated protein kinase 2 and the subsequent phosphorylation of the 27-kilodalton heat shock protein in monocytic cells. Mol Pharmacol 1994; 46:1077–1083.
123. Novogrodsky A, Vanichkin A, Patya M, Gazit A, Osherov N, Levitzki A. Prevention of lipopolysaccharide-induced lethal toxicity by tyrosine kinase inhibitors. Science 1994; 264:1319–1322.
124. Glaser KB, Sung A, Bauer J, Weichman BM. Regulation of eicosanoid biosynthesis in the macrophage. Involvement of protein tyrosine phosphorylation and modulation by selective protein tyrosine kinase inhibitors. Biochem Pharmacol 1993; 45: 711–721.
125. Iwasaki T, Uehara Y, Graves L, Rachie N, Bomsztyk K. Herbimycin A blocks IL-1-induced NF-kappa B DNA-binding activity in lymphoid cell lines. FEBS Lett 1992; 298:240–244.
126. Coyne DW, Morrison AR. Effect of the tyrosine kinase inhibitor, genistein, on interleukin-1 stimulated PGE_2 production in mesangial cells. Biochem Biophys Res Commun 1990; 173:718–724.
127. Ihle JN, Kerr IM. Jaks and stats in signaling by the cytokine receptor superfamily [Review]. Trends Genet 1995; 11:69–74.
128. Ihle JN. Janus kinases in cytokine signalling. Philos Trans R Soc Lond B Biol Sci 1996; 351:159–166.
129. Larner AC, Finbloom DS. Protein tyrosine phosphorylation as a mechanism which regulates cytokine activation of early response genes. Biochim Biophy Acta Mol Cell Res 1995; 1266:278–287.
130. DeFranco AL, Hambleton J, McMahon M, Weinstein SL. Examination of the role of MAP kinase in the response of macrophages to lipopolysaccharide. Prog Clin Biol Res 1995; 392:407–420.
131. Ding A, Sanchez E, Nathan CF. Taxol shares the ability of bacterial lipopolysaccharide to induce tyrosine phosphorylation of microtubule-associated protein kinase. J Immunol 1993; 151:5596–5602.
132. Dong Z, Qi X, Fidler IJ. Tyrosine phosphorylation of mitogen-activated protein kinases is necessary for activation of murine macrophages by natural and synthetic bacterial products. J Exp Med 1993; 177:1071–1077.
133. Blumer KJ, Johnson GL. Diversity in function and regulation of MAP kinase pathways. Trends Biochem Sci 1994; 19:236–240.
134. Marshall CJ. MAP kinase kinase kinase, MAP kinase kinase and MAP kinase. Curr Opin Genet Dev 1994; 4:82–89.
135. Chen F, Sun SC, Kuh DC, Gaydos LJ, Demers LM. Essential role of NF-kappa-B activation in silica-induced inflammatory mediator production in macrophages. Biochem Biophys Res Commun 1995; 214:985–992.

136. Geng Y, Zhang BP, Lotz M. Protein tyrosine kinase activation is required for lipopolysaccharide induction of cytokines in human blood monocytes. J Immunol 1993; 151:6692–6700.
137. Deng WL, Ohmori Y, Hamilton TA. LPS does not directly induce STAT activity in mouse macrophages. Cell Immunol 1996; 170:20–24.
138. Zhang SJ, Han JH, Sells MA, et al. Rho family GTPases regulate p38 mitogen-activated protein kinase through the downstream mediator PAK1. J Biol Chem 1995; 270:23934–23936.
139. Vallyathan V, Castranova V, Pack D, et al. Freshly fractured quartz inhalation leads to enhanced lung injury and inflammation. Potential role of free radicals. Am J Respir Crit Care Med 1995; 152:1003–1009.
140. Tuomala MH, Hirvonen MR, Savolainen KMP. Production of inositol phosphates and reactive oxygen metabolites in quartz-dust-stimulated human polymorphonuclear leukocytes. FEBS Lett 1992; 296:57–60.
141. Antonini JM, Murthy GGK, Brain JD. Responses to welding fumes—lung injury, inflammation, and the release of tumor necrosis factor-alpha and interleukin-1-beta. Exp Lung Res 1997; 23:205–227.
142. Hanneken A, Dejuan E, Lutty GA, Fox GM, Schiffer S, Hjelmeland LM. Altered distribution of basic fibroblast growth factor in diabetic retinopathy. Arch Ophthalmol 1991; 109:1005–1011.
143. Holley JA, Janssen YMW, Mossman BT, Taatjes DJ. Increased manganese superoxide dismutase protein in type-II epithelial cells of rat lungs after inhalation of crocidolite asbestos or cristobalite silica. Am J Pathol 1992; 141:475–485.
144. Quinlan T, Spivack S, Mossman BT. Regulation of antioxidant enzymes in lung after oxidant injury. Environ Health Perspect 1994; 102:79–87.
145. Deforge LE, Preston AM, Takeuchi E, Kenney J, Boxer LA, Remick DG. Regulation of interleukin-8 gene expression by oxidant stress. J Biol Chem 1993; 268: 25568–25576.
146. Dangio CT, Sinkin RA, Lomonaco MB, Finkelstein JN. Interleukin-8 and monocyte chemoattractant protein-1 mRNAS in oxygen-injured rabbit lung. Am J Physiol 1995; 12:L826–L831.
147. Feng L, Xia YY, Garcia GE, Hwang D, Wilson CB. Involvement of reactive oxygen intermediates in cyclooxygenase-2 expression induced by interleukin-1, tumor necrosis factor-alpha, and lipopolysaccharide. J Clin Invest 1995; 95:1669–1675.
148. Schreck R, Albermann K, Baeuerle PA. Nuclear factor kappa B: an oxidative stress-responsive transcription factor of eukaryotic cells (a review). Free Radical Res Communs 1992; 17:221–237.
149. Baeuerle PA, Rupec RA, Pahl HL. Reactive oxygen intermediates as second messengers of a general pathogen response. Pathol Biol 1996; 44:29–35.
150. Baeuerle PA, Henkel T. Function and activation of NF-kappa B in the immune system. Annu Rev Immunol 1994; 12:141–179.
151. Baeuml H, Behrends U, Peter RU, et al. Ionizing radiation induces, via generation of reactive oxygen intermediates, intercellular adhesion molecule-1 (ICAM-1) gene transcription and NF-kappa-B-like binding activity in the ICAM-1 transcriptional regulatory region. Free Radical Res 1997; 27:127–142.

152. Karin M. The regulation of AP-1 activity by mitogen-activated protein kinases. Philos Trans R Soc Lond B Biol Sci 1996; 351:127–134.
153. Karin M, Hunter T. Transcriptional control by protein phosphorylation—signal transmission from the cell surface to the nucleus. Curr Biol 1995; 5:747–757.
154. Finkelstein JN, Johnston C, Barrett T, Oberdorster G. Particulate–cell interactions and pulmonary epithelial gene expression. Environ Health Perspect 1997; 105: 1179–1182.
155. Sarih M, Souvannavong V, Brown SC, Adam A. Silica induces apoptosis in macrophages and the release of interleukin-1 alpha and interleukin-1 beta. J Leukoc Biol 1993; 54:407–413.
156. Absher M, Sjostrand M, Baldor LC, Hemenway DR, Kelley J. Patterns of secretion of transforming growth factor-alpha (TGF-alpha) in experimental silicosis. Acute and subacute effects of cristobalite exposure in the rat. Reg Immunol 1993; 5:225–231.
157. Williams AO, Flanders KC, Saffiotti U. Immunohistochemical localization of transforming growth factor-beta 1 in rats with experimental silicosis, alveolar type II hyperplasia, and lung cancer. Am J Pathol 1993; 142:1831–1840.
158. Koren HS, Joyce M, Devlin RB, Becker S, Driscoll K, Madden MC. Modulation of eicosanoid production by human alveolar macrophages exposed to silica in vitro. Environ Health Perspect 1992; 97:77–83.

9

Particle Uptake by Epithelial Cells

ANDREW CHURG

University of British Columbia
Vancouver, British Columbia, Canada

I. Introduction

Particles that are deposited on the airway mucosa or alveolar epithelium may be removed from the lung through a variety of mechanisms (see Chap. 3), or they may be taken up by airway and alveolar epithelial cells. This chapter is concerned with the interactions of mineral particles and epithelial cells and, in particular, the questions of what factors control the uptake of mineral particles by epithelial cells.

To approach this problem I have attempted to treat particle uptake as an independent function of airway and alveolar epithelium (which, in fact, it is to some extent) and largely ignored the effects of the inflammatory cells evoked by particle inhalation; the latter are covered in detail in Chapter 12. Similarly, I have mostly ignored the question of how interactions of particles with surfactants and the mucous layer affect uptake (but see Sec. VIII). The reader should, however, bear in mind that these simplifications, although providing some important mechanistic information, also ignore the complicated interactions that occur in vivo, and that undoubtedly influence particle uptake.

Even taking this approach, attempts to discern the general principles governing uptake are confounded by a variety of factors, particularly the wide range of experimental systems that have been studied. Minerals of every type, size, and shape have been employed in a variety of in vitro and in vivo systems, ranging from inhalation or intratracheal instillation in whole animals, to explants to monolayer cultures.

As much as possible I have relied on in vivo and tracheal explant experiments in writing this chapter, and devoted less emphasis to monolayer culture experiments. This choice reflects that, in terms of mechanisms controlling particle uptake, monolayer culture experiments are frequently hard to interpret. Perhaps most disconcerting is the observation that virtually every type of cell will take up particles in monolayer culture and, in fact, much of the data in the literature is not even based on lung-derived cells. Also, most cultured cells do not retain apical polarity or apical morphological specialization, and these appear to be important factors in controlling particle uptake (see following section). Furthermore, cultured cells sometimes have antioxidant capabilities quite different from their in vivo parents and, as discussed in Section VII, the interactions of oxidants and antioxidant defenses are important in particle uptake. Lastly, understanding particle uptake requires some type of quantitative measure of particle internalization, and these are difficult measurements to make when using monolayer cultures. Nonetheless, it is impossible to write about particle uptake without discussing monolayer culture experiments, and the reader should bear these limitations in mind.

II. Consequences of Particle Uptake

Particle uptake by pulmonary epithelial cells is, actually or potentially, associated with a variety of types of cell injury. The most common response to particle uptake is usually described under the widely used, but nonspecific term, of *cytotoxicity*, a label applied to everything from mild cellular dysfunction at one end of the spectrum, to cell death with epithelial ulceration at the other end (1–4). The mechanisms of particle-induced cytotoxicity are undoubtedly numerous, but one process common to many types of mineral particle in aqueous environments is the generation of active oxygen species (AOS) by reduction of molecular oxygen (reviewed in 5,6). Mineral-catalyzed formation of AOS leads to protein oxidation and lipid peroxidation, and lipid peroxidation itself generates further radicals and toxic species, producing additional injury (5–9). Induction of cell damage by mineral particle-derived AOS has been shown for various forms of asbestos, silica, and silicates, although the relative mineral-to-mineral severity of damage induced in vivo with these agents is poorly defined.

Some types of particles appear to be able to produce genotoxicity. At least in vitro, mineral fibers can cause DNA damage by direct physical interference with the mitotic apparatus or adhesion to individual chromosomes, with resulting aneuploidy, polyploidy, and chromosomal breakage and fragmentation. In tissue culture systems, where most such studies have been performed, these lesions are primarily an effect of fiber size, rather than fiber type and, in aggregate, these studies imply that any fiber is potentially carcinogenic (10–16). In addition, adsorption of fibers to chromosomes may be the mechanism by which asbestos produces large deletion mutations (17). Except for asbestos, these in vitro results, for the most part, are discordant with human epidemiological data and with much in vivo animal data, and they must be interpreted with extreme caution.

Particles that catalyze the formation of AOS can also cause oxidation of individual bases, as well as DNA strand breaks, if the particle enters the nucleus and is in close approximation to chromosomes. For the most part, this process is mediated by the iron-catalyzed formation of highly reactive species, such as hydroxyl radical, either using the surface iron on the particle itself as a Fenton catalyst, or using surface iron leached from the particle into the cytosol, where it acts in a fashion similar to a mobile source of hydroxyl radical formation (5,6).

Mineral fibers, particularly asbestos, can activate protein kinase C and increase expression of ornithine decarboxylase, the proto-oncogenes, c-*fos*, and c-*jun* (18–20), and the nuclear transcription factor, NF-κB (21). All these events are associated with cell proliferation and, potentially, with neoplastic transformation. Recently, Zanella et al. (22) have shown that asbestos activates the mitosis-associated kinase (MAP) system, apparently through interaction with the epidermal growth factor receptor, probably implying that some of these events are mediated by signal transduction pathways that start on the cell surface, rather than by fiber uptake, although this point needs to be directly examined.

Mineral particles may also adsorb other types of carcinogens and enhance their entry into cells, and there is some evidence that organic carcinogens adsorbed to particles are more readily metabolized to the active forms (23–26). Importantly, these observations apply both to particles, such as asbestos, that are classified as carcinogens and to atmospheric particles, such as iron oxide, that are classically considered "inert." Adsorption and enhanced transport of carcinogens in cigarette smoke might play a role in the markedly increased lung cancer rates seen in very heavily exposed asbestos workers who smoke (27).

Radioactive particles (e.g., ^{210}Po derived from cigarette smoke) that are translocated through epithelial cells (see later discussion) to the interstitium may come to lodge under the epithelial basement membrane and from there deliver carcinogenic doses of radiation to the overlying epithelium. It has been proposed that this process plays an important role in cigarette smoke carcinogenesis (28,29).

Exposure to dusts such as silica and asbestos is associated with expression of various proinflammatory and fibrogenic cytokines, some of which (e.g., macrophage inflammatory protein-2; MIP-2) may be produced in epithelial cells (30), although most are probably produced in alveolar macrophages. Exposure of rats to asbestos causes expression of transforming growth factor-alpha (TGF-α) and TGF-β in epithelial cells over the alveolar duct bifurcations where fibers deposit (31,32). But even when there is direct evidence of cytokine production in epithelial cells, it remains unclear whether this is caused by uptake of particles, or is driven by macrophage-derived cytokines or oxidant species.

Fibrosis of the walls of small airways and diffuse interstitial fibrosis are both associated with particle exposure. Several different mechanisms are probably operative. There is some evidence that exposure to asbestos and possibly other types of mineral particles causes increased permeability of the epithelium to small molecules (33); this process may allow particle-evoked, alveolar macrophage-derived growth factors and other cytokines to reach interstitial fibroblasts (30). The mechanism of increased permeability is disputed, with data extant that both support and deny a role for AOS (34,35).

Equally or perhaps even more importantly, some fraction of the particles that enter epithelial cells are translocated through the cells to the interstitium where they may be phagocytosed by interstitial macrophages. This process probably causes interstitial macrophages to release a variety of growth factors, eventually resulting in interstitial or airway wall fibrosis (1,2,36–41). Experimental data (42) suggest that interstitial generation of fibroblast growth factors is considerably more effective than alveolar production of growth factors in inducing fibroblast proliferation, although this conclusion is not universally accepted.

There is considerable evidence to suggest that coexposures to oxidants and particles may increase the severity of particle-induced interstitial fibrosis. Oxidants, such as cigarette smoke, greatly enhance both whole-lung particle retention and particle uptake by epithelia in experimental animals (43), and also increase the severity of particle-induced interstitial fibrosis (44). A variety of radiographic studies have shown that smoking increases the incidence of asbestosis in heavily exposed asbestos workers (45–47).

Lastly, there is increasing epidemiological data showing an association between atmospheric levels of the inhalable fraction of particulate air pollution (PM_{10}) and morbidity and mortality (see Chap. 2). The mechanisms behind these observations are a matter of intense speculation, and there is considerable dispute about which exact particulate species is involved. It has been proposed that very fine particles [possibly so-called ultrafine particles (48,49; see Sec. VI)] produce a particularly intense inflammatory reaction in the alveoli and also have the ability to penetrate into epithelial cells and to the interstitium in much greater numbers than larger particles, thereby producing more of the types of damage described in the foregoing (50; see Sec. VI).

III. Particle Uptake as a Function of Particle Type

In experimental systems, there is uptake of essentially every type of mineral particle (including particles, such as glass and latex spheres, that are not ordinarily thought of as minerals) by airway and epithelial cells in tracheal explants and in vivo (Table 1). Less information is available about human lungs, and much of this is indirect. Examination of light microscopic or electron microscopic sections from human lungs rarely, if ever, reveals particles in airway or alveolar epithelium, despite that ambient air contains a significant particulate load.

We approached this problem (82–84) by using analytical electron microscopy to evaluate microdissected pieces of human airway mucosa and parenchyma from nonsmokers and smokers in the general population and from dust-exposed workers (Table 2). In the autopsy lungs, airway mucosa is essentially airway wall (i.e., subepithelial connective tissue plus cartilage) because the airway epithelium is often lost postmortem. In the general population's lungs, the distribution of particles along the airways matched that expected from animal data and mathematical models of deposition (82,83), implying that the particles had been translocated through the epithelium after deposition on the cell surface. The airway particle burden, in terms of particle concentration, was surprisingly high, with typical values in the range of 10^7 particles per gram of dry tissue. In the paren-

Table 1 Types of Mineral Particles Reported to be Taken Up by Pulmonary Tracheobronchial and Alveolar Epithelial Cells in Experimental In Vivo and Tracheal Explant Systems

Mineral species	Refs.
Asbestos	4,40,43,44,51–61
Chrysotile	
Amosite	
Crocidolite	
Barium sulfate	62,63
Carbon	4,64–69
Carbonyl iron	70
Diesel exhaust	37
Glass fiber	71; Churg, unpublished
Iron oxide	54,72–74
Latex microspheres	64
Refractory ceramic fibers	Churg, unpublished
Rock and slag wool fibers	Churg, unpublished
Silicon carbide (compact particles)	53
Silicon carbide (fibers)	53
Silica	39,75–77
Talc	53
Copier toner	37,41
Titanium dioxide	49,78–81
Wollastonite	53
Uranium oxide	62,63

Table 2 Types of Mineral Particles in the Airway Walls in Human Autopsy Lungs

Aluminum oxide
Asbestos
Amosite
Chrysotile
Tremolite
Chromium oxide
Feldspars
Iron oxide
Kaolin
Lead
Mullite (fly ash)
Mica (muscovite)
Polonium
Silica
Talc
Titanium dioxide
Vermiculite

Source: Refs. 82–84.

chyma the burden was even higher, typically in a particle range of 10^7–10^8/g dry lung (85–88). The particles in the lungs of the general population were types commonly found in ambient air, implying that epithelial uptake, translocation, and subsequent interstitial retention of atmospheric particles are frequent events in the human lung.

All of the particles listed in Table 2 can also be found in bulk digests of the parenchyma in these same lungs (82,83) and, in persons with particular occupational exposures, additional particle types specific to the industry in question can be demonstrated. These data must be viewed with some caution because they are derived from bulk analyses, and this approach does not discriminate between particles in the alveolar interstitium and particles in alveolar macrophages. However, with either light or scanning electron microscopy, it is easy to find mineral particles in the interstitium in lungs from workers with occupational exposures, implying that particle uptake and translocation by alveolar epithelium must also be extremely common.

Probably the most important thing about Tables 1 and 2 is the apparent lack of specificity of uptake in terms of particle type and shape; indeed, Tables 1 and 2 suggest that particle uptake by pulmonary epithelial cells is, essentially, a universal phenomenon. But what these tables do not show is that there are marked differences in the extent to which different types of particles enter epithe-

Table 3 Relative Uptake of Two Types of Compact Particle by Tracheal Epithelial Cells[a]

Particle	Geometric mean diameter (μm)	Concentration administered	Uptake as volume proportion of epithelium
Iron oxide	0.45	4 mg/mL	0.31%
Titanium dioxide	0.51	5 mg/mL	0.87%

[a]Assuming the particles are spherical, the number of iron oxide particles applied is actually 16% greater than the number of titanium dioxide particles.
Source: Ref. 53.

lial cells. Table 3 provides an example of these differences: when compact particles of iron oxide or titanium dioxide of close to identical size were applied to tracheal explants at close to identical number concentrations (actually the iron oxide concentration was about 16% higher), uptake was 2.8 times greater for the titanium dioxide.

Subsequent sections of this chapter will attempt to outline some of the factors that contribute to the types of differences just illustrated, but the reader should understand that, as yet, there is little in the way of mechanistic explanations for these differences nor, as a general rule, even quantitative data on particle-to-particle variations in uptake.

IV. The Importance of Particle Clearance as a Defense Against Epithelial Particle Uptake

Contact with airway or alveolar epithelial cells is a prerequisite for particle uptake, and such contact depends on three factors: (1) particle deposition patterns (see Chap. 3); (2) penetration of particles through the surfactant and mucus layers that line the alveoli and airways (see Sec. VIII); and (3) removal or failure to remove particles by inflammatory cells. This section will concern itself with the relation between particle removal by inflammatory cells, particularly macrophages, and particle uptake by epithelial cells.

All inhaled particles evoke an inflammatory response in the lung. In most reported studies the initial inflammatory cells are polymorphonuclear leukocytes (PMNL), and these are followed by an influx of alveolar macrophages (1,41,49,64–68,78,89). In a few studies (55,70) only a macrophage response has been seen, at least when considering cells accumulating at the first alveolar duct bifurcations, the major site of particle impaction in these specific experiments. As a rule, and provided the point of overload (see following) is not reached, there is a reasonably good correlation between the number of particles deposited and the numbers of macrophages that appear as a response (64,78,89), although data (90) suggest that, at least under nonoverload conditions, only a small fraction of the evoked macrophages actually phagocytose particles.

Virtually all particles that deposit in the alveoli, and some portion of particles that deposit in the conducting airways, are phagocytosed by macrophages and either transported proximally along the airways, or transported through the pulmonary lymphatics to lymph nodes. But neither mucociliary clearance nor alveolar macrophages form a perfect defense (78), and even in the absence of overload (see following discussion) some, apparently quite small, fraction of deposited paticles is taken up by alveolar or airway epithelial cells, as can be deduced from Tables 1 and 2.

The importance of particle removal as a defense against particle uptake has been established by using experimental systems that manipulate macrophage numbers. If macrophage numbers are artificially decreased, then alveolar particle persistence is increased, along with epithelial particle uptake and translocation. In a classic experiment (65), mice were depleted of circulating monocytes (the source of the initial alveolar macrophage response) with radiation; the persistence of free carbon particles increased from 1 week in control mice to 3 weeks in radiated mice. This increase in alveolar persistence was accompanied by a substantial increase in type I cell particle uptake and translocation to the interstitium. Similar results were obtained with silica particles, with a marked increase in interstitial particles and in the degree of silica-induced fibrosis (39).

Another way of approaching the problem is to put the lung into *overload*, which for convenience, can be defined as a situation in which administration of sufficiently high loads of nontoxic insoluble dusts produces marked prolongation or even total failure of macrophage-mediated particle clearance (reviewed in 41,91). The mechanism of the overload effect is not entirely understood (see 91–94 for comments), but it is clear that, under overload conditions, the burden of free particles in the alveoli, the number of particles that are taken up by epithelial cells, and the number of particles translocated to the interstitium, all are greatly increased (41,91).

Experiments in which the lung is put into overload (40,41) also illustrate the deleterious effects of epithelial particle uptake, because under overload conditions, a variety of particles that are normally considered to be nonpathogenic (carbon black, titanium dioxide, copier toner, volcanic fly ash, and diesel exhaust) produce interstitial inflammation and fibrosis. Many also produce lung cancers in rats, although the latter phenomenon is probably restricted to rats (37,41,91,92) and appears not to occur in other species.

A different line of evidence for the idea that failure to remove particles from the lung leads to epithelial uptake comes from experiments using tracheal explants. Tracheal explants are, for practical purposes, free of inflammatory cells. If such explants are briefly exposed to a suspension of dust particles, the particles adhere to the epithelial surface (Fig. 1; and see Sec. VII). When the explants are maintained in air organ culture, there is slow uptake of the surface particles by the epithelial cells over time, and this is accompanied by transport of particles through the epithelial cells to the interstitium (3,4,51–53; see Fig. 1). Explant experiments also make the point that particle uptake is an intrinsic property of the pulmonary (here, specifically, airway) epithelium: neither inflammatory cells nor inflammatory cell products, such as active oxygen species or cytokines, are required for uptake to occur.

The major conclusion to be drawn from these studies is that persistence of free particles in the airspaces or in the airways is one of the major determinants of epithelial particle uptake (64,81,95). Particle clearance mechanisms thus serve as a defense against prolonged contact of particles with lung epithelial cells, and this defense is important, for once contact occurs, cell perturbation from surface

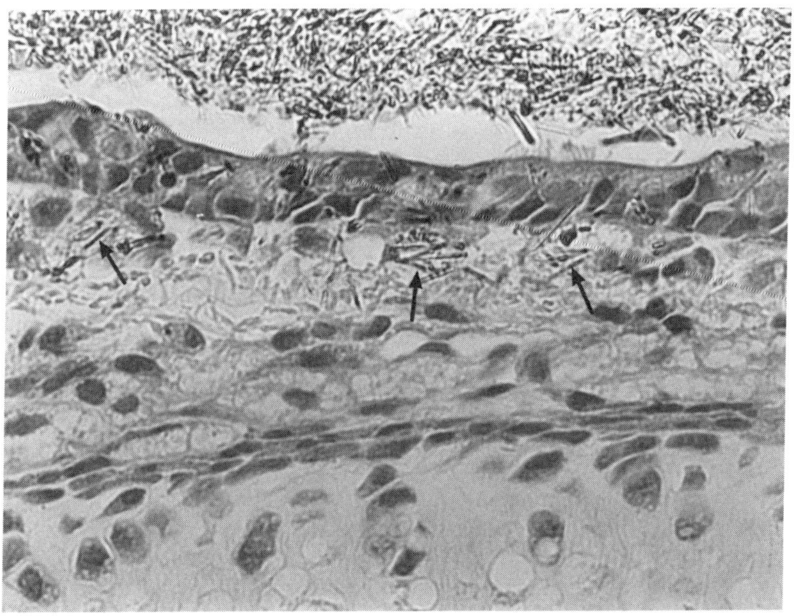

Figure 1 Micrograph of a rat tracheal explant: The explant was initially exposed to amosite asbestos for 1 hr, then maintained in air organ culture for 7 days, and fixed and processed for histological assessment. Note the adherent mass of fibers on the apical epithelial surface; some fibers have been taken up by the epithelium and some (arrows) have been translocated to the connective tissue layer beneath the epithelium. Cartilage is visible at the bottom of the field. Space between mass of fibers and apical surface is an artifact of cutting direction. (From Ref. 161.)

effects (e.g., generation of AOS or activation of MAP kinases) or particle internalization, with subsequent pathological reactions, may follow.

V. Particle Uptake as a Function of Anatomical Location and Cell Type

Little information is available about differences in particle uptake as a function of either anatomical location within the lung or as a function of cell type. In the mouse, all types of conducting airway cells, except mucous cells, phagocytosed 5-nm–iron oxide particles administered by inhalation (72,73). The iron oxide particles were translocated through the cell to the interstitium, and this phenomenon appeared to occur primarily in ciliated cells. In human bronchial explants, the ciliated cells took up both asbestos and glass fibers (71), but uptake occurred primarily in areas with relatively few cilia, apparently because areas with numerous actively beating cilia tended to move particles away from the cell surfaces. In hamster tracheal explants, there was a similar effect for long, but not short, fibers of both chrysotile and crocidolite.

Airway carinas have been the subject of considerable interest in terms of deposition models, because inertial motion in areas of high flow causes larger particles to impact at the carinas. Therefore, all other things being equal, carinas should accumulate greater numbers of particles than tubular segments. In fact, it has been suggested that accumulation of carcinogenic radioactive particles and particles with adsorbed carcinogens from cigarette smoke at airway carinas is a potentially important mechanism of human pulmonary carcinogenesis (28,29). In addition, animal studies suggest that clearance of particles from carinas is much slower than from tubular airway segments; although the mechanism of this effect is unknown, the net result is to further increase particle accumulation at carinas (62,96).

Enhanced deposition of particles on carinas has been demonstrated in animal models (72,96) and in human airway casts (97,98), and we have recently extended these observations to human autopsy lungs by microdissection of the mucosa of carinas and tubular segments in the large airways (99). When analyzing generations 1 to 4, we found that the median ratio of the concentration of particles in the mucosal tissues of the carinas to the mucosal tissues of the immediately preceding tubular segment was about 9:1 in a series of ten never-smoker lungs. Of particular note was the marked person-to-person variation, with some individuals having numerous carinal/tubular pairs with ratios higher than 100 (99). Whether these differences reflect individual-to-individual variations in deposition or clearance patterns, or abnormally high levels of epithelial particle uptake and translocation is unknown, but, at least in theory, such individuals may be particularly susceptible to the toxic effects of inhaled particles.

In experimental systems, accumulation of particles at carinas is also seen in the smaller airways including alveolar ducts (55,70,100), and in these models (e.g., asbestos exposure) small airway carinas show distinct localized pathological reactions.

Mathematical models of particle deposition predict that high levels of deposition will also be seen in the respiratory bronchioles (roughly Weibel generations 16–20; 101–103), and in fact, mural dust accumulation with fibrosis is commonly observed in the small airways in workers with heavy mineral dust exposure (104). The only quantitative human data addressing this question show that, in chrysotile asbestos miners with very heavy dust exposure, the number of particles in the walls of the more respiratory bronchioles (distal) is considerably higher than that in the membranous bronchioles (proximal; 105), as the models predict. It is possible that the fibrotic and inflammatory lesions of the membranous and respiratory bronchioles commonly seen in cigarette smokers and referred to as ''small airways disease'' (104) are also a reflection of high levels of deposition of smoke particles in this portion of the airway, as predicted by a recent model of cigarette smoke particle deposition (106).

High levels of deposition alone are probably not the complete explanation for the development of inflammatory and fibrotic lesions in the respiratory bronchioles, because administration of dust to experimental animals by intratracheal instillation still results in much greater epithelial uptake and interstitial transport of asbestos fibers and compact iron oxide particles in the respiratory bronchioles, compared with the more proximal membranous bronchioles (43,74). Lehnert (78) suggests that greater distal airway particle uptake may be caused by greater and more prolonged particle contact resulting from (1) a much less viscous mucous layer in the distal airways; (2) fewer ciliary beat frequencies and slower mucous transport rates in the distal airways (107–111). Some workers have reported areas of discontinuity in the distal mucous blanket, and such gaps would allow extensive contact of particles with the epithelium, but most investigators have not found discontinuities (78,112–114).

In the alveoli, illustrations showing uptake of particles by epithelial cells have been published for asbestos (40,55–61,70), silica (1,77), iron oxide (72,73), carbon (64,69), titanium dioxide (49), and latex spheres (64). This process appears to occur primarily in type I cells; uptake by type II cells has generally not been reported, or has been described as a minor effect (73). Actual quantitative data on the differences in uptake between type I and type II cells are scarce, but Pinkerton et al. (40) showed that, after 3 months exposure to chrysotile asbestos, the relative fiber density was about 13 times greater in type I compared with type II cells.

In general, particle uptake is a fairly rapid process, but again, there are site-to-site differences in the speed at which uptake occurs. Stirling and Patrick (63), using intratracheal instillation, noted that no instilled barium sulfate particles were found in the tracheal epithelium 2 hr after dust administration, but by 24 hr after administration, about 75% of the particles remaining in the trachea were in the epithelium, and by 7 days almost all the retained particles had traversed the epithelium to the subepithelial connective tissue. In rat tracheal explants, we observed uptake of asbestos, iron oxide, talc, titanium dioxide, and wollastonite particles by ciliated cells at 24 hr, which was the first time point sampled, and accumulation of particles beneath the epithelium by 1 week (51–53; and see Figs. 1 and 2). Similar results were reported by Mossman et al. (3,4,54), who studied the uptake of carbon, iron oxide, and asbestos fibers in hamster tracheal explants.

The limited data reporting uptake as a function of time suggest that alveolar epithelial uptake is probably faster than bronchiolar epithelial uptake. Watson and Brain found 5-nm–iron oxide particles within type I cells 1 hr after a 3-hr–inhalation exposure (73). Chrysotile fibers were visible within type I cells at the end of a 1 hr high-level inhalation exposure (55); by 5 hr after exposure, some fibers had been translocated to the interstitium. Carbon, latex, and silica particles have also been shown in type I cells within 24 hr of intratracheal or inhalation exposure (64,76,77).

These observations suggest that, for any given dust, there are quite marked differences in particle uptake and interstitial translocation in the various portions of the airways and between the airways and alveoli. Also, there are probably differences in uptake of any given particle among the different airway and alveolar eptihelial cells. However, quantitative data on the magnitude of these differences are few.

VI. Effects of Particle Size, Shape, and Dose on Particle Uptake

The issue of particle uptake as a function of particle size, which is of importance in itself, has taken on a new life as a result of recent observations on the uptake of ultrafine particles and the proposed relation of ultrafine particles to PM_{10} toxicity (50; also see following discussion).

The first proposition to be discussed in this section is the theory that, for any given type of compact particle, smaller particles are more readily phagocytosed by epithelial cells and also show greater rates of transport across the epithelium. A close corollary is the idea that uptake and transport are also affected by the rate of dust administration (4,38,49,64,78–81,114). The second part of the discussion will focus on the issue of size and uptake of fibrous particles.

At first glance the data on compact particles appear deceptively straightforward. Lehnert et al. (78) reported uptake of 2-µm polystyrene particles by rat airway epithelial cells, whereas Valasquez and Morrow (114) failed to find uptake of 7.9-µm particles by guinea pig airway cells. Adamson and Bowden (64) noted that 0.1-μm–latex spheres were readily seen in type I cells after intratracheal instillation, but in contrast, very few 1-μm spheres entered the cells. As the dose of administered particles increased, there was an increase in the number of particles entering alveolar epithelial cells. Mossman et al. (4), who used tracheal explants, found that 0.5- to 1.0-μm–carbon particles entered the epithelial cells, whereas 15- to 30-μm particles did not.

The issues of size and dose versus uptake have been investigated in considerable detail (38,53–55,85) using ultrafine (mean diameter approximately 0.020 μm) and fine (mean diameter 0.25 μm) titanium dioxide or similarly sized aluminum oxide particles. If equal particle masses were administered by intratracheal instillation and multiple lavages performed, the unlavageable mass (presumed to represent particles in epithelial cells, interstitium, lymphatics, and particles firmly bound in alveolar spaces) of ultrafine particles was about 50% greater after 1 day (Table 4) than the unlavageable mass of fine particles.

Different results were obtained by using a 12-week–inhalation experiment at equal mass doses (49). Until inhalation ceased, the unlavageable mass of dust was the same for both sizes of particle, but once inhalation ceased, the rate of (mass) clearance was significantly slower for the smaller particles ($t_{1/2}$ = 501 days) than with the larger ones ($t_{1/2}$ = 174 days). During exposure the particle content in the lymph nodes was considerably greater for the ultrafine particles, and the lymph node burden continued to increase much more rapidly than for the larger particles over 1 year. Administration of ultrafine particles was associated with a much more pronounced inflammatory response and with apparently greater histological evidence of translocation to the interstitium, although the latter does not appear to have been really quantified. An additional observation was that more rapid delivery of particles caused greater retention in the unlavageable compartment (49).

It was concluded from these experiments that translocation of particles is a function of delivered particle number, rate of particle delivery, and (inversely) particle size. The foregoing data were used with a multicompartment physiological model to calculate the rate of particle translocation (115). It was concluded

Table 4 Instilled and Unlavageable Amounts of Titanium Dioxide as a Function of Particle Size at 1 Day After Exposure

Particle type/size	Instilled mass (μg)	Instilled number	Unlavageable mass (μg)	Unlavageable number
Fine (0.250 μm)	500	1.6×10^{10}	66 ± 13	2.1×10^{9}
Ultrafine (0.021 μm)	500	2.7×10^{13}	102 ± 24	5.5×10^{12}
Ratio ultrafine/fine	1.00	1680	1.54	2620

Source: Ref. 49.

that the observed differences in retention would require an order of magnitude greater rate of translocation of ultrafine than of fine titanium dioxide particles.

On a second look, interpretation of these data is not straightforward. The simplest question, that of the relation of dose and uptake, is confounded because most of the experimental systems employed tend to put the lung into overload. Once overload is achieved, uptake is, in fact, related to number dose (although the relation is exponential: see 49,38,49,79,91), but below the point of overload the relation of dose and uptake is uncertain because the clearance efficiency for nontoxic particles is extremely high and few enter the interstitium. Because of the relation of particle uptake to overload, it is also difficult to determine whether uptake is really driven by delivery rate, as suggested by Ferin et al. (49), or more likely, the rate at which overload is achieved. This would be one explanation for the difference between the effects of a single intratracheal instillation and continuous inhalation exposure in the foregoing data of Oberdorster and colleagues (38,48,49,81).

The relation of uptake and particle size for compact particles is equally difficult. All of the studies (4,49,64,79,80,81) that claim greater uptake for smaller particles have used equal mass doses of smaller and larger particles, which means that the number of smaller particles administered is typically 3 or 4 orders of magnitude greater than the number of larger particles. Thus, apparently greater uptake of smaller particles may reflect not particle size, but particle number that, as noted in the previous paragraph, does drive uptake when particle number is great enough. This is well illustrated in the data (49) on the relation of unlavageable dose, particle size, and administered particle number: these data show that unlavageable dose remains about the same until a particle dose of about 10^{13} is reached, and then, it increases exponentially, and it does not matter whether the administered particles are fine or ultrafine titanium dioxide. The easiest explanation for these observations is that a dose of 10^{13} titanium dioxide particles puts the lung into overload, and that overload (or at least high particle number), rather than size, is really driving uptake. Entry into overload would also explain why the particle retention curve becomes exponential above 10^{13} particles, an observation that is quite difficult to explain on the basis of size alone.

The increase in lymph node burden seen with ultrafine titanium dioxide has also been cited as evidence of increased interstitial transport of small particles (49,91). The problem with this line of reasoning is that, although, in one sense, it is true by definition, increased lymph node burdens tell nothing of the route by which the particles reached the lymph nodes; certainly lymph node burdens provide no direct information about epithelial uptake and transport.

We (116) have recently used rat tracheal explants in an attempt to examine this problem in a simpler system. Explants were exposed to fine (0.12-μm) or ultrafine (0.021-μm) titanium dioxide at a particle number ratio of 1:200, and maintained in organ culture. Particle uptake was determined morphometrically using electron micrographs. Epithelial uptake showed small (at most twofold) differences that changed over time. However, at 7 days, the number of particles of each size in the interstitial space was exactly proportional to the number applied to the explant surface. These observations suggest that, in the absence of inflammatory cells, particle uptake is a function of particle number and not of particle size. Our data thus do not support the predictions of Stober et al. (115) described earlier.

The observation that the ultrafine particles elicit a numerically much greater inflammatory response than the fine particles (38,49) may, again, be a reflection of delivered particle number because, as indicated in Section IV, the inflammatory response closely matches the number of particles reaching the airways and alveoli. In addition, as Oberdorster points out (41), a marked increase in numbers of polymorphonuclear leukocytes is one of the most sensitive markers of overload.

In short, there is no doubt that, under certain circumstances, administration of smaller particles appears to result in greater epithelial and interstitial burdens than does administration of larger particles, along with a more intense inflammatory response, but the important question of whether this is a size effect, compared with a number effect or an overload effect, and what the role of inflammatory cells in this process might be, requires further study.

The relation of epithelial uptake to the size of fibrous, as opposed to compact particles is equally uncertain. In in vivo experiments long fibers (at least long asbestos fibers) tend to produce markedly greater degrees of interstitial fibrosis than short fibers (56,57,117,118), and these findings immediately suggest that long fibers reach the interstitium in greater numbers than short fibers. However, there are few quantitative data on fiber size and epithelial uptake and the available data are contradictory. Hesterberg et al. (16), who used Syrian hamster embryo cells in culture, found that although both long and short fibers of glass and asbestos adhered to the cell surface, long fibers of both types exhibited preferential uptake, with the result that the mean intracellular fiber length was about twice mean surface fiber length. In direct contradiction, it was observed (23,71) that shorter fibers of chrysotile, amosite, and crocidolite tended to be phagocytosed by the ciliated epithelium of tracheal explants, but longer fibers tend to be transported off the explant by ciliary motion. However, our own studies of tracheal explants maintained in organ culture show that asbestos, silicon carbide, and man-made mineral fibers up to 20 μm and sometimes up to 40 μm in length enter the epithelial cells (see Fig. 1; Churg A, unpublished data). Also, when tracheal explants were grown in media that promoted squamous metaplasia, then long and short fibers appear to be phagocytosed equally well (119), implying that different cells types may show different patterns of size-related uptake.

In whole animals, only short fibers were observed (53,54) in type I cells and in the interstitium of rats after inhalation or intratracheal instillation of chrysotile. Short crocidolite fibers entered type I cells and eventually reached the interstitium by transport through the cell (56), whereas long fibers of crocidolite reached the interstitium by causing epithelial ulceration and subsequent incorporation (57). Ulceration is typically seen in intratracheal instillation experiments with very high fiber or particle doses, and whether it occurs with inhalation is unknown, but very long fibers certainly do reach the interstitium after inhalation exposures, for interstitial asbestos bodies, which typically have mean lengths in the range of 30–40 μm, are easily observed in both humans and animals exposed to asbestos. Equally important, in vitro, both long and short crocidolite fibers induced alveolar macrophages and cultured interstitial macrophages to secrete fibroblast growth factors (36,42); this suggested that the greater ability of long fibers to enter the interstitium was why long fibers were more fibrogenic. Whether the differences between long and short fibers really reflect numbers of fibers reaching interstitial macrophages, a specific fiber length effect on interstitial macrophages, or some other parameter, remains unclear.

Analysis of human data is further complicated by the observation that common coexposures, such as ozone and cigarette smoke, can modify the uptake of both fibers and compact particles. Cigarette smoke increases the total uptake of asbestos fibers and iron oxide particles in rat tracheal explants in organ culture (see Sec. VII), and also increases both whole lung retention and bronchiolar epithelial uptake in laboratory animals (43,74,120; see Sec. VII). The relative increases in retention are much greater for short than long asbestos fibers (121). Increased retention is associated with increased interstitial fibrosis (asbestosis; 44). To show that smoke increases fiber retention in human lungs has proved difficult, but we recently demonstrated increased asbestos retention in the airway mucosa of smokers and also found that the fibers in the lungs of smokers were shorter than those in the lungs of nonsmokers (84), observations in accord with the experimental data just described. It is not known whether cigarette smoke modifies the size of a compact particle that is taken up by tracheobronchial epithelium, and whether smoke also affects particle uptake by alveolar epithelium.

VII. Effects of Active Oxygen Species on Particle Uptake

Many minerals can spontaneously catalyze the formation of active oxygen species (AOS) in aqueous systems, which in this context include both the cell surface and the cell cytoplasm (5). Most commonly, this process uses surface iron(II) or leachable iron(II) from the mineral particle to reduce molecular oxygen to superoxide anion; superoxide anion then dismutates to hydrogen peroxide and, in the presence of iron(II), the hydroxyl radical is formed via the Fenton reaction, along with iron(III). If iron(III) can be reduced (e.g., by additional superoxide anion or by cellular ascorbate), then continuous generation of AOS is possible (reviewed in 6). There is extensive evidence that asbestos produces AOS in this fashion (5–7), and the same is probably true of silica and silicates (116,117). As noted in Section II, AOS generated by mineral dusts are injurious to pulmonary epithelial cells (6,7,122,123).

We have used a rat tracheal explant system to examine the role of AOS in particle uptake. When tracheal explants are briefly immersed in a suspension of a mineral dust, dust particles adhere to the epithelial cell surfaces; if the explants are then maintained in organ culture in air, the epithelial cells slowly take up particles from the apical surface (see Fig. 1). The relative basal level of uptake of different types of particles is quite different (see Table 3), but every type of mineral particle thus far examined (asbestos, carbon, titanium dioxide, iron oxide, talc, wollastonite, or silicon carbide) enters the epithelial cells (3,4,51–54). This system offers several simplifying advantages for studying particle uptake, including lack of airspace inflammatory cells, maintenance of normal levels of intracellular antioxidant defense (Churg A, unpublished data), and retention of a polarized cell structure with normal apical differentiation.

In tracheal explants, the basal level of amosite asbestos uptake can be decreased by adding catalase, a scavenger of hydrogen peroxide, to the dust suspension, or by preincubating the dust with the iron chelator, deferoxamine (124), a chelator that prevents the reaction of iron with hydrogen peroxide to form a hydroxyl radical (6). The decreases in particle uptake are scavenger–chelator dose-dependent, but uptake cannot be reduced below about one-third to one-half the basal level (124). Conversely, uptake can be increased if amosite asbestos or titanium dioxide particles are preincubated with iron salt solutions to increase surface iron before they are applied to the explants (125).

Uptake can similarly be increased by exogenous sources of AOS. Brief exposure to whole cigarette smoke, which is a highly concentrated source of AOS and other radicals, and then to a mineral dust suspension produces considerably greater uptake of asbestos, titanium dioxide, fibrous silicon carbide, and talc (51–53; Fig. 2). The increase in uptake is proportional to the dose of cigarette smoke, and the smoke effect can be inhibited by catalase, superoxide dismutase (which destroys superoxide anion), or deferoxamine (see Fig. 2). The effects of low levels of ozone are similar (Fig. 3), but differ from cigarette smoke in that superoxide dismutase is not protective (126). Smoke also fails to enhance the uptake of nonfibrous silicon carbide or iron oxide (hematite; 53); the latter observation is particularly interesting because it was recently shown (127) that hematite does not catalyze the formation of AOS. This observation emphasizes the idea that redox-active surface iron, as opposed to compositional iron, is crucial to AOS formation and particle uptake.

These observations indicate that AOS can increase particle uptake by a direct effect on the tracheobronchial epithelium. The consistently inhibitory ef-

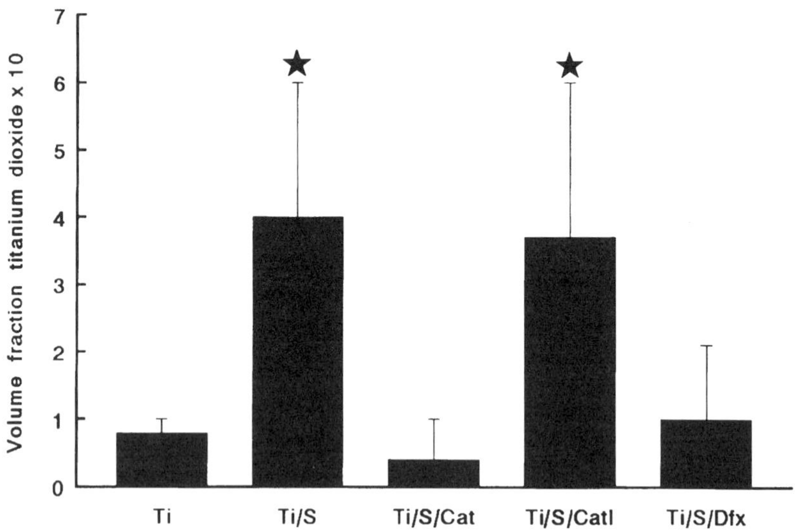

Figure 2 Effects of cigarette smoke and scavengers of active oxygen species on the uptake of titanium dioxide (Ti) in a rat tracheal explant system. Explants were exposed to smoke or air for 10 min and then submerged for 1 hr in a suspension of titanium dioxide, followed by 7 days of air organ culture. In some experiments, catalase (CAT) or inactivated catalase (CATI) was added to the dust suspension; in other experiments the dust was incubated overnight in deferoxamine (DFX). Smoke (S) markedly enhanced titanium dioxide uptake, and both catalase and deferoxamine completely abolished the smoke effect, suggesting that the hydrogen peroxide and the hydroxyl radical are involved. Inactivated catalase was not protective. (From Ref. 53.)

fects of catalase (51,53,124,126,128) indicate that hydrogen peroxide is involved, and this idea is supported by the simple observation that direct addition of hydrogen peroxide at low levels (e.g., 1 μM) to a suspension of amosite or titanium dioxide does result in increased dust uptake (Churg A, unpublished data). Similarly, the consistently inhibitory effects of deferoxamine and the observation that addition of iron to the fiber surfaces increases uptake (125) suggest a role for iron, either as the cation or as a catalyst for lipid peroxidation, in this process.

The use of a combination of scanning electron microscopy to examine surface adhesion and light microscopy to examine uptake, indicated that deferoxamine treatment decreased both the number of adherent fibers and the amount of fiber uptake, whereas catalase treatment decreased uptake with little effect on adhesion (Churg A, unpublished data), and reagent hydrogen peroxide increased

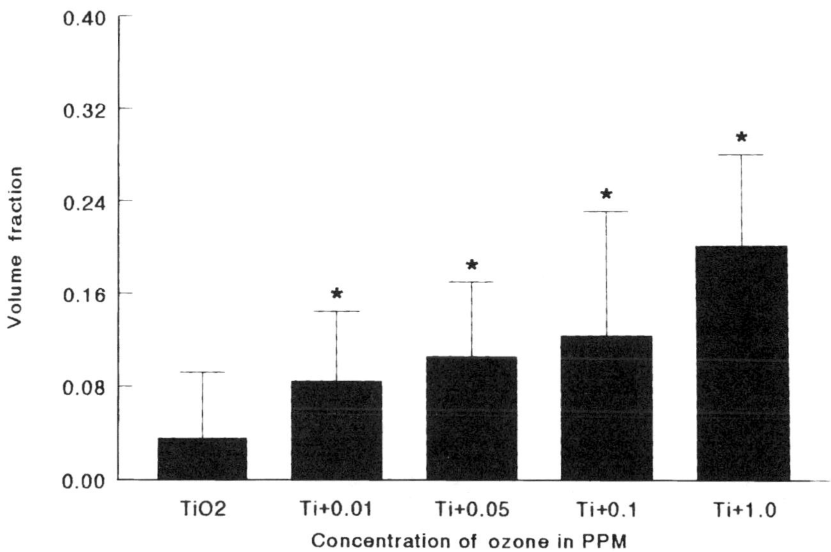

Figure 3 Effects of ozone on uptake of titanium dioxide particles: Explants were exposed to air or ozone at the concentrations indicated and then submerged in a suspension of titanium dioxide for 1 hr, followed by culture for 7 days. Even low concentrations (0.01 ppm) of ozone increase particle uptake, and there is a dose effect. (From Ref. 126.)

uptake without significantly increasing adhesion. These observations suggest either that there is iron-mediated hydroxyl radical-mediated binding of particles to the surface (as a result of lipid peroxidation?), but that the effect of hydrogen peroxide is to increase uptake without changing surface binding. These findings are in accord with other observations (129) that binding to the surface and uptake are two different processes that may proceed by two different mechanisms (see Sec. VIII).

Implicit in the data just described is the idea that AOS are exogenous to the lung. However, there are two additional endogenous sources of AOS that need to be considered. Both tracheobronchial epithelial cells and alveolar epithelial cells themselves produce and secrete small amounts of hydrogen peroxide on a constitutive basis (130,131); such endogenous AOS production could thus produce a type of autocrine mechanism of epithelial–cell-driven particle uptake. Equally, or even more important, the polymorphonuclear leukocytes and macrophages evoked by dusts produce superoxide anion, hydrogen peroxide, and hypochlorous anion as the usual physiological response to any substance they phagocytose (131). Thus, the inflammatory response to mineral particles might have the paradoxical effect of increasing particle uptake.

The observations appear to translate into effects on whole-lung particle retention and also on disease induction. There is evidence that smoke exposure increases dust retention in vivo in experimental animals, and this appears to be true in humans as well, although few data are available (83,132,133). In vivo, ozone also increases long-term (1 month) retention of asbestos fibers (134). The combination of smoking and asbestos exposure appears to increase the incidence of asbestosis in humans and animals, presumably because smoke-enhanced dust retention leads to a greater effective dose of fibers being retained in the lung (45–47).

VIII. Mechanisms of Binding of Particles to Epithelial Cells

Direct observation indicates that exposure of tracheal explants to a mineral dust suspension results in visible binding of the particles to the apical membrane of the tracheal epithelial cells (see Fig. 1). The same process probably occurs with alveolar epithelium. However, little is known about how particles bond to epithelial cells.

There is some evidence (135–137) that the alveolar and airway lining layers, and especially the surfactant components, play an indirect, but important, role in this process because experiments with latex particles have shown that surface tension effects cause particles to be displaced from the air into the lining layer, such that, once deposited, particles do not float on the surface, but instead, are completely submerged. Although this effect may help phagocytosis by macrophages, it also increases the chance of the particle making contact with the epithelial cell, and in fact, large enough particles actually indent the underlying epithelial cell. Surface tension effects act much more strongly on small than on large particles of the same composition (see Chap. 6).

Actual investigations of cell–particle binding have produced interesting but complex results. Brody et al. (138) examined asbestos fiber binding to red cells and found that binding of chrysotile fibers, which have a positive surface charge, could be greatly decreased by pretreatment of the cells with neuraminidase, an observation implying that the chrysotile fibers attached themselves to negatively charged sialic acid groups. Crocidolite, a negatively charged fiber, also bound to red cells, but neuraminidase treatment had no effect. The same group (139) then looked at binding of positively charged particles (chrysotile, carbonyl iron spheres, and aluminum spheres), or negatively charged particles (glass spheres or crocidolite fibers) to alveolar macrophages. Binding of the positively charged particles could be blocked with wheat germ agglutinin and limulus protein, both of which attach to sialic acid residues, but these agents did not affect binding of the negatively charged particles. Although these observations provide evidence for the importance of charge and of sialic acid binding in attachment of positively charged particles to red cells and macrophages, they do not explain attachment of negatively charged particles, nor is it known to what extent these findings apply to pulmonary epithelial cells.

There are also several reports that mineral particles adsorb serum proteins and surfactants and that this process appears to play a role in particle toxicity and particle uptake. Asbestos fibers are highly adsorptive and bind serum proteins in a very persistent fashion; this is true to a lesser extent of silica and titanium dioxide (140,141). The toxicity of amosite for cultured epithelial cells was increased by serum (142), and the effect was present with proteins having molecular weight ranges from 500 to 100,000 Da. Brown et al. (143) studied the binding of amosite and crocidolite, both negatively charged particles, as well as chrysotile to a variety of (nonpulmonary) cultured cells. Different cell lines showed distinct differences in binding, and the positively charged fibers bound quite differently from the negatively charged fibers. Amosite binding could be increased by increasing serum concentration in the medium or by addition of fibronectin to the medium, and could be decreased by blocking the cellular RGD receptor with an RGD-containing pentapeptide. Coating the amosite with poly-D-lysine, which gives the fibers a net positive charge, increased binding (144). The authors (143) came to the conclusion that binding of negatively charged fibers to cells was mediated through coating of the fibers with fibronectin and subsequent interaction between the fibronectin and the cell surface RGD receptors.

Boylan et al. (129) recently looked at the binding and internalization of crocidolite and the calcium silicate, wollastonite, by rabbit mesothelial cells in culture. Surface binding and particle internalization appeared to have different mechanisms; crocidolite internalization, but not binding, was mediated by vitronectin and the specific integrin $\alpha_v\beta_5$. Serum had the same effect, unless it was first depleted of vitronectin, but fibronectin had no effect on uptake or binding. However, vitronectin had no effect on the internalization of wollastonite.

The foregoing data are quite limited in scope and leave many questions unanswered. For practical purposes, nothing appears to be known of the binding of compact particles or fibers to pulmonary epithelial cells in vivo or in lung explant systems, and the rather scanty data on binding to tracheal explants was discussed earlier. The distinction among cell types is important, both because different cell types appear to have different binding properties [witness the data of Brown et al. (143) cited in the foregoing] and because the normally polarized cells of the intact lung or of explants probably function quite differently from nonpolarized cells in cell culture. It is also clear from these data that there are major discrepancies and contradictions from experiment to experiment and that, even within a given experiment, different minerals behave quite differently. Furthermore, as the data (129) make clear, there appears to be a distinction between binding and uptake.

IX. Mechanisms of Particle Uptake and Translocation

There is very little information and few morphological descriptions of how mineral particles actually enter cells. In polymorphonuclear leukocytes and macrophages, which are normally phagocytic, particle uptake requires that the particle in question (e.g., a bacterium) be coated with an opsonin such as fibronectin or immunoglobulin, or with surfactant (135). Uptake then proceeds by a mechanism in which cytoplasmic projections are extruded around the object to be phagocytosed until the projections meet and fuse (so-called zippering); it appears that binding of the opsonin to the advancing cell membrane is crucial to this process. In this context, enhancement of mineral particle uptake by vitronectin, fibronectin, and other opsonins, would make sense and would indicate that uptake of particles by pulmonary epithelial cells proceeds in a fashion analogous with ordinary macrophage-mediated phagocytosis.

The cytoskeleton appears to play an important role in transfer of mineral particles from the cell surface to the cell interior, and then in transport through the cell to the interstitium, but which cytoskeletal elements are involved in these processes are disputed issues. Moreover, there is some evidence that mineral particles can damage the cytoskeleton and such damage undoubtedly affects uptake.

The mechanisms behind particle uptake have been best studied in macrophages where phagocytosis, a term which is generally used to refer to uptake of relatively large particles, is largely mediated by actin filaments. Treatment of macrophages with cytochalasins, which cause actin depolymerization, will typically abolish phagocytosis (145,146). In contrast, smaller particles appear to be taken up by endocytosis, and experiments with cytochalasins suggest that apical endocytosis of substances that adhere to specific receptors and are internalized through pinching off of clathrin-coated vesicles is also a function of the actin cytoskeleton, although this issue has been disputed (for a brief review see 146). As cytochalasins do not interfere with binding of exogenous substances to the cell surface, it is likely that actin plays no role in surface attachment (146). It has also been proposed that microtubules play a role in the uptake of exogenous materials, but this point is unsettled (147).

Very little is known of how these principles apply to uptake of mineral particles by tracheobronchial, bronchiolar, and type I and II cells. Cytochalasin treatment abolished uptake of crocidolite fibers by cultured pleural mesothelial cells (129). On the basis of heavy meromyosin staining, it was concluded (148) that chrysotile fibers in alveolar type I cells of rats in tracheal explants were enmeshed in web-like actin complexes, and that actin filaments played a role in chrysotile fiber transport within the cells. Endocytosis of cationized ferritin (which serves as a model of a positively charged ultrafine particle) was examined (146) from the apical surface of MDCK cells, polarized kidney-derived cells; uptake could be abolished with cytochalasins, and specifically cytochalasins prevented pinching off of the endocytic vesicles from the cell surface. However, these are very limited observations, mostly made in nonlung epithelial cells, and whether mineral particle uptake by pulmonary epithelial cells in general is mediated by actin needs to be established.

In ordinary phagocytic cells most, but not all, exogenous substances that become internalized are incorporated into lysosomes. To what extent this applies to mineral particles and pulmonary epithelial cells is uncertain. Morphological studies have shown incorporation of at least some short fibers of chrysotile and crocidolite, and of fine iron oxide and carbon particles (3,4,23,55,61,59,60, 73,149) into lysosomes, but other fibers, particularly long asbestos fibers, have been reported to reside in the cytoplasm, with no membranous structures surrounding them (58,61,147).

In typical monolayer culture cells, lysosomes accumulate over time around the microtubule-organizing center near the nucleus, and disruption of microtubules with colchicine or nocodazole prevents this effect (149,150), whereas paclitaxel (Taxol) makes perinuclear lysosome accumulation more prominent. Perinuclear accumulation of asbestos and other fibrous minerals has been seen in monolayer culture cells (149,151,152), and the transport of crocidolite fibers toward the nucleus of cultured newt lung is microtubule-mediated (149,153). This observation (149) really applies only to relatively short ($< 5\ \mu m$) fibers that move in a saltatory fashion at a rate identical with non–fiber-containing lysosomes, whereas long fibers do not exhibit saltatory movements, perhaps because they are not enclosed within lysosomal membranes, or because their length produces contact with numerous microtubules and probably other cytoskeletal elements, and the fibers become enmeshed.

Whether these principles apply to other types of particles is unknown, nor is it clear whether actin also is important in intracellular particle transport. Brody et al. (148) concluded that central transport of chrysotile was actin mediated, and Gehr et al. (154), using cytomagnetometric measurements of magnetite particles in alveolar macrophages, were of the opinion that both actin and microtubules played a role.

Ordinary monolayer cultures may provide quite misleading information about these processes, because, in some types of polarized epithelial cells, the microtubules do not radiate from a single nucleating center, but run vertically through the cell to terminate in dense apical and less dense basal caps (155–158). The limited available information suggests that microtubules organized in this fashion play a major role on directing endocytosis and exocytosis (155–158). Again, whether the cytoskeleton of tracheobronchial and alveolar epithelial cells follows this pattern is unknown. Furthermore, there is evidence that basal endocytic processes are different from apical processes; in particular, basal processes may not be actin-dependent (146). This information is of potential importance in understanding the transport of particles phagocytosed at the apical surface to the basal pole of the cells with exocytosis into the interstitial space (so-called transcytosis; 159), and thus in understanding the potential of various particles to produce interstitial fibrosis (see Sec. II). How particle type, size, charge, and shape affect transcytosis is unknown.

Most experiments on particle uptake are based on the assumption that the particles are inert, but this may not be true of mineral particles, some of which can bind to chromosomes and cytoskeletal elements (see Sec. II) and many of which produce AOS. Thus, mineral particles that become internalized may be able to damage the cytoskeleton and change its functional properties. The evidence for this is contradictory. Brody et al. (148) observed that chrysotile fibers were associated with abnormal actin bundles, which they believed represented large aggregates of polymerized actin. Malorni et al. (141) and Aufderheide et al. (160) observed that internalization of asbestos fibers by monolayer-cultured cells resulted in loss of the normal filamentous structure of actin and microtubules. But Cole et al., using video-enhanced time-lapse microscopy of newt lung epithelial cells (149) exposed to crocidolite fibers, could not find evidence of microtubule damage (actin was apparently not examined). Similarly, Somers et al. (152) did not observe evidence of keratin, tubulin, or vimentin abnormalities in mesothelial cells exposed to amosite, and Peterson et al. (33) found no evidence of abnormal actin patterns in cells exposed to chrysotile. This area needs further study, both to determine whether, in fact, mineral particles damage the cytoskeleton and to determine how such damage affects particle uptake and transport.

X. Summary and Conclusions

The foregoing discussion makes it clear that uptake of mineral particles by tracheobronchial epithelial and alveolar epithelial cells is a universal phenomenon, and one that is potentially injurious. Unfortunately, the determinants of particle uptake remain poorly defined. The best understood and probably the most important mediator of uptake is free particle persistence on the airway surface or in the alveolar space; particles that are not rapidly removed by the mucociliary escalator or by macrophages are likely to enter epithelial cells. Although there is, in a general sense, a dose–response relation between numbers of particles reaching the airways and airspaces and the numbers of particles entering epithelial cells, this effect really has a threshold, because below the point at which overload occurs (and whether overload itself is driven by particle number, volume, or mass is still unsettled), most particles are cleared from the lung and few enter epithelial cells. Once overload has occurred, particle uptake increases with dose, probably in an exponential fashion.

That said, it is still impossible to provide any generalized explanation of the marked differences in uptake seen with different types of particles, and little is known of the mechanics of this process. Anatomical site and cell type (e.g., type I vs. type II cell) certainly play a role. Whether size really has an independent effect on uptake for compact particles is unclear, with the available data both supporting and denying a role for particle size. The relative uptake of short compared with long fibrous minerals is also unsettled, and this is an important issue, for long fibers appear to be more fibrogenic than short fibers.

In tracheal explant systems particles bind directly to epithelial cells, and this is probably true of the alveoli as well, although no direct data exist on this question. A variety of possible binding mechanisms exist, including particle charge, adherence to adhesion molecule receptors, and specific protein-mediated binding; limited data have been published to support all of these possibilities, and they are not mutually exclusive. Binding of particles to the cell surface and internalization of particles by the cell appear to operate through quite different mechanisms, some of which may involve integrins, others AOS, and others nonspecific phagocytosis. The cytoskeleton is certainly involved in particle uptake and transport through the cell. Most likely uptake initially requires a functional actin system. Some, but not all, internalized particles are incorporated into lysosomes. There are data to suggest that movement of particles through the cell may be mediated by the microtubule system, although this is not universally agreed on. How particles are extruded from the basal surface of the cell to the interstitium has not been investigated. Mineral particles may influence these processes in uncertain ways by either adhesive or oxidant damage to the cytoskeleton.

Active oxygen species, especially hydrogen peroxide and probably hydroxyl radical, play a role in particle uptake in the tracheobronchial epithelium and possibly in the alveolar epithelium. Surface iron on the particle is one important factor in this process. The normal production of small amounts of hydrogen peroxide by pulmonary epithelial cells may serve as an accidental autocrine mechanism that increases uptake, and release of AOS from particle-evoked inflammatory cells may well have the same effect. Exogenous sources of AOS (e.g., ozone and cigarette smoke) greatly enhance uptake of many particles and probably potentiate mineral dust-induced pathological reactions.

Acknowledgments

Supported by grant MA8051 from the Medical Research Council of Canada.

References

1. Adamson IYR, Bowden DH. Role of polymorphonuclear leukocytes in silica-induced pulmonary fibrosis. Am J Pathol 1984; 117:37–43.
2. Bowden DH, Adamson IYR. The role of cell injury and the continuing inflammatory response in the generation of silicotic pulmonary fibrosis. J Pathol 1984; 144: 149–161.
3. Mossman BT, Kessler MSJ, Ley BW, Craighead JE. Interaction of crocidolite asbestos with hamster respiratory mucosa in organ culture. Lab Invest 1977; 36:131–139.
4. Mossman BT, Adler KB, Craighead JE. Interaction of carbon particles with tracheal epithelium in organ culture. Environ Res 1978; 816:110–122.
5. Pezerat H, Zalma R, Guignard J, Jaurand MC. Production of oxygen radicals by the reduction of oxygen arising from the surface activity of mineral fibers. In: Bignon J, et al., eds. Biological Effects of Mineral Fibers in the Nonoccupational Environment. Lyon: IARC, 1989:100–111.
6. Hardy JA, Aust AE. Iron in asbestos chemistry and carcinogenicity. Chem Rev 1995; 95:97–118.
7. Mossman BT, Marsh JP. Evidence supporting a role for active oxygen species in asbestos-induced toxicity and lung disease. Environ Health Perspect 1989; 81:91–94.
8. Moyer VD, Cistulli AC, Vaslet CA, Kane AB. Oxygen radicals and asbestos carcinogenesis. Environ Health Perspect 1994; 102(suppl 10):131–136.
9. Farber JL, Kyle ME, Coleman JB. Mechanisms of cell injury by activated oxygen species. Lab Invest 1990; 62:670–679.
10. Hart GA, Kathman LM, Hesterberg TW. In vitro cytotoxicity of asbestos and man-made vitreous fibers: roles of fiber length, diameter and composition. Carcinogenesis 1994; 15:971–977.
11. Jaurand MC, Bastie-Sigeac I, Bignon J, Stoebner PP. Effect of chrysotile and crocidolite on the morphology and growth of rat pleural mesothelial cells. Environ Res 1983; 30:255–269.
12. Jaurand MC, Yegles M, Dong HY, Renier A, Stain Etiennne L, Kheuang L, Janson X, Bignon J. In vitro DNA and chromosome damage produced by some mineral and man made particles on rat pleural mesothelial cells. In: Davis JMG, Jaurand MC, eds. Cellular and Molecular Effects of Minerals and Synthetic Dusts and Fibres. Berlin: Springer-Verlag, 1994:184–188.
13. Yegles M, Saint-Etienne L, Renier A, Janson X, Jaurand MC. Induction of metaphase and anaphase/telophase abnormalities by asbestos fibers in rat pleural mesothelial cells in vitro. Am J Respir Cell Mol Biol 1993; 9:186–191.
14. Donaldson K, Golyasnya N, Davis JMG. Long and short amosite asbestos samples: comparison of their chromosome-damaging effects to cells in culture with the results of other in vitro and in vivo assays of toxicity. In: Davis JMG, Jaurand MC, eds. Cellular and Molecular Effects of Minerals and Synthetic Dusts and Fibres. Berlin, Springer-Verlag, 1994:221–226.
15. Hesterberg TW, Barrett CJ. Induction by asbestos-fibers of anaphase abnormalities:

mechanism for aneuploidy induction and possibly carcinogenesis. Carcinogenesis 1985; 3:473–475.
16. Hesterberg TW, Butterick CJ, Oshimura M, Brody AR, Barrett JC. Role of phagocytosis in Syrian hamster cell transformation and cytogenetic effects induced by asbestos and short and long glass fibers. Cancer Res 1986; 46:5795–5802.
17. Hei TK, Piao CQ, Vannais D, Waldren CA. Chrysotile fiber is a strong mutagen in mammalian cells. Cancer Res 1992; 52:6305–6309.
18. Perderiset M, Marsh JP, Mossman BT. Activation of protein kinase C by crocidolite asbestos in hamster tracheal epithelial cells. Carcinogenesis 1991; 12:1499–1502.
19. Marsh JP, Mossman BT. Role of asbestos and active oxygen species in activation and expression of omithine decarboxylase in hamster tracheal epithelial cells. Cancer Res 1991; 51:167–173.
20. Heintz NH, Janssen YM, Mossman BT. Persistent induction of c-*fos* and c-*jun* expression by asbestos. Proc Natl Acad Sci USA 1994; 90:3299–3303.
21. Janssen YMW, Barchowsky A, Treadwell M, Dircoll KE, Mossman BT. Asbestos induces nuclear factor κB (NF-κB) DNA-binding activity and NF-κB dependent gene expression in tracheal epithelial cells. Proc Natl Acad Sci USA 1995; 92: 8458–8462.
22. Zanella CL, Posada J, Tritton TR, Mossman BT. Asbestos causes stimulation of the extracellular signal-regulated kinase 1 mitogen-activated protein kinase cascade after phosphorylation of the epidermal growth factor receptor. Cancer Res 1996; 56:5334–5338.
23. Mossman BT, Eastman A, Landesman JM, Bresnick E. Effects of crocidolite and chrysotile asbestos on cellular uptake and metabolism of benzo(*a*)pyrene in hamster tracheal epithelial cells. Environ Health Perspect 1983; 51:331–335.
24. Saffiotti U, Stinson SF, Keenan KP, McDowell EM. Tumor enhancement factors and mechanisms in the hamster respiratory tract. In: Mass MJ, et al. eds. Carcinogenesis. vol 8. New York: Raven Press, 1985:63–92.
25. Stenback F, Rowland J, Sellakumar A. Carcinogenicity of benzo(*a*)pyrene and dusts in the hamster lung (instilled intratracheally with titanium oxide, aluminum oxide, carbon, and ferric oxide). Oncology 1976; 33:29–34.
26. Warshawsky D, Bingham E, Niemeier RW. Influence of airborne particulate on the metabolism of benzo(*a*)pyrene in the isolated perfused lung. J Toxicol Environ Health 1983; 11:503–517.
27. McDonald JC, McDonald AD. Epidemiology of asbestos-related lung cancer. In: Antman K, Aisner J, eds. Asbestos-Related Malignancy. New York: Grune & Stratton, 1986:57–79.
28. Martell EA. Radiation at bronchial bifurcations of smokers from indoor exposure to radon progeny. Proc Natl Acad Sci USA 1983; 80:1285–1289.
29. Martonen TB, Hofmann W, Lowe JE. Cigarette smoke and lung cancer. Health Phys 1987; 52:213–217.
30. Driscoll KE: The role of interleukin-1 and tumor necrosis factor in the lung's response to silica. In: Castranova V, Vallyathan V, Wallace WE, eds. Silica and Silica-Induced Lung Diseases. Boca Raton: CRC Press, 1995.
31. Perdue TD, Brody AR: Distribution of transforming growth factor-beta$_1$, fibronec-

tin, and smooth muscle actin in asbestos-induced pulmonary fibrosis in rats. J Histochem Cytochem 1994; 42:1061–1070.
32. Liu J, Morris GF, Lei W, Corti M, Brody AR. Up-regulated expression of transforming growth factor-alpha in the bronchiolar–alveolar duct regions of asbestos-exposed rats. Am J Pathol 1996; 149:205–217.
33. Peterson MW, Walter ME, Gross TJ. Asbestos directly increases lung epthelial permeability. Am J Physiol 1993; 265:L308–L317.
34. Mangum JB, Everitt JI, Bonne JC, Moore LR, Brody AR. Coculture of primary pulmonary cells to model alveolar injury and translocation of proteins in vitro. Cell Dev Biol 1990; 26:1135–1143.
35. Welsh MJ, Shasby DM, Husted RM, Karp P, Spory P. Oxidants increase paracellular permeability in a cultured epithelial cell line. J Clin Invest 1985; 76:1155–1168.
36. Adamson IYR, Letourneau HL, Bowden DH. Comparison of alveolar and interstitial macrophages in fibroblast stimulation after silica and long or short asbestos. Lab Invest 1991; 64:339–344.
37. Mermelstein R, Kilpper RW, Morrow PE, Muhle H. Lung overload, dosimetry of lung fibrosis and their implications to the respiratory dust standard. Ann Occup Hyg 1994; 38(suppl 1):313–322.
38. Oberdorster G, Ferin J, Soderholm S, Gelein R, Cox C, Baggs R, Morrow PE. Increased pulmonary toxicity of inhaled ultrafine particles: due to lung overload alone? Ann Occup Hyg 1994; 38(suppl 1):295–302.
39. Adamson IYR, Letourneau HL, Bowden DH. Enhanced macrophage–fibroblast interactions in the pulmonary interstitium increases fibrosis after silica injection to monocyte-depleted mice. Am J Pathol 1989; 134:411–418.
40. Pinkerton KE, Pratt PC, Brody AR, Crapo JD. Fiber localization and its relationship to lung reaction in rats after chronic inhalation of chrysotile asbestos. Am J Pathol 1984; 117:484–498.
41. Oberdorster G. Lung particle overload: implications for occupational exposures to particles. Regul Toxicol Pharmacol 1995; 27:123–135.
42. Adamson IYR, Bowden DH. Pulmonary reaction to long and short asbestos fibers is independent of fibroblast growth factor production by alveolar macrophages. Am J Pathol 1990; 137:523–529.
43. McFadden D, Wright JL, Wiggs B, Churg A. Smoking increases the penetration of asbestos fibres into airway walls. Am J Pathol 1986; 123:95–99.
44. Tron V, Wright JL, Harrison N, Wiggs B, Churg A. Cigarette smoke makes airway and early parenchymal asbestos-induced lung disease worse in the guinea pig. Am Rev Respir Dis 1987; 136:271–276.
45. Weiss W. Cigarette smoke, asbestos, and small irregular opacities. Am Rev Respir Dis 1984; 130:293–301.
46. Barnhart S, Thornquist M, Omenn GS, Goodman G, Feigl P, Rosenstock L. The degree of roentgenographic parenchymal opacities attributable to smoking among asbestos exposed subjects. Am Rev Respir Dis 1990; 141:1102–1106.
47. Jones RN, Diem JE, Hughes JM, Hammad YY, Glindmeyer HW, Weill H. Progression of asbestos effects: a prospective longitudinal study of chest radiographs and lung function. Br J Ind Med 1989; 46:97–105.
48. Oberdorster G, Gelein RM, Ferin J, Weiss B. Association of particulate air pollution

and acute mortality: involvement of ultrafine particles? Inhal Toxicol 1995; 7:111–124.
49. Ferin J, Oberdorster G, Penney DP. Pulmonary retention of ultrafine and fine particles in rats. Am J Respir Cell Mol Biol 1992; 6:535–542.
50. Seaton A, MacNee W, Donaldson K, Godden D. Particulate air pollution and acute health effects. Lancet 1995; 345:176–178.
51. Churg A, Hobson J, Wright JL. Effects of cigarette smoke dose and time after smoke exposure on uptake of asbestos fibers by rat tracheal epithelial cells. Am J Respir Cell Mol Biol 1990; 3:265–269.
52. Hobson J, Gilks B, Wright J, Churg A. Cigarette smoke directly enhances asbestos fiber penetration and asbestos induced epithelial proliferation in rat tracheal explants. J Natl Cancer Inst 1988; 80:518–521.
53. Keeling B, Hobson J, Churg A. Effects of cigarette smoke on tracheal epithelial uptake of non-asbestos mineral particles in organ culture. Am J Respir Cell Mol Biol 1993; 9:335–340.
54. Mossman BT, Craighead JE. Use of hamster tracheal organ cultures for assessing the cocarcinogenic effects of inorganic particulates on the respiratory epithelium. Prog Exp Tumor Res 1979; 24:37–47.
55. Brody AR, Hill LH, Adkins B, O'Connor RW. Chrysotile asbestos inhalation in rats: deposition pattern and reaction of alveolar epithelium and pulmonary macrophages. Am Rev Respir Dis 1981; 123:670–679.
56. Adamson IYR, Bowden DH. Response of mouse lung to crocidolite asbestos. 1. Minimal fibrotic reaction to short fibres. J Pathol 1987; 152:99–107.
57. Adamson IYR, Bowden DH. Response of mouse lung to crocidolite asbestos. 2. Pulmonary fibrosis after long fibres. J Pathol 1987; 109–117.
58. Fasske E. Pathogenesis of pulmonary fibrosis induced by chrysotile asbestos. Virchows Arch Pathol Anat 1986; 408:329–346.
59. Suzuki Y, Churg J, Ono T. Phagocytic activity of the alveolar epithelial cells in pulmonary asbestosis. Am J Pathol 1972; 69:373–388.
60. Suzuki Y. Interaction of asbestos with alveolar cells. Environ Health Perspect 1974; 9:241–252.
61. Brody AR, Hill LH. Interstitial accumulation of inhaled chrysotile asbestos fibers and consequent formation of microcalcifications. Am J Pathol 1982; 109:107–114.
62. Gore DJ, Patrick G. A quantitative study of the penetration of insoluble particles into the tissue of the conducting airways. Ann Occup Hyg 1982; 26:149–159.
63. Stirling C, Patrick G. The localization of particles retained in the trachea of the rat. Pathology 1980; 131:309–320.
64. Adamson IYR, Bowden DH. Dose response of the pulmonary macrophagic system to various particulates and its relationship to transepithelial passage of free particles. Exp Lung Res 1981; 2:165–175.
65. Adamson IYR, Bowden DH. Effects of irradiation on macrophagic response and transport of particles across the alveolar epithelium. Am J Pathol 1982; 106:40–46.
66. Adamson IYR, Bowden DH. Chemotactic and mitogenic components of the alveolar macrophage response to particles and neutrophil chemoattractant. Am J Pathol 1982; 109:71–77.

67. Bowden DH, Adamson IYR. Alveolar macrophage response to carbon in monocyte-depleted mice. Am Rev Respir Dis 1982; 126:708–711.
68. Bowden DH, Adamson IYR. Response of pulmonary macrophages to unilateral instillation of carbon. Am J Pathol 1984; 115:151–155.
69. Bowden DH, Adamson IYR. Pathways of cellular efflux and particulate clearance after carbon instillation to the lung. J Pathol 1984; 143:117–125.
70. Warheit DB, Overby LH, George G, Brody AR. Pulmonary macrophages are attracted to inhaled particles through complement activation. Exp Lung Res 1988; 14:51–66.
71. Haugen A, Schafer PQ, Lechner JF, Stoner GD, Trump BF, Harris CC. Cellular ingestion, toxic effects and lesions observed in human bronchial epithelial tissue and cells cultured with asbestos and glass fibers. Int J Cancer 1982; 30:265–272.
72. Sorokin SP, Brain JD. Pathways of clearance in mouse lungs exposed to iron oxide aerosols. Anat Rec 1974; 181:581–626.
73. Watson AY, Brain JD. Uptake of iron oxide aerosols by mouse airway epithelium. Lab Invest 1979; 40:450–459.
74. Gilks B, Wright JL, Churg A. Effects of cigarette smoke on tissue uptake and retention of iron oxide in the guinea pig. Am Rev Respir Dis 1988 137:1382–1384.
75. Adamson IYR, Prieditis H, Bowden DH. Instillation of chemotactic factor to silica-injected lungs lowers interstitial particle content and reduces pulmonary fibrosis. Am J Pathol 1992; 141:319–326.
76. Bowden DH, Adamson IYR. The role of cell injury and the continuing inflammatory response in the generation of silicotic pulmonary fibrosis. J Pathol 1984; 144: 149–161.
77. Brody AR, Roe MW, Evans JN, Davis GS. Deposition and translocation of inhaled silica in rats. Quantification of particle distribution, macrophage participation and function. Lab Invest 1982; 47:533–542.
78. Lehnert BE. Defense mechanisms against inhaled particles and associated particle-cell interactions. Rev Mineral 1993; 28:427–470.
79. Ferin J, Oberdorster G, Soderholm SC, Gelein R. Pulmonary tissue access of ultrafine particles. J Aerosol Med 1991; 4:57–68.
80. Ferin J, Oberdorster G, Soderholm SC, Gelein R. The rate of dose delivery affects pulmonary interstitialization of particles in rats. Ann Occup Hyg 1994; 38:289–293.
81. Ferin J, Oberdorster G, Penney DP, Soderholm SC, Gelein R, Piper HC. Increased pulmonary toxicity of ultrafine particles. 1. Particle clearance, translocation, morphology. J Aerosol Sci 1990; 21:381–384.
82. Churg A, Stevens B. Mineral particles in the human bronchial mucosa. II. Cigarette smokers without emphysema. Exp Lung Res 1992; 18:687–714.
83. Churg A, Wright JL, Stevens B. Exogenous mineral particles in the human bronchial mucosa and lung parenchyma. I. Nonsmokers in the general population. Exp Lung Res 1990; 16:169–175.
84. Churg A, Stevens B. Enhanced retention of asbestos fibers in the airways of human smokers. Am J Respir Crit Care Med 1995; 151:1409–1413.
85. Churg A, Wiggs B. Types, numbers, sizes, and distribution of mineral particles in the lungs of urban male cigarette smokers. Environ Res 1987; 42:121–129.

86. Stettler LE, Growth DH, Platek SF, Burg JR. Particulate concentrations in urban lungs. In: Ingram P, Shelburne JD, Roggli VL, eds. Microprobe Analysis in Medicine. New York: Hemisphere Press, 1989:133–146.
87. Kalliomaki PL, Taikina-aho O, Paakko P. Smoking and the pulmonary mineral particle burden. In: Bignon J, Peto J, Saracci R, eds. Non-occupational Exposure to Mineral Fibres. Lyon: IARC, 1989:323–329.
88. Paoletti L, Eibenschutz L, Cassano AM. Mineral fibres and dust in lungs of subjects living in an urban environment. In: Bignon J, Peto J, Saracci R, eds. Non-occupational Exposure to Mineral Fibres. Lyon: IARC, 1989:354–360.
89. Bowden DH. Macrophages, dust, and pulmonary disease. Exp Lung Res 1987; 12: 89–107.
90. Geiser M, Baumann M, Cruz-Orive LM, Im Hof V, Gehr P. The effect of particle inhalation on macrophage numbers and phagocytic activity in the intrapulmonary conducting airways of hamsters. Am J Respir Cell Mol Biol 1994; 10:594–603.
91. Morrow PE. Dust overloading of the lungs: update and appraisal. Toxicol Appl Pharmacol 1992; 113:1–12.
92. Vincent JH. The fate of inhaled aerosols: a review of observed trends and some generalizations. Ann Occup Hyg 1990; 34:623–637.
93. Morrow PE. Possible mechanism to explain dust overloading of the lungs. Fundam Appl Toxicol 1988; 10:369–384.
94. Oberdorster G, Ferin J, Morrow PE. Volumetric loading of alveolar macrophages (AM): a possible basis for diminished AM-mediated particle clearance. Exp Lung Res 1992; 18:87–104.
95. Brain JD. Macrophage damage in relation to the pathogenesis of lung diseases. Environ Health Perspect 1980; 35:21–28.
96. Svartengren M, Widtskiold-Olsson K, Philipson K, Camner P. Retention of particles on the first bifurcation and the trachea of rabbits. Bull Eur Physiopathol Respir 1981; 17:87–91.
97. Schlesinger B, Lippman M. Selective particle deposition and bronchogenic carcinoma. Environ Res 1978; 15:424–431.
98. Cohen BS, Harley NH, Schlesinger RB, Lippmann M. Nonuniform particle deposition on tracheobronchial airways: implications for lung dosimetry. Ann Occup Hyg 1988; 32:1045.
99. Churg A, Vedal S. Carinal and tubular airway particle concentration in the large airways of nonsmokers in the general population: evidence for high particle concentration at airway carinas. Occup Environ Med 1996; 53:553–558.
100. Warheit DB, Hartsky MA, Plopper CG. Regional alveolar deposition patterns of inhaled particles are dependent upon airway branching patterns. Ann Occup Hyg 1994; 38:55–61.
101. Bair WJ. Human respiratory tract model for radiological protection: a revision of the ICRP Dosimetric Model for the Respiratory System. Health Phys 1989; 57: 249–253.
102. Lippmann M, Yeates DB, Albert RE. Deposition, retention, and clearance of inhaled particles. Br J Ind Med 1980; 37:337–362.
103. Gerrity TR, Lee PS, Hass FJ. Calculated deposition of inhaled particles in the airway generations of normal subjects. J Appl Physiol 1979; 47:867–873.

104. Wright JL, Cagle P, Churg A, Colby TV, Myers J. State of the art: disease of the small airways. Am Rev Respir Dis 1992; 146:240–262.
105. Churg A, Wright JL. Mineral particles in the walls of small airways in long term chrysotile miners. Ann Occup Hyg 1988; 32:173–180.
106. Muller WJ, Hess GD, Scherer PW. A model of cigarette smoke particle deposition. Am Ind Hyg Assoc J 1990; 51:245–251.
107. Asmundsson T, Kilburn KH. Mucociliary clearance rates at various levels in dog lungs. J Aerosol Med 1970; 1:37–50.
108. Morrow PE, Gibb FR, Gazioglu KM. A study of particulate clearance from the human lung. Am Rev Respir Dis 1967; 96:1209–1221.
109. Yeates DB, Aspin N, Levison H, Jones MT, Bryan A. Mucociliary tracheal transport rates in man. J Appl Physiol 1975; 39:487–495.
110. Sleigh MA. The nature and action of respiratory tract cilia. In: Brain JD, Proctor DF, Reid LM, eds. Respiratory Defense Mechanisms. New York: Marcel Dekker, 1977:247–288.
111. van As A. Pulmonary airway defense mechanisms. Eur J Respir Dis 1980; 61(suppl 111):21–24.
112. Gil J, Weibel ER. Extracellular lining of bronchioles after perfusion fixation of rat lungs for electron microscopy. Anat Rec 1971; 169:185–200.
113. Luchtel DL. Mucociliary clearance interactions in rabbit intrapulmonary airways. Cell Motil Cytoskel 1982; 72(suppl):77–81.
114. Valasquez DJ, Morrow PE. Estimation of guinea pig tracheobronchial transport rates using a compartment model. Exp Lung Res 1984; 7:163–176.
115. Stober W, Morrow PE, Oberdorster G. Pulmonary retention of inhaled anatase (TiO_2) aerosols and lung tumor induction in rats simulated by a physiology-oriented model. Inhal Toxicol 1991; 7:1059–1074.
116. Churg A, Wright J, Stevens B. Comparison of the uptake of fine and ultrafine titanium dioxide in a tracheal explant system. Am J Physiol 1998; 274:281–286.
117. Davis JMG, Addison J, Bolton RE, Donaldson K. The pathogenicity of long vs short fibre samples of amosite asbestos administered to rats by inhalation and intraperitoneal injection. Br J Exp Pathol 1986; 67:415–430.
118. Davis JMG, Jones AD. Comparisons of the pathogenicity of long and short fibre chrysotile asbestos in rats. Br J Exp Pathol 1986; 69:717–737.
119. Woodworth CD, Mossman BT, Craighead JE. Interaction of asbestos with metaplastic squamous epithelium developing in organ cultures of hamster trachea. Environ Health Perspect 1983; 51:27–33.
120. McFadden D, Wright JL, Wiggs B, Churg A. Smoking inhibits asbestos clearance. Am Rev Respir Dis 1986; 133:372–374.
121. Churg A, Wright JL, Hobson J, Stevens B. Effects of cigarette smoke on the clearance of long and short asbestos fibers from the lung. Int J Exp Pathol 1991; 73: 287–297.
122. Ghio AJ, Kennedy TP, Whorton AR, Crumbliss AL, Hatch GE, Hoidal JR. Role of surface complexed iron in oxidant generation and lung inflammation induced by silicates. Am J Physiol 1992; 263:L511–L518.
123. Vallyathan V, Shi X, Dalal NS, Irr W, Castranova V. Generation of free radicals

from freshly fractured silica dust. Potential role in acute silica-induced lung injury. Am Rev Respir Dis 1988; 138:1213–1218.
124. Hobson J, Wright JL, Churg A. Active oxygen species mediate asbestos fiber uptake by tracheal epithelial cells. FASEB J 1990; 4:3135–3139.
125. Keeling B, Li KY, Churg A. Iron enhances uptake of mineral particles and increases lipid peroxidation in tracheal epithelial cells. Am J Respir Cell Mol Biol 1994; 10: 683–689.
126. Churg A, Brauer M, Keeling B. Ozone enhances the uptake of mineral particles by tracheobronchial epithelial cells in explant culture. Am J Respir Crit Care Med 1996; 153:1230–1234.
127. Fubini B, Mollo L, Giamello E. Free radical generation at the solid/liquid interface in iron containing minerals. Free Radic Res 1995; 23:593–614.
128. Churg A, Hobson J, Berean K, Wright J. Scavengers of active oxygen species prevent cigarette smoke induced asbestos fiber penetration in rat tracheal explants. Am J Pathol 1989; 135:599–603.
129. Boylan AM, Sanan DA, Sheppard D, Broaddus VC. Vitronectin enhances internalization of crocidolite asbestos by rabbit pleural mesothelial cells via the integrin avb5. J Clin Invest 1995; 96:1987–2001.
130. Kinnula VL, Adler KB, Ackley NJ, Crapo JD. Release of reactive oxygen species by guinea pig tracheal epithelial cells in vitro. Am J Physiol 1992; 262:L708–L712.
131. Kinnula VL, Crapo JD, Raivio KO. Generation and disposal of reactive oxygen metabolites in the lung. Lab Invest 1995; 73:3–19.
132. Cohen D, Arai SF, Brain JD. Smoking impairs long-term clearance from the lung. Science 1979; 204:514.
133. Freedman AP, Robinson SE, Street MR. Magnetopneumographic study of human alveolar clearance in health and disease. Ann Occup Hyg 1988; 32:809–820.
134. Pinkerton KE, Brody AR, Miller FJ, Crapo JD. Exposure to low levels of ozone results in enhanced pulmonary retention of inhaled asbestos fibers. Am Rev Respir Dis 1989; 140:1075–1081.
135. Gehr P, Green FHY, Geiser M, Im Hof V, Lee MM, Schurch S. Airway surfactant, a primary defense barrier: mechanical and immunological aspects. J Aerosol Med 1996; 9:163–181.
136. Gehr P, Schurch S, Berthiaume Y, Im Hof V, Geiser M. Particle retention in airways by surfactant. J Aerosol Med 1990; 3:27–43.
137. Schurch S, Gehr P, Im Hof V, Geiser M, Green F. Surfactant displaces particles toward the epithelium in airways and alveoli. Respir Physiol 1990; 80:17–32.
138. Brody AR, George G, Hill LH. Interactions of chrysotile and crocidolite asbestos with red blood cell membranes. Lab Invest 1983; 49:468–475.
139. Gallagher JE, George G, Brody AR. Sialic acid mediates the initial binding of positively charged inorganic particles to alveolar macrophage membranes. Am Rev Respir Dis 1987; 135:1345–1352.
140. Desai R, Richards RJ. The adsorption of biological macromolecules by mineral dusts. Environ Res 1978; 16:449–464.
141. Valerio F, Balducci D, Scarabelli L. Selective adsorption of serum proteins by chrysotile and crocidolite. Environ Res 1984; 41:432–439.

142. Kamp DW, Dunne M, Anderson JA, Weitzman SA, Dunn MV. Serum promotes asbestos-induced injury to human pulmonary epithelial cells. J Lab Clin Med 1990; 116:289–297.
143. Brown RC, Sara EA, Hoskins A, Evans CE. Factors affecting the interaction of asbestos fibres with mammalian cells: a study using cells in suspension. Ann Occup Hyg 1991; 35:25–34.
144. Brown RC, Sara EA, Hoskins JA, Houghton CE. Interaction between mineral fibres and cell surface receptors studied with amosite and surface derivatized amosite asbestos. Ann Occup Hyg 1994; 38:587–593.
145. Axline SG, Reaven EP. Inhibition of phagocytosis and plasma membrane mobility of the cultivated macrophage by cytochalasin B. J Cell Biol 1974; 62:647–659.
146. Gottlieb TA, Ivanov IE, Resnik M, Sabatini DD. Actin microfilaments play a critical role in endocytosis at the apical but not the basolateral surface of polarized epithelial cells. J Cell Biol 1993; 120:695–710.
147. Holtzman E. Lysosomes. New York: Plenum Press, 1989.
148. Brody AR, Hill LH, Stirewalt WS, Adler KB. Actin-containing microfilaments of pulmonary epithelial cells provide a mechanism for translocating asbestos to the interstitium. Chest 1993; 5:11–12.
149. Cole RW, Ault JG, Hayden JH, Rieder CL. Crocidolite asbestos fibers undergo size-dependent microtubule-mediated transport after endocytosis in vertebrate lung epithelial cells. Cancer Res 1991; 51:4942–4947.
150. Matteoni R, Kreis TE. Translocation and clustering of endosomes and lysosomes depends on microtubules. J Cell Biol 1987; 105:1253–1265.
151. Malorni W, Iosi F, Falchi M, Doneli G. On the mechanism of cell internalization of chrysotile fibers: an immunocytochemical and ultrastructural study. Environ Res 1990; 52:164–177.
152. Somers ANA, Mason EA, Gerwin BI, Harris CC, Lechner JF. Effects of amosite asbestos fibers on the filaments present in the cytoskeleton of primary human mesothelial cells. In: Brown RC, et al. eds. Mechanisms in Fibre Carcinogenisis. New York: Plenum Press, 1991:481–489.
153. Jensen CG, Jensen LCW, Ault JG, Osorio G, Cole R, Rieder CL. Time-lapse video light microscopic and electron microscopic observations of vertebrate epithelial cells exposed to crocidolite asbestos. In: Davis JMG, Jaurand MC, eds. Cellular and Molecular Effects of Mineral and Synthetic Dusts and Fibres. Berlin: Springer-Verlag, 1994:63–78.
154. Gehr P, Brain JD, Bloom SB, Valberg PA. Magnetic particles in the liver: a probe for intracellular movement. Nature 1983; 302:336–338.
155. Parton RG, Dotti CG, Bacallao R, Kurtz I, Simons K, Prydz K. pH-induced microtubule-dependent redistribution of late endosomes in neuronal and epithelial cells. J Cell Biol 1991; 113:261–274.
156. Vogl AW, Weis M, Pfeiffer DC. The perinclear centriole-containing centrosome is not the major microtubule organizing center in Sertoli cells. Eur J Cell Biol 1995; 66:165–179.
157. Achler C, Filmer D, Merte C, Drenckhahn D. Role of microtubules in polarized delivery of apical membrane proteins to the brush border of the intestinal epithelium. J Cell Biol 1989; 109:179–189.

158. Bre MH, Pepperkok R, Hill AM, Levilliers N, Ansorge W, Stelzer EHK, Karsenti E. Regulation of microtubule dynamics and nucleation during polarization in MDCK II cells. J Cell Biol 1990; 111:3013–3021.
159. Brown VI, Greene MI. Molecular and cellular mechanisms of receptor-mediated endocytosis. DNA Cell Biol 1991; 10:399–409.
160. Aufderheide M, Riebe-Imre M, Straub M, Emura M. A new in vitro approach to study cytotoxicity and carcinogenic effects of mineral fibres. Ann Occup Hyg 1994; 38:577–585.
161. Chung A. The uptake of mineral particles by pulmonary epithelial cells. Am J Respir Crit Care Med 1996; 154:1124–1140.

10

Responses of Inflammatory Cells

ROBERT B. DEVLIN, ANDREW J. GHIO, and DANIEL L. COSTA

U.S. Environmental Protection Agency
Research Triangle Park, North Carolina

I. Introduction

It is clear that inhaled particles have the capacity to cause acute lung damage and inflammation, and that transition metals play a major role in mediating this toxicity, particularly for occupationally derived substances, such as silica and asbestos. These compounds serve as solid-phase chelants for iron, and lung injury after silica and asbestos exposure is associated with the generation of oxygen-based free radicals, that is catalyzed by iron complexed to the dust. These oxidants can contribute to both cytotoxicity and release of mediators relevant to lung injury. The production of oxygen-based free radicals by mineral oxide particles can be observed after heating to high temperatures, grinding, dehydration, and coordination of transition metals (iron, copper, zinc, vanadium, and nickel) with two stable valence states at the solid–solution interface (1,2). Only the last of these can result in oxidant generation within a biological system.

Anthropogenic dusts derived from combustion have been associated with increased mortality and morbidity in numerous epidemiology studies. Despite these convincing associations, toxicological and controlled human exposure studies have not yet provided compelling evidence pointing to a specific biological mechanism that may be responsible for increased mortality and morbidity. Fine particles are known to cause inflammation, respiratory symptoms, and decrements in lung function. These events and others, such as bronchoconstriction, impaired diffusion, edema, and inflammation, can cause hypoxemia and lead to cardiac arrhythmias. In addition, the inhalable fraction of particulate matter in air pollution (PM_{10})-induced pulmonary inflammation, edema, and lung damage may not be perceptible to normal healthy individuals, but could lead to cardiopulmonary stress in elderly individuals or in those with underlying pulmonary disease. Combustion-derived particles are associated with concentrations of first-row transition metals, which have a capacity to support electron exchange and catalyze free radical production (3,4). Other potential active agents are acids, biological aerosols, ultrafine particles, and organic compounds.

A. Metals and Occupational Particles

In an aqueous environment, oxides and oxide minerals are covered with surface hydroxyl groups (5,6) and, subsequently, all silica and asbestos surfaces have some concentration of silanol groups (–SiOH). The open network of negatively charged silanol groups on the surface of silica and asbestos presents spaces large enough to accommodate adsorbed metal cations. Larger cations cannot approach this negative charge as closely as smaller cations, such as transition metals.

Iron is the second most abundant metal in the earth's crust and is an essential element for all forms of life. The ferric ion has a high affinity for oxygen donor ligands. This propensity is the result of the high charge and electropositivity of the ion (7). Iron-(III) (Fe^{3+}) complexes with both monomeric silicic acid and its polymers through interactions with the silanol groups (8,9). The critical stability constant of the coordination complex formed between silicic acid and iron cations is greater than those of any other metal cation (10). Ferric ions also react with surface silanol groups of silica and silicates to make a silicatoiron coordination complex (11).

$$Fe^{3+} + m(\text{–Si–OH}) \rightleftarrows Fe(\text{O–Si})_m^{(3-m)+} + mH^+$$

$$Fe^{3+} + e^- \rightleftarrows Fe^{2+}$$

Dose-dependent adsorption of inorganic iron has been demonstrated for crystalline silicates with critical stability constants approximating $1 \times 10^{17.15}$ (pK_{sc} = 17.15; 6,11–14). The relation between Fe^{3+} and the silicate surface is a true coordination, rather than cation exchange. The bond between the metal cation and the electron-donating silanol group is largely covalent, rather than ionic.

The lack of any pliancy by the inflexible crystal surface of silica and asbestos predicts that placement of electrons into the symmetrically located coordination sites around iron will be incomplete. Complexed iron, with at least one free or labile coordination site, can subsequently mediate electron exchange via the

Fenton reaction. Therefore, iron complexed to the surface of silica and asbestos can catalyze a generation of the hydroxyl radical:

$$Fe^{2+} + H_2O_2 \rightleftarrows Fe^{3+} + {}^{\bullet}OH + {}^{-}OH$$

The ability of mineral oxide particles to generate oxidants by the Fenton reaction has been established in vitro (15), thus supporting a role for complexed iron in oxidant generation by these dusts. Participation of this metal in free radical production and lipid peroxidation mediated by mineral oxides has also been demonstrated (16–20). Complexion of iron from both inorganic sources in the earth's crust and body sources onto the surface of these dusts with the resulting oxidant generation may be an essential aspect in their toxicity.

B. Metals and Anthropogenic Particles

Emission source and ambient air pollution particles also contain significant quantities of first-row transition metals that exist both complexed to insoluble components of the dust (e.g., mineral oxides, such as silica) and as soluble salts (e.g., sulfates and ammonium sulfates; 2,3). Iron is that metal cation in highest concentration among air pollution particles. The exception is fly ash produced by the combustion of oil. In this particular dust, vanadium and nickel are abundant. In atmospheric particles, quantities of iron can regularly be found in concentrations approximately tenfold higher than all others (21); therefore, this metal may assume greater importance. Iron can concentrate in the fogwater of urban settings, cloud droplets, and aerosol particles (22,23). Most of the iron exists in a soluble form, rather than the highly insoluble oxides and oxyhydroxides originally emitted (24). Some mass of iron oxides are photoreduced with dissolution in an aqueous medium (25). This solubilization is dependent on the presence of a suitable ligand for iron. Sulfate (SO_4^{2-}), a ligand available in the atmosphere in high concentrations, can complex both the ferrous and ferric ion; estimates of stability constants range between 10^2/M and 10^5/M (26). In addition, it is likely that other components included in anthropogenic particles coordinate metals. This could include hydroxyl groups of mineral oxides and the carboxylate and phenol groups of incompletely oxidized carbon fragments.

Emission source and ambient air pollution particles catalyze production of oxidants including the hydroxyl radical (3,4). This production of free radicals correlates with the concentrations of transition metals. As with silica and asbestos, it is likely that anthropogenic particles can present an oxidative stress to a living system with their exposure.

Lung injury after exposure to mineral oxide and anthropogenic particles has been postulated to advance through a release of either (1) toxic substances from cells damaged by particles and fibers (i.e., cytotoxicity); or (2) mediators that initiate and coordinate inflammatory and fibrotic responses. Both cytotoxicity and mediator release by pertinent lung cells can result from exposure to oxygen-based free radicals catalyzed by either iron complexed to silica and asbestos or transition metals associated with the anthropogenic particle.

II. Occupational Particles (Silica and Asbestos)

Occupational exposures to silica and asbestos are associated with lung injury in humans. This can include an irritant bronchitis, bronchiolitis, focal emphysema, pneumoconioses, an increased incidence of tuberculosis, bronchogenic carcinoma, pleural effusions and plaques, and mesothelioma. Industrialization greatly increased both the number of workers with a significant exposure to these mineral oxides and the incidence of disease after their exposure. Lung injury after silica and asbestos continues to result in a significant human morbidity and mortality, despite predictions of its pending elimination.

A. In Vitro Cytotoxicity

In selected studies, in vivo pulmonary injury after exposures of the lower respiratory tract to silica and asbestos can infrequently be predicted by in vitro measures of cytotoxicity (27,28). Subsequently, the mechanism(s) of this cytotoxicity has been investigated using diverse cells, both primary cells and cell lines, originating from numerous different animals. Indices of in vitro cytotoxicity have included such disparate measures as dye exclusion, quantification of cellular enzyme release, liberation of radiolabel from the cell, and inhibition of colony formation. Finally, investigations have employed different types of silica and asbestos, distinct doses of dusts, and dissimilar protocols, with varying strains and ages of animals. Predictably, results have varied and have not always been agreeable. Multiple mechanisms appear to contribute to the interaction between mineral oxide particles and cells. Most investigations have addressed the effects on cytotoxicity mediated by either the electrokinetic potential of the dusts or oxidant generation by the particle and fiber.

There is a relation between membranolysis by dusts with surface area and the negative electrokinetic potential of the particle and fiber (29–31). This is of particular importance in the cytotoxicity of these dusts with in vitro studies using erythrocytes. As a result of negative charges on the surfaces of silica and asbestos, a capacity for adsorption and exchange of both organic and inorganic cations is produced. The positive charge of quaternary ammonium groups on organic molecules is likely to result in their adsorption onto the particle and fiber (32). These molecules are normally held in a precise tertiary configuration by internal hydrogen bonding. If the particle is large, adsorption of the molecule onto the surface results in its uncoiling and flattening of the molecule, with breaking of hydrogen bonds. The structure of the molecule is irreversibly destroyed and, when involving the cell membrane, lysis can result immediately. However, if the molecule is brought into contact with particles smaller that 5 nm in diameter, the particles are adsorbed onto the surface of the protein, which will remain intact. The coating of particles will actually protect the molecule from damage by later contact with a larger dust surface (33,34). In vitro cytotoxicity, therefore, can be reduced by decreasing the negative surface charge. The addition of positively charged organic molecules, such as dipalmitoyl lecithin, proteins, immunoglobulins, erythrocyte membranes, and surfactant, diminishes both surface charge and in vitro toxicity (35). Similarly, saturating the surface of silica and asbestos with any metal cation should also reduce the negative charge and consequent cytotoxicity (36). Alternatively, displacement of positively charged cations off the silicate employing acid washings will increase surface electronegativity and the ability of the particle and fiber to damage or lyse target molecules and cells (37). Finally, heating a silicate to high temperature will dehydrate the surface by converting silanol groups to nonreactive siloxane bonds, decrease the surface charge, and in vitro membranolysis will be lessened (38):

$$2SiO^- + 2H^+ \rightleftarrows Si{-}O{-}Si + H_2O$$

Oxidant generation is a second mechanism that has been implicated in in vitro cytotoxicity (39). It is postulated that oxygen-based free radicals, catalyzed by iron associated with silica and asbestos, injure biomolecules in the environment immediately adjacent to the dust surface. This is assumed to ultimately result in cell injury and death. In support of a role for oxidant generation by mineral oxides, cytotoxicity can be decreased with the radical scavengers dimethylthiourea and mannitol (19). Investigations employing the antioxidant enzymes superoxide dismutase and catalase have similarly associated in vitro membranolysis with oxidant generation (19,40). However, the ability of antioxidants, including superoxide dismutase and catalase, to decrease membranolysis may also be associated with their positively charged functional groups that will decrease the electrokinetic potential after adsorption. If antioxidants are to be used in studies of oxidant generation and membranolysis, it may be necessary to measure the zeta potential both before and after intervention.

Correlations of in vivo injury with measures of in vitro cytotoxicity are likely to result from a dependence of both on silanol groups. Although in vivo injury is likely to be a function of oxidant production by complexed iron cations, in vitro cytotoxicity can be either (1) a mechanical disruption of the membrane resulting from attractive forces between the negatively charged surface groups of the dust (e.g., $-SiO^-$) and positively charged functional groups on the membrane, or (2) a product of oxidation of key biomolecules by free radicals catalyzed by iron cations complexed to silica and asbestos by surface functional groups (e.g., $-SiO^-$). The contribution of each mechanism to cytotoxicity depends on the specific exposure (particle and fiber) and the cell or cell line studied.

B. In Vitro Release of Mediators Associated with Acute Inflammation and Chronic Fibrosis

Most evidence supports that activation of cells to release inflammatory mediators after exposure to silica and asbestos is of greater importance than inherent cytotoxicity in lung injury associated with these dusts. Following exposures to silica and asbestos, the release of mediators relevant to both an acute inflammation and a chronic fibrosis has been demonstrated. That cell type responsible for this mediator release and, therefore, the coordination of the inflammatory and fibrotic responses to particles and fibers, has been assumed to be the alveolar macrophage. The designation of this specific cell as organizing lung injury after dust exposure has been made for two reasons: (1) there is an early chemotaxis of macrophages to the sites of particle and fiber deposition; and (2) the alveolar macrophage has a capacity both in vitro and ex vivo to release these mediators. However, cell types other than the macrophage have a capacity to release mediators after exposure to silica and asbestos. These include respiratory epithelial cells and fibroblasts. After in vitro exposures to silica and asbestos, the coordination of the inflammatory and fibrotic responses by respiratory epithelial cells is equally as probable as the alveolar macrophage performing this function.

Rather than affecting cellular damage after exposures, mineral oxide particles stimulate and activate cells resident in the lung without apparent cytotoxicity (41–43). These mediators include arachidonic acid products, cytokines, and growth factors. Among these, no single mediator has been convincingly demonstrated to be pivotal in the evolution of lung injury associated with particles and fibers.

Eicosanoid production by pertinent cells resident in the respiratory tract can participate in lung disease after particle exposure. These can include both cyclooxygenase products, such as prostaglandin D_2 (PGD_2), PGE_2, $PG_{F2\alpha}$, and thromboxane; and lipoxygenase products, including leukotriene B_4 (LTB_4) and hydroxyeicosatetraenoic acid derivatives (44–55). The release of cyclooxygenase products after dust exposure appears to predominate at lower doses of silica and asbestos, whereas lipoxygenase products predominate at higher doses. Specific prostaglandins can function in a proinflammatory manner as chemotactic agents to initiate an incursion of inflammatory cells (56,57). In addition, cyclooxygenase products can stimulate platelet activity and cause contraction of bronchial and vascular smooth muscle. Lipoxygenase products also have proinflammatory activities, such as chemotaxis and activation of neutrophils and monocytes (58–60). In addition to these effects, prostaglandins and leukotrienes can influence the release of other inflammatory mediators, including tumor necrosis factor (TNF-α), interferon gamma (IFN-γ), interleukin-1 (IL-1), and IL-2 (61–67).

Cytokines released by pertinent cell types after either in vitro or ex vivo exposures can include IL-1, IL-8, TNF-α, and (IFN-γ; 43,50,68,75). TNF-α is the mediator that is considered of greatest significance in lung injury after dust exposure (74). It has numerous proinflammatory activities, including chemotaxis and activation of inflammatory cells, expression of leukocyte adhesion molecules, and stimulation of other cytokines that contribute to acute inflammation. There is some evidence to support a role for TNF-α in the lung responses to silica and asbestos (74), and this includes (1) macrophages isolated from the lungs of humans with silicosis and asbestosis demonstrate an increased production and release of TNF-α; (2) following dust exposure, the concentration of TNF-α in the lavage fluid can correlate with neutrophil recruitment (50,69); (3) the in vivo administration of TNF-α can produce some of the biological responses observed after particle and fiber exposure; and (4) the passive immunization of mice with an anti-TNF-α antibody can diminish particle-induced increases in lung collagen (75).

It is difficult to categorize mediators as contributing specifically to either acute inflammation or chronic fibrosis because the primary mechanism by which lung fibrosis occurs is assumed to be persistent inflammation (76). Arachidonic acid metabolites and cytokines can both participate in pulmonary fibrosis after silica and asbestos exposure. In addition to these groups of mediators, in vitro exposures to mineral oxides are associated with the release of several growth factors by the alveolar macrophage. These molecules, which include the platelet-derived growth factor (PDGA)-like molecules, transforming growth factor (TGF), and insulin-like growth factor (IGF), are postulated to participate in chemotaxis and proliferation of fibroblasts (77–82).

Mediators of both the inflammatory and fibrotic responses have been associated with exposure to oxidants. Similarly, mediator release after incubation of cells with silica and asbestos can be the result of oxygen-based free radicals catalyzed by iron associated with the mineral oxide (Fig. 1). The increase in arachidonic acid metabolism after exposures of cells to particles and fibers can result from the cooxidation of arachidonate by metal-catalyzed oxidants. This is a lipid peroxidation that can be mediated by free radical production by the dust (83). In support of an association between metal-catalyzed oxidant generation and arachidonic acid products, the release of LTB_4 by alveolar macrophages can increase with the concentrations of iron complexed to the surface of silica and asbestos (84). Similarly, the cellular release of cytokines postulated to participate in the inflammatory and fibrotic responses can be associated with exposures to metal-dependent radicals (see Fig. 1). TNF-α production by alveolar macrophages after mineral oxide exposure can be inhibited by both the metal chelator deferoxamine and hydroxyl radical scavengers (74). The release of other cytokines pertinent to silica and asbestos exposure can also be responsive to oxidative stress (85,86). The release of these pertinent mediators after dust exposures is likely to be controlled by oxidant-sensitive promoters such as nuclear factor (NF)-κB (87). After exposure to silica and asbestos, NF-κB can function as a promoter

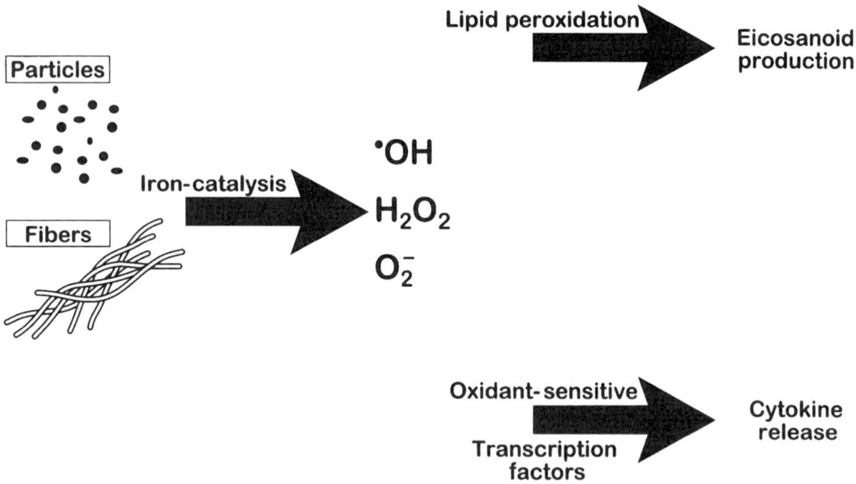

Figure 1 Schematic of an association between mediator release after silica and asbestos exposure and metal-catalyzed oxidant generation by the particles: Eicosanoid production can result from a co-oxidation of arachidonate by metal-catalyzed oxidants generated by the particles. Similarly, the release of other cytokines pertinent to silica and asbestos exposure can be responsive to oxidant-sensitive promoters.

for those cytokines (88–90) that have binding sites in the promoter region (91). Similarly, the nonenzymatic activation of the complement cascade by oxygen-based radicals can generate fragments that function as chemotactic factors for neutrophils (92). Such activation can be dependent on the binding of iron by the fifth component of complement (C5) and subsequent free radical generation. Therefore, mediator release after silica and asbestos exposure can be a result of the associated oxidative stress, which corresponds to an increased availability of catalytically active iron.

C. Extrapolation of In Vitro Mediator Release to In Vivo Injury

Mediator release is assumed to function to protect the host against the injurious effects of mineral oxides (101,102). Oxidant generation, which is catalyzed by complexed metal, is central in the injury after exposures to silica and asbestos (103–105). Therefore, arachidonic acid products, cytokines, and growth factors could protect the host against lung injury by influencing either oxidant generation or iron availability after silica and asbestos exposure. Mediators could contribute to such a defense through a myriad of interactions, which would include directing (1) an incursion of inflammatory cells to the site of particle and fiber deposition and (2) changes in iron metabolism in the host, resulting in the sequestration of the catalytically active iron associated with these dusts (Fig. 2).

All ligands, including mineral oxide dusts, have different affinities for Fe^{2+} and Fe^{3+}, with values of stability constants for ferrous ion often being considerably less than those for ferric ion. These dissimilarities offer a possible mechanism to remove ferric ion from the chelant (i.e., the particle and fiber). Parallel evolutionary development may account for similarities in the methods employed by all living organisms in the transport of iron. Bacteria, phytoplankton, and

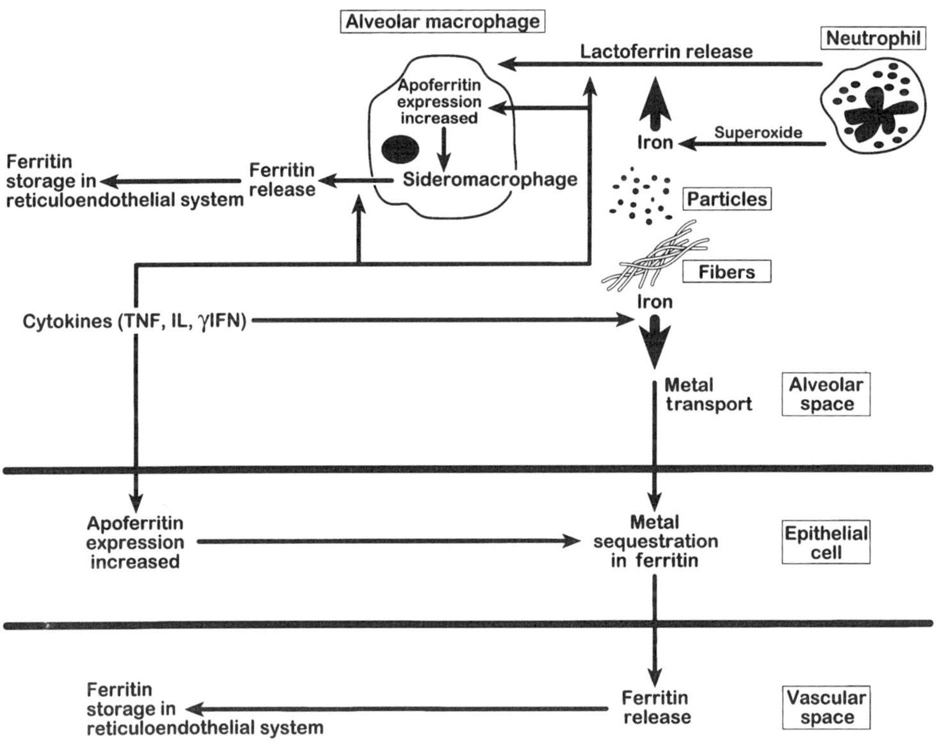

Figure 2 Schematic of the transport of metal associated with particles and fibers by the host: Mediators can function to protect the host by (1) directing an influx of inflammatory cells that have a capacity to isolate the iron by reducing the Fe^{3+} using superoxide; and (2) modifying iron metabolism in the host resulting in the sequestration of the catalytically active iron associated with these dusts. Mediator release after exposure to silica and asbestos may represent an attempt of the cell to coordinate the transport and sequestration of catalytically active iron. This response would diminish the oxidative stress associated with the particle and fiber and injury after their exposure.

plants most frequently procure requisite Fe^{3+} by reduction of the metal, using superoxide (106–108). The enzyme responsible for this reduction of iron is a NADPH oxidase, which catalyzes the reaction:

$$2NADPH + 2O_2 \leftrightarrows 2NADP + 2O_2^- + 2H^+$$

Neutrophils and macrophages perform the same enzymatic function with a NADPH oxidoreductase (109). The superoxide produced by this NADPH oxidoreductase reduces the metal complexed to silica and asbestos, dislodging it from the dust (26):

$$Fe^{3+}L + O_2^- \leftrightarrows Fe^{2+}L + O_2 \text{ (where L is the particle and fiber)}$$

$$Fe^{2+}L \leftrightarrows Fe^{2+} \text{ (aq.)} + L$$

Iron is then reoxidized to Fe^{3+} in an aerobic environment and coordinated by lactoferrin released from the secondary granules of neutrophils. The resultant lactoferrin–Fe^{3+} is taken up by specific receptors on macrophages (102,103). The transport of the iron, implicated as the target of neutrophilic inflammation, concludes as the metal is stored in ferritin (104,105). This deposition in the macrophage is histologically detected as a sideromacrophage and can be a reliable marker of neutrophilic inflammation (102,106,107).

Rather than being a maladaptive response, the inflammation initiated and coordinated by arachidonic acid products and cytokines after exposure to mineral oxides is absolutely essential for the survival of the host. The iron was initially complexed to the dust with a labile or reactive coordination site available. Consequently, the metal was capable of oxidant generation and injury to host tissues. After reduction by superoxide produced by NADPH oxidoreductase in the neutrophil, reaction with lactoferrin released by the neutrophil (108), and deposition in ferritin of the reticuloendothelial system (109), the iron is rendered catalytically less active.

The increased availability of catalytically active iron after silica and asbestos exposure presents a potential oxidative injury to a living system (110). Sequestration of this reactive iron, therefore, would confer a protective effect. The intracellular storage of iron by macrophages can limit the potential for the generation of free radicals and cellular injury resulting from exposure to a metal chelate (109). Ferritin is considered a safe form of storage for iron because metal sequestered in this protein infrequently participates in electron exchange and oxidant generation (109). The isolation of iron in this chemically less-reactive form within intracellular ferritin confers an antioxidant function to ferritin and, in certain cells, provides cytoprotection in vitro against oxidants (111–113).

Ferritin expression is regulated through a posttranscriptional mechanism (114–120). A specific sequence at the 5′-untranslated end of ferritin mRNA, called the iron responsive element, binds a cubane iron–sulfur cluster, the iron regulatory protein (IRP), when the IRP exists in the apoprotein form. Available iron reacts with the IRP to alter the conformation of this protein when it is complexed to the ferritin mRNA. The affinity of the protein to the mRNA is diminished, and it is displaced allowing translation of ferritin to proceed. This posttranscriptional regulation of ferritin allows the cell to respond rapidly to increased concentrations of iron by increasing the ferritin available to sequester the metal.

Employing superoxide, the alveolar macrophage mobilizes the iron from the surface of a mineral oxide by reducing it to the ferrous state (26). A higher concentration of reactive iron is likely to be the immediate result. Increased concentrations of available iron mobilize ferritin mRNA onto polysomes for translation by reacting with the apoprotein form of the IRP and displacing it from the IRE. Ferritin production increases. The metal can then be isolated in this storage protein. This allows a rapid sequestration of the metal in a chemically less-reactive state (i.e., ferritin) relative to its initial state (i.e., complexed to the silica surface). The result of ferritin regulation by iron is a decrease in the concentration of reactive iron in the cell, thereby preventing iron toxicity. This capacity to sequester iron in apoferritin is not unique to macrophages; it can be a property of many different cell types.

The surface of the mineral oxide retains the capacity to complex metal and appears to mobilize iron from both cells in vitro (121) and a living system (110). There are several possible sources for the iron that accumulates onto the silicate surface after its introduction into the lower respiratory tract. The most likely is the non–protein-bound cellular pool or iron associated with low molecular weight compounds, including ATP, ADP, GTP, citrate, and free amino acids (122). These are poorly characterized iron chelates, for which the critical stability constants with ferric ion are not yet quantified and may be important iron sources available to these dusts. The host will respond with continued attempts to sequester the metal by employing ferritin, which will accumulate locally. The product is recognized histologically as a ferruginous body, which is the particle, and the accumulated ferritin contiguous to the particle (e.g., the silica body). This formation of ferruginous bodies functions to protect the host by diminishing the oxidative injury mediated by metal complexed by mineral oxides. This is consistent with previous investigations that have demonstrated diminished in vitro cytotoxicity and in vivo injury by ferruginous bodies relative to uncoated particles (123,124).

Numerous cytokines can influence this sequestration of catalytically active iron and, subsequently, diminish an oxidative stress presented by the metal to a host. This regulation of iron availability can include changes in host concentrations of apoferritin, transferrin, or transferrin, receptors. Several cytokines induce an increased expression of ferritin, including TNF, IL-1, IL-6, and IL-8 (125–129). Once the ferritin is saturated with metal, release of this iron storage protein by lung cells with uptake by storage tissues (e.g., liver) would further diminish host iron available to the particle and fiber. IFN-γ can function to mediate such a ferritin release (130,131). Other cytokines can function to diminish iron availability by affecting changes in the cellular transport of the metal (131,132). The relative contributions of each cytokine to the resulting hypoferremia are unknown, but this decreased availability of iron is likely to result in a diminished toxicity of metal and, subsequently, decreased injury after exposure to silica and asbestos (133,134). Therefore, mediator release after exposure to silica and asbestos may represent an attempt of the cell to coordinate the transport and sequestration of catalytically active iron. This response would diminish the oxidative stress associated with the particle and fiber and injury after their exposure.

III. Particles Derived from Anthropogenic Sources

A. Epidemiology Studies Suggest an Association Between Urban Air Particles and Increased Mortality

Early epidemiology studies of severe air pollution episodes in the United States and Europe demonstrated that exposure to very high levels of urban air particles can result in increased mortality and morbidity (135–137). However, detailed measurements of air pollution during these episodes is unavailable; hence, it is difficult to attribute the effects to a specific component, such as PM_{10}. During the past decade, several epidemiological studies, using improved statistical techniques and more precise and extended particle monitoring data, have reported statistically significant positive correlations between daily (or several-day average) concentrations of PM_{10} and increased mortality and morbidity (138,141, 142). The observed increases in mortality and morbidity, although statistically significant, are still small compared with risks found in epidemiological studies of occupational or other risk factors. However, because of the large fraction of the population potentially exposed to elevated PM_{10} levels, it has been estimated that 60,000 excess mortalities in the United States each year may be attributable to PM_{10}. In addition to these studies, which demonstrate that increased mortality and morbidity are closely associated with acute changes in PM_{10} concentration, recent prospective cohort studies also provide evidence for an association between long-term exposure to PM_{10} and mortality and morbidity (139,140,143). Taken as a group, the epidemiology studies provide strong evidence linking increased cardiopulmonary mortality and morbidity with both short-term and long-term exposure to PM_{10} pollution and also suggest that the risks associated with long-term exposure are somewhat greater than the risks associated with daily exposure.

B. Risk Factors Associated with PM_{10}-Induced Increases in Mortality and Morbidity

It is important to examine specific causes of death in the epidemiology studies to determine if the excess deaths attributed to PM_{10} pollution could plausibly be contributed to by inhalation of PM_{10}. Analysis of mortality data from Philadelphia (144) reveals an increase in deaths of COPD, pneumonia, cardiovascular disease, and stroke. Increased numbers of asthma attacks (145), outpatient visits for asthma (146), and outpatient visits for bronchitis (147) are also associated with PM_{10}, as are small decrements in 1-sec forced expiratory volume (FEV_1) on days of high pollution (148,149). These studies and others lend plausibility to the idea that inhalation of PM_{10} results in cardiopulmonary problems that can trigger increased mortality or morbidity. Increased mortality is not likely due to a ''harvesting effect'' in which some at-risk people who would have died shortly anyway simply died a few days earlier, in which case there would be a decline in the mortality count in days immediately following a high PM_{10} exposure. For example, during the London episode of 1952, mortality remained somewhat elevated for several days after pollution levels returned to normal, despite the 4000 excess deaths that occurred during the episode (150). These studies and others point to persons with preexisting cardiopulmonary disease, the young, and the elderly as being especially susceptible to elevated levels of PM_{10}.

C. Possible Cellular Mechanisms of PM_{10}-Induced Lung Injury

Several potential mechanisms have been proposed to provide biological plausibility to the notion that acute exposure to relatively low levels of fine particles can result in a rapid increase in mortality and morbidity. PM_{10} has been reported to cause a variety of effects, including respiratory symptoms, inflammation, changes in mucociliary clearance of particles, decrements in lung function, and morphological changes in lung tissue. Many of these effects could contribute to pulmonary or cardiopulmonary events that could result in PM_{10}-associated mortality. Events that cause hypoxemia, such as bronchoconstriction, impaired diffusion, edema, and inflammation, can lead to cardiac arrhythmias. PM_{10}-induced acute inflammation can lead to production of numerous cytokines and other proinflammatory compounds, edema, and epithelial cell injury that may not be perceptible to normal healthy individuals, but could lead to cardiopulmonary stress in some elderly individuals or those with underlying pulmonary disease. Repeated induction of inflammation and lung injury could also lead to chronic lung injury, such as the initiation or progression of COPD. Acid aerosols present in PM_{10} cause slowing of mucociliary clearance, contributing to prolonged particle retention in the lung, including biologically active particles, such as bacteria and allergens (e.g., spores, fungi). Coupled with PM_{10}-impaired macrophage clearance and killing of microorganisms, susceptible individuals could be at greater risk for bacterial or viral infection, leading to pneumonia. PM_{10}-induced inflammation could sensitize the airways of allergic asthmatics, resulting in increased sensitivity to a subsequent challenge with bioaerosols containing allergens, as has been described for ozone and allergens (151,152).

D. Components of Urban Air Particles Responsible for Increased Lung Injury

Despite the impressive epidemiological evidence linking PM_{10} levels with increased mortality and morbidity, toxicological and controlled human exposure studies have not yet provided compelling evidence pointing to a specific component or components of PM_{10} that may be responsible for the health effects reported in the epidemiology literature. PM_{10} pollution is a complex mixture of organic and inorganic constituents the composition of which can vary widely depending on the time or year and geographic location. Particulate matter exists over a wide range of sizes and geometries. In general, however, it can be depicted as discrete solid particles, as agglomerated chains of such particles, or as dispersed liquid droplets. Because only those particles that are respirable are considered to be of health concern, attention is focused on particles nominally less than or equal to 10-μm mass median aerodynamic diameter (MMAD). The MMAD is a normalized diameter of a particle with equivalent aerodynamic properties of a sphere of unit density, and this size range is the basis of the current US regulation and WHO guideline for PM. This metric is used almost universally to characterize particles according to their probability of inhalation and deposition along the respiratory tract. However, although PM_{10} does provide insight into PM inhalability, it does not account for the distribution of particles within that inhalable range, which varies both in region and probability of deposition along the airways, thus, having differential bearings on health outcome.

Nevertheless, there are several properties or components of PM_{10} that may be responsible for increased mortality and morbidity:

Particle Size

Three frequency modes naturally exist within the ambient PM_{10} size distribution (Fig. 3). These size-based subdivisions are often referred to as the coarse, fine, and ultrafine PM modes. Generally, these modes also hold for other attributes of PM, such as their emission sources and mechanisms of formation, their chemical composition, and their physical or aerodynamic behaviors and inferred human dosimetry. The coarse mode comprises that distribution larger than 2.5-μm MMAD and derives almost totally from mechanical and abrasive processes (both anthropogenic and natural), including the entrainment of crustal surface dusts by wind. The PM of this mode is composed of various silicates and crustal metal

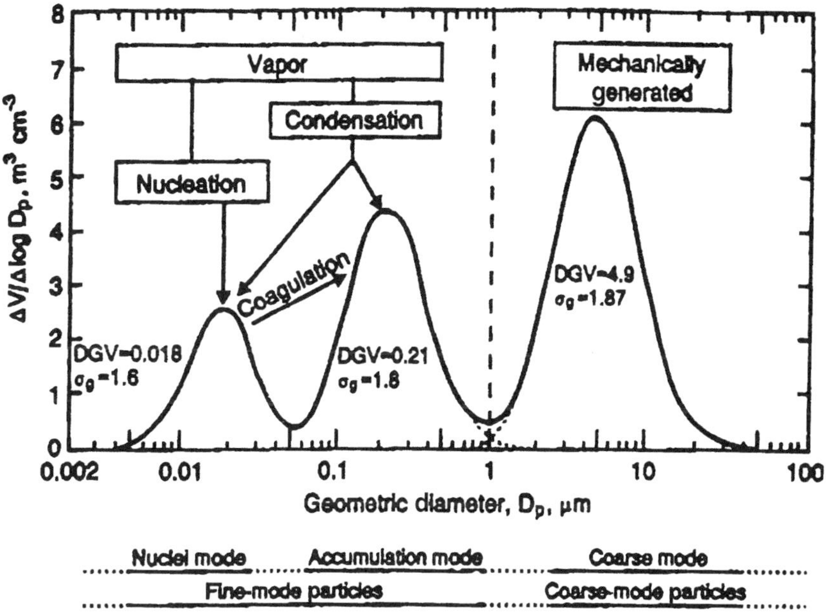

Figure 3 Measured volume–size distribution showing fine-mode and coarse-mode particles and the nuclei and accumulation modes within the fine-particle mode. DGV, geometric mean diameter by volume; equivalent to volume median diameter; and σ_g, geometric standard deviation, are shown for each mode. Also shown are transformation and growth mechanisms (e.g., nucleation, condensation, and coagulation). (From Ref. 138.)

oxides that are largely insoluble in water. Their life expectancy in the air is relatively short (minutes to hours), but they can constitute a major weight proportion of PM in agricultural areas (80–90% as opposed to 30% in urban areas). In these areas, coarse-mode PM are not considered to bear the major health risk of PM_{10}, although some coarse-mode particles can be irritant or possess unique toxic properties (e.g., pesticide and silica).

The deposition of coarse PM in the respiratory tract predominates in the nasopharynx and the conducting airways and, as such, could alter airway cell function (e.g., mucous secretion) or initiate a mild nonspecific inflammation, but the general lack of interest in this PM mode has left a void of information in this area. There is some concern, however, that windblown silicates that are inhaled and do reach the distal lung may have fibrogenic potential, but this claim still has little substantiation. On the other hand, recent speculation that fragments of biological material can be inhaled has drawn some attention because such materials are potentially antigenic and, were they to interact with presenting or other immune cells in the airways, they could initiate detrimental allergic responses (see later). Unfortunately, there is little direct evidence to support or refute any of these concerns about the potential health threats of coarse-mode PM and much work is needed.

The PM fine mode, quite in contrast with the coarse mode, is largely composed of particles derived directly or indirectly from anthropogenic combustion activities. Fossil fuel combustion emissions and coalescing photochemical products, which form by light-catalyzed interactions of gaseous SO_2 or volatile organic compounds, predominate in this mode. Because of their size and low individual mass, fine-mode PM can remain airborne for extended periods and thus can be transported over great distances by prevailing wind currents. These particles occupy the nominal size range of smaller than 2.5 μm, but larger than 0.1 μm, and may comprise substantial hygroscopic SO_4^- or NO_3^- ions, although frequently NH_4^+ coassociates and neutralizes the PM acidity (H^+). Elemental carbon (i.e., soot) and more complex organic compounds (e.g., polycyclic aromatic hydrocarbons), many of which are known carcinogens, also compose ambient PM, especially in urban areas. The combustion of fossil fuels also results in the volatilization of several trace metals and minerals that condense into the matrix of urban aerosols. The metals, in particular, although they exist typically in low concentrations, have been implicated in the inflammatory potency of this PM mode (discussed later). The concern for the fine-mode PM arises not only because of its composition, but also because it readily deposits throughout the respiratory tract, including the most distal lace-like structures of the lung, where any injury and disturbance of gas-exchange is of potential concern.

Last of the PM size modes is what is termed the ultrafine mode, perhaps the least understood PM fraction as a potential contributor to PM-ascribed human health effects. Similar to fine particles, ultrafine particles also arise from combustion and atmospheric photochemical processes, but rather represent a distribution of PM that is quite small, less than 0.1 μm. Being of such small diameter, they begin to approach the mean free path of gas molecules; hence, they move with vigorous brownian activity, colliding frequently with their surroundings as well as themselves. These collisions promote a steady agglomeration of ultrafines, which is thought to result in their rapid removal from the air as they grow in effective aerodynamic diameter into the fine mode distribution. But these PM are also being continuously generated in very large numbers, and although they occupy a small proportion of the PM mass for a given number of particles (e.g., a 2.0-μm particle can be made up of 2×10^6 0.020-μm particles), they can pose a significant threat if toxicity is related to particle number or overall surface area (153). The ultrafines are indeed inhalable and, in theory, deposit throughout the airways, including the nose, to the distal lung. However, there is considerable debate over the probability of human exposure beyond what may occur in the immediate area of PM generation (e.g., on a busy street where automobiles exhaust ultrafines). Furthermore, as PM pollution increases in any given area, there should, in theory, be more collisions of the ultrafines with the higher density of individual PM per given volume of air, and the amount of ultrafine particles should thereby be self-limiting. This would establish a ratio of ultrafines to total PM_{10} that would become increasingly disproportionate as pollution worsens and, thereby, belie correlation with adverse health. Yet, there are reports of single ultrafines particle densities in urban air of up to 5×10^4 to $3 \times 10^5/cm^3$ (154,155) as well as apparent biological evidence of exposure. Ultrafines have been identified in the alveolar macrophages of urban dwellers (156), and they have been correlated with health effects in at least one epidemiological study (157).

Although no toxicological studies with relevant ambient ultrafine particles have been performed, recent animal studies, using single ultrafine particles generated as polymer fumes, have been offered as confirmation that ultrafines can have unusual potency even at very low-mass–concentration exposure levels. In one study, rats exposed to ultrafine particles, generated from heating Teflon, had increased inflammation as evidenced by 80% polymorphoneutrophils (PMNs) in bronchoalveolar lavage (BAL) fluid, interstitial and alveolar edema, and epithelial cell damage (158). There were also increases in mRNAs coding for several proinflammatory cytokines (IL-1, IL-6, TNF-α), antioxidants (MnSOD, metallothionein), and inducible nitric oxide synthase (159). Hamsters exposed to ultrafine CuO particles also had a pulmonary inflammatory response, as evidenced by increased numbers of PMNs and eosinophils (160). Studies of humans exposed to soluble ultrafine acidic particles did not result in changes in pulmonary function or symptoms, suggesting that the soluble nature of the particles, or their tendency to aggregate, may account for their failure to elicit a response (161). The importance of particle size has been demonstrated by studies in which aggregated insoluble ultrafine carbon black (162), TiO_2 (153,163), or diesel soot particles (164) did not cause acute effects in animals.

Mechanisms responsible for ultrafine particle-induced toxicity could include (1) increased surface area available for reaction with other atmospheric components to produce free radicals or to act as a carrier for acids or organic compounds; (2) rapid penetration of epithelial layers into the interstitium (160); and (3) high pulmonary deposition efficiency and increased dose delivered to the alveolar regions of the lung.

Particle Acidity

Acid aerosols comprise those PM containing the strong acidic anions, SO_4^{-2} and NO_3^{-1}. Of the two, PM-associated SO_4^{-2} is generally considered the larger problem from the standpoint of geographic area affected and the sulfur oxide tonnage emitted each year. However, in urban environments with especially high density automobile traffic (e.g., Los Angeles), NO_3^{-1} can be a significant, if not the primary source of PM acidity. Although some sulfate is emitted from stationary fossil fuel combustors as well as from the exhaust of catalyst-equipped automobiles, most SO_4^{-2} is believed to arise from atmospheric transformation of SO_2 gas released from coal and oil combustion. Nitrate (as nitric acid) also is virtually entirely a photochemical by-product of NO_2 oxidation, catalyzed in aqueous aerosols. However, most SO_4^{-2} and NO_3^{-1} in PM do not exist in their highly acid forms (i.e., H_2SO_4 or HNO_3), but rather, exists as a partially or fully NH_4^+-neutralized product, which is considerably less irritating than the pure acids. As a result, concern typically is directed toward the actual concentration of H^+ rather than the anion in assessment of the irritant potential of an acidic aerosol exposure (138).

Acid aerosols (particularly SO_4^{-2}-based) are among the most studied air pollutants, with large databases in human epidemiology, controlled clinical studies, and animal toxicology (165). Field studies have shown positive correlations between asthma-related admissions and impairment of lung function in children with daily ambient acid aerosol concentrations (166). More than 20 controlled exposure studies of healthy human and asthmatic volunteers to acidic aerosols have been performed. They are in general agreement that healthy subjects and animals experience no decrements in lung function at levels up to 1000 $\mu g/m^3$ (an order of magnitude higher than ambient levels), although exposures at the highest concentrations were associated with mild increases in symptoms (reviewed in 165). It is possible that a large portion of the inhaled acid is neutralized by ammonia present in the mouth and respiratory tract. In human studies the size of the acidic aerosol was not a critical factor in response (167–169), although, in some studies with guinea pigs, smaller-sized droplets were more effective in eliciting responses (reviewed in 138). Several studies have suggested that persons with asthma are more sensitive than healthy subjects to acid aerosols (reviewed in 165), and that adolescents with asthma may experience small decrements in lung function, even at exposure levels less than 100 $\mu g/m^3$ (170,171).

Healthy subjects exposed to relatively modest concentrations of acidic aerosols experience accelerated clearance in large bronchi, but slower clearance in small airways (172–174). Interestingly, whereas macrophages from humans exposed to acidic aerosols have altered phagocytic function, acid exposures do not appear to induce an acute neutrophilic inflammation (175,176). Altered mucociliary clearance and phagocytic capability may render some individuals more susceptible to infections, and contribute to the observed increase in morbidity associated with PM.

Despite the extensive database indicting acid as an air pollutant of potential concern, the data have not been widely acknowledged as sufficient evidence to account for the mortality–morbidity effects recently ascribed to PM epidemiologically. Perhaps acid alone is too simple a metric for assessment. Guinea pigs exposed to acid-coated ZnO particles had significant reductions in total lung volume and vital capacity (177), airway responsiveness (178), and increased inflammatory mediators (179), compared with animals exposed to ZnO or acid alone. However, it remains to be seen whether humans respond in an analogous fashion, and whether such exposures are realistic in the general ambient environment.

Transition Metals

The prototypic transition metal Fe and its propensity to participate in redox chemistry were discussed in the foregoing in some detail in the context of mineral dusts. This property of Fe is not unique to that element, but is, in fact, a characteristic of several transition metals (V, Ni, Cu, Mn, Co, and others) that, similar to Fe, can exist in two stable valence states and participate in electron exchange. As cations, these transition metals can associate with various salts and other anions, such as SO_4^{-2}, which makes them quite water-soluble and bioavailable.

Mineral dusts, consisting of various metal-containing silicates (e.g., Al, Mg, and Fe) and metal oxides (e.g., Fe_2O_3), constitute a significant portion of PM_{10} (~20–35% by weight), although most reside in the coarse mode (~50% vs. ~5% in the fine mode; 138). The coordination sites of the metal cations are full and do not contribute to catalysis of free radicals; thus, the coarse-mode mineral dusts are not particularly active biologically (180). The metals that solubilize slowly do not appear to pose an inordinate risk when inhaled with the dust.

Other sources of metal in PM arise from anthropogenic combustion processes that volatilize an array of elements in both sulfated and oxide forms. Fugitive fly ashes from fossil and waste fuel combustion contribute more than 250×10^3 tons annually to the United States ambient PM burden (138), most of which is concentrated in urban areas. In contrast to the fly ash collected or settled in hoppers of air-cleaning systems, the fugitive fly ashes add to the fine-mode PM and can contribute metals to as much as 5% by mass (138). They can remain airborne for extended periods, and they are well within the respirable range (181). Although there is an occupational lung disease entity called "boilermakers lung" (182), which results from exposure to fly ash, the potential for fly ashes emitted into the ambient air as part of the PM environment to induce lung injury in humans is unknown.

Fly ashes from coal combustion have been used in various animal studies, with only modest effects (183). However, coal fly ash contrasts with fly ashes from oil combustion, from which the metals can be considerably more bioavailable (water- or acid-soluble). Early studies of residual oil fly ash have shown enhancement of pulmonary infections in mice and cytotoxicity to alveolar macrophages (180). The degree of acute inflammation (as measured by PMNs, lactic dehydrogenase [LDH], and protein in lavage) and nonspecific bronchial responsiveness was correlated with the surface-complexed iron found in three particle types (volcanic ash, residual oil fly ash, and urban ambient air particles) (184). The inflammatory potential (as measured by BAL neutrophil influx and lavage protein) of ten different metal-containing dusts was related to the amount of total acid-soluble metal, the oxidant-generating potential of the PM extract, and toxicity (185,186). Mortality in mice after instillation of particles and exposure to bacteria was also correlated with metal concentrations.

In vitro studies with alveolar macrophages and airway epithelial cells provide further evidence for the involvement of transition metals in lung injury and inflammation and also yield some insight into the mechanisms by which inflammation is induced. Rabbit alveolar macrophages exposed to fly ash, with or without surface coatings of metal oxides, showed evidence of injury only with metal-coated particles (187). The release of hydrogen peroxide by bovine alveolar macrophages correlated with the amount of metals present in six different samples of metal-containing dusts (188). Oil fly ash caused a strong and immediate chemiluminescence response by human and rat alveolar macrophages, which was inhibitable by the iron chelator deferoxamine, whereas particles with few transition metals were much less active (189). Interestingly, oil fly ash did not stimulate the production of inflammatory mediators by macrophages in this study; rather the production of these mediators was stimulated by dusts high in biological components. In contrast, airway epithelial cells exposed to oil fly ash produced large amounts of IL-6, IL-8, and TNF protein and mRNA (190), as well as prostaglandin E_2 and cyclooxygenase-2 mRNA (191). Production of these proteins and mRNAs was inhibited by deferoxamine and the antioxidant dimethylthiourea (DMTU). NF-κB likely contributes to the induction of the cytokine genes, as demonstrated by electromobility gel shift assays using nuclear extracts from oil fly ash-stimulated cells and NF-κB sequences adjacent to the IL-6 and IL-8 genes (192). Promotor reporter assays also showed that mutations in the NF-κB region ablated oil fly ash stimulation of IL-6 and IL-8 (192).

Although studies at relevant inhalation doses of these PM are needed to further explore the metal hypothesis of lung injury, there is a plausible link to the recent ambient air PM epidemiological findings. Transition metals are found in highest concentration in urban air PM when compared with those of more rural regions (193) and, similar to the sulfate and H^+ content, the concentration of transition metals in ambient air PM increases with decreasing size (181). In summary, several recent studies have reported a significant correlation between the metal content of urban air PM and acute lung injury, and a potential role for metals as causative agents in PM_{10}-induced effects seems likely.

Biological Agents

The PM_{10} contains bioaerosols that include bacteria, viruses, endotoxin, pollen, fungal spores, and animal debris. The smaller bacteria, viruses, and endotoxin are primarily attached to other particles, whereas fungal spores, pollen, and animal debris are usually separate particles. Bioaerosols represented about 30% of the total particles collected on a single day in Mainz, Germany (194), and they were more heavily distributed toward the fine-particle mode. In Brisbane, Australia, fungal spores were the primary bioaerosol component in the coarse fraction (larger than 2.5 μm) (195), and, their the overall contribution of bioaerosols to PM_{10} mass was 5–10%. The amounts of bioaerosols vary seasonally, depending on the source, but are generally lowest in the winter.

Bioaerosols can contribute to increased mortality and morbidity. Asthma mortality has been associated with levels of fungal spores (OR = 2.1/1000 spores per cubic meter) (196), and shows a seasonal peak in Scotland that is associated with ambient pollen levels (197). Fungal spores have also been a precipitating factor in respiratory arrest in persons with asthma (198). Increased morbidity has also been associated with fungal spores. Healthy individuals can develop hypersensitivity pneumonitis after exposure to spores (199). Although actual induction usually requires exposure to higher concentrations than are present in ambient air, responses of already-sensitized individuals requires much lower concentrations. There is also an association between exacerbations of asthma or allergic rhinitis and fungal spores or pollen (200).

Other biological agents in PM_{10}, besides fungal spores and pollen, can also exacerbate asthma and cause pulmonary effects, even in healthy individuals. Anto and Sunyer (201) reported an association between airborne dust derived from soybean husks and increased emergency room visits in Barcelona, Spain. There is also an association between levels of endotoxin in grain dust and the severity of response in grain workers who experience symptoms, decrements in lung function, and airway hyperresponsiveness (202). The concentration of inhaled endotoxin is associated with the development of airflow obstruction among poultry workers (203) and workers exposed to cotton dust (204). Volunteers who inhaled grain dust extract had significant airflow obstruction and increased numbers of PMNs in bronchoalveolar lavage fluid, as well as increased levels of IL-1β, IL-6, IL-8, and TNF-α in lavage fluid (205). mRNAs for these cytokines were also increased in cells recovered in BAL fluid.

Bioaerosol concentrations in these studies are generally considerably higher than observed in the ambient air, especially in the winter months, when notable PM_{10} effects have been observed; consequently, their contribution to PM_{10}-induced mortality and morbidity is unclear. However, although not present in enough quantity to cause noticeable effects on healthy individuals, even the low concentrations measured in ambient air may be sufficient to exacerbate airways injury in persons with chronic lung disease, such as asthma or COPD. Furthermore, bioaerosol concentrations are frequently much higher indoors than outdoors, and exposure to relatively high levels of indoor bioaerosols could exacerbate lung injury or inflammation induced by previous exposure to other toxic agents found in ambient PM_{10} outdoors, such as transition metals or acids.

Organic Constituents

Very little is known about the acute nongenotoxic effects of organic compounds associated with PM_{10} pollution. Nearly 3000 different compounds have been associated with fine particles (206), and in the United States, organic compounds account for 20–50% of total fine-particle mass (207). Organic extracts from particulates recovered from an urban setting using a high-volume–air sampler were mutagenic in a *Salmonella* assay system; when instilled into rat tracheas, they resulted in the formation of adducts to lung DNA. The instilled extracts also resulted in an increase in PMNs and ciliated epithelial cells in lavage fluid (208). Diesel exhaust particles have been reported to stimulate increased IgE production following instillation into nasal passages of volunteers (209); it was suggested that polyaromatic hydrocarbons (PAHs) present on the particles were responsible for the response.

Some mechanisms have been proposed for increasing the toxicity of particles through particle interactions with atmospheric organics. For instance, decreased lung host defense against a variety of infectious agents was observed in mice coexposed to acrolein and carbon black, whereas no immunotoxicity was observed from exposures to either toxicant alone (210). A possible mechanism for this enhanced effect of coexposure was proposed to be due to particles being a carrier for more distal deposition of the carbonyl. Increased lung inflammation and decreased alveolar macrophage phagocytosis was observed in mice coexposed to ozone and carbon black, compared with exposure to either agent alone (211). The enhanced toxicity of the particulate was attributed to an ozone-induced alteration of the physicochemical properties of the carbon black, which is primarily organic. There is evidence for reactive oxygen species (ROS) production derived from reactions of iron with ozone and atmospheric water droplets, and ROS formation is also promoted by the presence of formaldehyde and formate. Similar chemical interactions of gaseous ozone, water droplet organic, and particulate iron (leading to ROS formation) could occur on particle surfaces.

IV. Summary

Inhaled particles have the capacity to cause acute lung damage and inflammation. Transition metals may play a major role in mediating toxicity of occupationally derived substances, such as silica and asbestos. These compounds serve as solid-phase chelants for iron, and lung injury after silica and asbestos exposure is associated with the generation of oxygen-based free radicals catalyzed by iron complexed to the dust. These oxidants can contribute to both cytotoxicity and release of mediators relevant to lung injury. They can also function to protect the host by directing an influx of inflammatory cells that have a capacity to isolate iron by reducing the Fe^{3+} using superoxide, and by modifying iron metabolism in the host, resulting in sequestration of the catalytically active iron associated with the particles.

There are statistically significant associations between combustion-derived particles and elevations in mortality and morbidity, particularly among elderly persons with cardiopulmonary disease. The mechanism(s) by which these particles exert their effect is unknown, but may also involve generation of oxidants from transition metals present on these particles. Additionally, the size and acidity of PM_{10} may contribute to its toxicity, as may organic or biological compounds found on the surface of these particles.

References

1. Iler RK. The Chemistry of Silica. New York: John Wiley & Sons, 1979:622–727.
2. Solomon DH. Clay minerals as electron acceptors and/or electron donors in organic reactions. Clays Clay Miner 1968; 16:31–39.
3. Pritchard RJ, Ghio AJ, Park P, Gilmour MI, Lehmann J, Winsett DW, Costa DL. Oxidant generation and lung injury after exposure to particulate air pollutants are associated with concentrations of complexed iron. Inhal Toxicol 1996; 8:457–477.
4. Ghio AJ, Stonehuerner J, Pritchard RJ, Piantadosi CA, Quigley DR Dreher KL, Costa DL. Humic-like substances in air pollution particulates correlate with concentrations of transition metals and oxidant generation. Inhal Toxicol 1996; 8:4479–4494.
5. Stumm W, Morgan JJ. Aquatic Chemistry. An Introduction Emphasizing Chemical Equilibria in Natural Waters. New York: John Wiley & Sons, 1981:599–684.
6. Schindler PW, Stumm W. The surface chemistry of oxides, hydroxides, and oxide minerals. In: Stumm W, ed. Aquatic Surface Chemistry. Chemical Processes at the Particle–Water Interface. New York: John Wiley & Sons, 1987:83–110.
7. Crumbliss AL, Garrison JM. A comparison of some aspects of the aqueous coordination chemistry of aluminum(III) and iron(III). Comm Inorg Chem 1988; 8:1–26.
8. Olson LL, O'Melia CR. The interactions of Fe(III) with $Si(OH)_4$. J Inorg Nucl Chem 1973; 35:1977–1985.
9. Hazel F, Schock U, Gordon M. Interaction of ferric ions with silicic acid. J Am Chem Soc 1949; 71:2256–2257.
10. Dugger DL, Stanton JH, Irby BN, McConnell BL, Cummings WW, Maatman RW. The exchange of twenty metal ions with the weakly acidic silanol group of silica gel. J Phys Chem 1964; 68:757–760.
11. Fordham AW. Sorption and precipitation of iron on kaolinite. Factors involved in sorption equilibria. Aust J Soil Res 1969; 7:185–197.
12. Rees LVC. Mossbauer spectroscopic studies of ferrous ion exchange in zeolite A. In: Jacobs PA, Jaeger NI, Jiru P, Schulz-Ekloff G, eds. Metal Microstructures in Zeolites. Preparation—Properties—Applications. Proceedings of a Workshop, Bremen, September 22–24, 1982. New York: Elsevier Scientific, 1982:55–59.

13. Herrara R, Peech M. Reaction of montmorillonite with iron(III). Soil Sci Soc Am Proc 1970; 34:740–745.
14. Whittig LD, Page AL. Iron adsorption by montmorillonite systems: preliminary studies. Soil Sci Soc Proc 1961; 25:278–281.
15. Kennedy TP, Dodson R, Rao NV, Ky H, Hopkins C, Baser M, Tolley E, Hoidal JR. Dusts causing pneumoconiosis generate ·OH and produce hemolysis by acting as Fenton catalysts. Arch Biochem Biophys 1989; 269:359–364.
16. Gabor S, Anca Z. Effect of asbestos on lipid peroxidation in the red cells. Bri J Ind Med 1975; 32:39–41.
17. Gulumian M, Sardianos F, Kilroe-Smith T, Ockerse G. Lipid peroxidation in microsomes induced by crocidolite fibers. Chem Biol Interact 1983; 44:111–118.
18. Weitzman SA, Graceffa P Asbestos catalyzes hydroxyl and superoxide radical generation from hydrogen peroxide. Arch Biochem Biophys 1984; 228:373–376.
19. Fontecave M, Mansuy D, Jauen M, Pezerat H. The stimulatory effects of asbestos on NADPH-dependent lipid peroxidation in rat liver microsomes. Biochem J 1987; 241:561–565.
20. Dalal NS, Shi XL, Vallyathan V. Role of free radicals in the mechanisms of hemolysis and lipid peroxidation by silica: comparative ESR and cytotoxicity studies. J Toxicol Environ Health 1990; 29:307–316.
21. Jacob DJ, Gottlieb EW. Chemistry of a polluted cloudy boundary layer. J Geophys Res 1989; 94:12975–13002.
22. Munger JW, Jacob DJ, Waldman JM, Hoffmann MR. Fogwater chemistry in an urban atmosphere. J Geophys Res 1983; 88:5109–5121.
23. Weschler CJ, Mandich ML, Graedel TE. Speciation, photosensitivity, and reactions of transition metal ions in atmospheric droplets. J Geophys Res 1986; 91:5189–5204.
24. Faust BC, Hoffmann MR. Photoinduced reductive dissolution of alpha-Fe_2O_3 by bisulfite. Environ Sci Technol 1986; 20:943–948.
25. Waite TD, Morel FMM. Photoreductive dissolution of colloidal iron oxide: effect of citrate. J Colloid Interface Sci 1984; 102:121–137.
26. Perrin DD. Stability Constants of Metal–Ion Complexes. New York: Pergamon Press, 1979.
27. Chamberlain M, Brown RC, Daview R, Griffiths DM. In vitro prediction of the pathogenicity of mineral dusts. Br J Exp Pathol 1979; 60:320–327.
28. Vallyathan V, Schwegler D, Reasor M, Stettler L, Clere J, Green FHY. Comparative in vitro cytotoxicity and relative pathogenicity of mineral dusts. Ann Occup Hyg 1988; 32:279–289.
29. Nolans RP, Langer AM, Harington JS, Oster G, Selikoff IJ. Quartz hemolysis as related to its surface functionalities. Environ Res 1981; 26:503–520.
30. Light WG, Wei ET. Surface charge and hemolytic activity of asbestos. Environ Res 1977; 13:135–145.
31. Ottery J, Gormley IP. Some factors affecting the haemolytic activity of silicate minerals. Ann Occup Hyg 1978; 21:131–139.
32. Cao CJ, Liu SJ, Lin KC. Raman spectroscopic study on the mechanism of membrane damage induced by quartz. Abstracts of Communications of the 7th International Pneumoconioses Conference. Pittsburgh PA, NIOSH, 1988:135.

33. Haley JD, Margolis J. Haemolytic activity of colloidal silica. Nature 1961; 189: 1010–1011.
34. Charache P, MacLeod CM, White P. Effects of silicate polymers on erthrocytes in the presence and absence of complement. J Gen Physiol 1962; 45:1117–1143.
35. Heppleston AG. Pulmonary toxicology of silica, coal and asbestos. Environ Health Perspect 1984; 55:111–127.
36. Langer AM, Nolan RP. Physicochemical properties of quartz controlling biological activity. In: Goldsmith DF, Winn DM, Shy CM, eds. Silica, Silicosis, and Cancer. New York: Praeger, 1986:125–135.
37. Clark SG, Holt PF. Dissolution of chrysotile asbestos in water, acid, and alkali. Nature 1960; 185:237.
38. Kriegseis W, Biederbick R, Boese J, Robock K, Scharmann A. Investigations into the determination of the cytotoxicity of quartz dust by physical methods. In: Walton WH, ed. Inhaled Particles IV. Oxford: Pergamon Press, 1977:345–359.
39. Razzaboni BL, Bolsaitis P. Evidence of an oxidative mechanism for the hemolytic activity of silica particles. Environ Health Perspect 1990; 87:337–341.
40. Goodglick LA, Kane AB. Role of reactive oxygen metabolites in crocidolite asbestos toxicity to mouse macrophages. Cancer Res 1986; 46:5558–5566.
41. Mohr C, Davis GS, Graebner C, Hemenway DR, Gemsa D. Enhanced release of prostaglandin E_2 from macrophages of rats with silicosis. Am J Respir Cell Mol Biol 1992; 6:390–396.
42. Leikauf GD, Fink SP, Miller ML, Lockey JE, Driscoll KE. Refractory ceramic fibers activate alveolar macrophage eicosanoid and cytokine release. J Appl Physiol 1995; 78:164–171.
43. Claudio E, Segade F, Wrobel K, Ramos S, Lazo PS. Activation of murine macrophages by silica particles in vitro is a process independent of silica-induced cell death. Am J Respir Cell Mol Biol 1995; 13:547–554.
44. Gabor S, Anca Z, Zugravu E. In vitro action of quartz on alveolar macrophage lipid peroxides. Arch Environ Health 1975; 30:499–501.
45. Brown RC, Poole A. Arachidonic acid release and prostaglandin synthesis in a macrophage-like cell line exposed to asbestos. Agents Actions 1984; 15:336–340.
46. Rom WN, Bitterman PB, Rennard SI, Cantin A, Crystal RG. Characterization of the lower respiratory tract inflammation of nonsmoking individuals with interstitial lung disease associated with chronic inhalation of inorganic dusts. Am Rev Respir Dis 1987; 136:1429–1434.
47. Englen MD, Taylor SM, Laegreid WW, Denny Liggitt H, Silflow RM, Breeze RG, Wes Leid R. Stimulation of arachidonic acid metabolism in silica-exposed alveolar macrophages. Exp Lung Res 1989; 15:511–526.
48. Garcia JGN, Griffith DE, Cohen AB, Callahan KS. Alveolar macrophages from patients with asbestos exposure release increased levels of leukotriene B_4. Am Rev Respir Dis 1989; 139:1494–1501.
49. Klien JH, Adamson IYR. Fibroblast inhibition and prostaglandin secretion by alveolar epithelial cells exposed to silica. Lab Invest 1989; 60:808–813.
50. Driscoll KE, Higgins JM, Leytart MJ, Crosby LL. Differential effects of mineral dusts on the in vitro activation of alveolar macrophage eicosanoid and cytokine release. Toxicol In Vitro 1990; 4:284–288.

51. Driscoll KE, Lindenschmidt RC, Maurer JK, Higgins JM, Ridder G. Pulmonary response to silica or titanium dioxide: inflammatory cells, alveolar macrophage-derived cytokines, and histopathology. Am J Respir Cell Mol Biol 1990; 2:381–390.
52. Kuhn DC, Demers LM. Influence of mineral dust surface chemistry on eicosanoid production by the alveolar macrophage. J Toxicol Environ Health 1992; 35:39–50.
53. Mohr C, Davis GS, Graebner C, Hemenway DR, Gemsa D. Enhanced release of prostaglandin E_2 from macrophages of rats with silicosis. Am J Respir Cell Mol Biol 1992; 6:390–396.
54. Panos RJ, Voelkel NF, Cott GR, Mason RJ, Westcott JY. Alterations in eicosanoid production by rat alveolar type II cells isolated after silica-induced lung injury. Am J Respir Cell Mol Biol 1992; 6:430–438.
55. Kuhn DC, Griffith JW, Stauffer JL, Riling S, Demers LM. Characterization of alveolar macrophage eicosanoid production in a non-human primate model of mineral dust exposure. Prostaglandins 1993; 46:207–220.
56. Campbell PB, Tolson TA. Modulation of human monocyte leukotactic responsiveness by thromboxane A_2 and 12-hydroxyheptadecatrienoic acid (12-HHT). J Leukoc Biol 1988; 43:117–124.
57. Downey GP, Gumbay RS, Doherty DE, LaBrecque JF, Henson JE, Henson PM, Worthen GS. Enhancement of pulmonary inflammation by PGE_2: evidence for a vasodilator effect. J Appl Physiol 1988; 64:728–741.
58. Kalmar JR, Van Dyke TE. Effect of bacterial products on neutrophil chemotaxis. Methods Enzymol 1994; 236:58–87.
59. Oda H, Kadota J, Kohno S, Hara K. Leukotriene B_4 in bronchoalveolar lavage fluid of patients with diffuse panbronchiolitis. Chest 1995; 108:116–122.
60. Turner CR, Breslow R, Conklyn MJ, Andresen CJ, Patterson DK, Lopez-Anaya A, Owens B, Lee P, Watson JW, Showell HJ. In vitro and in vivo effects of leukotriene B_4 antagonism in a primate model of asthma. J Clin Invest 1996; 97:381–387.
61. Renz H, Gong J-H, Schmidt A, Nain M, Gemsa D. Release of tumor necrosis factor-α from macrophages. Enhancement and suppression are dose-dependently regulated by prostaglandin E_2 and cyclic nucleotides. J Immunol 1988; 141:2388–2393.
62. Kassis S, Lee JC, Hanna N. Effects of prostaglandins and cAMP levels on monocyte IL-1 production. Agents Actions 1989; 27:274–276.
63. Scales WE, Chensue SW, Otterness I, Kunkel SL. Regulation of monokine gene expression: Prostaglandin E_2 suppresses tumor necrosis factor but not interleukin-1B-mRNA and cell-associated bioactivity. J Leuk Biol 1989; 45:416–421.
64. Dubois CM, Bissonnette E, Rola-Pleszczynski M. Asbestos fibers and silica particles stimulate rat alveolar macrophages to release tumor necrosis factor. Autoregulatory role of leukotriene B_4. Am Rev Respir Dis 1989; 139:1257–1264.
65. Lemaire I, Beaudoin H, Dubois C. Cytokine regulation of lung fibroblast proliferation: pulmonary and systemic changes in asbestos-induced pulmonary fibrosis. Am Rev Respir Dis 1986; 134:653–658.
66. Oghiso Y, Kubota Y. Interleukin 1 production and accessory cell function of rat

alveolar macrophages exposed to mineral dust particles. Microbiol Immunol 1987; 31:275–287.
67. Rola-Pleszczynski M, Bouvrette L, Gingras D, Girard M. Identification of interferon as the lymphokine that mediates leukotriene B_4 induced immunoregulation. J Immunol 1987; 139:513–517.
68. Driscoll KE, Lindenschmidt RC, Maurer JK, Higgins JM, Ridder G. Pulmonary response to silica or titanium dioxide: inflammatory cells, alveolar macrophage-derived cytokines, and histopathology. Am J Respir Cell Mol Biol 1990; 2:381–390.
69. Driscoll KE, Maurer JK. Cytokine and growth factor release alveolar macrophages: potential biomarkers of pulmonary toxicity. Toxicol Pathol 1991; 19:398–407.
70. Mohr C, Gemsa D, Graebner C, Hemenway DR, Leslie KO, Absher PM, Davis GS. Systemic macrophage stimulation in rats with silicosis: enhanced release of tumor necrosis factor-α from alveolar and peritoneal macrophages. Am J Respir Cell Mol Biol 1991; 5:395–402.
71. Perkins RC, Scheule RK, Hamilton R, Gomes G, Freidman G, Holian A. Human alveolar macrophage cytokine release in response to in vitro and in vivo asbestos exposure. Exp Lung Res 1993; 19:55–65.
72. Rosenthal GJ, Germolec DR, Blazka ME, Corsini E, Simeonova P, Pollock P, Kong LY, Kwon J, Luster MI. Asbestos simulates IL-8 production from human lung epithelial cells. J Immunol 1994; 153:3237–3244.
73. Savici D, He B, Geist LJ, Monick MM, Hunninghake GW. Silica increases tumor necrosis factor (TNF) production, in part, by upregulating the TNF promoter. Exp Lung Res 1994; 20:613–625.
74. Simeonova PP, Luster MI. Iron and reactive oxygen species in the asbestos-induced tumor necrosis factor-α response from alveolar macrophages. Am J Respir Cell Mol Biol 1995; 12:676–683.
75. Piguet PF, Collart MA, Grau GE, Sappino AP, Vassalli P. Requirement for tumor necrosis factor for development of silica-induced pulmonary fibrosis. Nature 1990; 344:245–247.
76. Harris JA, Hyde DM, Wang Q, Stovall MY, Giri SN. Repeated episodes of C5a-induced neutrophil influx do not result in pulmonary fibrosis. Inflammation 1991; 15:233–250.
77. Lasky JA, Bonner JC, Brody AR. The pathobiology of asbestos-induced lung disease: a proposed role for macrophage-derived growth factors. Ann NY Acad Sci 1991; 643:239–244.
78. Adamson IY, Letourneau HL, Bowden DH. Comparison of alveolar and interstitial macrophages in fibroblast stimulation after silica and long or short asbestos. Lab Invest 1991; 64:339–344.
79. Bonner JC, Goodell AL, Coin PG, Brody AR. Chrysotile asbestos upregulates gene expression and production of alpha-receptors for platelet-derived growth factor (PDGF-AA) on rat lung fibroblasts. J Clin Invest 1993; 92:425–430.
80. Lasky JA, Coin PG, Lindroos PM, Ostrowski LE, Brody AR, Bonner JC. Chrysotile asbestos stimulates platelet-derived growth factor-AA production by rat lung fibroblasts in vitro: evidence for an autocrine loop. Am J Respir Cell Mol Biol 1995; 12:162–170.

81. Osornio-Vargas AR, Goodell AL, Hernandez-Rodriguez NA, Brody AR, Coin PG, Badgett A, Bonner JC. Platelet-derived growth factor (PDGF)-AA, -AB, and -BB induce differential chemotaxis of early passage rat lung fibroblasts in vitro. Am J Respir Cell Mol Biol 1995; 12:33–40.
82. Walker C, Everitt J, Ferriola PC, Stewart W, Manjum J, Bermudez E. Autocrine growth stimulation by transforming growth factor alpha in asbestos-transformed rat mesothelial cells. Cancer Res 1995; 55:530–536.
83. Shi X, Dalal NS, Vallyathan V. ESR evidence for the hydroxyl radical formation in aqueous suspensions of quartz particles and its possible significances to lipid peroxidation in silicosis. J Tox Environ Health 1988; 25:237–245.
84. Ghio AJ, Kennedy TP, Whorton AR, Crumbliss AL, Hatch GE, Hoidal JR. Role of surface complexed iron in oxidant generation and lung inflammation induced by silicates. Am J Physiol 1992; L511–L518.
85. Ala Y, Palluy O, Favero J, Bonne C, Modat G, Dornand J. Hypoxia/reoxygenation stimulates endothelial cells to promote interleukin-1 and interleukin-6 production. Effects of free radical scavengers. Agents Actions 1992; 37:134–139.
86. DeForge LE, Preston AM, Takeuchi E, Kenney J, Boxer LA, Remick DG. Regulation of interleukin 8 gene expression by oxidant stress. J Biol Chem 1993; 268: 25568–25576.
87. Hayashi T, Ueno Y, Okamato T. Oxidoreductive regulation of nuclear factor κB. J Biol Chem 1993; 268:11380–11388.
88. Chen R, Kuhn DC, Sun SC, Gaydos LJ, Demers LM. Dependence and reversal of nitric oxide production on NF-kappa B in silica and lipopolysaccharide-induced macrophages. Biochem Biophys Res Commun 1995; 214:839–846.
89. Chen R, Sun SC, Kuh DC, Gaydos LJ, Demers LM. Essential role of NF-kappa B activation in silica-induced inflammatory mediatory production in macrophages. Biochem Biophys Res Commun 1995; 214:985–992.
90. Janssen YM, Barchowsky A, Treadwell M, Driscoll KE, Mossman BT. Asbestos induces nuclear factor kappa R (NF-kappa B) DNA-binding activity and NF-kappa B-dependent gene expression in tracheal epithelial cells. Proc Natl Acad Sci USA 1995; 92:8458–8462.
91. Collart MA, Baeuerle P, Vassalli P. Regulation of tumor necrosis factor alpha transcription in macrophages: involvement of four κB-like motifs and of constitutive and inducible forms of NF-κB. Mol Cell Biol 1990; 10:1498–1506.
92. Vogt W, Nolte R, Brunahl D. Binding of iron to the 5th component of human complement directs oxygen radical-mediated conversion to specific sites and causes nonenzymatic activation. Complement Inflamm 1991; 8:313–319.
93. Kuhn DC, Demers LM. Influence of mineral dust surface chemistry on eicosanoid production by the alveolar macrophage. J Toxicol Environ Health 1992; 35:39–50.
94. Driscoll KE, Hassenbein DG, Carter JM, Kunkel SL, Quinlan TR, Mossman BT. TNF-α and increased chemokine expression in rat lung after particle exposure. Toxicol Lett 1995; 82/83:483–489.
95. Mossman BT, Marsh JP, Sesko A, Hill S, Shatos MA, Doherty J, Petruska J, Adler KB, Hemenway D, Mickey R, Vacek P, Kagan E. Inhibition of lung injury, inflammation, and interstitial pulmonary fibrosis by polyethylene glycol-conjugated

catalase in a rapid inhalation model of asbestosis. Am Rev Respir Dis 1990; 141: 1266–1271.
96. Schapira RM, Ghio AJ, Effros RM, Morrisey J, Dawson CA, Hacker AD. Am J Respir Cell Mol Biol 1994; 10:573–579.
97. Schapira RM, Ghio AJ, Effros RM, Morrisey J, Almagro UA, Dawson CA, Hacker AD. Hydroxyl radical production and injury in the rat lung following silica or titanium dioxide instillation. Am J Respir Cell Mol Biol 1995; 12:220–226.
98. Bienfait HF, Bino RJ, van der Bliek AM, Duivenvoorden JF, Fontaine JM. Characterization of ferric reducing activity in roots of Fe-deficient *Phaseolus vulgaris*. Physiol Plant 1983; 59:196–202.
99. Jones GJ, Palenik BP, Morel FMM. Trace metal reduction by phytoplankton: the role of plasmalemma redox enzymes. J Phycol 1987; 23:237–244.
100. Dancis A, Roman DG, Anderson GJ, Hinnebusch AG, Klausner RD. Ferric reductase of *Saccharomyces cerevisiae*: molecular characterization, role in iron uptake, and transcriptional control by iron. Proc Natl Acad Sci USA 1992; 89:3869–3873.
101. Bellavite P. The superoxide-forming enzymatic system of phagocytes. Free Radic Biol Med 1988; 4:225–261.
102. van Snick J, Masson PL, Heremans JF. The affinity of lactoferrin for the reticuloendothelial system (RES) as the molecular basis for the hyposideraemia of inflammation. In: Crichton RR, ed. Proteins of Iron Storage and Transport in Biochemistry and Medicine. Amsterdam: North Holland Publishing, 1975:433–438.
103. Markowetz B, van Snick JI, Masson PL. Binding and ingestion of human lactoferrin by mouse alveolar macrophages. Thorax 1979; 34:209–212.
104. Birgens HS. The interaction of lactoferrin with human macrophages. Dan Med Bull 1991; 38:244–252.
105. Birgens HS, Kristensen LO, Borregaard N, Karle H, Hansen NE, Lactoferrin-mediated transfer of iron to intracellular ferritin in human monocytes. Eur J Haematol 1988; 41:52–57.
106. Konijn AM, Hershko C. Ferritin synthesis in inflammation. Pathogenesis of impaired iron release. Br J Haematol 1977; 37:7–16.
107. Birgegard G, Caro J. Increased ferritin synthesis and iron uptake in inflammatory mouse macrophages. Scand J Haemotol 1984; 33:43–48.
108. Britigan BE, Hassett DJ, Rosen GM, Hamill DR, Cohen MS. Neutrophil degranulation inhibits potential hydroxyl-radical formation. Relative impact of myeloperoxidase and lactoferrin release on hydroxyl-radical production by iron-supplemented neutrophils assessed by spin-trapping techniques. Biochem J 1989; 264:447–455.
109. Olakanmi O, McGowan SE, Hayek MB, Britigan BE. Iron sequestration by macrophages decreases the potential for extracellular hydroxyl radical formation. J Clin Invest 1993; 91:889–899.
110. Ghio AJ, Jaskot RH, Hatch GE. Collagen deposition after intratracheal instillation of silica is associated with an accumulation of non-heme iron in the rat lung. Am J Physiol 1994; 267:L686–L692.
111. Cozzi A, Santambrogio P, Levi S, Arosio P. Iron detoxifying activity of ferritin. Effects of H and L human apoferritins on lipid peroxidation in vitro. FEBS Lett 1990; 277:119–122.
112. Balla G, Jacob HS, Balla J, Rosenberg M, Nath K, Apple F, Eaton JW, Vercellotti

GM. Ferritin: a cytoprotective antioxidant strategem of endothelium. J Biol Chem 1992; 267:18148–18153.
113. Balla J, Nath DA, Balla G, Juckett MB, Jacob HS, Vercellotti GM. Endothelial cell heme oxygenase and ferritin induction in rat lung by hemoglobin in vivo. Am J Physiol 1995; 268:L321–L327.
114. Leibold EA, Munro HN. Cytoplasmic protein binds in vitro to a highly conserved sequence in the 5′ untranslated region of ferritin heavy- and light-subunit mRNAs. Proc Natl Acad Sci USA 1988; 85:2171–2175.
115. Rouault TA, Hentze MW, Wright-Caughman S, Harford JB, Klausner RD. Binding of a cytosolic protein to the iron-responsive element of human ferritin messenger RNA. Science 1988; 241:1207–1210.
116. Kaptain S, Downey WE, Tang C, Philpott C, Haile D, Orloff DG, Harford JB, Rouault TA, Klausner RD. A regulated RNA binding protein also possesses aconitase activity. Proc Natl Acad Sci USA 1991; 88:10109–10113.
117. Haile DJ, Rouault TA, Harford JB, Kennedy MC, Blondin GA, Beinert H, Klausner RD. Cellular regulation of the iron-responsive element binding protein: disassembly of the cubane iron–sulfur cluster results in high-affinity RNA binding. Proc Natl Acad Sci USA 1992; 89:11735–11739.
118. Kennedy MC, Mende-Mueller L, Blondin GA, Beinert H. Purification and characterization of cytosolic aconitase from beef liver and its relationship to the iron-responsive element binding protein. Proc Natl Acad Sci USA 1992; 89:11730–11734.
119. Beinert H, Kennedy MC. Aconitase, a two-faced protein: enzyme and iron regulatory factor. FASEB J 1993; 7:1442–1449.
120. Basilion JP, Rouault TA, Massinople CM, Klausner RD, Burgess WH. The iron-responsive element-binding protein: localization of the RNA-binding site to the aconitase active-site cleft. Proc Natl Acad Sci USA 1994; 91:574–578.
121. Koerten HK, de Brujin JD, Daems WTH. The formation of asbestos bodies by mouse peritoneal macrophages. An in vitro study. Am J Pathol 1990; 137:121–134.
122. Jacobs A. Low molecular weight intracellular iron transport compounds. Blood 1977; 50:433–439.
123. Vorwald AJ, Durkan TM, Pratt PC. Experimental studies of asbestosis. Arch Ind Hyg Occup Med 1951; 3:1–43.
124. McLemore TL, Mace ML, Roggli V, Marshall MV, Lawrence EC, Wilson RK, Martin RR, Brinkley BR, Greenberg SD. Asbestos body phagocytosis by human free alveolar macrophages. Cancer Lett 1980; 9:85–93.
125. Fahmy M, Young SP. Modulation of iron metabolism in monocyte cell line U937 by inflammatory cytokines: changes in transferrin uptake, iron handling and ferritin mRNA. Biochem J 1993; 296:175–181.
126. Lissoni P, Cazzaniga M, Ardizzoia A, Rossini F, Fiorelli G, Tancini G, Pittalis S, Barni S. Cytokine regulation of iron metabolism: effect of low-dose interleukin-2 subcutaneous therapy on ferritin, transferrin and iron blood concentrations in cancer patients. J Biol Regul Homeost Agents 1993; 7:31–33.
127. Kobune M, Kohgo Y, Kato J, Miyazaki E, Niitsu Y. Interleukin-6 enhances hepatic transferrin uptake and ferritin expression in rats. Hepatology 1994; 19:1468–1475.

128. Rogers JT, Andriotakis JL, Lacroix L, Durmowicz GP, Kasschau KD, Bridges KR. Translational enhancement of H-ferritin mRNA by interleukin-1 beta acts through 5′ leader sequences distinct from the iron responsive element. Nucleic Acids Res 1994; 22:2678–2686.
129. Rogers JT. Ferritin translation by interleukin-6: the role of sequences upstream of the start codons of the heavy and light subunit genes. Blood 1996; 87:2525–2537.
130. Byrd TF, Horwitz MA. Regulation of transferrin receptor expression and ferritin content in human mononuclear phagocytes. Coordinate upregulation by iron transferrin and downregulation by interferon gamma. J Clin Invest 1993; 91:969–976.
131. Caraglia M, Libroia AM, Corradino S, Coppola V, Guarrasi R, Barile C, Genua G, Bianco AR, Tagliaferri P. Alpha-interferon induces depletion of intracellular iron content and upregulation of functional transferrin receptors on human epidermoid cancer KB cells. Biochem Biophys Res Commun 1994; 203:281–288.
132. Lu J, Kaur C, Ling EA. Expression and upregulation of transferrin receptors and iron uptake in the epiplexus cells of different aged rats injected with lipopolysaccharide and interferon-gamma. J Anat 1995; 187:603–611.
133. Hirayama M, Kohgo Y, Kondo H, Shintani N, Fujikawa K, Sasaki K, Kato J, Niitsu Y. Regulation of iron metabolism in HepG2 cells: a possible role for cytokines in the hepatic deposition of iron. Hepatology 1993; 18:874–880.
134. Warren S, Torti SV, Torti FM. The role of iron in the cytotoxicity of tumor necrosis factor. Lymphokine Cytokine Res 1993; 12:75–80.
135. Firket J. The causes of accidents which occurred in the Meuse Valley during the fogs of December 1930. Bull Acad R Med Belg 1931; 11:683–741.
136. Schrenk HH, Heimann H, Clayton GD, Gafafer WM, Wexler H. Air pollution in Donora, PA. Epidemiology of the unusual smog episode of October 1948: preliminary report. Washington, DC: Public Health Service; Public Health Service Bulletin 306; 1949.
137. Martin AE. Mortality and morbidity statistics and air pollution. Proc R Soc Med 1964; 57:969–975.
138. U.S. Environmental Protection Agency. Air Quality Criteria for Particulate Matter. Vol I. Office of Research and Development. April, 1996; EPA/600/P-95/001cF.
139. Dockery DW, Pope CA, Xu X, Spengler JD, Ware JH, Fay ME, Ferris BG, Speizer JE. An association between air pollution and mortality in six U.S. cities. N Engl J Med 1993; 329:1753–1759.
140. Pope CA, Thun MJ, Namboodiri MM, Dockery DW, Evans JS, Speizer FE, Heath CW. Particulate air pollution as a predictor of mortality in a prospective study of U.S. adults. Am J Respir Crit Care Med 1995; 151:669–674.
141. Schwartz J. Air pollution and hospital admissions for the elderly in Birmingham, AL. Am J Epidemiol 1994; 139:589–598.
142. Pope CA. Respiratory hospital admissions associated with PM_{10} pollution in Utah, Salt Lake, and Cache Valleys. Arch Environ Health 1991; 46:90–97.
143. Dockery DW, Cunningham J, Damokosh AI, Neas LM, Spengler JD, Koutrakis P, Ware JH, Raizenne M, Speizer FE. Health effects of acid aerosols on North American children: respiratory symptoms. Environ Health Perspect 1996. In press.
144. Schwartz J. What are people dying of on high air pollution days? Environ Res 1994; 64:26–35.

145. Ponka A. Asthma and low level air pollution in Helsinki. Arch Environ Health 1991; 46:262–220.
146. Gordian ME, Ozkaynak H, Xue J, Morris SS, Spengler JD. Particulate air pollution and respiratory disease in Anchorage, Alaska. Environ Health Perspect 1996; 104: 290–297.
147. Hefflin BJ, Jalaludin B, McClure E, Cobb N, Johnson CA, Jecha L, Etzel RA. Survelliance for dust storms and respiratory diseases in Washington State. Arch Environ Health 1991; 49:170–174.
148. Pope CA, Kanner RE. Acute effects of PM_{10} pollution on pulmonary function of smokers with mild to moderate chronic obstructive pulmonary disease. Am Rev Respir Dis 1993; 147:1336–1340.
149. Chestnut LG, Schwartz J, Savitz DA, Burchfiel CM. Pulmonary function and ambient particulate matter: epidemiological evidence from NHANES I. Arch Environ Health 1991; 46:135–144.
150. Logan WPD. Mortality in the London fog incident, 1952. Lancet 1953; Feb 14th: 336–339.
151. Molfino NA, Wright SC, Katz I, Tarlo S, Silverman F, McClean PA, Szalai JP, Raizenne M, Slutsky AS, Zamel N. Effect of low concentrations of ozone on inhaled allergen responses in asthmatic subjects. Lancet 1991; 338:199–201.
152. Jorres R, Nowak D, Magnussen H. The effect of ozone exposure on allergen responsiveness in subjects with asthma or rhinitis. Am J Respir Crit Care Med 1996; 153: 56–64.
153. Oberdorster G, Ferin J, Soderholm SC, Finkelstein J. Role of the alveolar macrophage in lung injury: studies with ultrafine particles. Environ Health Perspect 1992; 97:193–199.
154. Brand P, Ruob K, Gebhart J. Performance of a mobile aerosol spectrometer for an in situ characterization of environmental aerosols in Frankfurt city. Atmos Environ 1992; 26:2451–2457.
155. Castellani CM. Characterization of the atmospheric aerosol in an urban area and the vicinity of a main highway. In: ENEA Environment Department Meetings and Seminars; Bologna and Rome, Italy. INTO 1993; 7(93):35–55.
156. Hatch V, Hauser R, Hayes GB, Stearns R, Christiani D, Godleski JJ. Detection of ultrafine particles in the lung macrophages of healthy people. In: Bailey GW, Garrant-Reed AJ, eds. Proceedings of the 52nd Annual Meeting, Microscopy of America, New Orleans, LA, 1994:1004–1005.
157. Peters A, Neas L, Tuch T, Heinrich J, Heyder J, Wichmann HE. Contribution of ultra-fine particles to short-term effects of air polution on asthmatics. Am J Respir Crit Care Med 1996; 153:A16.
158. Oberdorster G, Gelein RM, Ferin J, Weiss B. Association of particulate air pollution and acute mortality: involvement of ultrafine particles? Inhal Toxicol 1994; 7:111–124.
159. Johnson CJ, Finkelstein JN, Gelein R, Baggs R, Oberdorster G. Characterization of the early pulmonary inflammatory response associated with ultrafine PTFE particle exposure. Toxicol Appl Pharmacol 1996. In press.
160. Stearns RC, Murphy GGK, Skornik W, Hatch V, Katler M, Godleski JJ. Detection of ultrafine copper oxide particles in the lungs of hamsters by electron spectroscopic

imaging. Proceedings of International Conference on Electron Microscopy, Paris: ICEM 13, July 1994:763–764.

161. Horvath SM, Folinsbee LJ, Bedi JF. Combined effect of ozone and sulfuric acid on pulmonary function in man. Am Ind Hyg Assoc J 1987; 48:94–98.
162. Mauderly JL. Noncancer pulmonary effects of chronic inhalation exposure of animals to solid particles. In:Mohr U, Dungworth DL, Mauderly JL, Oberdorster G, eds. Toxic and Carcinogenic Effects of Solid Particles in the Respiratory Tract. Proceedings of the 4th International Inhalation Symposium, March 1993; Hannover, Ger: International Life Sciences Institute Press, 1993:355–365.
163. Ferin J, Oberdorster G, Penney DP. Pulmonary retention of ultrafine and fine particles in rats. Am J Respir Cell Mol Biol 1992; 6:535–542.
164. White HJ, Garg BD. Early pulmonary response of the rat lung to inhalation of high concentration of diesel particles. J Appl Toxicol 1981; 1:104–110.
165. Bascom R, Bromber PA, Costa DL, Devlin R, Dockery DW, Frampton MW, Lambert W, Samet JM, Speizer FE, Utell M. Health effects of air pollution: parts I. Am J Respir Crit Care Med 1996; 153:3–50.
166. Bates D, Sizto R. The Ontario Air Pollution Study: identification of the causative agent. Environ Health Perspect 1989; 79:69–72.
167. Avol EL, Linn WS, Whynot JD, Anderson KR, Shamoo DA, Valencia LM, Little DE, Hackney JD. Respiratory dose–response study of normal and asthmatic volunteers exposed to sulfuric acid aerosol in the sub-micrometer size range. Toxicol Ind Health 1988; 4:173–180.
168. Avol EL, Linn WS, Wightman LH, Whynot JD, Anderson KR, Hackney JD. Short-term respiratory effects of sulfuric acid in fog: a laboratory study of healthy and asthmatic volunteers. JAPCA 1988; 38:258–263.
169. Linn WS, Avol EL, Anderson KR, Shamoo DA, Peng RC, Hackney JD. Effect of droplet size on respiratory responses to inhaled sulfuric acid in normal and asthmatic volunteers. Am Rev Respir Dis 1989; 140:161–166.
170. Koenig JQ, Pierson WE, Horike M. The effects of inhaled sulfuric acid on pulmonary function in adolescent asthmatics. Am Rev Respir Dis 1983; 128:221–225.
171. Koenig JQ, Covert DS, Pierson WE. Effects of inhalation of acidic components on pulmonary function in allergic adolescent subjects. Environ Health Perspect 1989; 79:173–178.
172. Leikauf GD, Yeates DB, Wales KA, Spektor D, Albert RE, Lippmann M. Effects of sulfuric acid aerosol on respiratory mechanics and mucociliary particle clearance in healthy nonsmoking adults. Am Ind Hyg Assoc J 1981; 42:273–282.
173. Leikauf GD, Spektor DM, Albert RE, Lippman M. Dose-dependent effects of submicrometer sulfuric acid aerosol on particle clearance from ciliated human lung airways. Am Ind Hyg Assoc J 1984; 45:285–292.
174. Spektor DM, Yen BM, Lippmann M. Effect of concentration and cumulative exposure of inhaled sulfuric acid on tracheobronchial particle clearance in healthy humans. Environ Health Perspect 1989; 79:167–172.
175. Frampton MW, Morrow PE, Cox C, Levy PC, Condemi JJ, Speers D, Gibb FR, Utell MJ. Sulfuric acid aerosol followed by ozone exposure in healthy and asthmatic subjects. Environ Res 1992; 69:1–14.

176. Becker S, Devlin RB, Koren HS, Roger LB. Exposure of humans to HNO_3 causes alveolar macrophage activation. Inhal Toxicol 1996; 8:185–200.
177. Amdur MO, Chen LC. Furnace-generated acid aerosols: speciation and pulmonary effects. Environ Health Perspect 1989: 79:147–150.
178. Chen LC, Miller PD, Amdur MO, Gordon T. Airway hyperresponsiveness in guinea pigs exposed to acid-coated ultrafine particles. J Toxicol Environ Health 1992; 35: 165–174.
179. Chen LC, Miller PD, Amdur MO. Effects of sulfur oxides on eicosanoids. J Toxicol Environ Health 1989; 28:99–109.
180. Hatch GE, Boykin E, Graham JA, Lewtas J, Pott F, Loud K, Mumford JL. Inhalable particles and pulmonary host defense: in vivo and in vitro effects of ambient air and combustion particles. Environ Res 1985; 36:67–80.
181. Natusch DFS, Wallace JR, Evans CA Jr. Toxic trace elements: preferential concentration in respirable particles. Science 1974; 183:202–204.
182. Hauser R, Elreedy S, Hoppin JA, Christiani DC. Airway obstruction in boilermakers exposed to fuel oil ash: a prospective study. Am J Respir Crit Care Med 1995; 152:1478–1484.
183. Alarie YC, Krumm AA, Busey WM. Long term exposure to sulfur dioxide, sulfuric acid mist, fly ash and their mixtures: results of studies in monkeys and guinea pigs. Arch Environ Health 1975; 30:254–262.
184. Costa DL, Dreher KL. Bioavailable transition metals in particulate matter mediate cardiopulmonary injury in healthy and compromised animal models. Environ Health Perspect 1997; 105(5):1053–1060.
185. Pritchard RJ, Ghio AJ, Lehmann JR, Winsett DW, Park P, Gilmore I, Dreher K, Costa DL. Oxidant generation and lung injury after particulate air pollutant exposure increases with the concentration of associated metals. Inhal Toxicol 1996; 8: 457–477.
186. Dreher KL, Jaskot RH, Lehmann JR, Richards JH, McGee JK, Ghio AJ, Costa DL. Soluble transition metals mediate residual oil fly ash induced acute lung injury. J Toxicol Environ Health 1997; 50:285–305.
187. Garrett NE, Campbell JA, Stack HF, Waters MD, Lewtas J. The utilization of the rabbit alveolar macrophage and Chinese hamster ovary cell for evaluation for the toxicity of particulate materials: I. Model compounds and metal-coated fly ash. Environ Res 1981; 24:345–365.
188. Berg I, Schulter T, Gercken G. Increase of bovine alveolar macrophage superoxide anion and hydrogen peroxide release by dusts of different origin. J Toxicol Environ Health 1993;39:241–354.
189. Becker S, Soukup JM, Gilmour IM, Devlin RB. Stimulation of human and rat alveolar macrophages with urban air particulates: effects on oxidant radical generation and cytokine production. Toxicol Appl Pharmacol 1996; 141:637–648.
190. Carter J, Ghio AJ, Samet JM, Devlin RB. Residual oil fly ash induces increases in mRNAs and proteins for IL-6, IL-8, and TNF in human airway epithelial cells. Am J Physiol 1997; 146:180–188.
191. Samet JM, Reed W, Ghio AJ, Devlin RB, Carter J, Dailey LM, Bromberg PA, Madden MC. Induction of prostaglandin H synthase 2 in cultured airway epithelial cells exposed to residual oil fly ash. Toxicol Appl Pharmocol 1996; 141:159–168.

192. Quay J, Reed W, Devlin RB. Residual oil fly ash upregulates IL-6 gene expression by processes involving NF-κB. Am J Cell Respir Mol Biol 1998; 19:98–106.
193. Schroeder WH, Dobson D, Kane DM, Johnson ND. Toxic trace elements associated with airborne particulate matter: a review. Environ Sci Technol 1987; 9:838–845.
194. Mathias-Maser S, Jaenicke R. Examination of atmospheric bioaerosol particles with radii > 0.2 μm. J Aerosol Sci 1994; 25:1605–1613.
195. Glikson M, Rutherford S, Simpson RW, Mitchell CA, Yago A. Microscopic and submicron components of atmospheric particulate matter during high asthma periods in Brisbane, Queensland, Australia. Atmos Environ 1995; 29:549–562.
196. Targonski PV, Persky VW, Ramekrishan V. Effect of environmental molds on risk of death from asthma during the pollen season. J Allergy Clin Immunol 1995; 95: 955–961.
197. Mackay TW, Wather CG, Sudlow MF, Elton RA, Caulton E. Factors affecting asthma mortality in Scotland. Scott Med 1992;37:5–7.
198. O'Hallaren MT, Yunginger JW, Offord KP, Somers MJ, O'Connell EJ, Ballard DJ, Sachs MI. Exposure to an aeroallergen as a possible precipitating factor in respiratory arrest in young patients with asthma. N Engl J Med 1991; 324:359–363.
199. Lacey J, Dutkiewicz J. Bioaerosols and occupational lung disease. J Aerosol Sci 1994; 25:1371–1404.
200. Ayres JG. Trends in asthma and hay fever in general practice in the United Kingdom 1876–83. Thorax 1986;41:111–116.
201. Anto JM, Sunyer J. Epidemiologic studies of asthma epidemics in Barcelona. Chest 1990; 90:185S–190S.
202. Schwartz DA, Thorne PS, Yagla SI, Burmeister LF, Olenchock SA, Watt JL, Quinn TJ. The role of endotoxin in grain dust-inducing lung disease. Am J Respir Crit Care Med 1995; 152:603–608.
203. Thelin A, Tegler O, Rylander R. Lung reactions during poultry handling related to dust and bacterial endotoxin levels. Eur J Respir Dis 1984; 65:266–271.
204. Kennedy SM, Christiani DC, Eisen EA, Wegman DH, Greaves IA, Olenchock SA, Ye T, Lu P. Cotton dust and endotoxin exposure–response relationships in cotton textile workers. Am Rev Respir Dis 1987;135:194–200.
205. Clapp WD, Becker S, Quay J, Watt JL, Thorne PS, Frees KL, Zhang X, Koren HS, Lux CR, Schwartz DA. Grain dust-induced airflow obstruction and inflammation of the lower respiratory tract. Am J Respir Crit Care Med 1994; 150:611–617.
206. Tomatis L, ed. Air Pollution and Human Cancer Berlin: Springer-Verlag, 1990.
207. Gray HA, Cass GR, Huntzicker JJ, Heyerdahl EK, Rau JA. Characteristics of atmospheric organic and elemental carbon particle concentrations in Los Angeles. Environ Sci Technol 1986; 20:580–589.
208. Izzotti A, Camoirano A, D'Agostini F, Sciacca S, De Naro Papa F, Cesarone CF, De Flora S. Biomarker alterations produced in rat lung by intratracheal instillations of air particulate extracts and chemoprevention with oral *N*-acetylcysteine. Cancer Res 1996; 56:1533–1538.
209. Diaz-Sanchez D, Dotson AR, Takenaka H, Saxon A. Diesel exhaust particles induce local IgE production in vivo and alter the pattern of IgE messenger RNA isoforms. J Clin Invest 1994; 94:1417–1425.

210. Jakob GJ. The toxicological interactions resulting from inhalation of carbon black and acrolein on pulmonary antibacterial and antiviral defenses. Toxicol Appl Pharmacol 1993;121:167–175.
211. Jakob GJ, Hemenway DR. Concomitant exposure to carbon black particulates enhance ozone-induced lung inflammation and suppression of alveolar macrophage phagocytosis. J Toxicol Environ Health 1994; 41:221–231.

11

Dendritic Cells as Sentinels of Immune Surveillance in the Airways

ANDREW S. McWILLIAM

University of Western Australia
Nedlands, Western Australia, Australia

PATRICK G. HOLT

TVW Telethon Institute for Child Health Research
West Perth, Western Australia, Australia

PETER GEHR

University of Bern
Bern, Switzerland

I. Introduction

Although they are anatomically connected, the conducting airways and the gas-exchange region of the respiratory tract clearly have a number of different functions to fulfill. Primarily, the conducting airways must provide a conduit for the transport of air, whereas the gas-exchange region (lungs) must provide a surface for gas exchange. In providing these functions they must also provide a barrier between the tissues of the body and an external environment that is often hazardous. In an average human this surface barrier may comprise up to 140 m^2 of epithelial surface (1) that may be exposed to as much as 15,000 L of air per day. To highlight the potential for damage to this surface, it has been estimated (2) that, in humans, the airways may be exposed to more than 7 kg of pollutant per year, compared with 1.4 kg in the gastrointestinal tract. During this exposure, it is critically important for survival that airway function is maintained and that the constant barrage of damaging pollutants is dealt with in a rapid and efficient manner. The consequences of inadequate response to environmental insults may vary considerably between the gas-exchange region and the conducting airways. Thus, inflammation of the airways may give rise to bronchoconstriction, as in asthma, whereas fibrosis may be induced in the lung parenchyma.

The range of materials to which the respiratory tract may be exposed and which must be contained or eliminated is enormous, and in an increasingly industrialized society this number is growing constantly. The apparent anatomical simplicity of the respiratory tract belies the complex and numerous mechanisms that are in constant use to defend these tissues. Other chapters in this book have covered, in some detail, the range of materials to which the airways may be exposed and have described the mechanical and physical processes of particle clearance and some of the cell types involved in homeostatic and inflammatory situations. Although these processes are extremely important, they are essentially nonspecific and entail no elements of a memory or anamnestic response. At another level, it is important to the host organism to generate specific cognate responses that can be brought into play and amplified immediately on a second encounter with antigen.

In this chapter we will describe the process by which immune responses may be initiated against any foreign antigens that threaten functional mucosal integrity and specifically review the role of the dendritic cell (DC) in this process.

II. Antigen Presentation: An Overview

The alveolar macrophage is undoubtedly of extreme importance in the frontline-defense mechanisms of the respiratory tract. As a result of their location and versatile responses to many stimuli they are able to phagocytose particulate material and release numerous proinflammatory mediators that initiate inflammatory or immune responses. However, before a more prolonged and specific immune response can be initiated, other elements of the immune system, such as T lymphocytes, must be employed. Unfortunately, T cells are somewhat limited in that they cannot by themselves initiate immune responses, nor can they respond to antigen without the intercession of a second or accessory cell. Because pulmonary alveolar macrophages (PAM) are able to express surface class II molecules, they were, for many years, considered to be the major antigen-presenting cells in the airways and lungs. Clearly PAM are capable of functioning as antigen-presenting cells; however, there are several studies (3) suggesting that PAM are, in fact, poor accessory cells. This has been clearly demonstrated by Thepen (4), who used the so-called liposome-suicide technique to ablate the PAM population. In the absence of PAM, animals were still able to mount an immune response to intratracheally administered antigen, suggesting that PAM are not essential for antigen presentation in the lung, but indeed, that they may be inhibitory to the process. The role of the so-called accessory cells in initiating T-cell responses is commonly placed under the umbrella term of *antigen presentation* (AP). This process may be considered to be composed of a series of sequential, but related, events.

First, our concept of AP necessitates that incoming antigens must be broken down or dismantled into smaller peptide-sized fragments. This process is still not clearly understood, but reason suggests that it may occur either extracellularly, as a result of enzymatic degradation, or intracellularly within phagocytes, such as macrophages or neutrophils, which may release the digested peptides before uptake by the antigen-presenting cell. The alternative to this scenario is that the antigen-presenting cell may itself be capable of internalization and degradation of the antigen. Thus, although DC are able to phagocytose selected particles, they appear to be relatively unskilled at this, and there is still much missing from our understanding of this part of their biology. Second, the antigen-presenting cell must process the internalized material in such a way that it becomes associated with major histocompatibility complex (MHC) molecules (HLA in humans) and is then transported to a final location on the surface of the cell. Once this association with polymorphic MHC molecules occurs, then the essential element of restriction has been introduced. Third, the accessory cell must have the capacity to migrate from peripheral sites of antigen uptake to regional lymph nodes where sufficient numbers of naive T lymphocytes must be found. Finally, the accessory cell bearing its load of peptide–MHC complex, must physically couple with a receptive T lymphocyte by surface T-cell–antigen receptor complex (TCR) and set in process an activation cascade that ultimately results in antigen specific T-cell effector functions, such as cytotoxicity and cytokine production.

Within the respiratory tract, several cell types are capable (based on their expression of surface class II MHC) of antigen presentation. These may be broadly categorized as either *professional* APC, which may include B cells, macrophages, and DC, or *opportunistic* APC, such as fibroblasts and epithelial cells, either ciliated or type II pneumonocytes. The potential for each of these populations to contribute to T-cell activation is dependent on factors such as the host's existing immune status, degree of local inflammation, and physicochemical properties of the inhaled particle or antigen.

By their very nature, larger, insoluble particulate material may be restricted in their access to cell populations located below the epithelial cell surface; therefore, the participation of active phagocytic cells at the airway luminal surface may be mandatory. In contrast, soluble materials are readily translocated to intraepithelial or submucosal microenvironments by pinocytotic or receptor-mediated pathways, and thereby gain access to DC populations. The mechanisms by which environmental antigens may breach the epithelial barrier have been extensively reviewed elsewhere (5,6).

III. Distribution of Airway Dendritic Cells

Analogous with the mononuclear phagocyte system, there appears to be an extensive network of DC present within most tissues and organs of the body, and they may be linked by common pathways of migration (7). The individual population elements of this network have historically been ascribed different names, depending on the tissue of discovery; for example, epidermal DC are known as Langerhans cells (LC), whereas those in lymph are known as veiled cells, and in lymph nodes as interdigitating cells. The terms DC or LC are largely interchangeable and we will use the term DC within this chapter. Although arising from a common bone marrow precursor population, the relation between these different DC populations is still far from clear, and the role of microenvironmentally induced differentiation and maturation is still a largely unexplored area. DC populations within the lung, were first described in inflammatory granulomatous and fibrotic tissues (8–12) and, since these descriptions, several studies have demonstrated that DC are constitutive residents of normal human airway epithelium, alveolar parenchyma, and nasal mucosa (13–17). In addition, they can be found, albeit in small numbers, on the human alveolar surface and, therefore, they may be present in bronchoalveolar lavage fluid (18). In laboratory animals, DC have been identified in sections of parenchymal lung and airway mucosa (19–23).

In addition to constitutive expression of surface class II molecules, some DC also contain an organelle, unique to DC/LC, known as the Birbeck granule (BG). The function of BG is unknown; however, the observations that 10–15% of granules in human DC are acidic, and that acidic endosomes and BG disappear from DC at times when there is a concomitant reduction in antigen-processing capacity, suggest that they are involved in antigen processing by DC (24). Furthermore, membrane-bound molecules reach intracellular BG after endocytosis (25).

In sections of lung and airway tissue, the relatively large size and pleomorphic morphology of DC have posed a significant hurdle to their visualization and accurate quantitation. Sections that are cut either transversely or parallel to the lumen either fail to show any staining for MHC class II antigen (Ia) or only succeed in sectioning isolated portions of those arborizing processes that are the hallmark of these DC. Work from this laboratory has approached the problem of accurately quantifying the population of DC within the airway epithelium. It was reasoned that by cutting tracheal segments in a tangential sectional plane,

---

Figure 1 A view of the rat tracheal epithelium taken from a tangential section stained with the monoclonal antibody Ox6, which is directed against rat MHC class II antigen. (A) This clearly demonstrates both the number and morphology of dendritic cells within the airway epithelium. (B) A higher magnification micrograph illustrating the nature of the "dendritic" processes. (C) When isolated airway dendritic cells are stained with Ox6, they are seen to be complexed with several lymphocytes, and the extended nature of their processes is revealed.

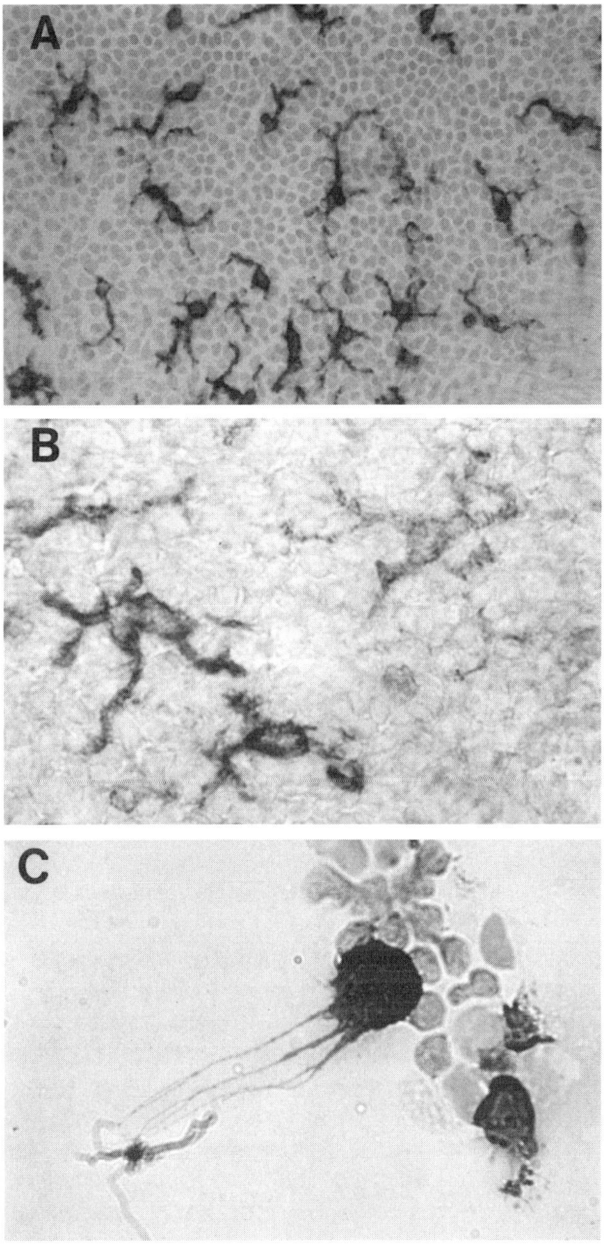
A
B
C

this would produce some sections passing through the epithelial lining in a plane parallel to the underlying basement membrane. Thus, on immunohistochemical staining of these tangential sections a ''planar'' view of the DC population would expose the full extent of the epithelial network of cells in a fashion similar to that seen with staining of LC on epidermal sheets. Indeed, staining of these sections for the presence of class II antigen revealed an extensive network of intraepithelial DC that appear morphologically identical with those present in the epidermis of both rat and humans (17,26,27). Ox6-stained tangential sections and isolated Ox6-positive dendritic cells are shown in Figure 1. With normal transverse sections, these cells have often been mislabeled as class II-positive epithelial cells or monocytes; however within the tracheal epithelium there are very few ED2-positive macrophages, and it is clear that all of the class II-positive staining is associated with epithelial DC. This sectioning and staining protocol has been used in several studies aimed at understanding the biology and significance of these cells. The position and spatial relation of these airway DC in relation to the epithelial layer and airway macrophages is depicted schematically in Figure 2.

In normal animals, the number of DC is higher on the dorsal surface of the airways than on the ventral surface (881/mm^2, compared to 675/mm^2; 26).

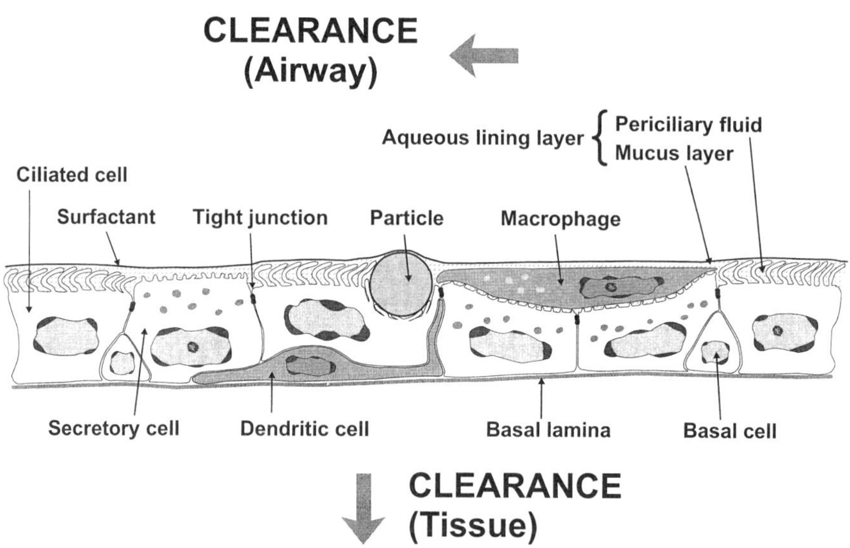

Figure 2 A schematic drawing of the airway epithelial layer showing the close association of dendritic cells, airway macrophages, epithelial cells, and particulate matter.

If it proves true that these DC are essential for the processing and presentation of airway-exposed antigens, then we may be correct in assuming that the higher dorsal density is a consequence of the greater deposition of material on that surface because of the aerodynamics of inhalation.

In the same study, DC epithelial density was compared within the different airway generations. DC numbers were highest in the upper airways (600–800/mm^2) and declined progressively down the respiratory tract, until only 75/mm^2 are present in the peripheral lung. This pattern of distribution is highly suggestive of microenvironmental control of DC numbers and shows that numbers are higher in the upper part of the airways where the highest antigen deposition occurs.

IV. Ontogeny of Airway Dendritic Cells

The relatively naive status of the immune system during the first few weeks or months of life places newborn animals at much higher risk for infection or sensitization to foreign antigenic material. The DC network within the respiratory tract may play a critical role in the development of immunity; hence, it may influence the nature of future responses (i.e., protective or damaging). Information on the development of respiratory tract DC populations in humans is very limited; however, there is considerable work being published for rat DC development. By examining the respiratory tract DC network in animals that have been born and raised in conditions of minimal exposure to inhaled dust, we have been able to show that airway class II-positive DC are usually not detectable until 2–3 days after birth, and that adult-staining patterns are evident only on weaning at day 21 after birth (28). Staining with a monoclonal antibody Ox62, which visualizes DC in the rat, showed that large numbers of Ox62-positive DC are present in fetal, infant, and adult rat airway epithelium. Costaining experiments determined that Ox62-positive DCs that also express Ia antigen are rare in neonatal animals, but increase steadily until weaning, when 65% of the Ox62-positive cells are also Ia-positive. These Ia-positive DCs can be detected first at the base of the nasal turbinates, which is the anatomical site where inhaled material is first deposited. This pattern of development is consistent with the notion that it is inflammatory stimuli that drive the maturation of the airway DC system. Densitometric analysis of the amount of Ia antigen present on individual cells again confirmed that the nasal epithelial DC Ia expression evident 2–3 days after birth was comparable with that found on epidermal Langerhans cells from adjacent facial skin. By comparison, Ia levels on tracheal DCs remained low until several weeks after birth, when levels begin to rise to achieve adult levels at weaning. Administration of interferon gamma (IFN-γ) was able to significantly accelerate the development of this Ia expression and, similarly, aerosol exposure to topical steroids, such as fluticasone, was able to retard its development. These studies highlight the concept that development and maturation of a fully functional antigen presentation system is largely dependent on local factors and may be modulated in either a positive or negative fashion. The full implications of neonatal exposure to environmental factors, such as dusts and gases, remains to be determined.

V. Turnover of Airway Dendritic Cells

The paradigms of DC function have so far envisioned a model in which DC function may change or alter, depending on the histological location or the particular stage in the life cycle of the individual cell. In this model, the antigen recognition and uptake that is taking place at peripheral sites of exposure, such as skin, airways, and gut, gives way to an increased presentational capacity as the DC migrates to central lymphoid tissues. During this sojourn, the DC acts as a courier for delivery of antigen to T-cell–rich sites. If this concept is accurate, it would be a logical progression to assume that net flow of DCs from peripheral sites to lymphoid destinations may be dependent on the particular level of antigenic exposure at each peripheral tissue, and this may be reflected in the steady-state levels of DC turnover for each of these particular tissues. To date most of the available data has been derived for DC turnover within lymphoid organs, where primary exposure to antigen is infrequent. The airways offer an ideal situation in which to examine DC turnover in a position characterized by continuous antigenic exposure. As it is now accepted that DCs are hematopoietic in origin, we attempted to interrupt the flow of precursor cells from the bone marrow by ablation of bone marrow using whole-body irradiation of 1000 rad. After this procedure, resident tracheal DC numbers declined by 85% during the ensuing 72 hr (29). Similar experiments were performed in which bone marrow was repopulated with donor cells from CD45 congenic animals, thus permitting identification and differentiation of host and donor DCs. This approach demonstrated very clearly that, in the rat, airway DCs have a half-life within the epithelium of approximately 2 days and that this contrasts with the published data for epidermal Langerhans cells of 15 days or more. Similar comparisons produced a figure for lung parenchymal DC that was intermediate between airway and skin DC. Because DC turnover time within the gastrointestinal tract epithelium is similar to that of airway epithelium (30), the conclusion may be drawn that those DC populations associated with mucosal surfaces are turning over at a constantly faster rate than those in other tissues, and this may be a consequence of the requirement to be able to cope with larger persistent loads of foreign material.

VI. Inflammatory Changes in Airway Dendritic Cell Populations

The hypothesis that DC population dynamics is influenced by inflammatory stimuli was initially tested in experiments involving brief aerosol exposure to bacterial lipopolysaccharide (LPS; 24). This resulted in a transient 50% increase in the density of DCs within the tracheal epithelium during 24–48 hr after exposure. In an extension of this work, normal rats were exposed to an aerosol of heat-killed *Moraxella catarrhalis* (31) bacteria, which was chosen as a result of its clinical association with acute purulent tracheitis in children and, hence, its ability to induce a rapid inflammatory response. From this model it was apparent that one of the earliest detectable cellular changes within the inflamed trachea is the recruitment of small, round, MHC class II-positive, putative DC precursors into the epithelium. These cells were detectable shortly before the influx of neutrophils, and although the inflammatory neutrophils are able to pass through the epithelium and enter the lumen of the airway, presumably in response to chemotactic signals generated by macrophages, the DC remain within the epithelium and appear to maintain a foothold onto the basement membrane, thereby permitting their subsequent egress to regional lymph nodes. In the epithelium, DC numbers reached a maximum within 1 hr after exposure; numbers that ultimately exceeded three times the steady-state population. In contrast with neutrophil numbers, which remained high for approximately 8 hr, DC numbers remained elevated for over 24 hr. During this time, the DC continued to differentiate morphologically into the typically dendriform cells found in the steady state. The signal that induces this differentiation is unknown, but it is presumably derived from the local environment. Within 48 hr after exposure, it was possible to detect a 200% increase in the number of DCs within the draining lymph nodes, again reflecting the movement of DCs from surface epithelium to T-cell–rich lymph nodes. In a series of related studies (32) several different inflammatory models were examined for their capacity to alter airway DC numbers. These inflammatory stimuli included a viral infection (Sendai), infection with a live bacteria (*Bordetella pertussis*), and a soluble antigen (ovalbumin) aerosol sensitization model. Each of these systems was examined for the nature of the cellular influx that they were able to generate within the airway epithelium. The nature of the cellular influx was always quite separate and distinct (i.e., restricted to neutrophils in the *Moraxella* model, eosinophils in the ovalbumin model, T cells and NK cells in the Sendai model, and neutrophils and some T cells in the *Bordetella* model). Despite the differing cellular influx associated with each model, the one common factor was the influx of DCs that represented the first cell to appear within the airways. If recruitment of DCs into the mucosa is a universal feature of the inflammatory response in these areas, then, this suggests that the rapid amplification of antigen surveillance mechanisms at challenge sites may actually be an integral part of the innate immune response at mucosal surfaces; hence, it may represent a form of ''early-warning system'' to signal the adaptive or cognate arm of the immune system to incoming pathogens.

VII. Antigen Uptake and Processing by Airway Dendritic Cells

Our picture of the function of airway DCs then, has these cells occupying a central role in sampling both particulate and soluble antigens from their immediate environment. We must then consider the mechanisms by which this uptake occurs. Until relatively recently it has been considered that DCs in regional tissues were very poor at antigen uptake by phagocytic processes and, instead, relied on endocytic uptake of soluble material. Detailed studies have now changed this view, and we now appreciate that DCs can use both phagocytosis and endocytosis to take up antigen.

As with macrophages, phagocytosis represents a mechanism used primarily for the uptake of large particulate material such as bacteria, inert particles, yeast, fungal spores, and perhaps also pollens. This appears to be restricted to immature or freshly isolated tissue DC and is ultimately lost, either in culture or en route to lymphoid tissue. Phagocytosis of bacteria and the subsequent presentation of bacterial peptides to T cells have been demonstrated by mouse bone marrow-derived DC (33,34). Phagocytosis of both bacteria and inert particles by freshly isolated epidermal Langerhans cells (35) and Peyers' patch DCs (36) has also been shown. In an effort to demonstrate phagocytic uptake by human DCs prepared by culture of blood monocytes in granulocyte–macrophage colony-stimulating factor (GM-CSF) and interleukin (IL)-4, we have exposed these cells (unpublished observations) to polystyrene particles of various sizes, ranging from 0.2 to 6.0 μm. The DC nature of these cells has been established by flow cytometric analysis with a panel of monoclonal antibodies (Smith W, personal communication). After appropriate incubation, the cells were fixed in glutaraldehyde and prepared for transmission electron microscopy. Several electron micrographs from this series of experiments are shown in Figure 3. In Figure 3A we can see several of these cells in the process of surrounding 6-μm particles, with thin pseudopod layers of cell membrane, presumably in the first stages of phagocytosis. Figure 3B shows subsequent total internalization of one of these particles. Other studies have demonstrated uptake of carbon particles by liver-derived DCs (37).

Uptake of small particulate material or soluble material is primarily the domain of pinocytosis or receptor-mediated endocytosis. Thus, mouse splenic DCs are actively endocytic (38) and can induce both T- and B-cell–specific in

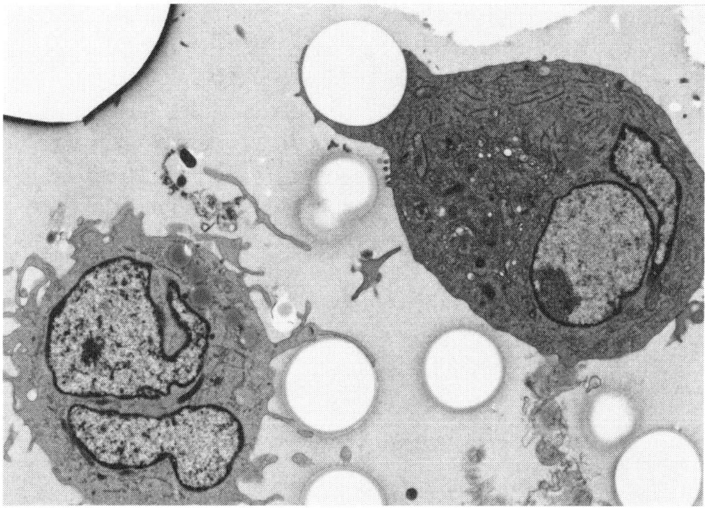

(a)

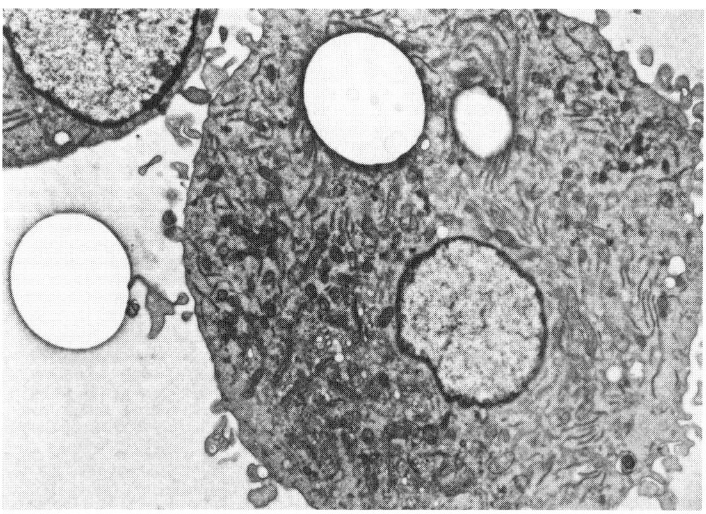

(b)

Figure 3 (a) Transmission electron micrograph of dendritic cells that have been incubated with 6-μm–diameter polystyrene spheres. It illustrates how two cells are each in the process of engulfing one of the particles (P). Magnification × 6000. (b) Transmission electron micrograph of the same cell culture showing part of a dendritic cell with an internalized polystyrene sphere (P). Magnification × 8000.

vivo responses following in vitro antigen pulsing (39,40). In vivo endocytosis by DCs has also been demonstrated in various systems (41–43).

It now seems that many of the uptake mechanisms used by macrophages have also been adopted by DCs. Thus, most of the work to date on DC receptor-mediated endocytosis of soluble antigen has centered around the mannose receptor (44,45), although DCs also express surface DEC 205 (46), FcεRI (47), and FcγR (45). Recently, several studies have highlighted the importance of the mannose receptor in DC-mediated endocytosis (48,49). We (McWilliam and Gehr) have preliminary evidence suggesting that monocyte-derived DCs have surface receptors specific for surfactant proteins A and D. This observation also suggests another mechanism by which particulate material, such as bacteria and viruses, can be taken up by DCs and allows an element of opsonization to be included.

VIII. Migration and Recruitment of Airway Dendritic Cells

The life cycle of the DC involves several changes of location. To accomplish this there must be a unique set of signals that call on DC precursors to set down in specific locations, such as mucosal surfaces, and an equally important, but distinct, set that induces migration to T-cell areas of draining lymph nodes through the afferent lymph. Systemic administration of LPS reduces by over 95% the number of Ia-positive DCs present in mouse hearts and kidneys within 1–3 hr of administration (50). The effects of LPS are modulated by production of inflammatory cytokines; therefore the authors of this study administered systemic TNF-α and noted a profound decrease in DCs within nonlymphoid organs, such as heart, kidney, and epidermis, whereas similar administration of IL-1α resulted in a decrease from only the renal medulla. These results suggest that migration from specific tissues may be controlled by different patterns of cytokines; however, it is unclear whether these cytokines were acting directly or indirectly. The nature of the signals that attract DCs to sites of inflammation are beginning to be examined. Thus, DCs have a receptor for C5a and will migrate in chemotaxis assays to concentrations of C5a as small as 10^{-8} M (51). Monocyte chemoattractant protein 1 (MCP-1) is capable of recruiting dendritic and Langerhans cells to skin (52), and fMLP, C5a, and the C-C chemokines MCP-3, MIP-1α/LD78, and RANTES, were chemotactic for human blood-derived DCs (53). We (32) have also demonstrated that C-C chemokines are chemotactic in vitro for rat bone marrow-derived DCs.

IX. Steroidal Modulation of Airway Dendritic Cells

Immunomodulating drugs, such as inhaled corticosteroids, are the most potent and commonly used forms of treatment for inflammatory diseases of the airways, such as asthma and allergic rhinitis. Because DCs are the major resident APC within the airways, we have examined the effects of exposure to both inhaled steroids and to systemic steroids on the DC population (54). Aerosol administration of several of the most frequently prescribed steroids to adult rats resulted in a decline in the number of epithelial DCs within 24 hr of administration. This reduction continued for 5 days, when numbers were reduced by between 30 and 60% of steady-state levels. Numbers remained at this low level as long as steroid administration continued; however, within 24 hr of cessation of steroid administration, DC numbers had started to increase and had returned to normal within 48–72 hr. In comparison, systemic administration of dexamethasone at 10 mg/kg reduced numbers by 80% after 24 hr. In light of our argument that the progressive development of the DC population after birth is governed by the degree of exposure to inflammatory stimuli, exposure of rats to aerosols of steroids from birth until weaning succeeded in reducing the natural increase in DC numbers by as much as 50%, compared with littermates not exposed to the steroids. Interestingly, removal of steroids allowed adult levels to be rapidly achieved. These studies suggest that steroid treatments will delay the development of APC function within the airways. The implications for respiratory tract immunity in children who are receiving long-term steroid treatments may be important and should be examined further.

X. Conclusions

There is continuing evidence pointing to the conclusion that DCs within the respiratory tract occupy a unique part of the immune surveillance system both in terms of initiating immune responses and as an early-warning component of the innate immune system. There is still much to learn about the function of these cells, particularly relative to infectious diseases and the possibility of harnessing DC functions to improve local immune responses to infectious agents.

References

1. Gehr P, Bachofen M, Weibel ER. The normal human lung: ultrastructure and morphometric estimation of diffusion capacity. Respir Physiol 1978; 32:121–140.
2. Phalen RF. Basic morphology and physiology of the respiratory tract. In: Inhalation Studies: Foundations and Techniques. Boca Raton, FL: CRC Press, 1984:61–65.
3. Hance AJ. Accessory-cell/lymphocyte interactions. In: Crystal RG, West LB, eds. The Lung: Scientific Foundations. New York: Raven Press, 1991:483–498.
4. Thepen T, Van Rooijen N, Kraal G. Alveolar macrophage elimination in vivo is associated with an increase in pulmonary immune response in mice. J Exp Med 1989; 170:499–509.

5. Stewart GA, Thomson PJ, McWilliam AS. Biochemical properties of aeroallergens: contributory factors in allergic sensitization? Pediatr Allergy Immunol 1993; 4:163–172.
6. Folkesson H, Matthay MA, Weström BR, Kim KJ, Karlsson BW, Hastings RH. Alveolar epithelia clearance of protein. J Appl Physiol 1996; 80:1431–1445.
7. Steinman RM. The dendritic cell system and its role in immunogenicity. Annu Rev Immunol 1991; 9:271–296.
8. Cagle FT, Mattioli CA, Truong LD, Greenberg SD. Immunohistochemical diagnosis of pulmonary eosinophilic granuloma on lung biopsy. Chest 1988; 94:1133–1137.
9. Kawanami O, Basset F, Ferrans VJ, Soler P, Crystal RG. Pulmonary Langerhans' cells in patients with fibrotic lung disorders. Lab Invest 1981; 44:227–233.
10. Webber D, Tron V, Askin F, Churg S. S-100 staining in the diagnosis of eosinophilic granuloma of lung. Am J Clin Pathol 1985; 84:447–453.
11. Soler P, Chollet S, Jacque C, Fukuda Y, Ferrans VJ, Basset F. Immunochemical characterization of pulmonary histiocytosis X, cells in lung biopsies. Am J Pathol 1985; 118:439–451.
12. Hamman S, Brockus D, Remmington S, Bartha M. The widespread distribution of Langerhans' cells in pathological tissues. An ultrastructural and immunohistochemical study. Hum Pathol 1986; 17:894–905.
13. Sertl K, Takemura T, Tschachler E, Ferrans VJ, Kaliner MA, Shevach EM. Dendritic cells with antigen-presenting capability reside in airway epithelium, lung parenchyma and visceral pleura. J Exp Med 1986; 163:436–451.
14. Soler P, Moreau A, Basset F, Hance AJ. Cigarette smoking induced changes in the number and differentiated state of pulmonary dendritic cells/Langerhans' cells. Am Rev Respir Dis 1989; 139:1112–1117.
15. Fokkens WJ, Vroom TMA, Rijnijes E, Mulder PGH. $CD1^+$ (T6) HLA-DR–expressing cells, presumably Langerhans' cells in nasal mucosa. Allergy 1989; 44:67–172.
16. Richard S, Barbey S, Pfister A, Scheinmann P, Jaubert F, Nezelof C. Demonstration of Langerhans cells in the human bronchial epithelium. CR Acad Sci Paris Ser III 1987; 305:35–39.
17. Holt PG, Schon-Hegrad MA, Oliver J, Holt BJ, McMenamin PG. A contiguous network of dendritic antigen-presenting cells within the respiratory epithelium. Int Arch Allergy Appl Immunol 1990; 91:155–159.
18. Casolaro MA, Bernaudin JF, Saltini C, Ferrans VJ, Crystal RG. Accumulation of Langerhans' cells on the epithelial surface of the lower respiratory tract in normal subjects in association with cigarette smoking. Am Rev Respir Dis 1988; 137:406–411.
19. Simecka JW, Davis JK, Cassell GH. Distribution of Ia antigens and T lymphocyte subpopulations in rat lungs. Immunology 1986; 57:93–98
20. Breel M, Van der Ende M, Siminia T, Kraal G. Subpopulations of lymphoid and non-lymphoid cells in bronchus-associated lymphoid tissue (BALT) of the mouse. Immunology 1988; 63:657–662.
21. Holt PG, Schon-Hegrad MA, Oliver J. MHC class II antigen-bearing dendritic cells in pulmonary tissues of the rat. Regulation of antigen presenting activity by endogenous macrophage populations. J Exp Med 1988; 167:262–274.
22. Kradin RL, McCarthy KM, Xia W, Lazarus D, Schneeberger EE. Accessory cells

of the lung. I. Interferon-gamma increases Ia$^+$ dendritic cells in the lung without augmenting their accessory activities. Am J Respir Cell Mol Biol 1991; 4:210–218.
23. Holt PG, Schon-Hegrad MA. Localization of T-cells, macrophages and dendritic cells in respiratory tract tissue: implications for immune function studies. Immunology 1987; 62:349–356.
24. Stössel H, Koch F, Kämpgen E, Stöger P, Lenz A, Heufler C, Romani N, Schuler G. Disappearance of certain acidic organelles (endosomes and Langerhans' cell granules) accompanies loss of antigenic processing capacity upon culture of epidermal Langerhans' cells. J Exp Med 1990; 172:1471–1482.
25. Schuler G, Romani N, Stössel H, Wolff K. Structural organization and biological properties of langerhans cells. In: Schuler G, ed. Epidermal Langerhans Cells. Boca Raton, FL: CRC Press, 1990:87–137.
26. Schon-Hegrad MA, Oliver J, McMenamin PG, Holt PG. Studies on the density, distribution, and surface phenotype of intraepithelial class II major histocompatibility complex antigen (Ia)-bearing dendritic cells (DC) in the conducting airways. J Exp Med 1991; 173:1345–1356.
27. Holt PG, Schon-Hegrad MA, Phillips MJ, McMenamin PG. Ia-positive dendritic cells form a tightly meshed network within the human airway epithelium. Clin Exp Allergy 1989; 19:597–601.
28. Nelson DJ, McMenamin C, McWilliam AS, Brenan M, Holt PG. Development of the airway epithelial dendritic cell network in the rat from class II major histocompatibility (Ia)-negative precursors: differential regulation of Ia expression at different levels of the respiratory tract. J Exp Med 1994; 179:203–212.
29. Holt PG, Haining S, Nelson D, Sedgwick JD. Origin and steady-state turnover of class II MHC-bearing dendritic cells in the epithelium of the conducting airways. J Immunol 1994; 153:256–261.
30. Fossum S. Dendritic leukocytes: features of their in vivo physiology. Res Immunol 1989; 140:883–891.
31. McWilliam AS, Nelson D, Thomas JA, Holt PG. Rapid dendritic cell recruitment is a hallmark of the acute inflammatory response at mucosal surfaces. J Exp Med 1994; 179:331–336.
32. McWilliam AS, Napoli S, Marsh AM, Pember L, Nelson DJ, Pimm CL, Stumbles PA, Wells TNC, Holt PG. Dendritic cells are recruited into the airway epithelium during the inflammatory response to a broad spectrum of stimuli. J Exp Med 1996; 184:2429–2432.
33. Svensson M, Stockinger B, Wick MJ. Bone marrow-derived dendritic cells can process bacteria for MHC-I and MHC-II presentation to T cells. J Immunol 1997; 158: 4229–4236.
34. Inaba K, Inaba M, Naito M, Steinman RM. Dendritic cell progenitors phagocytose particulates, including bacillus Calmette-Guerin organisms, and sensitize mice to mycobacterial antigens in vivo. J Exp Med 1993; 178:479–488.
35. Reis E, Sousa C, Stahl PD, Austyn JM. Phagocytosis of antigens by Langerhans cells in vitro. J Exp Med 1993; 178:509–519.
36. Ruedl C, Hubele S. Maturation of Peyer's patch dendritic cells in vitro upon stimulation via cytokines or CD40 triggering. Eur J Immunol 1997; 27:1325–1330.
37. Matsuno K, Ezaki T, Kudo S, Uehara Y. A life stage of particle-laden rat dendritic

cells in vivo: their terminal division, active phagocytosis, and translocation from the liver to the draining lymph. J Exp Med 1996; 183:1865–1878.
38. Levine TP, Chain BM. Endocytosis by antigen presenting cells: dendritic cells are as endocytically active as other antigen presenting cells. Proc Natl Acad Sci USA 1992; 89:8342–8346.
39. Sallusto F, Lanzavecchia A. Efficient presentation of soluble antigen by cultured human dendritic cells is maintained by granulocyte/macrophage colony-stimulating factor plus interleukin 4 and downregulated by tumor necrosis factor alpha. J Exp Med 1994; 179:1109–1118.
40. Inaba K, Metlay JP, Crowley MT, Steinman RM. Dendritic cells pulsed with protein antigens in vitro can prime antigen-specific, MHC-restricted T cells in situ. J Exp Med 1990; 172:631–640.
41. Crowley M, Inaba K, Steinman RM. Dendritic cells are the principal cells in mouse spleen bearing immunogenic fragments of foreign peptides. J Exp Med 1990; 172: 383–386.
42. Macatonia SE, Edwards AJ, Knight SC. Dendritic cells and the initiation of contact sensitivity to fluorescein isothiocyanate. Immunology 1986; 59:509–514.
43. Bujdoso R, Hopkins J, Dutia BM, Young P, McConnell I. Characterization of sheep afferent lymph dendritic cells and their role in antigen carriage. J Exp Med 1989; 170:1285–1301.
44. Sallusto F, Cella M, Danieli C, Lanzavecchia A. Dendritic cells use macropinocytosis and the mannose receptor to concentrate macromolecules in the major histocompatibility complex class II compartment: downregulation by cytokines and bacterial products. J Exp Med 1995; 182:389–400.
45. Sallusto F, Lanzavecchia A. Efficient presentation of soluble antigen by cultured human dendritic cells is maintained by granulocyte/macrophage colony-stimulating factor plus interleukin 4 and downregulated by tumor necrosis factor alpha. J Exp Med 1994; 179:1109–1118.
46. Jiang W, Swiggard WJ, Heufler C, Peng M, Mirza A, Steinman RM, Nussenzweig MC. The receptor DEC-205 expressed by dendritic cells and thymic epithelial cells is involved in antigen processing. Nature 1995; 375:151–155.
47. Maurer D, Stingl G. Immunoglobulin E-binding structures on antigen-presenting cells present in skin and blood. J Invest Dermatol 1995; 10:707–710.
48. Tan MCAA, Mommaas AM, Drijfhout JW, Jordens R, Onderwater JJM, Verwoerd D, Mulder AA, Vanderheiden AN, Scheidegger D, Oomen LCJM, Ottenhoff THM, Tulp A, Neefjes JJ, Koning F. Mannose receptor-mediated uptake of antigens strongly enhances HLA class II-restricted antigen presentation by cultured dendritic cells. Eur J Immunol 1997; 27:2426–2435.
49. Engering AJ, Cella M, Fluitsma D, Brockhaus M, Hoefsmit ECM, Lanzavecchia A, Pieters J. The mannose receptor functions as a high capacity and broad specificity antigen receptor in human dendritic cells. Eur J Immunol 1997; 27:2417–2425.
50. Roake JA, Rao AS, Morris PJ, Larsen CP, Hankins DF, Austyn JM. Dendritic cell loss from nonlymphoid tissues after systemic administration of lipopolysaccharide, tumor necrosis factor, and interleukin 1. J Exp Med 1995; 181:2237–2247.
51. Morelli A, Larregina E, Chuluyan E, Kolkowski E, Fainboim L. Expression and

modulation of C5a receptor (CD88) on skin dendritic cells. Chemotactic effect of C5a on skin migratory dendritic cells. Immunology 1996; 89:126–134.
52. Nakamura K, Willjams IR, Kupper TS. Keratinocyte-derived monocyte chemoattractant protein 1 (MCP-1): analysis in atransgenic model demonstrates MCP-1 can recruit dendritic and Langerhans cells to skin. J Invest Dermatol 1995; 105:635–643.
53. Sozzani S, Luini W, Borsatti A, Polentarutti N, Zhou D, Piemonti L, D'Amico G, Power CA, Wells TN, Gobbi M, Allavena P, Mantovani A. Receptor expression and responsiveness of human dendritic cells to a defined set of CC and CXC chemokines. J Immunol 1997; 159:1993–2000.
54. Nelson DJ, McWilliam AS, Haining S, Holt PG. Modulation of airway intraepithelial dendritic cells following exposure to steroids. Am J Respir Crit Care Med 1995; 151:475–481.

12

Potential Consequences of Interactions Between Aeroallergens and Cells Within the Respiratory Tree

GEOFFREY A. STEWART, ANDREW S. McWILLIAM, and PHILIP J. THOMPSON

University of Western Australia
Nedlands, Western Australia, Australia

CECILE M. KING

The Scripps Research Institute
La Jolla, California

CLIVE ROBINSON

St. George's Hospital Medical School
London, England

I. Introduction

The respiratory system is continually exposed to particles in the form of organic and inorganic dusts, pollens, fungal and bacterial spores, and viruses, despite a range of physiological adaptations within the respiratory tree. Some of the inhaled particles will be benign, but others will have the capacity to irritate mucous membranes, induce inflammation, with or without the concomitant induction of an immune response, or infect the host. Individuals may present with frank disease if infectious, or if noninfectious, with a variety of acute local symptoms, which may range from cough, airflow limitation, bronchial hyperreactivity, and immunity, depending on a variety of factors, such as dose, duration of exposure, genetic background, and "foreignness." In some circumstances, generalized symptoms, including toxic fever, influenza-like symptoms, joint pains, dermatitis, and neurological symptoms may also appear. Such symptoms may then be associated with the clinical syndromes of asthma, occupational asthma, allergic alveolitis, and chronic bronchitis (1).

In this chapter, we will examine the potential consequences resulting from the interaction of cells within the respiratory tree with a particular group of inhaled particles (i.e., domestic or occupational allergens). Their interaction with respiratory epithelium and luminal and subepithelial cells, such as macrophages, lymphocytes, and dendritic cells, will be emphasized, because these cells represent the interface between the outside world and the host, and are of paramount importance in the generation of immune responses (2,3). Previously, allergens were considered to be benign, with little likelihood of interacting with cells within the lung other than by their initial interaction with antigen-presenting cells to produce IgE, and then subsequent interaction with sensitized mast cells to produce the symptoms associated with immediate hypersensitivity. However, recent data from several laboratories indicate that allergens possess biochemical properties with the potential to influence the biology of a range of cell types in the lung, with concomitant implications for immunogenicity (4–6).

II. Aeroallergens

Allergens possess a varied range of properties and can be divided into several broad groupings appropriate for proteins (4). They include enzymatically active allergens, those allergens possessing or showing homology with known enzyme inhibitors, those allergens possessing or showing homology with low molecular weight ligand-transporting proteins, and allergens possessing regulatory properties (Table 1). Although various allergens do not, as yet, fall into any of these groups, it is likely that most allergens will ultimately fall within one or another of these divisions. It is still unclear whether any of these biochemical properties are important once inhaled. However, many of the physicochemical and biochemical properties of aeroallergens are similar to those displayed by pathogens or their virulence factors (5) that are recognized by components of the innate immune defense system within the respiratory system; for example, macrophage receptor-mediated endocytosis (5). In support of this, several investigators have shown that cells, such as mast cells and respiratory epithelial cells, respond to allergen challenge in a non–IgE-dependent manner (7–9).

A. Enzymatically Active Allergens

A significant number of allergens possess enzymatic activity and include many of the important domestic and occupational allergens from plants, bacteria, fungi, and dust mite (4,10). They include hydrolytic enzymes, such as proteases (cysteine, serine, and aspartate), carbohydrases, and ribonucleases. Of particular importance are the house dust mite, cockroach, and bacterial proteases; the fungal carbohydrases, such as amylase and the grass and tree pollen; and fungal ribonucleases. In addition to the hydrolytic enzymes, several nonhydrolytic enzymes have been described. These include the pectin-degrading enzymes, such as pectin lyase from tree pollen; the glycolytic enzymes from fungi, such as enolase, alco-

Table 1 A Summary of the Major Groups of Biochemically Active Allergens

Biochemical activity	Allergens
Hydrolytic enzymes	
Proteases	
Serine proteases	Group 3 mite trypsins, group 6 mite chymotrypsins, group 9 mite proteases, mammalian trypsin, mammalian chymotrypsin, bacterial subtilisins
Cysteine protease	Group 1 mite allergens, papain, bromelain
Aspartate protease	Mammalian pepsin, fungal protease, renin, Bla g 2
Metalloprotease	Bacterial collagenase
Carbohydrases	Egg white lysozyme, mite group 4 amylase, plant, fungal, bacterial and mammalian amylases, cellulase, xylanase, fungal pectinase, fungal glucoamylase, Cry j 2[a]
Ribonucleases	Asp f 1, group 5 grass pollen allergens, group 1 tree pollen allergens
Nonhydrolytic enzymes	Soybean lipoxygenase, fungal aldolase, enolase, alcohol dehydrogenase, phosphoglycerate kinase, mite and cockroach glutathione transferases, Amb a 1[a], Amb a 2[a], and Cry j 1[a] pectate lyases
Enzyme inhibitors	Ric c 1, wheat CM16, wheat WMAI-1, barley CMb, BMAI-1, BDAI-1, Ory s 1, ragweed cystatin, Gal d 1, Gal d 2, soybean trypsin inhibitor, Lol p 11[a], Ole e 1[a]
Transport proteins	Group 10 grass pollen cytochrome c allergens, Amb a 3[a], Amb a 6[a], Amb a 7[a], Mus m 1, Rat n 2, Fel d 1[a], Gal d 3, midge hemoglobins, Bla g 4, animal serum albumins
Regulatory proteins	Grass, weed, and tree pollen profilins, tree pollen calmodulin, mite and fungal tropomyosins, mite and fungal heat shock proteins, ribosomal p2 proteins, bovine oligomycin, sensitivity-conferring protein
Miscellaneous	Wheat lectin, pollen lectin, latex lectin (prohevein) allergen

[a]Indicates that allergens possess activity or show homology with proteins that do so.
Source: Ref. 4.

hol dehydrogenase, aldolase, and phosphoglycerate kinase; and glutathione transferases from cockroach and dust mites.

B. Enzyme Inhibitors

Several occupational and domestic allergens have been described that show enzyme inhibitory activity or demonstrate marked sequence homology with known inhibitors (4,10). They are either derived from plant seeds, pollen, or hen egg white, and usually inhibit protease or amylase activity. They include the 2S albumins or napins, the 14-kDa–subunit proteins known to inhibit both trypsin and α-amylase, and the Kunitz-type protease inhibitors from seeds, as well as the serine and cysteine protease inhibitors from pollen or egg white.

C. Proteins Involved in Transport

A variety of allergens demonstrate significant homology with proteins involved in the transport of ligands, such as lipids, pheromones, electrons, oxygen, and iron (4,10). They include allergens from grass and weed pollen, animal tissue, cockroaches, and hen egg white. Of these, the most important are the lipocalin allergens from animals, such as rodents, dogs, cows, and horses. These proteins show marked structural and sequence similarities to proteins, such as odorant-binding proteins, retinol-binding protein, and α_1-microglobin, which are termed the lipocalins or calycins. Several pollen allergens also demonstrate homology with proteins known to transport a variety of ligands, such as electrons, iron, oxygen, and lipid.

D. Regulatory Proteins

Some allergens are similar to a disparate but ubiquitous group of proteins known or considered to possess regulatory properties (4,10). These allergens are often encountered in food allergy, parasite infection, and autoimmunity. They include tree, weed, and grass pollen profilins; tree pollen calmodulin; the cytoskeletal protein tropomyosin from mites and fungi; and mite heat-shock proteins. Although their regulatory properties are varied, several appear to be associated with actin.

E. Aerobiology of Allergens

Exposure to aeroallergen occurs by the inhalation of allergen in the form of pollens from wind-pollinated (rather than insect-pollinated) plants, fecal pellets, dusts, or spores. Pollens range in size from 17 to 58 μm, whereas fecal pellets from sources, such as mites, are 10–50 μm, and fungal spores are often smaller than 10 μm. These allergen carriers contain many allergens, and some, such as pollen and fecal pellets, release their contents when deposited on mucosal surfaces in the respiratory tree. That this occurs reflects their natural function. For example, pollens release enzymes that play a role in the fertilization process, and mite fecal pellets consist of a semipermeable peritrophic membrane that allows the egress of nutrients and digestive enzymes.

The pollen grains of grass release a large number of starch granules (approximately 3 μm in diameter) containing allergens such as Lol p1 and 5 on contact with water (Fig. 1; 11). These grains have been implicated in the provocation of asthma in grass pollen allergic individuals, and they likely account partly

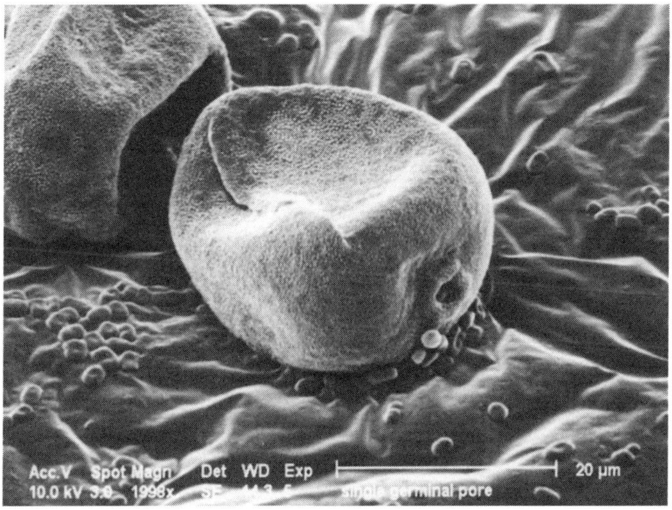

(a)

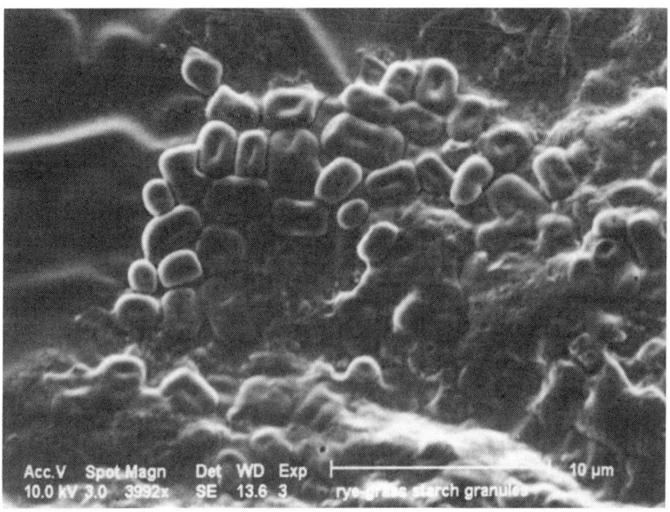

(b)

Figure 1 Scanning electron micrographs of (a) rye grass (*Lolium perenne*) pollen surrounded by starch granules and (b) starch granules. (Courtesy of Prof. Frank Murray, Murdoch University, Perth, Western Australia, Australia.)

for the submicronic form of allergen demonstrated for grass, weed, and tree pollens (12,13), although the number entering the lung has not yet been determined. Similarly, a significant amount of cat allergen is present on particles smaller than 5 μm in diameter and can be easily detected in undisturbed air (14). In contrast, mite and cockroach allergens are carried on particles larger than 10 μm, and air must be disturbed before it can be detected in aerosols (14,15). Interestingly, however, the mite allergen Der p 1 is relatively easily detected in bronchoalveolar lavage fluid (BAL) from individuals exposed to house dust (16).

With both pollens and fecal pellets, the focal concentration of total protein (allergens) eluted onto the mucosal surface may be in the order of milligrams per milliliter (15,17). As such, allergens released into the vicinity of cells within the respiratory tree are likely to be present in sufficient concentration to be physiologically or physicochemically potent. The relative importance and role of each cell type remains speculative but cells, such as epithelial cells, macrophages, mast cells, and dendritic cells, are obvious candidates and will be discussed in the following sections.

III. The Respiratory Epithelium

The major function of the respiratory epithelium was once thought to be primarily that of a physical barrier, but recent studies clearly indicate that it is metabolically very active, with the capacity to modulate a variety of inflammatory processes through the agency of an array of receptor-mediated events (18–21). On activation, it has the capacity to produce several proinflammatory cytokines (22); proinflammatory or regulatory mediators, such as nitric oxide and prostanoids (23); together with a variety of other proteins associated with inflammatory processes, such as glutathione (24), fibrinogen (25), endothelin (26), complement components (27), Clara cell CC16 protein (28), matrix metalloproteases (29), and protease inhibitors (30–32; Table 2). Each of these plays a major role in inflammation (see Chap. 10), and modulation of their synthesis may occur in response to a variety of stimuli, including a variety of enzymes, bacterial toxins, viruses, pollutants, and more recently, allergens (Table 3; Fig. 2).

In addition to producing a range of pharmacologically and immunologically active agents, the respiratory epithelium also plays a major role in the recruitment of inflammatory cells (see Chap. 10) from the circulation, through the expression of adhesion molecules that are upregulated in response to stimuli, such as cytokines (33–36). There are several families of adhesion molecules, including those belonging to the selectin family (P- and E-selectin), the immunoglobulin superfamily (VCAM-1 and ICAM-1), and the integrin family (LFA-1), as well as various adhesion molecules belonging to the cadherin family, the major role of which is maintaining cellular architecture, and CD44. Of these, ICAM-1 (CD54) appears

Table 2 Cytokines, Mediators, Proteins, and Peptides Released from or Induced in Respiratory Epithelium in Response to Inflammatory Insults

Arachidonic acid metabolites	Cytokines
15-HETE	IL-1
Prostaglandins	IL-2
Leukotrienes	IL-3
Cyclooxygenase enzymes	IL-4
PGSH-1	IL-5
PGSH-2	IL-6
Cytokeratin 19	IL-10
Fibrinogen	IL-12
α-Chain	IL-13
β-Chain	IL-16
γ-Chain	IFN-γ
Endothelin	TNF-α
Glutathione	TGB-β
Clara cell CC16 protein	LIF
Fibronectin	Chemokines
Nitric oxide	IL-8
Gelatinases A and B	RANTES
Collagenase	Eotaxin
Protease inhibitors	MIP-1
α_1-Protease inhibitor	MCP-3
α_1-Antichymotrypsin	MCP-4
Secretory leukocyte protease inhibitor	
	Colony-stimulating factors
Elafin	G-CSF
Nitric oxide synthase	GM-CSF

to be the most important inducible adhesion molecule expressed on respiratory epithelial cells involved in cell recruitment, but others, such as CD44 appear to be associated with epithelial repair (32–36). As a result of inflammatory cell recruitment, some of the responses observed in the respiratory epithelium will derive from the activation of cells, such as T cells, mast cells, macrophages, eosinophils, and neutrophils, and their release of a range of physiologically important products. Some, such as histamine, prostanoids, leukotrienes, and platelet-activating factor, will modulate respiratory epithelial function and play a major role in the acute phase of inflammation observed in the lung, whereas others are likely to be involved in the more chronic inflammatory phases.

Table 3 Agents Known to Stimulate Cytokine or Inflammatory Mediator Release from Respiratory Epithelium or Mucosa

Endogenous	Exogenous
Endothelin	Bacteria and their products
Eosinophil peroxidase	*Bordetella pertussus* (e.g., tracheal toxin)
Neutrophil elastase	*Haemophilus influenzae* (e.g., endotoxin)
Mast cell tryptase	*Pseudomonas aeruginosa* (e.g., nitrite reductase)
Cytokines	
Nitric oxide	Viruses
	Influenza virus A
	Respiratory syncytial virus
	Adenovirus
	Fungi
	Aspergillus fumigatus protease
	Occupational and environmental agents
	Allergens
	Der p 1
	Der p 9
	Toluene diisocyanate
	Diesel exhaust particles
	Ozone
	Wood chip mulch
	Swine dust

A. Epithelium and Cytokines

Data are accumulating that suggest cytokines play a major role in both acute and chronic respiratory diseases owing to their capacity to recruit inflammatory cells into the lung (22). On the basis of BAL and sputum samples from patients with quiescent or active diseases, such as asthma, bronchitis, and other lung diseases (37–42), or from BAL and biopsy studies employing experimental instillation of agents, such as allergens, in sensitized individuals, it has been shown that cytokines such as IL-1, IL-5, IL-6, IL-11, TNF-α, and granulocyte–macrophage colony-stimulating factor (GM-CSF); chemokines, such as IL-8, eotaxin, MIP-1-α, and RANTES; and LIF are easily demonstrable (43–46). These cytokines, individually or in combination, have the capacity to stimulate the proliferation of cells, such as T cells; activate and chemoattract inflammatory cells, such as neutrophils and eosinophils; induce the expression of adhesion molecules; alter tissue permeability; and induce the synthesis of cytokines and mediators, such as prostaglandins and nitric oxide. They are produced by a variety of cells, includ-

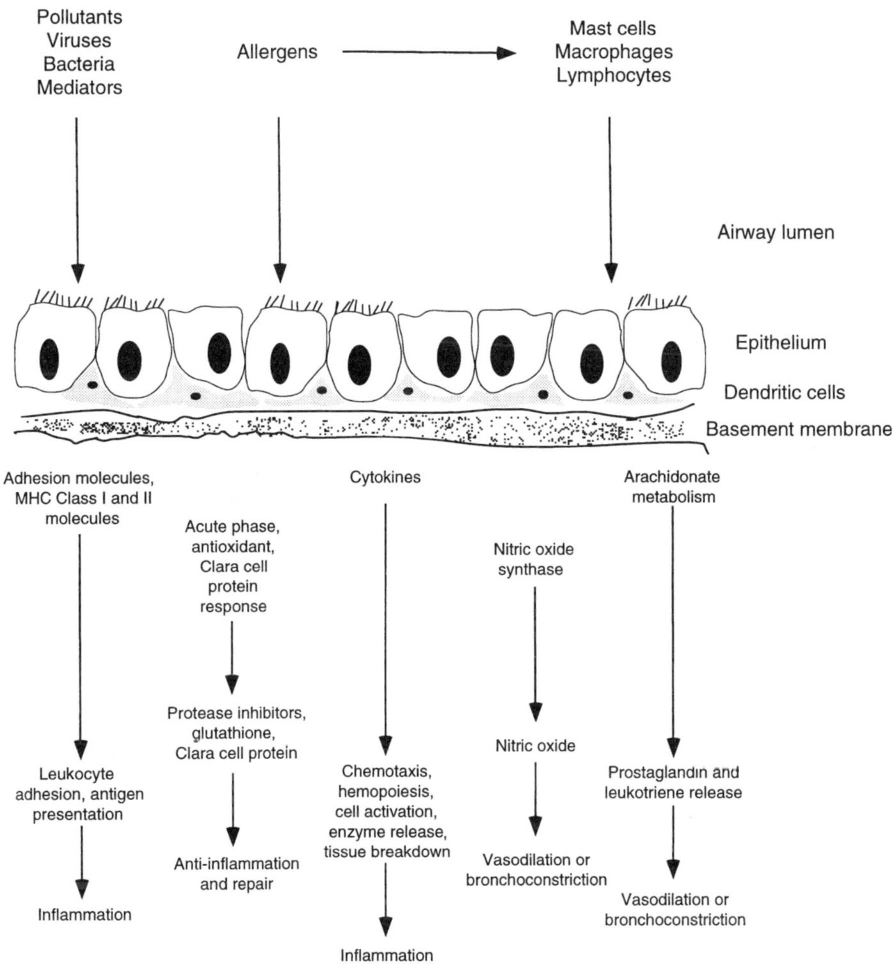

Figure 2 Schematic representation of the potential interactions with, and consequences of, inhaled allergens and respiratory epithelium.

ing T cells, macrophages, mast cells, and monocytes, that are likely to be attracted to or resident in the lung. More recently, however, studies have shown bronchial epithelium to be a significant source of a wide range of cytokines, such as IL-1β, IL-6, IL-8, IL-11, TGF-β, RANTES, eotaxin, and GM-CSF (see Table 2; 47–51). The release of several of these appears to involve the common transcription factor, NF-κB (52,53).

B. Importance of Respiratory Epithelium-Derived Cytokines

The importance of individual epithelial-derived cytokines in the lung is unclear, but each has the potential to play a role. For example, IL-8, either alone or synergistically with GM-CSF and RANTES, is chemotactic for neutrophils and eosinophils, with IL-8 concentrations correlating with both cell types and their proinflammatory products (54,55). The precise roles of IL-6 and TNF-α in the lung are yet to be determined, but both cytokines are pleiotropic and important in a variety of inflammatory and immunological processes occurring in this tissue. For example, IL-6 is associated with $CD4^+$ and $CD8^+$ T-cell hyperplasia, as well as driving $CD4^+$ T cells toward a Th2 effector type (56–58); whereas TNF-α may be associated with airway hyperresponsiveness and ICAM-1 expression (59–61). In addition, epithelium-derived cytokines may also be important in the autocrine and paracrine regulation of mediator synthesis and cell surface marker expression. For example, the synthesis of prostanoid mediators and nitric oxide may be upregulated owing to the induction of prostaglandin G/H synthase (cyclooxygenase 2) and nitric oxide synthase (iNOS), respectively, by cytokines, such as IL-1β and TNF-α (23). Similarly, cytokines upregulate the expression of the major histocompatibility complex (MHC) class II and ICAM-1 expressed on respiratory epithelium (33).

C. Modulation of Respiratory Epithelial Function

Many stimuli modulate the release of all of the foregoing agents from respiratory epithelium, including both endogenous and exogenous, agents (see Table 3). For example, a variety of inflammatory cell-derived enzymes (e.g., neutrophil and mast cell proteases and eosinophil peroxidase), endothelin, nitric oxide, and cytokines, modulate respiratory epithelial function (62–67). Similarly, several bacterial products (e.g., *Haemophilus influenzae* endotoxin from typable and nontypable strains and nitrite reductase from *Pseudomonas aeruginosa*; 68,69), and respiratory viruses (influenza virus A, rhinovirus, respiratory syncytial virus, and adenovirus; 70–72), also stimulate the release of cytokines and upregulate cell surface marker expression. Finally, a variety of occupational and environmental agents also cause cytokine release from epithelium, including toluene diisocyanate, ozone, and diesel exhaust particles (74–76), and more recently, allergens (8).

D. Endogenous Proteases and Epithelial Cell Function

Neutrophil and mast cell proteases are important in initiating cytokine and mediator release from epithelium (62,63) and in modulating epithelial permeability (77). Similarly, proteases from inflammatory cells, such as eosinophils, as well as from elsewhere within the lung may also be important in respiratory disease

(78–83). Proteases are important in lung diseases, such as cystic fibrosis and bronchiectasis, in which neutrophils are prominent. However, their role in other lung diseases, such as asthma and allergic rhinitis, are based on circumstantial data. For example, proteases have been demonstrated in BAL fluid from asthmatic patients (84), and bronchoconstriction may be induced by aerosolized human neutrophil elastase (85) and prevented by pretreatment with protease inhibitors (85,86). Similarly, mast cell tryptase inhibitors markedly attenuate early- and late-phase immediate hypersensitivity responses in a sheep model, and kallikrein inhibitors inhibit nasal airway resistance in allergen-challenged patients (87,88). These data suggest that tryptase or tryptase-like enzymes (e.g., thrombin, Clara cell tryptase, and kallikrein) that cleave to the carboxy-terminal side of arginine residues play a significant role in allergic inflammation. Further indirect evidence for the role of proteases in asthma and allergic diseases has been obtained from studies showing that, in some asthmatic patients, there may be reduced or defective antiprotease screen and that α_1-antiprotease may be of value in steroid unresponsive atopic dermatitis (89–91). Together, these data suggest that any imbalance in the concentration of protease inhibitor in favor of protease is likely to enhance inflammatory processes. In addition, proteases, such as neutrophil elastase, chymase (but not tryptase), and cathepsin G, that cleave at the carboxy-terminal side of amino acids such as leucine and phenylalanine are potent mucous secretogogues (92,93). Finally, in diseases for which glucocorticoids are used to modulate inflammation in the lung, cytokine synthesis not only is downregulated, but also the production of several protease inhibitors is upregulated (94–96).

E. Allergens and Epithelial Cell Function

In addition to endogenous proteins that modulate respiratory epithelial function, the lung may also be exposed to exogenous proteins in the form of aeroallergens, both domestic and occupational. However, of particular interest to this chapter are the proteolytically active allergens that appear to be associated with sources considered to be significant risk factors for the development of asthma, such as house dust mite (97), cockroach (98), and pollen (99). This interest has developed because of the findings from mite studies and from a review of the occupational asthma literature that clearly show that allergenic proteases not only bear structural similarities with the proinflammatory proteases discussed in Section III.D, but also demonstrate similar substrate specificities (Table 4). These findings suggest the possibility that proteolytically active allergens modulate respiratory epithelial function in a manner similar to that discussed for endogenous proteases. The potential importance of proteolytically active allergens from fecally enriched mite extracts derived from mites belonging to the genus *Dermatophagoides* is currently being investigated. The proteases of interest include the cysteine protease (e.g., Der p 1) and the serine proteases trypsin (e.g., Der p 3), chymotrypsin (e.g., Der p 6) and a collagenolytic enzyme (e.g., Der p 9) (97,100–105).

Table 4 NH_2-Terminal Sequences[a] of Mammalian Proinflammatory Serine Proteases and Mite Proteases

Protease	Sequence																			
Lysine–arginine-specific																				
	1																			20
Der f 3	**I**	**V**	**G**	**G**	**V**	**K**	**A**	**Q**	**A**	**G**	**D**	**C**	**P**	**Y**	**Q**	**I**	**S**	**L**	**Q**	**S**
Der p 3	**I**	**V**	**G**	**G**	E	**K**	**A**	**L**	**A**	**G**	**E**	**C**	**P**	**Y**	**Q**	**I**	**S**	**L**	**Q**	**S**
Human kallikrein	**I**	**V**	**G**	**G**	T	**N**	S	**S**	W	**G**	**E**	W	**P**	W	**Q**	V	**S**	**L**	**Q**	**V**
Dog tryptase	**I**	**V**	**G**	**G**	R	E	**A**	P	G	S	K	W	**P**	W	**Q**	V	**S**	**L**	R	L
Human tryptase	**I**	**V**	**G**	**G**	**Q**	E	**A**	P	R	S	K	W	**P**	W	**Q**	V	**S**	**L**	R	**V**
Tyrosine–leucine–phenylalanine-specific																				
Der p 6	V	I	**G**	**G**	**Q**	**D**	**A**	A	E	**A**	**E**	**A**	**P**	F	**Q**	**I**	**S**	**L**	M	**K**
Der f 6	(A)	**V**	**G**	**G**	**Q**	**D**	**A**	D	L	**A**	**E**	**A**	**P**	F	**Q**	**I**	**S**	**L**	L	**K**
Rat chymase	**I**	I	**G**	**G**	**V**	E	S	R	**P**	H	S	R	**P**	**Y**	M	A	H	**L**	E	I
Human cathepsin G	**I**	I	**G**	**G**	R	E	S	R	**P**	H	S	R	**P**	**Y**	M	A	Y	**L**	**Q**	I
Der p 9	**I**	**V**	**G**	**G**	S	**N**	**A**	**S**	**P**	**G**	**D**	**A**	V	**Y**	**Q**	**I**	A	**L**	**Q**	**S**

[a] One-letter code used throughout. Residues showing identity within the group 3, 6, or 9 mite allergens with nonmite proteases are indicated by bold type, whereas those residues considered to be chemically similar (A,S,T; D,E; N,Q; I,L,M,V; F,Y,W) are underlined.
Source: Refs. 100–105.

F. Proteolytically Active Allergens and Epithelial Cell Function

Proteolytically active allergens have the potential to modulate epithelial cell function and, in support of this, studies have shown that the group 1 mite cysteine protease allergen Der p 1, can affect mucosal integrity (7). These studies showed that exposure of the apical surface of bovine bronchial mucosa to either proteolytically active Der p 1 or fecally enriched growth medium at concentrations within the anticipated physiological range (1–10 mg/mL; 15) significantly increased the apical-basolateral flux of a high molecular weight protein marker, but the mechanism was not determined. However, it did not appear to be necrotic in origin, suggesting some interaction with tight junction proteins. These studies also demonstrated that the mite proteases were capable of detaching a variety of epithelial cells, including canine tracheal epithelium, canine kidney epithelial cells, transformed human respiratory cells (BEAS-2B), and primary explant epithelial cells from collagen or Matrigel-coated plastic substrata (7). In addition, Der p 1, as well as the collagenolytic mite protease Der p 9 induce IL-6, IL-8, and GM-CSF release from primary epithelial cell cultures and BEAS-2B (106,107) together with upregulating NF-κB activity (108). Furthermore, these proteases upregulated respiratory epithelial cell class II and ICAM-1 expression (102). Similar findings have been reported for proteases derived from the allergenic fungus *Aspergillus fumigatus* (109).

IV. Allergens and Mast Cells

Mast cells are capable of degranulating in a non–IgE-dependent manner in response to various stimuli. For example, degranulation has been observed with both endogenous proteases, such as mast cell-derived chymase, together with exogenous mammalian serine proteases, such as α-chymotrypsin and trypsin (110,111), and the collagenolytic mite protease allergen Der p 9 was also capable of degranulating rat peritoneal mast cells (112). Similarly, the phospholipase A_2 allergen from bee venom also degranulates mast cells in a non–IgE-dependent manner (9,113). These data suggest that local histamine release may occur on allergen deposition or injection of allergens in the vicinity of mast cells, without the involvement of antigen-specific IgE, and have a significant effect on epithelial permeability.

V. Allergens and Macrophages

Of central importance to immunogenicity is the recognition of foreign proteins by appropriate antigen-presenting cells, and various cell types of the respiratory system, such as dendritic cells and alveolar macrophages are likely to be involved (2–4). Of these, current evidence suggests that dendritic cells may be particularly important because they present antigen to naive T cells (2), in contrast with resident lung macrophages. However, once activated, cells such as macrophages are also likely to be able to efficiently present antigen in vivo. Interestingly, cells such as the macrophage possess receptors that bind many different kinds of ligand. These receptors are thought to have evolved before the development of adaptive immune recognition systems to cope either with invasion by pathogenic microorganisms or the release of host hydrolytic enzymes, occurring as a result of inflammatory stimuli (114,115). The receptors characterized so far recognize either carbohydrates, lipopolysaccharide, proteases, lipids, matrix components, humoral immune components, cytokines, or transport proteins (116). Once bound, receptor–ligand complexes are endocytosed and proceed to intracellular compartments where dissociation may occur. Following endocytosis, cells become activated, resulting in the release of mediators, such as cytokines, hydrolytic enzymes, and superoxide. As many allergens possess many of these described characteristics, it is feasible that endocytosis plays a role in the processing or presentation of allergen, thus contributing to immunogenicity. Such a concept is consistent with a substantial body of data that show that antigen capture and presentation (i.e., immunogenicity) is increased by several orders of magnitude if mediated by cell surface receptors or by intermediary molecules, including IgG and IgE (117–119).

A. Protease Inhibitor Receptors

The respiratory system produces several protease inhibitors, such as the serine protease inhibitors α_1-antiprotease and secretory leukocyte protease inhibitor, the cysteine protease inhibitor, cystatin C, and if extravasation occurs, the serine and cysteine protease inhibitor, α_2-macroglobulin. Several cell types, including macrophages and monocytes, possess at least three different high-affinity receptors that recognize protease-inhibitor complexes, with subsequent endocytosis, and include the serpin receptor I (which binds a variety of serine protease inhibitors, such as α_1-antiprotease, antithrombin III, and α_1-antichymotrypsin), the anti-plasmin receptor, and the α_2-macroglobulin receptor (120–122). Once bound to protease, all inhibitors undergo conformational change that results in the exposure of specific sites recognized by receptors on phagocytic cells (123–125). Thus, it is plausible that such a mechanism could serve to direct allergens expressing proteolytic activity to relevant immunocompetent cells within the respiratory tree. Interestingly, mite proteases may degrade inhibitors such as α_1-antiprotease (126,127), arguing against such a mechanism occurring in vivo. However, in model studies using elastase (which also degrades this inhibitor) secreted from neutrophils, although this may occur in close proximity to the source of enzyme, the protease is eventually inhibited (128). In addition to the binding of protease–protease inhibitor complexes to potential antigen-presenting cells, allergens possessing protease-inhibitory activity may also bind directly to cell surface membranes. This binding is due to the direct interaction between the inhibitor and membrane-bound proteases, which are thought to play an important role in cell proliferation (129). Again, the end result of this process is endocytosis. This finding is of particular significance, given that the major occupational wheat and barley allergens (CM16 and CMb, respectively) possess trypsin inhibitory activity (130), and seed-derived allergens, such as the 2S napin-related proteins from mustard seed (Sin a I) and castor bean (Ric c I), and the rye grass pollen allergen, *Lol p* 11, show sequence homology with known plant-derived protease inhibitors (131–133).

B. Lectin Receptors

Macrophages also possess a variety of receptors that recognize terminal sugars comprising the *N*-linked oligosaccharide moieties of glycoproteins (114,116). As with the protease–protease inhibitor complexes, interaction between glycoprotein and receptor results in endocytosis. Several receptors have been described that bind sugars, such as mannose, fucose, galactose, and glucose, and they are particularly important in host defense, in which they play a role in the removal of bacteria, soluble bacterial proteins, and host glycoproteins, such as lysosomal enzymes. The binding of glycosylated proteins to receptors, such as the macrophage mannose receptor, stimulates the release of cytokines (134). It is unclear whether phagocytic cells endocytose glycoprotein allergens by lectin-like receptors, or if such interactions can result in enhanced antigen presentation. However, both biochemical and sequence analyses show that many allergens, such as the pollen and fungal allergens, contain carbohydrate or appropriate glycosylation sites (135–139), and unpublished observations from our laboratory have shown that alveolar macrophages phagocytose allergen that contains starch granules from rye grass pollen. This process is inhibited by free carbohydrate and neoglycoproteins, indicating the involvement of carbohydrate in binding to cells. Thus, binding to sugar receptors on macrophages may represent a potent mechanism by which allergens can also be directed to relevant immunocompetent cells or, alternatively, initiate the production and release of proinflammatory cytokines.

VI. Allergens and Dendritic Cells

Dendritic cells form a contiguous network within the epithelium and are found in both the upper and lower respiratory tree, where they interdigitate with epithelial cells in a manner analogous to that described for Langerhans cells in the skin (2; see Chap. 11). Their dendritic processes do not appear to protrude through the epithelium, but are limited by the tight junctions connecting each cell. Therefore, it is currently thought that, to fulfill their antigen-presenting role, allergen must cross the mucous layer and penetrate the tight junctions between epithelial cells to contact immunocompetent cells. The precise mechanisms are unclear, but given that the junctions are relatively impermeable to proteins, it is feasible that proteolysis of respiratory epithelium could have a marked influence on the recognition of inspired antigens. Thus, proteolytically active allergens, such as those from the mites, have the potential to reach dendritic cells in this manner. Whether allergens have the potential to interact with dendritic cells by specific cell surface receptors, as described for macrophages and monocytes, remains to be determined.

VII. Allergens and Noncellular Respiratory Components

In addition to interacting with cells in the respiratory system, it is also possible that allergens interact with a variety of acellular components within the respiratory tract owing to electrostatic properties, enzymatic activity, or carbohydrate content. For example, basic proteins bind to the sialic acid-rich mucins present in high concentration in respiratory secretions owing to electrostatic interactions

(140,141) and, on this basis, it is possible that many basic allergens might also bind in this manner and, subsequently, interact with phagocytic cells. Enzymatic activity, proteolytically active allergens, such as those from mites and pollen, generate the anaphylatoxins C3a and C5a from complement components C3 and C5, to activate the kinin-generating cascade, with subsequent effect on vascular permeability, to activate fibrinolysis, and to cleave angiotensin II (142–145). In addition, the mite allergen Der p 1 cleaves CD23 from the surface of B cells, suggesting that the soluble form of this protein may upregulate IgE synthesis (146,147). It is also feasible that any allergen with carbohydrase activity, such as mite and fungal amylases, could bind to specific carbohydrate moieties that compose the respiratory mucins owing to enzyme–substrate interactions and enhance phagocytosis. In a similar fashion, the lectin-like lung surfactant proteins A and D bind to allergens, such as pollen and mite allergens, by carbohydrate moieties (148).

In addition to these properties, it is also possible that the physicochemical properties of allergens may enhance interactions with appropriate cells. Allergens, such as the occupational allergen hen egg white lysozyme, the cat allergen Fel d 1, and the rodent urinary allergens (lipocalins), all are similar to proteins that are normally found in respiratory mucosa per se (4). These proteins are all highly soluble and diffuse easily within respiratory secretions, and it would be anticipated that allergens with similar structures would behave accordingly and be immunogenic.

VIII. Summary

The data described in this chapter indicate that the biochemical properties of aeroallergens have the potential to interact with a variety of cell types and molecules in the respiratory tree, the end result of which may be manifest either in sensitization in genetically susceptible individuals or, alternatively, contribute to ongoing inflammation. Such properties include enzymatic activity, physicochemical properties, and receptor–ligand interactions (Table 5). As sensitization is thought to occur in the neonatal period, such properties may facilitate interaction with innate immune mechanisms at a time when the cognate immune system is developing. In the clinical situation, only limited and circumstantial in vivo data exist to support this, and most relate to proteolytically active allergens. For example, studies have demonstrated Der p 1 concentrations in mattress dust from newborn infants correlated with increased airway responsiveness, but not lung function, and was unrelated to family history of asthma, atopy, or parental smoking; in sensitized asthmatic subjects some, but not all, studies have demonstrated a relation between asthma severity and mite allergen concentration unrelated to the degree of sensitization, as judged by dust mite allergen skin test reactivity; a

Table 5 Physicochemical and Biochemical Properties of Allergens and Their Potential Biological Consequences

Property of allergen	Potential consequence
Protease activity	Epithelial permeability owing to
	Mast cell degranulation
	Tight junction degradation
	Kinin generation
	Macrophage–monocyte receptor interaction
	Cytokine release
	Adhesion molecule upregulation
	Complement activation
Protease inhibitor	Macrophage–monocyte receptor interaction
Glycosylation	Macrophage–monocyte receptor interaction
High focal concentration	Epithelial permeability owing to osmotic effects

reported correlation between protease activity in dust and cough, wheeze and breathlessness, in an elderly population; and the demonstration of a primary irritant effect in the lung of exposed workers, and a reported correlation between the concentration of airborne proteases and chronic bronchitis and byssinosis (149–151). Whether such observations reflect a causal link between asthma and the properties of particular allergen source known to represent an independent risk factor for the development of the disease is unclear, but warrants further study. Despite this uncertainty, it is clear that allergens should not be considered to be just benign particles entering the lung.

Nomenclature

CD	cluster of differentiation
Der p 1	*Dermatophagoides pteronyssinus* cysteine protease
Der p 3	*D. pteronyssinus* trypsin
Der p 6	*D. pteronyssinus* chymotrypsin
Der p 9	*D. pteronyssinus* collagenolytic serine protease
GM-CSF	granulocyte–macrophage colony-stimulating factor
ICAM-1	intercellular adhesion molecule
iNOS	inducible nitric oxide synthase
IL	interleukin
LFA-1	lymphocyte function associated antigen
LIF	leukemia inhibitory factor
MCP	monocyte chemotactic protein
MIP	macrophage inflammatory protein

NF-κB	nuclear factor κB
PGHS	prostaglandin G/H synthase
RANTES	regulated on activation, normal T-expressed and secreted
TGF	transforming growth factor
TNF	tumor necrosis factor
VCAM-1	vascular cell adhesion molecule

Acknowledgments

The authors' work was supported by grants from the Asthma Foundation of W A Inc Ltd and the Australian National Health and Medical Research Council. The secretarial assistance of Mrs. Sylvia German is gratefully acknowledged.

References

1. Rylander R. Symptoms and mechanisms—inflammation of the lung. Am J Ind Med 1994; 25:19–23.
2. Steinman RM. The dendritic cell system and its role in immunogenicity. Annu Rev Immunol 1991; 9:271–296.
3. Holt PG. Regulation of antigen-presenting cell function(s) in lung and airway tissue. Eur Respir J 1993; 6:120–129.
4. Stewart GA, Thompson PJ. The biochemistry of common aeroallergens. Clin Exp Allergy 1996; 26:1020–1044.
5. Stewart GA, Thompson PJ, McWilliam AS. Biochemical properties of aeroallergens: contributory factors in allergic sensitization? Pediatr Allergy Immunol 1993; 4:163–172.
6. Robinson C, Kalsheker NA, Srinivasan N, King CM, Garrod DR, Thompson PJ, Stewart GA. On the potential significance of the enzymatic activity of mite allergens to immunogenicity. Clues to structure and function revealed by molecular characterization. Clin Exp Allergy 1997; 27:10–21.
7. Herbert CA, King CM, Ring PC, Holgate ST, Stewart GA, Thompson PJ, Robinson C. Augmentation of permeability in the bronchial epithelium by the house dust mite allergen Der p 1. Am J Respir Cell Mol Biol 1995; 12: 369–378.
8. King C, Brennan S, Thompson PJ, Stewart GA. Dust mite proteolytic allergens induce cytokine release from cultured airway epithelium. J Immunol 1998; 161:3645–3651.
9. Dudler T, Machado DC, Kolbe L, Annand RR, Rhodes N, Gelb MH, Koelsch E, Suter M, Helm BA. A link between catalytic activity, IgE-independent mast cell activation, and allergenicity of bee venom phospholipase a(2). J Immunol 1995; 155: 2605–2613.
10. Stewart GA. Molecular Biology of Allergens. In: Busse WW, Holgate ST, eds. Asthma and Rhinitis. Oxford: Blackwell Scientific, 1995:898–932.
11. Suphioglu C, Singh MB, Taylor P, Bellomo R, Holmes P, Puy R, Knox RB. Mechanism of grass-pollen-induced asthma. Lancet 1992; 339:569–572.
12. Habenicht HA, Burge HA, Muilenberg ML, Solomon WR. Allergen carriage by

atmospheric aerosol. II. Ragweed-pollen determinants in submicronic atmospheric fractions. J Allergy Clin Immunol 1984; 74:64–67.
13. Stewart GA, Holt PG. Submicronic airborne allergens. Med J Aust 1985; 143:426–427.
14. Deblay F, Sanchez J, Plattsmills T, Chapman M, Pauli G. The metrology of airborne particles carrying the principal aeroallergens. Rev Mal Respir 1995; 12:343–352.
15. Tovey ER, Chapman MD, Wells CW, Platts MT. The distribution of dust mite allergen in the houses of patients with asthma. Am Rev Respir Dis 1981; 124:630–635.
16. Ferguson P, Broide DH. Environmental and bronchoalveolar lavage *Dermatophagoides pteronyssinus* antigen levels in atopic asthmatics. Am J Respir Crit Care Med 1995; 151:71–74.
17. Baraniuk JN, Bolick M, Esch R, Buckley C. Quantification of pollen solute release using pollen grain column chromatography. Allergy 1992; 47:411–417.
18. Devalia JL, Davies RJ. Airway epithelial cells and mediators of inflammation. Respir Med 1993; 87:405–408.
19. Knight DA, Stewart GA, Thompson PJ. The respiratory epithelium and airway smooth muscle homeostasis: its relevance to asthma. Clin Exp Allergy 1994; 24: 698–706.
20. Martin LD, Rochelle LG, Fischer BM, Krunkosky TM, Adler KB. Airway epithelium as an effector of inflammation—molecular regulation of secondary mediators. Eur Respir J 1997; 10:2139–2146.
21. Campbell AM. Bronchial epithelial cells in asthma. Allergy 1997; 52:483–489.
22. Stadnyk AW. Cytokine production by epithelial cells. FASEB J 1994; 8:1041–1047.
23. Robbins RA, Barnes PJ, Springall DR, Warren JB, Kwon OJ, Buttery LD, Wilson AJ, Geller DA, Polak JM. Expression of inducible nitric oxide in human lung epithelial cells. Biochem Biophys Res Commun 1994; 203:209–218.
24. Cantin AM, North SL, Hubbard RC, Crystal RG. Normal alveolar epithelial lining fluid contains high levels of glutathione. J Appl Physiol 1987; 63:152–157.
25. Haidaris PJ. Induction of fibrinogen biosynthesis and secretion from cultured pulmonary epithelial cells. Blood 1997; 89:873–882.
26. Sun G, De AG, Nucci F, Ackerman V, Bellini A, Mattoli S. Functional analysis of the preproendothelin-1 gene promoter in pulmonary epithelial cells and monocytes. Biochem Biophys Res Commun 1996; 221:647–652.
27. Saunders NA, Smith RJ, Jetten AM. Differential responsiveness of human bronchial epithelial cells, lung carcinoma cells, and bronchial fibroblasts to interferon-gamma in vitro. Am J Respir Cell Mol Biol 1994; 11:147–152.
28. Singh G, Katyal SL, Brown WE, Kennedy AL, Singh U, Wong CM. Clara cell 10 kDa protein (CC10): comparison of structure and function to uteroglobin. Biochim Biophys Acta 1990; 1039:348–355.
29. Pardo A, Ridge K, Uhal B, Iasha Sznajder J, Selman M. Lung alveolar epithelial cells synthesise interstitial collagenase and gelatinases A and B in vitro. Int J Biochem 1997; 29:901–910.
30. Cichy J, Potempa J, Travis J. Biosynthesis of alphal-proteinase inhibitor by human lung-derived epithelial cells. J Biol Chem 1997; 272:8250–8255.
31. Sallenave JM, Shulmann J, Crossley J, Jordana M, Gauldie J. Regulation of secre-

tory leukocyte proteinase inhibitor (SLPI) and elastase-specific inhibitor (ESI/elafin) in human airway epithelial cells by cytokines and neutrophilic enzymes. Am J Respir Cell Mol Biol 1994; 11:733–741.
32. Cichy J, Potempa J, Chawla RK, Travis J. Stimulatory effect of inflammatory cytokines on alpha 1-antichymotrypsin expression in human lung-derived epithelial cells. J Clin Invest 1995; 95:2729–2733.
33. Vignola AM, Campbell AM, Chanez P, Bousquet J, Paul LP, Michel FB, Godard P. HLA-DR and ICAM-1 expression on bronchial epithelial cells in asthma and chronic bronchitis. Am Rev Respir Dis 1993; 148:689–694.
34. Bloemen PG, van den Tweel Mc, Henricks PA, Engels F, Wagenaar SS, Rutten AA, Nijkamp FP. Expression and modulation of adhesion molecules on human bronchial epithelial cells. Am J Respir Cell Mol Biol 1993; 9:586–593.
35. Papi A. Epithelial ICAM-1 regulation and its role in allergy. Clin Exp Allergy 1997; 27:721–724.
36. Lackie PM, Baker JE, Gunthert U, Holgate ST. Expression of CD44 isoforms is increased in the airway epithelium of asthmatic subjects. Am J Respir Cell Mol Biol 1997; 16:14–22.
37. Robinson DS, Hamid Q, Ying S, Tsicopoulos A, Barkans J, Bentley AM, Corrigan C, Durham SR, Kay AB. Predominant TH2-like bronchoalveolar T-lymphocyte population in atopic asthma. N Engl J Med 1992; 326:298–304.
38. Berkman N, Krishnan VL, Gilbey T, Newton R, O'Connor B, Barnes PJ, Chung KF. Expression of RANTES mRNA and protein in airways of patients with mild asthma. Am J Respir Crit Care Med 1996; 154:1804–1811.
39. Jahnz RK, Plusa T, Faber M, Stepnowski L, Pirozynska E, Pojda Z. Interleukin-6 and interleukin-8 in bronchoalveolar lavage fluid material from patients with chronic bronchitis. Pol Merkuriusz Lekarski 1996; 1:383–385.
40. Wang Z, Larsson K, Palmberg L, Malmberg P, Larsson P, Larsson L. Inhalation of swine dust induces cytokine release in the upper and lower airways. Eur Respir J 1997; 10:381–387.
41. Wintermeyer SF, Kuschner WG, Wong H, D'Alessandro A, Blanc PD. Pulmonary responses after wood chip mulch exposure. J Occup Environ Med 1997; 39:308–314.
42. Jorens PG, De JR, Bossaert LL, De BW, Herman AG, Pollet H, Bosmans E, Taupin JL, Moreau JF. High levels of leukaemia inhibitory factor in ARDS. Cytokine 1996; 8:873–876.
43. Kato M, Liu MC, Stealey BA, Friedman B, Lichtenstein LM, Permutt S, Schleimer RP. Production of granulocyte/macrophage colony-stimulating factor in human airways during allergen-induced late-phase reactions in atopic subjects. Lymphokine Cytokine Res 1992; 11:287–292.
44. Virchow JJ, Walker C, Hafner D, Kortsik C, Werner P, Matthys H, Kroegel C. T cells and cytokines in bronchoalveolar lavage fluid after segmental allergen provocation in atopic asthma. Am J Respir Crit Care Med 1995; 151:960–968.
45. Robinson D, Hamid Q Bentley A, Ying S, Kay AB, Durham SR. Activation of $CD4^+$ T cells, increased TH2-type cytokine mRNA expression, and eosinophil recruitment in bronchoalveolar lavage after allergen inhalation challenge in patients with atopic asthma. J Allergy Clin Immunol 1993; 92:313–324.

46. Huang SK, Xiao HQ, Kleine TJ, Paciotti G, Marsh DG, Lichtenstein LM, Liu MC. IL-13 expression at the sites of allergen challenge in patients with asthma. J Immunol 1995; 155:2688–2694.
47. Cromwell O, Hamid Q, Corrigan CJ, Barkans J, Meng Q, Collins PD, Kay AB. Expression and generation of interleukin-8, IL-6 and granulocyte–macrophage colony-stimulating factor by bronchial epithelial cells and enhancement by IL-1 beta and tumour necrosis factor-alpha. Immunology 1992; 77:330–337.
48. Stellato C, Beck LA, Gorgone GA, Proud D, Schall TJ, Ono SJ, Lichtenstein LM, Schleimer RP. Expression of the chemokine RANTES by a human bronchial epithelial cell line. Modulation by cytokines and glucocorticoids. J Immunol 1995; 155: 410–418.
49. Garcia ZE, Rothenberg ME, Ownbey RT, Celestin J, Leder P, Luster AD. Human eotaxin is a specific chemoattractant for eosinophil cells and provides a new mechanism to explain tissue eosinophilia. Nat Med 1996; 2:449–456.
50. Stellato C, Collins P, Ponath PD, Soler D, Newman W, La RG, Li H, White J, Schwiebert LM, Bickel C, Liu M, Bochner BS, Williams T, Schleimer RP. Production of the novel C-C chemokine MCP-4 by airway cells and comparison of its biological activity to other C-C chemokines. J Clin Invest 1997; 99:926–936.
51. Taipale J, Lohi J, Saarinen J, Kovanen PT, Keski OJ. Human mast cell chymase and leukocyte elastase release latent transforming growth factor-beta 1 from the extracellular matrix of cultured human epithelial and endothelial cells. J Biol Chem 1995; 270:4689–4696.
52. Blackwell TS, Christman JW. The role of nuclear factor-kappa B in cytokine gene regulation. Am J Respir Cell Mol Biol 1997; 17:3–9.
53. Bitko V, Velazquez A, Yang L, Yang YC, Barik S. Transcriptional induction of multiple cytokines by human respiratory syncytial virus requires activation of NF-kappa B and is inhibited by sodium salicylate and aspirin. Virology 1997; 232: 369–378.
54. Erger RA, Casale TB. Interleukin-8 is a potent mediator of eosinophil chemotaxis through endothelium and epithelium. Am J Physiol 1995; 268:L117–122.
55. Baggiolini M, Clark LI. Interleukin-8, a chemotactic and inflammatory cytokine. FEBS Lett 1992; 307:97–101.
56. Galandrini R, Cernetti C, Albi N, Dembech C, Terenzi A, Grignani F, Velardi A. Interleukin-6 is constitutively produced by human CTL clones and is required to maintain their cytolytic function. Cell Immunol 1991; 138:11–23.
57. Vink A, Uyttenhove C, Wauters P, Van SJ. Accessory factors involved in murine T cell activation. Distinct roles of interleukin 6, interleukin 1 and tumor necrosis factor. Eur J Immunol 1990; 20:1–6.
58. Rincon M, Anguita J, Nakamura T, Fikrig E, Flavell RA. Interleukin (IL)-6 directs the differentiation of IL-4-producing $CD4^+$ T cells. J Exp Med 1997; 185:461–469.
59. Godding V, Stark JM, Sedgwick JB, Busse WW. Adhesion of activated eosinophils to respiratory epithelial cells is enhanced by tumor necrosis factor-alpha and interleukin-1 beta. Am J Respir Cell Mol Biol 1995; 13:555–562.
60. Burke GA, Hellewell PG. Tumour necrosis factor-alpha-induced ICAM-1 expres-

sion in human vascular endothelial and lung epithelial cells: modulation by tyrosine kinase inhibitors. Br J Pharmacol 1996; 119:1149–1158.
61. Amrani Y, Martinet N, Bronner C. Potentiation by tumour necrosis factor-alpha of calcium signals induced by bradykinin and carbachol in human tracheal smooth muscle cells. Br J Pharmacol 1995; 114:4–5.
62. Ruef C, Jefferson DM, Schlegel HS, Suter S. Regulation of cytokine secretion by cystic fibrosis airway epithelial cells. Eur Respir J 1993; 6:1429–1436.
63. Cairns JA, Walls AF. Mast cell tryptase is a mitogen for epithelial cells. Stimulation of IL-8 production and intercellular adhesion molecule-1 expression. J Immunol 1996; 156:275–283.
64. Harkonen E, Virtanen I, Linnala A, Laitinen LL, Kinnula VL. Modulation of fibronectin and tenascin production in human bronchial epithelial cells by inflammatory cytokines in vitro. Am J Respir Cell Mol Biol 1995; 13:109–115.
65. Lilly CM, Nakamura H, Kesselman H, Nagleranderson C, Asano K, Garciazepeda EA, Rothenberg ME, Drazen JM, Luster AD. Expression of eotaxin by human lung epithelial cells—induction by cytokines and inhibition by glucocorticoids. J Clin Invest 1997; 99:1767–1773.
66. Mullol J, Baraniuk JN, Logun C, Benfield T, Picado C, Shelhamer JH. Endothelin-1 induces GM-CSF, IL-6 and IL-8 but not G-CSF release from a human bronchial epithelial cell line (BEAS-2B). Neuropeptides 1996; 30:551–556.
67. Motojima S, Adachi T, Manaka K, Arima M, Fukuda T, Makino S. Eosinophil peroxidase stimulates the release of granulocyte–macrophage colony-stimulating factor from bronchial epithelial cells. J Allergy Clin Immunol 1996; 98:S216–S223.
68. Khair OA, Davies RJ, Devalia JL. Bacterial-induced release of inflammatory mediators by bronchial epithelial cells. Eur Respir J 1996; 9:1913–1922.
69. Oishi K, Sar B, Wada A, Hidaka Y, Matsumoto S, Amano H, Sonoda F, Kobayashi S, Hirayama T, Nagatake T, Matsushima K. Nitrite reductase from *Pseudomonas aeruginosa* induces inflammatory cytokines in cultured respiratory cells. Infect Immun 1997; 65:2648–2655.
70. Terajima M, Yamaya M, Sekizawa K, Okinaga S, Suzuki T, Yamada N, Nakayama K, Ohrui T, Oshima T, Numazaki Y, Sasaki H. Rhinovirus infection of primary cultures of human tracheal epithelium— role of ICAM-1 and IL-1-beta. Am J Physiol 1997; 17:749–759.
71. Noah TL, Becker S. Respiratory syncytial virus-induced cytokine production by a human bronchial epithelial cell line. Am J Physiol 1993; 265:1472–1478.
72. Becker S, Reed W, Henderson FW, Noah TL. RSV infection of human airway epithelial cells causes production of the beta-chemokine RANTES. Am J Physiol 1997; 272:L512–L520.
73. Stark JM, Amin RS, Trapnell BC. Infection of A549 cells with a recombinant adenovirus vector induces ICAM-1 expression and increased CD-18-dependent adhesion of activated neutrophils. Hum Gene Ther 1996; 7:1669–1681.
74. Mattoli S, Colotta F, Fincato G, Mezzetti M, Mantovani A, Patalano F, Fasoli A. Time course of IL1 and IL6 synthesis and release in human bronchial epithelial cell cultures exposed to toluene diisocyanate. J Cell Physiol 1991; 149:260–268.

75. Devlin RB, McKinnon KP, Noah T, Becker S, Koren HS. Ozone-induced release of cytokines and fibronectin by alveolar macrophages and airway epithelial cells. Am J Physiol 1994; 266:L612–L619.
76. Devalia JL, Bayram H, Rusznak C, Calderon M, Sapsford RJ, Abdelaziz MA, Wang J, Davies RJ. Mechanisms of pollution-induced airway disease: in vitro studies in the upper and lower airways. Allergy 1997; 52:45–51.
77. Peterson MW, Walter ME, Nygaard SD. Effect of neutrophil mediators on epithelial permeability. Am J Respir Cell Mol Biol 1995; 13:719–727.
78. Matsunaga Y, Kido H, Kawaji K, Kamoshita K, Katunuma N, Ogura T. Inhibitors of chymotrypsin-like proteases inhibit eosinophil peroxidase release from activated human eosinophils. Archs Biochem Biophy 1994; 312:67–74.
79. Herbert CA, Edwards D, Boot JR, Robinson C. Stimulated eosinophils and proteinases augment the transepithelial flux of albumin in bovine bronchial mucosa. Br J Pharmacol 1993; 110:840–846.
80. Herbert CA, Arthur MJ, Robinson C. Augmentation by eosinophils of gelatinase activity in the airway mucosa: comparative effects as a putative mediator of epithelial injury. Br J Pharmacol 1996; 117:667–674.
81. Yasuoka S, Tsuchihashi S, Kurokawa M, Terao T, Yoshinaga T, Kawano S, Takekawa Y, Nakayama T, Doi H, Ogawara M. Comparison of biochemical properties of human airway tryptase isolated from mucoid sputum with those of lung mast cell tryptase. Jpn J Thorac Dis 1996; 34:678–684.
82. Heidtmann HH, Travis J. A novel chymotrypsin-like serine proteinase from human lung. Biol Chem Hoppe Seyler 1993; 374:871–875.
83. Caughey GH. Of mites and men: trypsin-like proteases in the lungs. Am J Respir Cell Mol Biol 1997; 16:621–628.
84. Plusa T, Tchorzewski H, Raczka A. Interaction of lysosomal enzymes and their natural inhibitors in bronchoalveolar lavage fluid and serum in atopic bronchial asthma. Arch Immunol Ther Exp 1987; 35:49–55.
85. Suzuki T, Wang W, Lin JT, Shirato K, Mitsuhashi H, Inoue H. Aerosolized human neutrophil elastase induces airway constriction and hyperresponsiveness with protection by intravenous pretreatment with half-length secretory leukoprotease inhibitor. Am J Respir Crit Care Med 1996; 153:1405–1411.
86. Slapke J, Hummel S, Wischnewsky GG, Winkler J. Protease inhibitor prevents bronchoconstriction in man. Eur J Respir Dis 1986; 68:29–34.
87. Clark JM, Abraham WM, Fishman CE, Forteza R, Ahmed A, Cortes A, Warne RL, Moore WR, Tanaka RD. Tryptase inhibitors block allergen-induced airway and inflammatory responses in allergic sheep. Am J Respir Crit Care Med 1995; 152:2076–2083.
88. Katori M, Nishiyama K, Iguchi Y, Majima M, Yao K. Reduction by a kallikrein inhibitor of the increased nasal airway resistance of allergic patients after antigen challenge. Immunopharmacology 1996; 33:308–310.
89. Pina JS, Horan MP. alpha-1-Antitrypsin deficiency and asthma. The continuing search for the relationship. Postgrad Med 1997; 101:153–156.
90. Lindmark B. Asthma and heterozygous alpha 1-antichymotrypsin deficiency: a possible association. J Intern Med 1990; 227:115–118.
91. Lindmark B, Svenonius E, Eriksson S. Heterozygous alpha 1-antichymotrypsin and

PiZ alpha 1-antitrypsin deficiency. Prevalence and clinical spectrum in asthmatic children. Allergy 1990; 45:197–203.

92. Lundgren JD, Rieves RD, Mullol J, Logun C, Shelhamer JH. The effect of neutrophil proteinase enzymes on the release of mucus from feline and human airway cultures. Respir Med 1994; 88:511–518.
93. Sommerhoff CP, Fang KC, Nadel JA, Caughey GH. Classical second messengers are not involved in proteinase-induced degranulation of airway gland cells. Am J Physiol 1996; 271:L796–L803.
94. Abbinante NJ, Simpson LG, Leikauf GD. Corticosteroids increase secretory leukocyte protease inhibitor transcript levels in airway epithelial cells. Am J Physiol 1995; 268:1601–1606.
95. Cichy J, Potempa J, Chawla RK, Travis J. Regulation of alpha 1-antichymotrypsin synthesis in cells of epithelial origin. FEBS Lett 1995; 359:262–266.
96. Cichy J, Potempa J, Travis J. Biosynthesis of alpha$_1$-proteinase inhibitor by human lung-derived epithelial cells. J Biol Chem 1997; 272:8250–8255.
97. Chua KY, Stewart GA, Thomas WR, Simpson RJ, Dilworth RJ, Plozza TM, Turner KJ. Sequence analysis of cDNA coding for a major house dust mite allergen, *Der p* I. Homology with cysteine proteases. J Exp Med 1988; 167:175–182.
98. Arruda LK, Vailes LD, Mann BJ, Shannon J, Fox JW, Vedvick TS, Hayden ML, Chapman MD. Molecular cloning of a major cockroach (*Blattella germanica*) allergen, Bla g 2. Sequence homology to the aspartic proteases. J Biol Chem 1995; 270: 19563–19568.
99. Bagarozzi DA, Pike R, Potempa J, Travis J. Purification and characterization of a novel endopeptidase in ragweed (*Ambrosia artemisiifolia*) pollen. J Biol Chem 1996; 271:26227–26232.
100. Stewart GA, Ward LD, Simpson RJ, Thompson PJ. The group III allergen from the house dust mite *Dermatophagoides pteronyssinus* is a trypsin-like enzyme. Immunology 1992; 75:29–35.
101. Yasueda H, Mita H, Akiyama K, Shida T, Ando T, Sugiyama S, Yamakawa H. Allergens from *Dermatophagoides* mites with chymotryptic activity. Clin Exp Allergy 1993; 23:384–390.
102. Nishiyama C, Yasuhara T, Yuuki T, Okumura Y. Cloning and expression in *Escherichia coli* of cDNA encoding house dust mite allergen Der f 3, serine protease from *Dermatophagoides farinae*. FEBS Lett 1995; 377:62–66.
103. Smith WA, Chua KY, Kuo MC, Rogers BL, Thomas WR. Cloning and sequencing of the *Dermatophagoides pteronyssinus* group III allergen, *Der p* III. Clin Exp Allergy 1994; 24:220–228.
104. Bennett BJ, Thomas WR. Cloning and sequencing of the group 6 allergen of *Dermatophagoides pteronyssinus*. Clin Exp Allergy 1996; 26:1150–1154.
105. King CM, Simpson RJ, Moritz RL, Reed GE, Thompson PJ, Stewart GA. The isolation and characterization of a novel collagenolytic serine protease allergen (Der p 9) from the dust mite *Dermatophagoides pteronyssinus*. J Allergy Clin Immunol 1996; 98:739–747.
106. King CM, Thompson PJ, Stewart GA. Dust mite proteolytic allergens induce cytokine release from cultured airway epithelium. Am J Respir Crit Care Med 1995; 151:A191.

107. Mori L, Kleimberg J, Mancini C, Bellini A, Marini M, Mattoli S. Bronchial epithelial cells of atopic patients with asthma lack the ability to inactivate allergens. Biochem Biophys Res Commun 1995; 217:817–824.
108. Stacey MA, Sun G, Vassalli G, Marini M, Bellini A, Mattoli S. The allergen Der p 1 induces NF-kappaB activation through interference with IkappaB alpha function in asthmatic bronchial epithelial cells. Biochem Biophys Res Commun 1997; 236: 522–526.
109. Tomee J, Wierenga A, Hiemstra PS, Kauffman HF. Proteases from *Aspergillus fumigatus* induce release of proinflammatory cytokines and cell detachment in airway epithelial cell lines. J Infect Dis 1997; 176:300–303.
110. Lagunoff D, Chi EY, Wan H. Effects of chymotrypsin and trypsin on rat peritoneal mast cells. Biochem Pharmacol 1975; 24:1573–1578.
111. Sasaki J. Mechanism of histamine release by alpha-chymotrypsin from isolated rat mast cells. Jpn J Pharmacol 1975; 25:311–324.
112. Stewart GA, Boyd SM, Bird CH, Krska KD, Kollinger MR, Thompson PJ. Immunobiology of the serine protease allergens from house dust mites. Am J Ind Med 1994; 25:105–107.
113. Machado DC, Horton D, Harrop R, Peachell PT, Helm BA. Potential allergens stimulate the release of mediators of the allergic response from cells of mast cell lineage in the absence of sensitization with antigen-specific IgE. Eur J Immunol 1996; 26:2972–2980.
114. Stahl PD. The macrophage mannose receptor: current status. Am J Respir Cell Mol Biol 1990; 2:317–318.
115. Janeway CJ. The immune system evolved to discriminate infectious nonself from noninfectious self. Immunol Today 1992; 13:11–16.
116. McWilliam AS, Tree P, Gordon S. Carbohydrate recognition receptors of the macrophage and their regulation. In: van Furth R, ed. Mononuclear Phagocytes. Biology of Monocytes and Macrophages. Dordrecht: Kluwer Academic, 1992:224–232.
117. Lanzavecchia A. Receptor-mediated antigen uptake and its presentation to class II-restricted T lymphocytes. Annu Rev Immunol 1990; 8:773–793.
118. Manca F, Fenoglio D, Pira GL, Kunkl A, Celada F. Effect of antigen/antibody ratio on macrophage uptake, processing, and presentation to T cells of antigen complexed with polyclonal antibodies. J Exp Med 1991; 173:37–48.
119. Mudde GC, Bheekha R, Bruijnzeel KC. IgE-mediated antigen presentation. Allergy 1995; 50:193–199.
120. Fuchs HE, Shifman MA, Pizzo SV. In vivo catabolism of alpha$_1$-proteinase inhibitor–trypsin, antithrombin III–thrombin and alpha$_2$-macroglobulin-methylamine. Biochim Biophys Acta 1982; 716:151–157.
121. Pizzo SV, Mast AE, Feldman SR, Salvesen G. In vivo catabolism of alpha$_1$-antichymotrypsin is mediated by the serpin receptor which binds alpha$_1$-protease inhibitor, antithrombin III and heparin cofactor II. Biochim Biophys Acta 1988; 967:158–162.
122. Pizzo, SV. Serpin receptor I: a hepatic receptor that mediates the-clearance of antithrombin III-proteinase complexes. Am J Med 1989; 87:10S–14S.
123. Debanne MT, Bell R, Dolovich J. Uptake of proteinase-α_2-macroglobulin complexes by macrophages. Biochim Biophys Acta 1975; 411:295–304.

124. Joslin G, Fallon RJ, Bullock J, Adams SP, Perlmutter DH. The SEC receptor recognizes a pentapeptide neodomain of α_1-antitrypsin-protease complexes. J Biol Chem 1991; 266:11282–11288.
125. Barrett AJ, Starkey PM. The interaction of α_2-macroglobulin with proteinases. Characteristics and specificity of the reaction, and a hypothesis concerning its molecular mechanism. Biochem J 1973; 133:709–723.
126. Schulz O, Laing P, Sewell HF, Shakib F. Der p I, a major allergen of the house dust mite, proteolytically cleaves the low-affinity receptor for human IgE (CD23). Eur J Immunol 1995; 25:3191–3194.
127. Kalsheker NA, Deam S, Chambers L, Sreedharan S, Brocklehurst K, Lomas DA. The house dust mite allergen Der p 1 catalytically inactivates alpha 1-antitrypsin by specific reactive centre loop cleavage: a mechanism that promotes airway inflammation and asthma. Biochem Biophys Res Commun 1996; 221:59–61.
128. Liou TG, Campbell EJ. Quantum proteolysis resulting from release of single granules by human neutrophils. J Immunol 1996; 157:2624–2631.
129. Scott GK. Proteinases and proteinase inhibitors as modulators of animal cell growth. Comp Biochem Physiol 1992; 103:785–793.
130. Gómez L, Martín E, Hernández D, Sanchez-Monge R, Barber D, del Pozo V, de Andrés B, Armentia A, Lahoz C, Salcedo G, Palomino P. Members of the alpha-amylase inhibitors family from wheat endosperm are major allergens associated with baker's asthma. FEBS Lett 1990; 261:85–88.
131. Menendez AL, Moneo I, Dominguez J, Rodriguez R. Primary structure of the major allergen of yellow mustard (*Sinapis alba* L.) seed, *Sin a* I. Eur J Biochem 1988; 177:159–166.
132. Thorpe SC, Kemeny DM, Panzani RC, McGurl B, Lord M. Allergy to castor bean. II. Identification of the major allergens in castor bean seeds. J Allergy Clin Immunol 1988; 82:67–72.
133. Vanree R, Hoffman DR, Vandijk W, Brodard V, Mahieu K, Koeleman C, Grande M, Vanleeuwen WA, Aalberse RC. Lol p XI, a new major grass pollen allergen, is a member of a family of soybean trypsin inhibitor-related proteins. J Allergy Clin Immunol 1995; 95:970–978.
134. Lefkowitz DL, Mills K, Castro A, Lefkowitz SS. Induction of tumor necrosis factor and macrophage-mediated cytotoxicity by horseradish peroxidase and other glycosylated proteins. J Leukoc Biol 1991; 50:615–623.
135. de la Hoz F, Polo F, Moscoso DPJ, Selles JG, Lombardero M, Carreira J. Purification of *Art v* I, a relevant allergen of *Artemisia vulgaris* pollen. Mol Immunol 1990; 27:651–657.
136. Matthiesen F, Schumacher MJ, Lowenstein H. Characterization of the major allergen of *Cynodon dactylon* (Bermuda grass) pollen, *Cyn d* I. J Allergy Clin Immunol 1991; 88:763–774.
137. Nilsen BM, Sletten K, Paulsen BS, O'Neill M, Van HH. Structural analysis of the glycoprotein allergen *Art v* II from the pollen of mugwort (*Artemisia vulgaris* L.). J Biol Chem 1991; 266:2660–2668.
138. Yunginger JW, Jones RT, Nesheim ME, Geller M. Studies on *Alternaria* allergens (III) Isolation of a major allergenic fraction (ALT-1). J Allergy Clin Immunol 1980; 66:138–147.

139. Sward-Nordmo M, Smestad PB, Wold JK. Immunological studies of the glycoprotein allergen Ag 54 (*Cla h* II) in *Cladosporium herbarum* with special attention to the carbohydrate and protein moieties. Int Arch Allergy Appl Immunol 1989; 90: 155–161.
140. Creeth JM, Bridge JL, Horton JR. An interaction between lysozyme and mucus glycoproteins. Biochem J 1979; 181:717–724.
141. Snyder CE, Nadziejko CE, Herp A. Binding of basic proteins to glycoproteins in human bronchial secretions. Int J Biochem 1982; 14:895–898.
142. Maruo K, Akaike T, Ono T, Okamoto T, Maeda H. Generation of anaphylatoxins through proteolytic processing of C3 and C5 by house dust mite protease. J Allergy Clin Immunol 1997; 100:253–260.
143. Maruo K, Akaike T, Matsumura Y, Kohmoto S, Inada Y, Ono T, Arao T, Maeda H. Triggering of the vascular permeability reaction by activation of the Hageman factor–prekallikrein system by house dust mite proteinase. Biochim Biophys Acta 1991; 1074:62–68.
144. Matsushima A, Shioya K, Kobayashi M, Kodera Y, Inada Y. Activation of blood coagulation system with the protease from *Dermatophagoides farinae*. Thromb Haemost 1993; 69:531–532.
145. Matheson N, Schmidt J, Travis J. Isolation and properties of an angiotensin II-cleaving peptidase from mesquite pollen. Am J Respir Cell Mol Biol 1995; 12: 441–448.
146. Hewitt C, Brown AP, Hart BJ, Pritchard DI. A major house dust mite allergen disrupts the immunoglobulin E network by selectively cleaving CD23—innate protection by antiproteases. J Exp Med 1995; 182:1537–1544.
147. Schulz O, Sutton BJ, Beavil RL, Shi J, Sewell HF, Gould HJ, Laing P, Shakib F. Cleavage of the low-affinity receptor for human IgE (CD23) by a mite cysteine protease: nature of the cleaved fragment in relation to the structure and function of CD23. Eur J Immunol 1997; 27:584–588.
148. Wang JY, Kishore U, Lim BL, Strong P, Reid KB. Interaction of human lung surfactant proteins A and D with mite (*Dermatophagoides pteronyssinus*) allergens. Clin Exp Immunol 1996; 106:367–373.
149. O'Keeffe PT, Young S, Arnott J, Henderson J, Stewart GA, LeSouef PN, Landau, LI. *Der p* I exposure and increased airway responsiveness in early infancy. Aust NZ J Med 1994; 24:475.
150. Shamssain MH, Rowell FJ. Indoor level of proteases as a marker of respiratory illness in elderly population. Chest 1996; 110:10S.
151. Chapman MD, Heymann PW, Sporik RB, Platts-Mills TAE. Monitoring allergen exposure in asthma: new treatment strategies. Allergy 1995; 50:29–33.

Part Five

SYSTEMIC RESPONSES OF THE LUNG TO INHALED PARTICLES

13

Effect of Particles on Mucus and Mucociliary Clearance

MALCOLM KING

University of Alberta
Edmonton, Alberta, Canada

I. Introduction

This chapter will deal with how the mucus reacts to particles and particulate loads, thereby altering its rate of clearance. Particles can stimulate secretion and modulate ciliary function, either by mechanical factors or irritation, or by the chemicals they contain or are capable of releasing. Particles have a direct effect on the physical properties of mucus, even when acting as a "neutral filler," for which their contribution to viscoelasticity is a simple function of their volume fraction. Beyond this, particles may interact with the mucous gel network, and add multiple cross-link points.

Living particles, such as bacteria and leukocytes, can have profound effects on the mucus through the macromolecules and mediators they release. Particles may also disturb the osmotic balance, thereby altering the mucus, and indirectly or directly enhancing or depressing clearance.

The chapter will begin with a brief introduction to the mechanical properties of mucus and how they relate to clearance.

II. Viscoelastic Properties of Airway Mucus

Because of the cross-linking of glycoproteins, mucus's rheological behavior is described as viscoelastic, having characteristics of both a liquid and solid (1,2). Viscosity is the resistance to flow, reflecting the absorption of energy from an object, such as a solid particle, moving through a substance. Elasticity is the recoil energy transmitted back to this object. With ideal fluids, viscosity is independent of the applied stress. With viscoelastic liquids, such as mucus, viscosity decreases with increasing stress or rate of strain (shear rate). Mucus responds to stress with an initial solid-like deformation, followed by a viscoelastic deformation, and finally, by a period of steady flow in which the rate of deformation is constant. Only partial recovery of the strain follows removal of the stress, indicating a permanent deformation of its gel structure. This type of viscoelastic behavior is illustrated in Figure 1.

Mucus exhibits shear thinning (i.e., following exposure to high shear forces, it shows a decreased viscosity at low shear rates). Some shear thinning may be permanent, with a permanently reduced viscosity (altered molecular structure), whereas other shear thinning may be reversible (thixotropy). When sputum is obtained by aspiration under pressure, it undergoes shear thinning, dilution by irrigation fluids, and incorporation of air bubbles.

Water can bind to mucous glycoprotein (MGP) macromolecules and influence viscosity. Viscosity can be increased by dehydration of the mucus, as can adhesion of mucus–epithelium. In purulent sputum, the correlation between viscosity and dry weight of solids is poor and may explain why mucous glycoprotein content is a poor index of viscoelasticity in chronic bronchitis, bronchiectasis, and cystic fibrosis. Mucus's viscoelasticity increases with acidic pH (3), causing reduced mucociliary clearance. Its viscoelasticity is also dependent on the content of low molecular weight electrolytes. These properties reflect the polyelectrolyte nature of mucins (4–6).

Changes in the mucus's viscosity and elasticity are generally interrelated (3,7), although interventions that break or add cross-links can alter the close relation (8,9). Optimum mucociliary clearance of airway mucus is located at the low end of the normal range of viscoelasticity (1,10,11). A decrease in clearance rate (transport) occurs with increasing elasticity of mucus and with increasing viscosity. Increasing viscosity with constant elasticity causes a pronounced decrease in the mucociliary transport rate (12). Decreasing the viscosity of mucus alone results in an increased transport rate and may explain the improvement in sputum mobilization following hydration or mucolytic drug therapy.

Another measure of elasticity is the spinnability (*Spinnbarkeit*, *filance*)—the thread-forming ability of mucus under the influence of large-amplitude elastic deformation. Spinnability has been correlated positively with mucociliary clear-

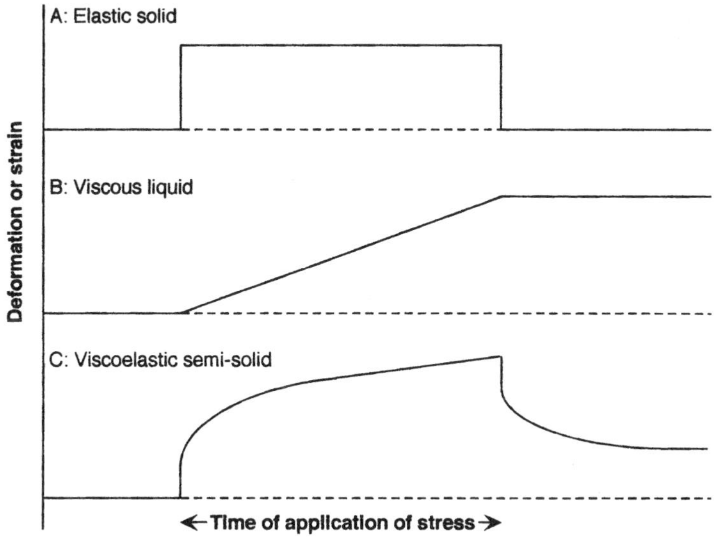

Figure 1 Diagram showing the viscoelastic behavior of a mucous gel. The first two panels illustrate stress–strain relations in idealized materials, namely an elastic solid, for which the displacement or strain is proportional to the applied force or stress, and a viscous liquid, for which the rate of strain (displacement/time) is proportional to the stress. Mucus is a viscoelastic semisolid. It responds instantaneously as a solid, with a very rapid displacement in response to an applied force. This is followed by a transition to a liquid-like response, in which the rate of strain is constant with time. Finally a zone of viscous response is reached, in which the rate of displacement is constant with time. After release of the applied force, the mucous gel recoils only partially to its initial position.

ance (13) and negatively with cough clearance (14). Adhesivity is the ability of mucus to bond to a solid surface, measured as the force of separation between one or more solid surfaces and the adhesive material. This is dependent on mucus's surface tension, hydration, wettability, and contact (dwell) time. Adhesivity correlates inversely with both mucociliary clearance and cough clearance (14,15).

III. Role of Mucus's Viscoelasticity in Mucociliary and Cough Clearance

Mucociliary clearance can be measured by visualizing the movement of particles, such as Teflon disks, tantalum powder, or charcoal powder, placed on the airway during bronchoscopy. An inert, radiolabeled tracer can also be placed on the airway, and its clearance monitored with scintillation counters or a gamma-camera. Whole-lung clearance is measured by having the subject inhale an aerosol of radiolabeled tracer and then scanning over defined regions in the proximal and distal lung.

A decrease in mucous transport velocity occurs with increasing airway generation (16); otherwise stated, the rate of mucus's transport accelerates from the peripheral airways to the larynx. For example, in excised dog lungs, the rate of particle clearance increases from 1.6 mm/min in the subsegmental bronchi to 8.3 mm/min in the mainstem, and 12.6 mm/min in the trachea (16). Impaired mucociliary transport leads to retained secretions in the airways and increased susceptibility to infection. Accumulation of mucus could increase the risk of destructive, inflammatory and neoplastic lung diseases by prolonging the contact time between inhaled materials and the airway mucosa (17). Because cough clearance is ineffective in peripheral airways (18), mucociliary clearance is relatively more important in cleansing and protecting these lung regions.

The structure and function of the epithelial cilia have been the subject of excellent reviews (19,20). The periciliary fluid appears to be regulated by various mechanisms, the most important of which are active water and ion transport across the airway surface epithelium (21,22). If the depth of the periciliary fluid is too shallow, the cilia are unable to beat effectively and may become entangled in the mucous gel layer. On the other hand, a fluid layer too deep may not allow the cilia to make contact with the mucous gel layer, thereby decreasing mucociliary clearance. The depth of the periciliary layer may be regulated by homeostatic mechanisms.

The viscoelasticity of the mucous layer contributes to the effectiveness of the mucociliary interaction, but the surface interaction between mucus and cilia, perhaps through the influence of surfactant (23,24), also plays a critical role. Ion and water transport across the surface epithelium appear to be crucial to this interaction. By generating local osmotic gradients, epithelial ion transport processes regulate the depth and composition of the periciliary sol layer (21,25). Ion transport is regulated by neurohumoral mechanisms, cholinergic and adrenergic agonists prostaglandins, substance P, vasoactive intestinal peptide (VIP), and bradykinin (26; see Chap. 13).

The transport velocity of mucus-simulant gels is directly related to mucus's elasticity and the depth of the periciliary fluid, and it is inversely related to mucus' viscosity (1). An ideal viscoelastic ratio may exist for optimal mucociliary interaction; an increase in viscosity or a decrease in elasticity would result in a reduced transport rate. Transport by cough or airflow interaction depends inversely on viscosity, elasticity (spinnability), and adhesivity (1). Mucus that is elastic, rather than viscous is transported well by ciliary action, but less well by coughing (2).

IV. Stimulation of Secretion and Modulation of Mucociliary Function by Particles

Particles can stimulate secretion and modulate ciliary function either by mechanical factors or irritation, or by the chemicals they contain or are capable of releasing. Even neutral particles can represent a burden on the mucociliary system. Although there is some evidence that the completely unloaded mucociliary system may be quiescent, it is apparent over a wide range of loads that mucociliary systems are relatively insensitive to the particulate burden they bear. This has long been recognized for the frog palate mucociliary system (27,28), and this also appears to be true for normal mammalian mucociliary clearance (29), whereas a particle's clearance velocity in healthy dogs was independent of the depth of tracheal mucus, up to apparent depths of about 100 μm. The same is not true for clearance by airflow mechanisms, for which increasing the particulate or fluid burden can stimulate cough clearance (30,31).

V. Effects of Particles as a Mechanical Filler

The effect of cellular debris, and other particulate matter, on the mechanical properties of mucus depends on the strength of the interaction. It has generally been assumed that cells act as a neutral filler, adding relatively little to the viscoelastic properties of mucus in comparison with other sources of variation in mucous gel viscoelasticity.

The contribution of cellular debris to the mechanical properties of mucus has been considered as follows (32): For an ideal gel loaded with noninteracting rigid particles, the elasticity is predicted to increase by the factor $(1 - f/f_m)^{-2.5}$, where f is the volume fraction of particles (independent of particle size) and $(f_m$ is the maximum volume fraction corresponding to close packing (about 0.8). For a viscoelastic gel, G' and η' are reportedly both increased by about the same factor (7). In simpler terms, the contribution of a neutral filler varies as the volume fraction to the 2.5-power. Thus, a cellular content of 2%, if weakly interacting, would only increase G' and η' by about 6%, and even doubling the number of cells would change these parameters by less than 15%, below the precision level for most rheological methods for mucous gel viscoelasticity.

Tracheal mucous samples obtained by scraping, for which the cellularity is high, show little variation in viscoelastic properties from samples obtained by more gentle approaches (7). In the referenced study, the cellular contents of the samples of mucus were not measured; however, the fraction of cellular debris in the samples obtained by tracheal scraping was probably higher than in those obtained from the cytology brush. In nonpurulent sputum, the nondispersable dry weight fraction, presumably cellular debris, is about 0.3–0.4% (33), which would correspond to about 1.5–2 vol% cellular debris, assuming a cellular water content of approximately 80%. If the interaction between particles were strong, the particles could act as additional cross-links and increase G' and η'. However, that no significant differences were found between the two sampling techniques suggests that epithelial cells contribute relatively little to cross-linking of mucus, other than perhaps their role as noninteracting filler. The same can be said of erythrocytes, which again show little effect on rheology up to 5–10% admixture (King M, 1995, technical report to Kimberly-Clark),

VI. Contributions of Living Particles to the Rheology of Mucus and Its Clearance

Some living particles, such as bacteria and leukocytes, can have profound effects on the mucus through the macromolecules and mediators they release. Thus, the foregoing considerations about particles as neutral filler may not extend to leukocytes, particularly eosinophils, which are numerous in asthma and bronchopulmonary asperillogosis. The main protein output of eosinophils include highly basic proteins, such as major basic protein (MBP) and eosinophil cationic protein (ECP) (34), which are highly charged cations, and could be expected to contribute to cross-linking by interacting with the anionically charged mucin macromolecules. Leukocytes can also contribute to mucus's viscoelasticity through the release of DNA and actin proteins, both occurring as inflammatory cells die during infections (35). For example, neutrophil DNA and F-actin are believed to contribute significantly to the viscoelasticity of mucus in cystic fibrosis lung disease, by providing extra cross-linked networks parallel to the basic mucin network (36,37). The inadequacy of native levels of DNase and actin-limiting proteins has led to new therapeutic approaches to reduce the hyperviscoelasticity of infected sputum (e.g., rhDNase, gelsolin, or thymosin b4); (9,38). Some of these approaches are illustrated in Figure 2.

However, neutrophils also release large quantities of proteases, such as elastase and cathepsin G. These proteases are the most potent secretagogues known (39). Not only do they stimulate the output of mucus from secretory cells, but they are also capable of degrading mucous glycoproteins, particularly when the DNA and actin that accompany the mucins in purulent secretions become degraded (40). Thus the net effect of the by-products of infection on mucus's rheology is rather unpredictable.

VII. Effects of Particles as an Osmotic Load

Particles may also disturb the osmotic balance, thereby altering the mucus, and indirectly or directly enhancing or depressing clearance. This possibility is illus-

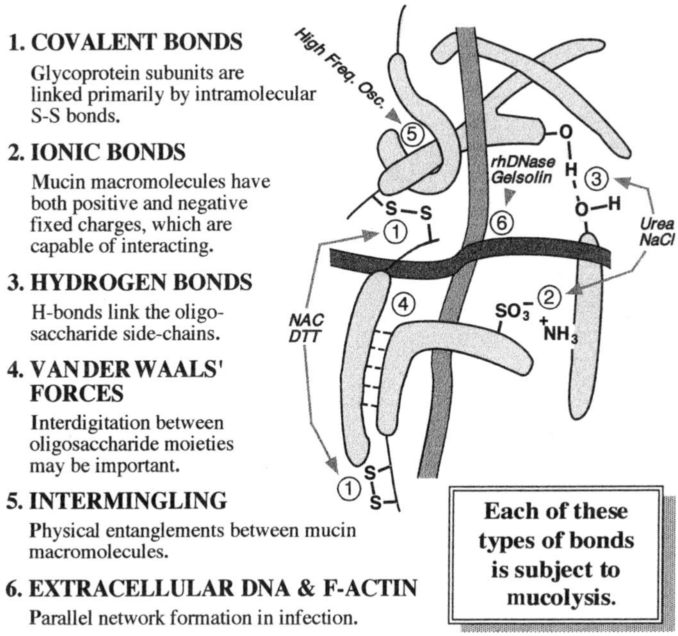

Figure 2 Diagram illustrating the types of bonding in a mucous gel, and the site of interaction with various mucolytic treatments, and of potential interaction with active particles. DTT, dithiothreitol; NAC, *N* acetylcysteine; rhDNase, recombinant human DNase. The mucous glycoproteins (mucins) consist of highly glycosylated subunits of about 500/ kDa ("sausages") linked by nonglycosylated regions ("ribbons") containing cysteines that stabilize the structure by intramolecular bonds. The oligosaccharide side chains are composed mainly of *N*-acetylglucosamine, *N*-acetylgalactosamine, galactose, fucose, and sialic acid. These glycosidic units contain numerous sites for hydrogen bonds, as well as ionic interactions. The blood-group specificity of the terminal saccharide units allow specific interactions with surface antigens on "particles," such as leukocytes and bacteria. In infection, additional large macromolecules, such as undergraded DNA and actin filaments released from leukocytes and bacteria, participate extensively in the three-dimensional structure of the gel. (From Ref. 6.)

trated in Figure 3, indicating the polyelectrolyte nature of mucins. Increasing the ionic content of the mucus could result in reducing the size of the macromolecules, thereby reducing entanglement cross-linking (3,41). Several recent studies have indicated a positive effect of hypertonic saline aerosols on mucociliary clearance (42,43), and at least part of the effect appears to occur through altering the cross-link density of the mucus. These effects could be of particular importance in chronic airway diseases, during which the mucins become typically more acidic and more highly charged (4,33).

Incorporation of charged particles into the mucous gel could also affect its viscoelastic behavior; positively charged particles could interact with the anionic macromolecules, resulting in increased cross-link density. Indeed, negatively charged sulfur colloid is transported consistently faster than albumin (neutral) or anion-exchange particles (44). Normally, this effect of particle charge on mucociliary clearance appears to be relatively minor, but the effect of particles could become more important in airway disease, when the mucins become more anionic and could interact more strongly with positively charged particles. Further studies are needed in this area.

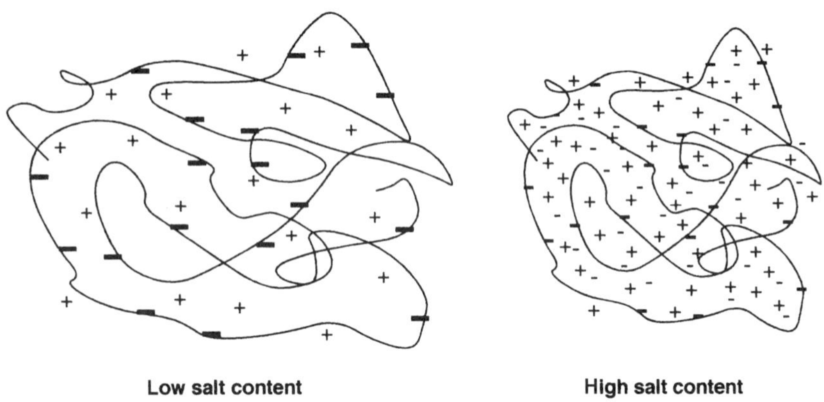

Figure 3 Diagram illustrating the polyelectrolyte nature of mucous glycoproteins (mucins). The excess of fixed negative charges along the macromolecular chain is indicated by the solid bars. Mobile ions are indicated by + and − symbols. At low ionic strength, the fixed charges along the macromolecule are poorly shielded by the mobile counterions, and the polymer is in a highly expanded conformation owing to the ionic repulsion. This permits excess entanglements (cross-linking) between neighboring macromolecules. At higher ionic strength, the excess numbers of mobile ions solvate and shield the fixed charges, reducing the effective size of the mucin macromolecules, resulting in fewer entanglement cross-links.

References

1. King M. Mucus, mucociliary clearance and coughing. In: Bates DV, ed. Respiratory Function in Disease. 3rd ed. Philadelphia: WB Saunders, 1989:69–78.
2. King M, Rubin BK. Rheology of airway mucus: relationship with clearance function. In: Takashima T, Shimura S, eds. Airway Secretion: Physiological Bases for the Control of Mucous Hypersecretion. New York: Marcel Dekker, 1994:283–314.
3. Lutz RJ, Litt M, Chakrin LW. Physical–chemical factors in mucus rheology. In: Gabelnick HL, Litt M, eds. Rheology of Biological Systems. Springfield, IL: Charles C Thomas, 1973:158–194.
4. Lamblin G, Aubert JP, Perini JM, Klein N, Porchet N, Degand P, Roussel P. Human respiratory mucins. Eur Respir J 1992; 5:247–256.
5. Bansil R, Stanley E, LaMont JT. Mucin biophysics. Annu Rev Physiol 1995; 57: 635–657.
6. Dasgupta B, King M. Molecular basis for mucolytic therapy. Can Respir J 1995; 2: 223–230.
7. King M, Macklem PT. Rheological properties of microliter quantities of normal mucus. J Appl Physiol 1977; 42:797–802.
8. Meyer FA, Gelman RA. Mucociliary transference rate and mucus viscoelasticity: Dependence on dynamic storage and loss modulus. Am Rev Respir Dis 1979; 120: 553–557.
9. Dasgupta B, Tomkiewicz RP, De Sanctis GT, Boyd WA, King M. Rheological properties in cystic fibrosis airway secretions with combined rhDNase and gelsolin treatment. In: Singh M, Saxena VP, eds. Advances in Physiological Fluid Dynamics. New Delhi: Narosa, 1996:74–78.
10. Dulfano MJ, Adler KB. Physical properties of sputum. VII. Rheologic properties and mucociliary transport. Am Rev Respir Dis 1975; 112:341–347.
11. Shih CK, Litt M, Khan MA, Wolf DP. Effect of nondialyzable solids concentration and viscoelasticity on ciliary transport of tracheal mucus. Am Rev Respir Dis 1975; 115:989–995.
12. King M. Relationship between mucus viscoelasticity and ciliary transport in guaran gel/frog palate model system. Biorheology 1980; 17:249–254.
13. Puchelle E, Zahm JM, Duvivier C. Spinnability of bronchial mucus: relationship with viscoelasticity and mucus transport properties. Biorheology 1993; 20:239–249.
14. King M, Zahm JM, Pierrot D, Vaquez-Girod S, Puchelle E. The role of mucus gel viscosity, spinnability, and adhesive properties in clearance by simulated cough. Biorheology 1989; 26:737–745.
15. Puchelle E, Zahm JM, Jacquot J, Plotkowski C, Duvivier C. A simple technique for measuring adhesion tension properties of human bronchial secretions. Eur J Respir Dis 1987; 71(suppl 153):281–282.
16. Asmundsson T, Kilburn KH. Mucociliary clearance rates at various lengths in dog lungs. Arch Environ Health 1970; 29:290–293.
17. Hilding AC. Ciliary streaming in the bronchial tree and the time element in carcinogenesis. N Engl J Med 1957; 256:634–640.

18. Clarke SW. The role of two-phase flow in bronchial clearance. Bull Eur Physiopathol Respir 1973; 9:359–372.
19. Blake JR, Winet H. On the mechanics of mucociliary transport. Biorheology 1980; 17:125–134.
20. Sleigh MA, Blake JR, Liron N. The propulsion of mucus by cilia. Am Rev Respir Dis 1988; 137:726–741.
21. Boucher RC, Stutts MJ, Bromberg PA, Gatzy JT. Regional differences in airway surface liquid composition. J Appl Physiol 1981; 50:613–620.
22. Nadel JA, Widdicombe JH, Peatfield AC. Regulation of airway secretions, ion transport, and water movement. In: Handbook of Physiology: The Respiratory System I. Bethesda, MD: American Physiological Society, 1985:419–445.
23. Jacquot J, Hayem A, Galabert C. Functions of proteins and lipids in airway secretions. Eur Respir J 1992; 5:343–358.
24. De Sanctis GT, Tomkiewicz RP, Rubin BK, Schürch S, King M. Exogenous surfactant enhances mucociliary clearance in the anesthetized dog. Eur Respir J 1994; 7: 1616–1621.
25. Al-Bazzaz FJ. Regulation of salt and water transport across airway mucosa. Clin Chest Med 1986; 7:259–272.
26. Widdicombe JH. Ion and fluid transport by airway epithelium. In: Takashima T, Shimura S, eds. Airway Secretion: Physiological Bases for the Control of Mucus Hypersecretion. New York: Marcel Dekker, 1994:399–431.
27. Sadé J, Eliezer N, Silberberg A, Nevo AC. The role of mucus in transport by cilia. Am Rev Respir Dis 1970; 102:48–52.
28. Stewart WC. Weight-carrying capacity and excitability of excised ciliated epithelium. Am J Physiol 1948; 152:1–10.
29. King M, Kelly S, Cosio M. Alteration of airway reactivity by mucus. Respir Physiol 1985; 62:47–59.
30. King M. Role of mucus viscoelasticity in cough clearance. Biorheology 1987; 24: 589–597.
31. Camner P. Studies on the removal of inhaled particles from the lungs by voluntary coughing. Chest 1981; 80:824–827.
32. Ferry JD. Cross-linked and filled polymers. In: Viscoelastic Properties of Polymers. 2nd ed. New York: Wiley, 1970:455–461.
33. Lopata M, Barton AD, Lourenço RV. Biochemical characteristics of bronchial secretions in chronic obstructive pulmonary disease. Am Rev Respir Dis 1974; 110:730–739.
34. Wardlaw AJ, Moqbel R, Kay AB. Eosinophils: biology and role in disease. Adv Immunol 1995; 60:151–266.
35. Lethem MI, James SL, Marriott C, Burke JF. The origin of DNA associated with mucus glycoproteins in cystic fibrosis sputum. Eur Respir J 1990; 3:19–23.
36. Shak S, Capon DJ, Hellmiss R, Marsters SA, Baker CL. Recombinant human DNase I reduces the viscosity of cystic fibrosis sputum. Proc Natl Acad Sci USA 1990; 87: 9188–9192.
37. Vasconcellos CA, Allen PG, Wohl ME, Drazen JM, Janmey PA, Stossel TP. Reduction in viscosity of cystic fibrosis sputum in vitro by gelsolin. Science 1994; 263: 969–971.

38. Rubin BK, Kater AP, Dian T, Ramirez O, Tomkiewicz RP, Goldstein AL. Thymosin b4 is synergistic with DNase in reducing sputum bulk and surface viscoelasticity. Pediatr Pulmonol 1995; 125:134–135.
39. Schuster A, Ueki I, Nadel JA. Neutrophil elastase stimulates tracheal submucosal gland secretion that is inhibited by ICI 200,355. Am J Physiol 1992; 262:L86–L91.
40. Lieberman J. Inhibition of protease activity in purulent sputum by DNA. J Lab Clin Med 1967; 70:595–605.
41. McCullagh CM, Jamieson AM, Blackwell J, Gupta R. Viscoelastic properties of human tracheobronchial mucin in aqueous solution. Biopolymers 1995; 35:149–159.
42. Robinson M, Regnis JA, Bailey DL, King M, Bautovich GJ, Bye PTP. Effect of hypertonic saline, amiloride, and cough on mucociliary clearance in patients with cystic fibrosis. Am J Respir Crit Care Med 1996; 153:1503–1509.
43. Tomkiewicz RP, Boyd WA, Feng W, App EM, Rubin BK, King M. Tracheal clearance and rheology of mucus after aerosolization of 3 and 7% hypertonic saline in healthy dogs. Am J Respir Crit Care Med 1997; 155:A780.
44. Lee TK, Man SFP, Connolly TP, Noujaim AA. Simultaneous comparison of canine tracheal transport of anion exchange resin particles to albumin macroaggregates and sulfur colloid. Am Rev Respir Dis 1980; 121:487–494.

14

The Role of Surfactant in Disease Associated with Particle Exposure

FRANCIS H. Y. GREEN and SAMUEL SCHÜRCH

University of Calgary
Calgary, Alberta, Canada

PETER GEHR

University of Bern
Bern, Switzerland

MARTIN M. LEE

Harvard Medical School and
Brigham and Women's Hospital
Boston, Massachusetts

I. Introduction

The extracellular fluid lining the respiratory tract and airspaces exists as a continuum from larynx to alveolus. It has a complex composition and a structure that varies from site to site that reflects its many functions. In the airways it consists of sol and gel layers surmounted by a surfactant film of unknown composition at the air–liquid interface. In the alveolus, the extracellular fluid consists of a thin hypophase covered by a dipalmitoyl phosphatidylcholine (DPPC)-rich surfactant film. These surfactant films are the first point of interaction between inhaled particles and the host and influence their deposition, clearance, and toxicity (1).

The direct demonstration of a surfactant film in the airways is relatively recent (2–4), although a surface-active film had been inferred from physiological (5) and electron microscopic studies (6) many years before. The surface tension in large airways has been measured directly with a bronchoscope from the spreading behavior of oil droplets placed onto the tracheal walls or bronchi of anesthetized sheep and horses (7,8). A surface tension of approximately 32 mN/m has been recorded at the mucus–air interface in these animals. This relatively low surface tension suggests the presence of a surface film in large airways, because proteins, surface polymers of blood cells, polysaccharides, and other biopolymers, all have surface tensions between 45 and 60 mN/m (9,10). The concept that surface forces are generated by a surface-active film at the air–aqueous interface is also supported by the observation that the film promotes the displacement of particles into the aqueous phase (2–4,11). These observations, together with in vitro experiments of particle displacement (12) suggest that particles are pulled into the extracellular layer by surface tension forces. Improvements in lung fixation have led to better preservation of the mucous layer and the demonstration of a multilamellated osmiophilic film at the air–liquid interface (13–15). Thus, both the direct measurement of surface tension and the results of electron microscopy support the concept of a surfactant film existing at the air–liquid interface in the airways.

II. Alveolar Surfactant

Alveolar surfactant consists of approximately 85–90% lipids, 10% proteins, and 2% carbohydrates (16,17). The most abundant phospholipid (PL) in surfactant is phosphatidylcholine (PC), in particular the dipalmitoylated form, dipalmitoyl phosphatidylcholine (DPPC). Smaller amounts of phosphatidylglycerol, phosphatidylinositol, phosphatidylethanolamine, and sphingomyelin are also present. On the alveolar surface, pulmonary surfactant forms a thin film that is capable of reducing both the tendency of alveoli to collapse at the end of expiration and the transudation of fluid from the capillaries to airspaces. During expiration the surfactant film is thought to be enriched in DPPC by film compression and preferential adsorption (18,19), which accounts for the low surface tension observed. If surfactant were not present, the alveoli would collapse on expiration, and an enormous force would have to be supplied by the respiratory muscles to reinflate the lungs. Surface tension in the normal lung is between values close to zero (end-expiration) to 25 mN/m (end-inspiration) during the respiratory cycle. In addition to lipids, pulmonary surfactant contains two hydrophobic proteins; surfactant protein-B (SP-B) and SP-C, and two hydrophilic proteins; SP-A and SP-D. SP-A regulates the amount of surfactant secreted through a receptor-mediated process and, together with SP-B, is essential for the formation of tubular myelin in the hypophase. When combined with SP-B and SP-C, SP-A has the capacity of accelerating the adsorption process and enriching the film with DPPC, thereby reducing the compression requirement and stabilizing the film (20–22). Thus, SP-A plays an important role in maintaining mechanical stability of the lung's terminal airspaces (23). SP-B and SP-C are responsible for the low surface tension, by facilitating the transfer of surfactant lipids to the surface film.

The formation of tubular myelin requires the presence of phosphatidylglycerol and both SP-A and SP-B (24,25). Gene knockout studies indicate that SP-B is essential for the functioning of normal surfactant (26,27). SP-A is essential when surfactant concentrations are limited, such as in severe neonatal respiratory distress syndrome (RDS), or when the surfactant is compromised by the presence of inhibitory serum proteins (28,29).

Surfactant lipids and apoproteins are synthesized by the type-II pneumonocytes. The proteins are formed on the rough endoplasmic reticulum, whereas the lipids are synthesized inside the Golgi apparatus. The lipids are transported to lamellar bodies where they are stored (Fig. 1). Here they are organized in the form of concentrically arranged and tightly packed phospholipid bilayers. Lamellar bodies contain most of the lipid constituents of surfactant (30). The lipids are arrayed into bilayers that form concentric onion-like layers, as revealed by morphological techniques (31). A close investigation of the ultrastructure of a lamellar body shows that each lamellar body comprises proteins and lipids. In addition, lamellar bodies contain lysozyme and SP-A (32), but lack SP-D (33).

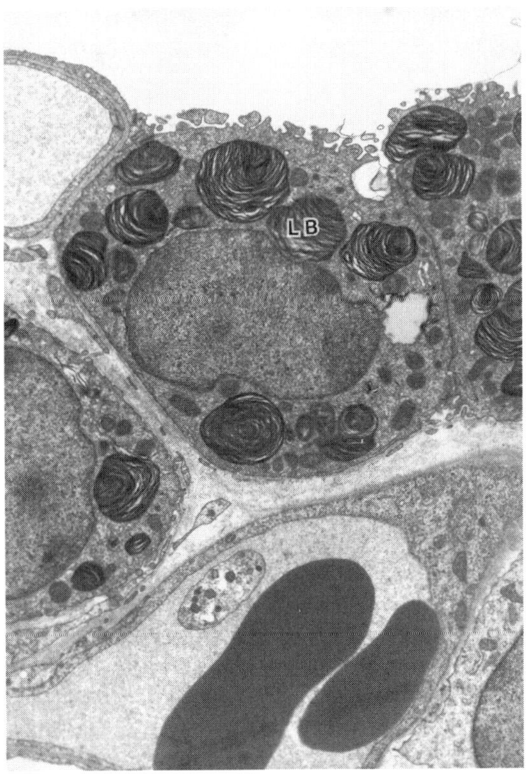

Figure 1 Transmission electron micrograph showing characteristic features of lamellar bodies (LB) within type II cells of a guinea pig lung (magnification × 10,000).

The concentration of calcium ions is quite high within the lamellar bodies, and these ions are bound to phospholipid (34).

The lamellar body contents are secreted from the apices of the type II cells into the alveoli. Secretion appears to involve membrane fusion and exocytosis into the hypophase between the cell and the air surface. After their release, the lamellar bodies become hydrated in the aqueous subphase and unravel into a matrix of tubular myelin (Fig. 2). Tubular myelin is hypothesized to release phospholipid spontaneously to the air–liquid interface where the phospholipids reside in thermodynamically favorable orientation with the acyl chains extending into the air phase, whereas the head groups remain submerged in the aqueous phase. After one or several respiratory cycles, the surfactant material is then forced back into the aqueous phase, where the surfactant forms bilayer vesicles. The vesicles may then enter into either a recycling or degradative pathway (31).

Tubular myelin is often observed in alveolar spaces and is one of the most interesting forms of surfactant. This form is characterized by a highly ordered lattice structure that consists of long tubules, each a square when viewed in cross section (see Fig. 2). Under high-power electron microscopy, the tubules appear

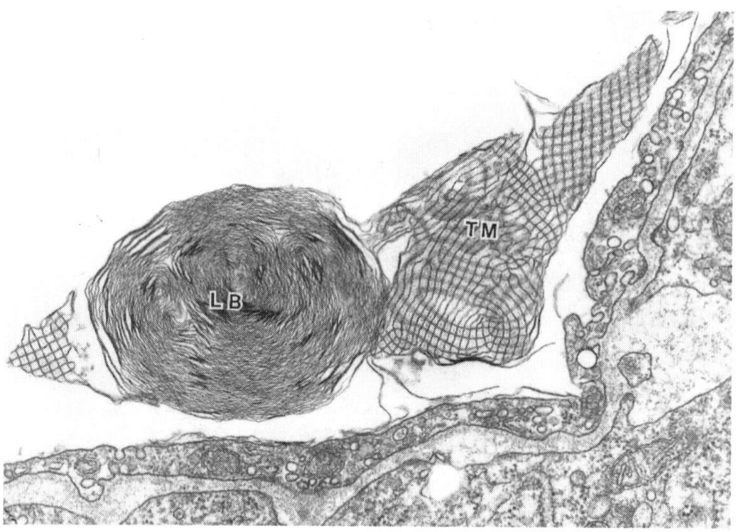

Figure 2 Transmission electron micrograph showing the formation of tubular myelin (TM) from a secreted lamellar body (LB) in the alveolar space of a guinea pig: The unravelling of the lamellar body to form the tubular myelin can be seen. There is a fuzzy zone within each interstice of the lattices, which has been shown to contain SP-A (magnification × 40,000).

to be composed of intersecting bilayer membranes. The lattice dimensions are about 45–55 nm (31). Tubular myelin is also characterized by rod-like extramembranous particles that extend from the corner of the tubule to the center (35,36). In vitro experiments using reconstituted lipid–protein systems, with well-defined composition, have shown that the aforementioned particles are SP-A apoproteins. Furthermore, the tubular myelin structures require millimolar concentrations of calcium ions for the lattice network to form, as well as to maintain the integrity of this structure (37). When tubular myelin is placed in EDTA-containing solutions (which chelate calcium), tubular myelin tends to lose its lattice structure and is subsequently converted into a structure that comprises multiple membrane layers separated with a wide intermembrane spacing of about 20–30 nm. The spaces are filled with a filamentous and fuzzy material that does not appear to be particle-like. Further analysis, using immunocytochemistry on frozen thin sections (prepared for electron microscopy), revealed that the fuzzy material is SP-A (31). This observation suggests that SP-A is only partially dissociated from the altered form of tubular myelin when placed in a calcium-chelating solution, or that there might be other molecular species interacting with SP-A inside the tubular myelin, working to maintain the lattice network. Williams et al. (38) have shown in an in vitro experiment using reconstituted SP-A, SP-B, DPPC, PG, and calcium, that tubular myelin can be formed. Although the mechanisms of formation of tubular myelin in vitro may be quite different from those in vivo, the end products are morphologically identical.

Although SP-A is important for the formation of tubular myelin, it is not essential for the formation of the surface film at the air–liquid interface. Other surfactant materials (i.e., SP-B or SP-C–lipid mixtures) can generate surfactant films at the air–liquid interface, with rapid adsorption times and high surface pressures (low surface tension) that closely resemble the characteristics of natural pulmonary surfactant (39).

In the alveolus, surfactant is recycled through reuptake into type II cells (major route, about 90%), or degraded in alveolar macrophages after phagocytosis (about 10%). A smaller fraction (about 1%) is lost to the airways (40,41).

III. Airway Surfactant

Biochemical studies have demonstrated the presence of surface-active components, predominantly phospholipids, in airway secretions (42). Bernhard et al. (43,44) studied the conductive airway phospholipids in the tracheobronchial secretions of adult pigs and compared their results with analyses of bronchoalveolar lavage (BAL) fluid, tracheobronchial epithelium, and lung parenchyma. The composition of the PC and PL molecular species of the tracheal aspirates was similar to that of BAL and lung parenchyma, but differed considerably from that of airway epithelium. Surfactant protein A was decreased in the tracheal aspirates compared with BAL, and SP-B and SP-C were absent, whereas total protein was increased.

Slomiany et al. (45) reported the lipid and protein composition in tracheobronchial secretions from normal individuals and patients with cystic fibrosis. In the normal bronchial secretions, the total phospholipid was only about half as much as has been reported for normal alveolar surfactant (46). The largest differences were in the amounts of lysophosphatidylcholine, 29.5 versus 0.4%, sphingomyelin, 15.8 versus 3.7%, and phosphatidylethanolamine, 12.4 versus 2.6%, respectively. The differences in the surfactant composition between alveolar and airway surfactant may be due to the addition of mucus from goblet cells and submucosal mucous glands (47), and the contribution of Clara cells (48).

In contrast with alveolar surfactant, the source of airway surfactant is less clear (49). Since surfactant material is presumed to leave the tracheal surface by mucociliary transport, the surfactant film has to be replenished by local secretion or from the alveolar region. The two options for the origin of airway surfactant are not mutually exclusive, and it is likely that airway surfactant is derived from both alveolar and local sources.

Clements et al. (50) provided indirect evidence that surface-active material from the alveoli may reach the large airways. They showed that when phospholipid-labeled liposomes were deposited in rabbit alveoli, about 1% reached the trachea, whereas 50–60% remained in the lung.

The tendency of surfactant to flow from areas of low surface tension (such as exist in the alveoli at the end of expiration) to areas of high surface tension was recently studied by Grotberg et al. (51), who used a mathematical model of fluid dynamics: Exogenous surfactant would be carried along a surface tension gradient by a net force acting to pull the surface film in the direction of the higher surface tension. This motion is resisted by a viscous shear stress acting in the liquid layer just beneath the surface. This shear stress, in turn, drags the liquid within the entire liquid layer in the direction of the higher surface tension, producing a bulk convection. This bulk convection caused by a surface tension gradient is called the ''Marangoni effect'' (52). Expansion and contraction of the surface film during respiration will probably assist in the clearance of particles deposited on the airways (53–55).

If local production of surfactant components occurs in the airways, which cells are involved? One candidate is the Clara cell. Clara cells are nonciliated, nonmucous secretory cells, located in the surface epithelium of the airways (48,56). They are usually found in the bronchioles (56). Occasionally, cells resembling Clara cells morphologically are found in larger airways, including the trachea. There is variability in the cellular and organellar distribution among different species. In the adult human, they are restricted to the terminal bronchioles, where they bulge into the airway lumen. They contain electron-dense granules, approximately 500–600 nm in diameter. The function of Clara cells is thought to involve secretion of a hypophase constituent of mucus (6,57). They contain the surfactant-associated proteins SP-A, -B, and -D (33), and are reported to secrete a leukocyte protease inhibitor and a trypsin-like protease (56,58). They may also act as stem cells for the small airways (59).

Another source of airway lipids may be airway secretory cells, such as mucous and serous cells (60). Explants of human bronchi that include mucous glands synthesize cholesterol, phosphatidylcholine, and phosphatidylethanolamine (42). Phospholipids are found in the secretory granules of airway submucosal glands, suggesting local production of phospholipids at these sites (47). The breakdown of cellular membrane material from epithelial cells and macrophages could also be a source of surface-active lipids, and some lipids may be derived from plasma. Plasma-rich exudates containing lipid and lamellar material have been demonstrated by electron microscopy in the airway secretions of the guinea pig when injured by an acid aerosol (14). Cellular and plasma sources of lipid (phospholipid) may be more important in damaged than in healthy airways. Epithelial cells of the tracheobronchial tree of the human also have the capacity to synthesize SP-A (61,62), SP-B, and SP-C (63). The fate of airway surfactant is unknown, but it is more likely that it is expectorated or swallowed than recycled.

IV. Determination of Surface Tension of Airway Surfactant

The technique used for measuring surface tension of the alveolar surface film has been used to measure surface tension in the larger airways. The method is based on the spreading properties of oil droplets; for example, a mixture of dimethylphthalate and normal octanol (DMP/O) pigmented with crystal violet (64). The oil droplets have negligible solubility in water and when placed onto surfactant films in the Langmuir–Wilhelmy balance change their diameter with changing film surface tension in a reversible fashion. As the film surface tension increases, the droplet diameter increases, and with decreasing film surface tension, the droplet diameter decreases. The computation of the surface tension of the air–water interface at the surface of a trachea, denoted as $\gamma_{A/W}$ has been described (14).

With this method, the tracheal surface tension has been measured in sheep and rodents in vitro and in sheep and horses in vivo. The latter experiments involved placing oil droplets onto the tracheas or bronchi of anesthetized sheep and horses or onto the tracheas of nonanesthetized horses through a bronchoscope

(7,8). The surface tension of the tracheal wall in the normal rat, guinea pig, sheep, and horse is approximately 32–33 mN/m, substantially more than the plateau surface tension (23–25 mN/m) of alveolar surfactant extracts from mammalian lungs. These data are consistent with recent studies in the pig, using relatively pure extracts of tracheal fluid, that have shown that the surface tension properties of tracheal fluid are considerably less than those of BAL fluid (44).

The reason(s) for the difference in equilibrium surface tensions of airway and alveolus are unknown, but they may reflect differences in the composition, concentration, or both, of the surfactant of the two compartments. As the rate of adsorption of lipids to the film interface depends on both the composition and concentration of the surfactant phospholipids and the associated surfactant proteins (23,65), the low SP-A and absent SP-B and SP-C in the pig tracheal fluid in the foregoing experiments (44) may account for the higher static adsorptions observed in the tracheal fluids from this species.

V. Structure of the Surface Film

A. Preservation of the Surface Film

Ultrastructural studies of airway mucus and alveolar surfactant have been compromised by difficulties of preservation. By conventional aqueous fixation methods, the extracellular fluid lining is dissolved in the fixative more quickly than it can be stabilized. These techniques consist of either instilling the aqueous fixatives through the airways or by immersing small sections of tissue directly into the solution. This process causes the surface film to break up and to be washed away. Better preservation of the surface film was achieved by Weibel and Gil (66), who fixed the tissue by perfusion of the vasculature at controlled pressures. All of these methods used glutaraldehyde as the primary fixative; however, glutaraldehyde may remove structured layers of adsorbed surface-active phospholipid (67). Fixatives using tannic acid in conjunction with reduced amounts of glutaraldehyde may be preferable for preserving lamellated phospholipid structures (67–70), because tannic acid interacts with the choline component of phosphatidylcholine (71).

Other preservation techniques that have achieved success involve freeze–fracture (72), freeze–substitution (73), low-temperature scanning electron microscopy (74), and use of fixative vapors (6); however, these methods are not widely employed in view of their technical complexity. Sims et al. (15,75) and others (14) have used a nonaqueous fixative technique (76) to preserve mucus in bovine, guinea pig, and rat trachea. Adapted from methods originally designed to maintain inflation of lungs through reduction of surface tension, the technique involves dissolving fixative (osmium tetroxide) in a nonaqueous fluorocarbon

(FC) solvent, with the aim of stabilizing mucous glycoprotein and glycosaminoglycan molecules, as well as phospholipids in the surfactant material, before dilution in aqueous fixative can occur.

B. Structure of the Alveolar Surface Film

The precise structure of the film is still in question. The results obtained from the nonaqueous techniques indicate that the fluid lining the alveolus is continuous, varies in thickness from 0.09 μm over protruding features to 0.14 μm over relatively flat areas (74) and may have a variable number of lipid layers at its surface (69). This concept is supported by surface-activity studies, using the captive bubble surfactometer, which indicate that the film can form a reservoir of surface-active material (77).

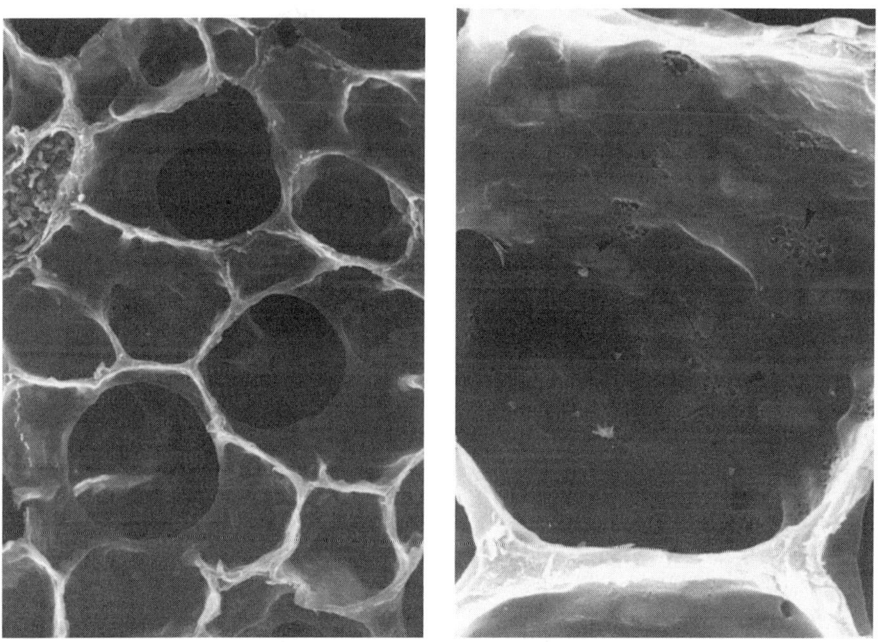

Figure 3 Scanning electron micrograph of a rat lung following fixation with a nonaqueous osmium–fluorocarbon mixture. Surface details of the alveoli, for example microvilli on type II cells or pores of Kohn, are not seen because of the preservation of the surfactant and associated hypophase as a continuous film (magnification × 1000).

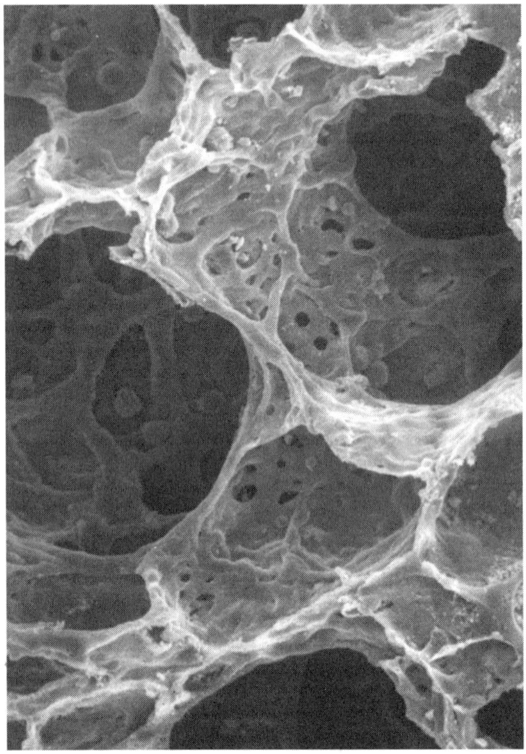

Figure 4 Scanning electron micrograph of alveolar region from rat fixed with aqueous glutaraldehyde: With this preparation the surfactant film is lost and details of the epithelial cells and pores of Kohn can be seen (magnification × 1000).

An aqueous hypophase lies beneath the surface film and above the epithelium. Its thickness may vary depending on its location within the alveolus (74). The hypophase has an amorphous structure and contains proteins, proteoglycans, lipoproteins, lipid micelles, and tubular myelin (78).

The film appears continuous over the alveolar surface and covers the pores of Kohn (74; Figs. 3 and 4). By transmission electron microscopy (TEM) the surface film is seen to be multilayered (Fig. 5), consistent with the concept of a surfactant reservoir. The mechanism of formation of this multilayered film and the ways in which respiratory forces interact with it are not understood. One model proposed by Ries and Swift (79) is shown in Figure 6.

C. Structure of the Airway Surface Film

The aqueous layer covering the walls of the airways is thought to consist of two phases, a less viscous sol phase, in which the cilia beat and, above, a more viscous gel phase, the mucous blanket (6,80; Fig. 7). The relatively low viscosity of the sol layer allows the cilia to beat freely. This blanket, containing trapped particles, is moved toward the pharynx by ciliary action. Its total thickness varies from 5–30 μm in the trachea (75) to less than 1 μm in the peripheral airways, and shows

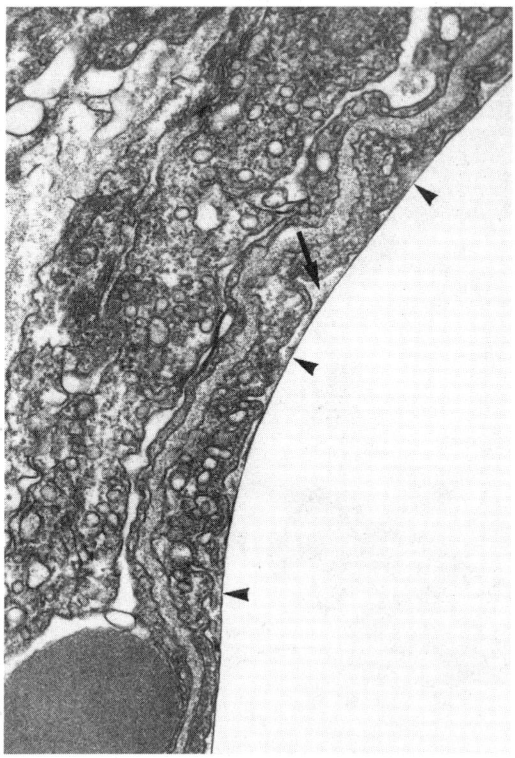

(a)

Figure 5 (a) Transmission electron micrograph from guinea pig lung following fixation with nonaqueous osmium–fluorocarbon mixture. The surfactant film (arrowheads) is preserved and continuous, and overlies a thin hypophase (arrow) above the type I epithelium. (b) Higher magnification of the alveolar surface film from a guinea pig showing that it is multilaminated. (c) Close-up of boxed area showing variation in the number of lamellae from two to seven (magnification: a, × 6000; b, × 100,000; c, × 200,000).

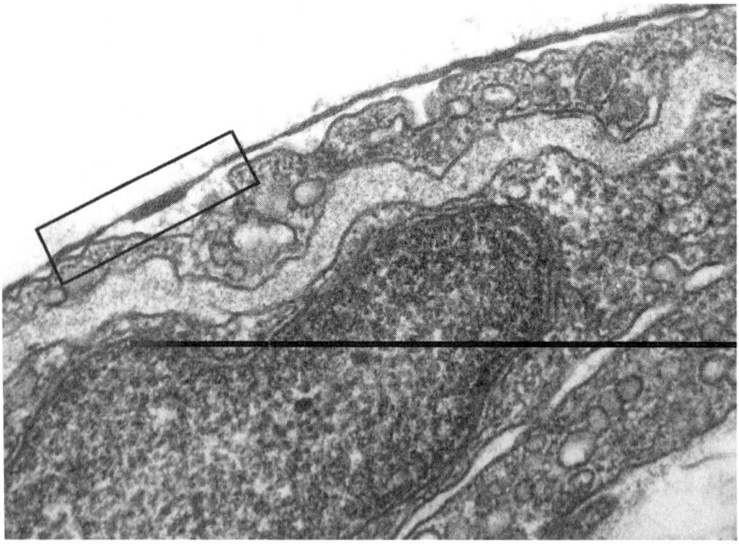

(b)

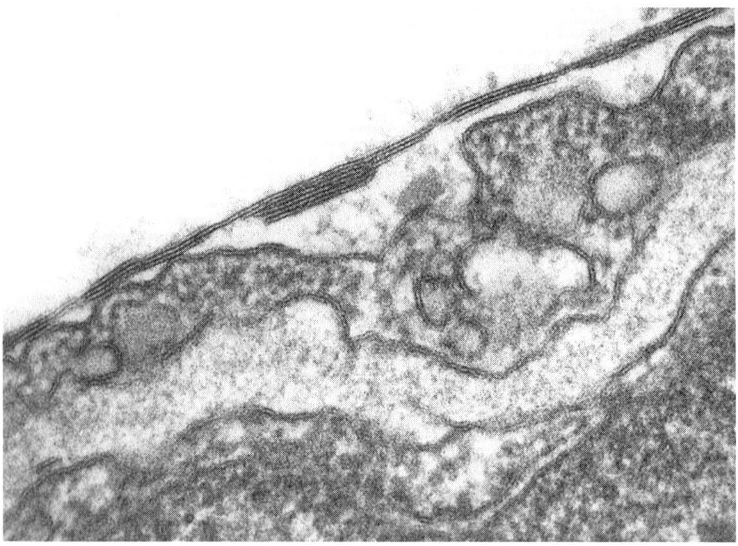

(c)

Figure 5 Continued

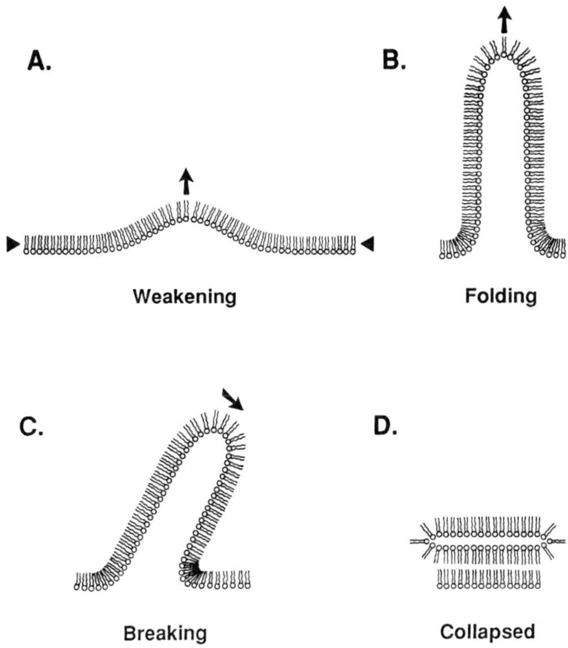

Figure 6 Schematic showing a possible mechanism whereby a multilayer of surfactant can be formed: The monolayer of the surfactant film A is being compressed (arrowheads) slightly beyond the closest packing configuration allowed by DPPC molecules. In this configuration, some DPPC molecules begin to lift off from the interface in the Z direction. This is called the weakening state. The configuration in B shows the folding state in which some film material exists in a bilayer configuration in the airphase. On further compression, the breaking state C sets in and the folding film surface begins to topple back onto the monolayer. Finally, after the bilayer breaks, the film is in the collapsed state D in which a triple layer is formed. This process can repeat itself to form multilayers. (From Ref. 79.)

variations in thickness with changes in lung volume (81,82). Sturgess (83) reported that the extracellular layer of mucus in the human trachea appears as a smooth, cohesive blanket overlaying the tips of ciliated cells. This smooth layer occasionally shows series of overlapping sheets or plaques of mucus (13,6,84).

There is general agreement that a surfactant film exists at the air–aqueous interface. It appears as a continuous amorphous or multilayered structure (13,14,75). The sol and gel phases have also been reported to be separated by osmiophilic membranes that are thought to consist of surfactant and may act as a lubricant to facilitate sliding of the mucous blanket on the sol phase (6,85–

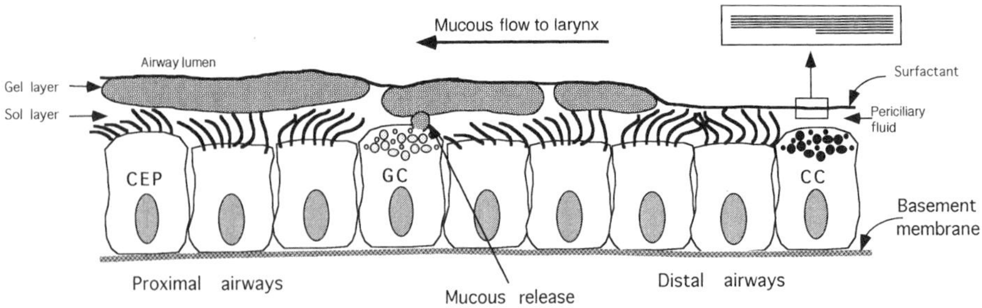

Figure 7 Diagram of mucous blanket of the conducting airways: Although the exact structure of the mucous layer of the airways is unknown, the diagram shows some of the features that have been demonstrated in recent light and electron microscopic studies. An osmiophilic film is seen at the air–liquid interface, which has a multilaminated appearance and exists in various degrees of thickness (see inset). Beneath this surfactant film lies an aqueous hypophase, again of variable thickness, in which are found macrophages, mucus, and osmiophilic lamellar structures. CC, Clara cell; CEP, ciliated epithelial cell; GC, goblet cell.

87). Although such, structures have been observed occasionally in tissue preparations from different species (3,88,89), complete information about their continuity and function is lacking.

When the mucous layer is appropriately preserved, it shows a smooth or slightly undulating surface, as shown in scanning electron micrographs (Fig. 8). By transmission electron microscopy, the top-most layer can be seen to be coated with an osmiophilic film (Fig. 9), which may appear multilayered (Fig. 10). Lamellar bodies and other lipid structures may be present in the sol layer (6,86; Fig. 11). The periodicity of these osmiophilic lamellae has been measured at approximately 40 Å (6), suggesting structural homology with the alveolar lining layer.

Figure 8 (a) Scanning electron micrograph of rat tracheal surface following fixation with osmium–fluorocarbon mixture: The surface film is preserved as a continuous, gently undulating, and smooth-surfaced structure; (b) scanning electron micrograph of rat tracheal surface following aqueous fixation. The mucus layer is lost, revealing ciliated and nonciliated epithelial cells (magnification: a and b, × 3000).

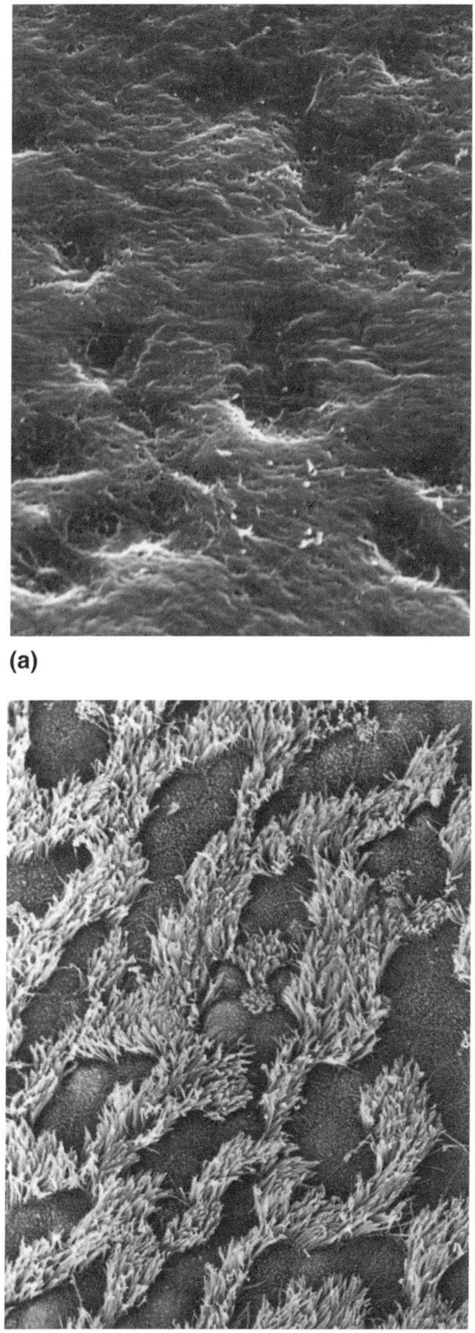

(a)

(b)

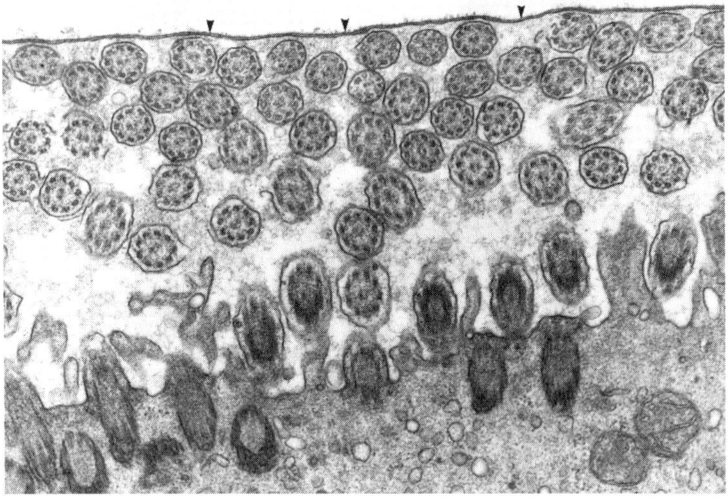

Figure 9 Transmission electron micrograph of the osmiophilic film (arrowheads) in the trachea of a normal guinea pig: The osmiophilic film in this area consists of a bilayer (magnification × 40,000).

VI. Properties of the Surfactant Film

A. Alveolar and Airway Stability

The function of the surfactant film lining the alveolar airspaces in preventing alveolar collapse and in keeping the alveolus relatively dry has been well documented (90). It is also recognized that airway surfactant may confer important mechanical properties, but these have been less studied. The surface tension of airway surfactant is lower than that of other secretions (21). This relatively low surface tension decreases the tendency for small airways to collapse during expiration (5). Liu et al. (91) have studied this function of surfactant in narrow glass pipettes (ID = 400 μm). When 1-μL of saline was deposited in these micropipettes, the apposing surfaces of the liquid inside the glass pipet tended to minimize the excessive surface free energy between the air–liquid interface by forming a ''liquid column.'' This blocked the passage of air through the lumen of the pipette. Calf lung surfactant extract added to the suspension (1 mg/mL) prevented this column from forming, whereas plasma proteins, such as albumin, promoted the formation of a liquid column. The investigators suggested that surfactant was important in maintaining small-airway patency. These findings are supported by theoretical analyses of small-airway closure (92).

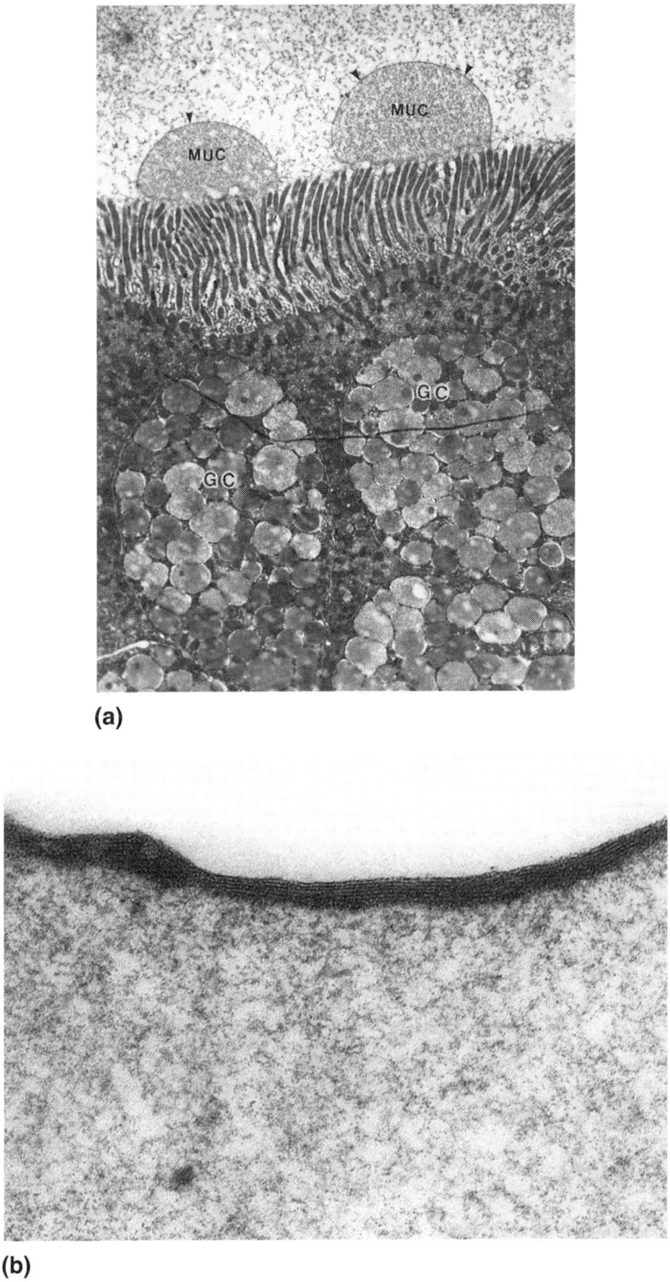

(a)

(b)

Figure 10 (a) Transmission electron micrograph showing mucus (MUC) release from goblet cells (GC) in the mainstem bronchus of a guinea pig induced by an aerosol of hexadecane. Note that the envelope of the bolus of mucus is covered by an osmiophilic film (arrowheads). (b) High-magnification view of the osmiophilic film at the air–liquid interface. The surfactant film is thickened and shows a multilaminated structure (magnification: a, × 7000; b, × 160,000).

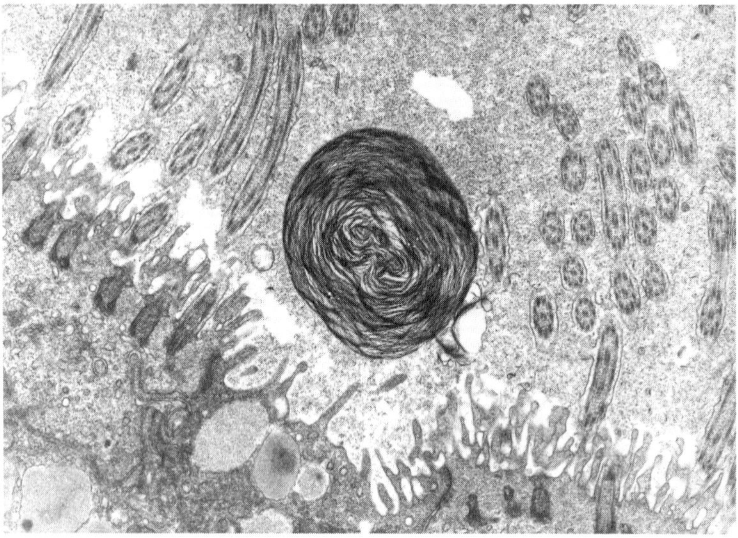

Figure 11 Transmission electron micrograph of area of normal guinea pig trachea showing a lamellar body in the hypophase of the mucus: The source of these lipid structures is unknown. An alveolar origin as well as local secretion have both been proposed (see text; magnification × 20,000).

B. Fluid Balance and Mucus' Viscosity

The surfactant film at the air–mucus interface is probably important for the rheological properties of the extracellular layer by stabilizing the aqueous layer mechanically and by reducing the evaporation of water (54,93). These are well-known functions of surfactant films if spread on top of a water surface (94). Fluid balance in the airway lining layer may also be influenced by the recently demonstrated effect of surfactant in stimulating chloride secretion by airway epithelial cells (95).

VII. Particle–Surfactant Interactions

A. Particle Deposition and Retention

Sneezing, coughing, as well as aerodynamic filtration and bronchoconstriction, serve to protect the gas-exchange surface from the deposition of particles. Particles deposited along the airways stimulate nonspecific and specific defense mechanisms that supplement these structural and mechanical defense mechanisms. The cellular defense components include phagocytes and other immune-competent cells. They are supported by humoral defense components, which include immunoglobulins, factors of the complement system, α_1-antitrypsin, antioxidants, fibronectin, lactoferrin, and surfactant (96–98). Together these components interact to maintain the integrity and sterility of the smaller conducting airways and gas-exchange regions of the lung.

Particles deposited onto the alveolar and airway surfaces are coated with surfactant and displaced into the subphase (2). This film may appear as a multilayered structure. That this film is organized in such a structure at the interface between a fluid or solid particle and the wall of the airway is interesting. The generation of multilayered structures might be related to the movement of surfactant molecules owing to a surface tension gradient related to the Marangoni effect (99,100). This effect involves the surface movement of molecules of an interfacial film (surfactant in our particular example) in the presence of a surface tension gradient. Figure 12 illustrates this phenomenon. The surface tension gradient can be induced by either a contraction or extension of the interface. For either a droplet or a particle deposited onto the tracheal wall surface, the interface will be expanded, causing a surface tension gradient. The surface tension gradient may decrease in two ways: (1) through a process whereby the moving surface (deformed surface) pulls along with it a given amount of surface film, and (2) the deformed surface can adsorb from the bulk phase new surfactant material. Of the two mechanisms, the first one occurs much more rapidly than the second.

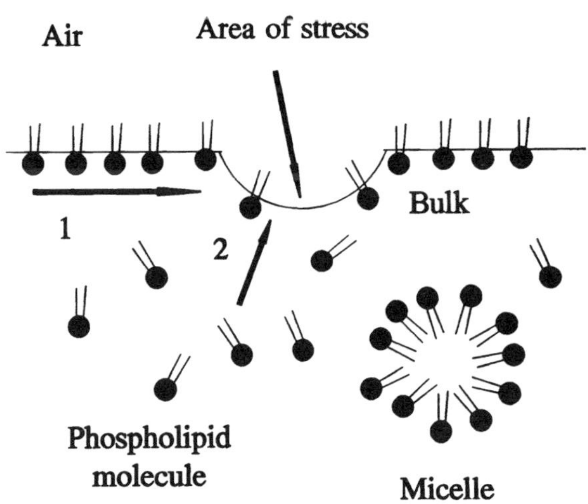

Figure 12 Schematic of the plateau–Marangoni–Gibbs effect: As the surface area of the air interface is impacted, a surface tension gradient is created locally resulting in the movement of phospholipid molecules toward areas of stress. (From Ref. 99.)

Another property of the surface film is to displace particles into the aqueous phase toward the epithelium (1,4). The extent of particle immersion depends on the surface tension of the surface film. The lower the surface tension, the greater the immersion into the subphase (21). As can be seen from the force analysis in Figure 13, the surface tension force generated by the surfactant film during the immersion of a small particle is orders of magnitude greater than the forces related to gravity. The magnitude of the surface forces that can be exerted on a particle depend on the surface chemistry of the particle, its geometry, and the surface tension of the surfactant film. More specifically, the surface tension force promoting particle immersion depends on the magnitude of the film tension and the wetting contact angle which, in turn, depends on the film surface tension and the free energies between particle and air and particle and fluid. Thus, particles having a relatively low surface free energy (e.g., Teflon) will generally be immersed less than high-energy particles (e.g., glass) for a given film surface tension. Hydrated particles, such as bacteria, with a surface free energy of approximately 70 mJ/m^2 would be displaced forcefully into the aqueous layer below the surfactant film.

Small particles, a few microns in diameter or less, are displaced to a greater extent than larger ones of the same surface chemistry. This is likely a consequence of line tension acting on the three-phase line between the air, particle, and film, during the immersion process (101–103; Figs. 13 and 14). For relatively large particles this effect is negligible, but it plays a significant role for small particles in the micrometer or submicrometer range (21). For discussion of line tension effects, see Chapter 6.

Furthermore, the wetting properties of particles with sharp edges is different from those of smooth, spherical particles. Oliver et al. (104) have shown theoretically and experimentally, using a circular sapphire disk with a 90° edge, that sharp edges inhibit the spreading of liquid. Other experiments reported by Lay et al. (105) have shown that submicron sulfur colloid particles with sharp edges, when instilled into the dog bronchus, were cleared rapidly (within 24 hr) by mucociliary transport, rather than by transepithelial adsorption. As might be expected from the effect of line tension on the displacement of small particles, submicron particles should be submersed mainly by line tension and brought into close proximity to the epithelial cells and cleared slowly. The fact that clearance was relatively fast supports the notion that the sharp edges on the sulfur colloid particles resisted wetting. Thus, the particles may not have come into close contact with the epithelium for transepithelial adsorption. Studies on wetting of talc particles in the modified Wilhelmy balance lends support to the concept that sharp edges resist wetting (106).

B. Particle Clearance

Clearance of insoluble particles from the airways and respiratory surfaces in the lungs is thought to take place in two phases (107–109). Respirable particles de-

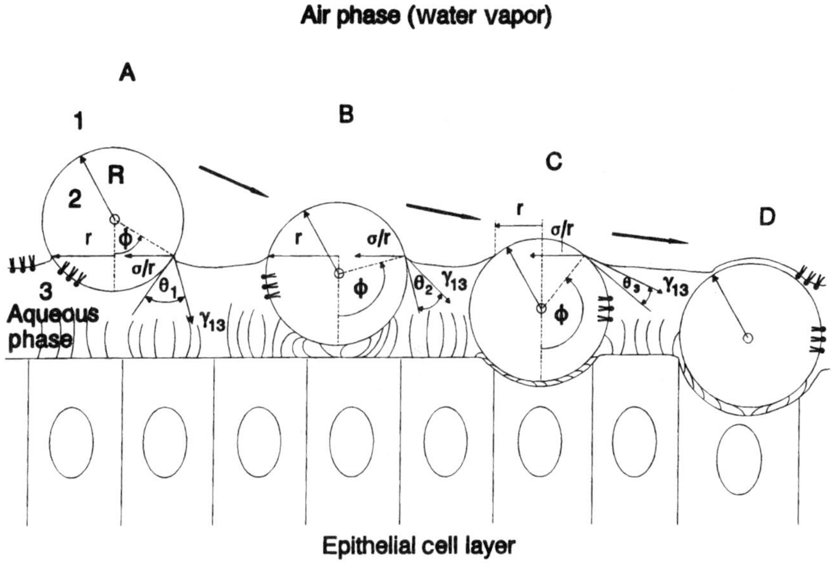

Figure 13 Schematic of particle displacement into the epithelium. The solid spherical particle under consideration has a radius, R. In addition to the interfacial tension γ, the line tension contribution to the mechanical equilibrium, σ/r (two-dimensional pressure), is considered. Line tension is the one-dimensional analogue of surface tension or the excess free energy density associated with the linear phase (three-phase line) where the phases vapor (1), fluid + film (3), and solid (2) join. The contact angle θ is determined by the three interfacial tensions and the two-dimensional pressure σ/r, directed toward the center of the three-phase line, σ is the line tension and r represents the radius of the three-phase line. ϕ indicates the position of the three-phase line. (A) The particle immediately after deposition onto the surfactant film. Here the particle equator is above the water level and σ/r tends to prevent wetting. However, the vertical component of γ_{13} (not shown) is dominant here. (B) The particle is further displaced until contact with the epithelial cell layer is established. The line tension promotes wetting because the particle equator is below the water level. The effect of line tension is to reduce the length of the three-phase line and, thereby, reduces the contact angle to a smaller value, θ_2. (C) The surface tension γ_{13}, in conjunction with the line tension σ promotes further particle displacement; the cell layer is deformed by the particle. The value of θ_3 is substantially lower than the original contact angle θ_1, because of the line tension contribution. (D) The particle is sitting below the surfactant film, which may be considered as an elastic skin keeping the particle submerged. Here, there is no longer an air–particle–water three-phase line and thus no line tension. Note: In (B) and (C) only σ/r is drawn.

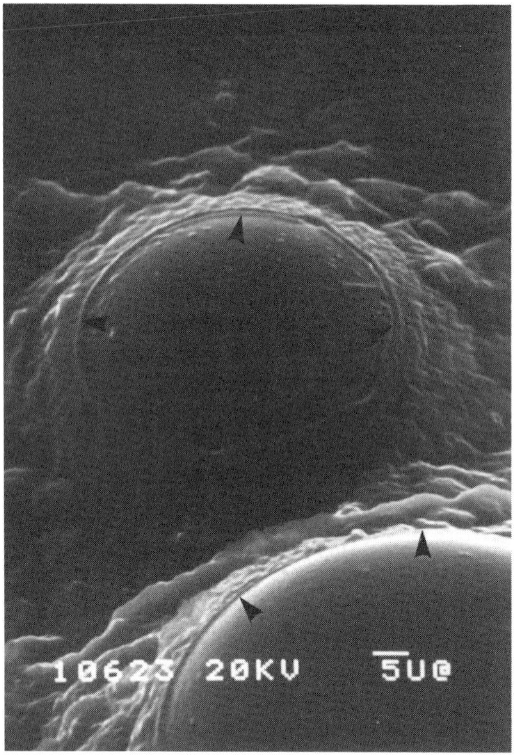

Figure 14 Scanning electron micrograph showing two (50-μm) polymethacrylate acetate (PMMA) particles partially submerged in the mucous layer of a rat trachea: The three-phase line (air–particle–liquid), where line tension has its effect, is shown by the arrowheads (magnification × 3000).

posited in the conducting airways are generally cleared within 24 hr (105,110). However a proportion of the smaller particles may be retained for an extended period (3,11,111). Clearance of particles deposited in the gas-exchange region is slow by comparison; may last for months or years; and involves phagocytosis by alveolar macrophages, macrophage migration, and eventually, mucociliary transportation. Mucociliary clearance maintains the sterility of the distal airways and lung parenchyma by the constant sweeping of the mucosal surface of foreign substances, such as bacteria and respired particles.

The direction of flow of mucus is from the small airways to the larynx. To prevent drowning in mucus, the ciliary beat frequency and mucus's velocity increase from distal to proximal airways (112). At the pharynx, the mucus is either swallowed or expectorated. Particle deposition appears to trigger the rapid release of mucus from goblet cells and submucosal mucous glands (14,113,114), which serves to dilute the particle concentration per unit volume. The mechanism for this response is unknown, but may involve both local mechanisms and vagal reflexes (114–116; see also Chap. 13). Changes in surface tension caused by expansion and contraction of the surface film during respiration, and surface tension gradients along the airways may enhance particle clearance (54,55,82). Surfactant also enhances particle clearance by accelerating ciliary beat frequency (85,117,118) and by conditioning the viscosity of the mucus (119,120). These latter effects might be mediated by the stimulatory effects of surfactant on chloride ion transport across airway epithelium (95).

The lipid fraction of airway surfactant may also modify the rheology of mucus (49). The addition of combinations of mixtures of lipids or exogenous surfactant to mucus reduces its viscosity (49,121) and enhances mucociliary clearance (118). One reason for this effect could be the higher surface pressure of the surfactant film because of the decrease in surface tension (increase in surface pressure) from higher than 30 mN/m to 23–25 mN/m. An increase in surface pressure may result in damping of the high-frequency surface waves (ripples) at the interface between air and liquid owing to the adsorbed surface film (122). This inhibition of wave motion might reduce energy dissipation and thereby, allow a more efficient transfer of the ciliary kinetic energy to the mucous layer.

There is a strong interaction between retained particles and macrophages residing in the aqueous phase of the surface mucus (108,123,124). Most airway macrophages are probably eliminated by mucociliary clearance; however, a small percentage of the macrophages may reenter the pulmonary tissue to join the interstitial macrophage populations or may be further cleared through the lymphatics into other lung compartments, including the pleura, perivascular and peribronchial–bronchiolar connective tissue, or into the regional lymph nodes, where they could be retained for months or years (125).

Uptake of particles by the epithelium is likely to be enhanced by airway surfactant and could account for the delayed clearance of fine and ultrafine particles from the airways noted in some studies (126,127). Forces from the free energy at interfaces and dividing lines might also contribute substantially to particle–cell interactions. These interactions are considered nonspecific, in contrast with the specific receptor–ligand interactions. Thus, nonspecific interactions could contribute to the uptake of particles by cells that are not professional phagocytes, such as epithelial cells. Epithelial cells of the airways take up particles such as silica and asbestos (128,129).

Within the epithelium resides a population of bone marrow–derived phagocytic cells (airway dendritic cells or Langerhans cells) that constitute the principal population of antigen-presenting cells in the airways (130,131). They extend long cytoplasmic filaments between the epithelial cells to form a continuous network of extensions in the horizontal plane of the mucosa. Stimulation of the airway mucosa by particulate antigen leads to rapid recruitment of dendritic cells to the airway mucosa (132). Following immune stimulation, they can rapidly withdraw their cytoplasmic extensions and migrate to the regional lymph nodes. Particles within their cytoplasm would also be transported to these sites (see also Chap. 11).

C. Particle Toxicity

The initial contact between inhaled particles and the host will occur at the air–liquid interface of the conducting airways and alveoli, where they will become coated with surfactant. The amount of a surfactant adsorbed to the surface of particles of quartz or kaolin after mild saline rinsing amounted to the equivalent of a bilayer, in which one monolayer coats the particle with their zwitterionic headgroups toward the dust's surface and the ionic phosphorylcholine heads of the second layer orientated toward the aqueous phase (133). These in vitro observations are in keeping with the observations of deposited particles studied by electron microscopy, which show coating with a bilamellar film (2).

In vitro studies with DPPC, a primary component of surfactant, absorbed to mineral and organic particles have shown a marked suppression of their cytotoxic activity (134–136). This effect was demonstrated as long ago as 1957 (136), when it was demonstrated that quartz cytotoxicity was reduced following the adsorption of surfactant.

In vivo, most inhaled mineral dust particles are rapidly phagocytosed into macrophages and incorporated into secondary lysosomes; surfactant coating enhances this process (137). In the intracellular environment, particles are exposed to hydrolytic lysosomal enzymes, including phospholipase A_2. In vitro studies modeling this process have shown that removal of the lipid coating by phospholipase A_2 restores the cytotoxicity of mineral dusts (133). The rate of removal of the surfactant coating by macrophages is different for kaolin and quartz; the coating being removed more slowly from kaolin than from quartz (138). Thus, the strength of adsorption of surfactant to the particle surface and the kinetics of desorption in the lysosome may account for the differences in cytotoxicity between these dusts (139). These models are consistent with the prompt neutralization of particle toxicity by adsorbed surfactant and a gradual retoxification within the macrophage (140).

The reduced cytotoxicity of surfactant-coated particles may be related to a suppression of surface free radical activity (141) by surfactant. Natural surfactant is capable of scavenging hydrogen peroxide (H_2O_2), the oxygen free radicals ($O^\bullet$ and $OH^\bullet$), and radical species derived from peroxynitrite (142). In the process, peroxidation of unsaturated lipids in surfactant and degradation of surfactant proteins may occur with impairment of surfactant function (98,143–148), and type II cell metabolism (149).

Alveolar lining fluid (98,150–152) and airway mucus (153–155) also contain potent antioxidants, including catalase, superoxide dismutase, peroxidases, and glutathione. These enzymes are physically associated with airway and alveolar surfactant and may serve to protect surfactant from oxidative injury.

Prolonged inhalation of dusts by humans (156), rodents (157,158), and other species (159,160) is associated with an increase in the number of type II cells and increased secretion of surfactant. The stimulation of surfactant appears to be directly related to the toxicity of the dust. It may be so florid, as in acute silicosis, that flooding of the alveolar spaces with surfactant lipids and associated proteins may occur, a condition known as alveolar lipoproteinosis (156). In experimental lipoproteinosis in the rat, the major lipid component is disaturated phosphatidylcholine (157), but all lipid fractions are increased. In the sheep model of experimental silicosis, phosphatidylglycerol, phosphatidylethanolamine, and phosphatidylinositol, showed the greatest increases following silica exposure (159). The excess production of surfactant in response to silica dust may be an adaptive response, perhaps to reduce particle cytotoxicity or to compensate for oxidant-induced lipid peroxidation (147,161).

The adsorption of surfactant to particles could also affect the surface tension in the conducting airways or alveoli. Ma et al. (162) noted a significant increase in surface tension when kaolin and other particles were sprinkled onto a surfactant-rich film in a Wilhelmy balance. This phenomenon has also been reported for the bronchographic agent tantalum (163) and for particles of coal and silica (164). A significant biological effect would probably be seen in vivo only for fine and ultrafine particles, such as fumes and smoke (165), which have high surface areas relative to their mass. Abnormalities of surfactant function have also been reported in BAL fluid from cigarette smokers (165–170).

The adsorption of surfactant to porous particles, such as diesel exhaust soot, containing absorbed mutagens (171) might affect their genotoxic activity. Particle-free surfactant extracts of diesel soot are not mutagenic in vitro (171,172). However, particles dispersed in surfactant show greater genotoxic activity in a variety of assays than particles dispersed in saline (173,174). The increased genotoxicity of surfactant-coated particles in microbial and eukaryotic cell systems may be related to trapping of mutagens within the particle, or to changes in the surface free energies of surfactant-coated particles with enhanced cellular uptake.

By contrast, surfactant coating of nonporous particles, such as silica and asbestos (175), may result in a decrease in genotoxicity. This effect may be due to a masking of surface-active sites by surfactant lipids and is in keeping with the ability of surfactant to reduce particle cytotoxicity.

D. Surfactant Interactions with Infectious Agents

Antimicrobial Activity

Adherence of a microbe to the mucosal surface precedes its colonization and subsequent proliferation (176). The mechanical properties of surfactant that promote particle displacement (see Fig. 14) may have the unwanted effect of increasing epithelial cell–particle contact. Fortunately, surfactant may be capable of impeding adherence of a microbe to an epithelial cell (97). By coating microbial agents, surfactants can also enhance phagocytosis and subsequent intracellular killing by alveolar macrophages (177–179). Surfactant has direct antimicrobial properties (96); the long chain free fatty acids in rat BAL fluid are able to kill pneumococci extracellularly (180). These properties of surfactant appear to reside in specific components of whole surfactant.

Surfactant Proteins

The most abundant surfactant protein, SP-A, appears to play a major role in macrophage function (181). SP-A binds with high affinity to alveolar macrophages through a specific cell surface receptor, probably by its collagen-like tail (182,183). SP-A potentiates the antimicrobial functions of alveolar macrophages, suggesting that it acts as an opsonin (184–186). The collagen-like domain of SP-A also plays a role in the chemotactic migration of alveolar macrophages to sites of inflammation (187). The abundance of SP-A in tracheal and bronchial glands and in epithelium of airways, at all levels of the lung, supports the concept that SP-A provides an important nonimmune mechanism for control of airway infection.

The hydrophilic surfactant proteins, SP-A and SP-D, appear to function as collectins, a group of proteins that selectively recognize and bind to configurations of carbohydrates and lipopolysaccharides on the surface of viral and bacterial pathogens in the presence of Ca^{2+} and enhance their phagocytosis (17,188–191). This occurs with organisms, such as group B hemolytic streptococci and *Pneumocystis carinii*, that have oligosaccharides in their surface membranes or capsular material (192). Because this process does not require specific immune recognition, it elicits a response within minutes of exposure, providing a rapid first-line defense against invading microorganisms. The ability of SP-A to bind to both microorganisms and macrophages may be a disadvantage to the immunocompromised host: Elevated levels of SP-A in the lungs of HIV-infected individuals increased the attachment of tubercle bacilli to alveolar macrophages (193).

The enhanced killing of bacteria by macrophages in the presence of SP-A and SP-D involves chemotaxis (187), opsonization (184,186), activation of complement (185), and the stimulation of superoxide radical and proteolytic enzymes (184,185). SP-A may also regulate cytokine release from alveolar type II cells (194).

Surfactant Lipids

Unlike surfactant proteins, which appear to stimulate cellular defense mechanisms, the lipid component of surfactant may dampen inflammatory reactions (97). Surfactant lipids suppress the release of inflammatory cytokines (195,196) and prostanoids (197) by monocytes, and inhibit fibrogenesis (161). Surfactant phospholipids also appear to inhibit activation of both T and B lymphocytes (97,198–201).

VIII. Implications for Disease States

A. Particle-Induced Acute Lung Injury

Adverse effects on pulmonary surfactant have been demonstrated after experimental exposures to wood smoke (165), hydrochloric acid (202), hypochlorous acid (203), and toxic gases, such as hydrogen sulfide (36,204), nitrogen dioxide (205), nitric oxide (147), ozone (206), sulfur dioxide (53), and other particles (207).

Impairment of lung surfactant activity is a frequent finding in models of lung injury involving the alveolar capillary membrane at which there is leakage of blood components into the alveoli. Plasma proteins, including immunoglobulins, albumin, fibrinogen, and fibrin monomer; matrix molecules, for example, elastin; and components of erythrocytes, all functionally impair the surface tension properties of natural surfactant (208–215).

Recent evidence indicates that the mechanisms of inhibition by proteins may involve competition between the surfactant phospholipids and proteins for space at the air–liquid interface (210–212). In certain systems, the inhibitory effect of a protein on surfactant activity can be reduced by increasing the surfactant concentraton in the assay (210,211).

Mechanisms involving inflammatory cells or their products could also account for the dysfunction of surfactant in acute lung injury. Inhaled particles, such as asbestos and silica, stimulate macrophages to release reactive oxygen metabolites (216,217). Activated neutrophils also release proteolytic enzymes, such as elastase and lysozyme (218,219). Activated polymorphonuclear leukocytes impair surfactant function through a process that involves proteolysis of surfactant proteins (148,220). SP-A also has antioxidant properties of its own (220,221).

Loss of alveolar surfactant activity is likely to have pathophysiological consequences. These might include an increase in the work of breathing, owing to focal or widespread atelectasis (222); augmentation of pulmonary edema, consequent to a reduction in interstitial hydrostatic pressure (223); and increased susceptibility to infection, owing to loss of the antibacterial properties of surfactant (97). Because many of the adverse effects of surfactant deficiency can be reversed in the experimental model by intratracheal instillations of natural and artificial surfactants (224–226) and surfactant-associated proteins (28), it may be appropriate to treat acute lung injury with these preparations.

The effect of particle-induced injury on airway surfactant has been studied in the guinea pig. Animals were exposed to sulfuric acid aerosol at high concentration (43 mg/m^3) for 4 hr (14). The aqueous lining of the airways was preserved using an osmium fluorocarbon fixative (15). Following exposure, the surface of the mucous layer was covered with a granular protein-like material. TEM revealed irregular thickening of the osmiophilic film at the air–mucus interface. The surface tension of the acid-treated tracheas (~32 mN/m) was similar to that of the control animals, and the ability of the mucus to submerge particles was not compromised, indicating that the surface film was functionally normal. It is possible that the known inhibitory effects of tissue injury and protein leakage on surfactant activity were mitigated by an excess of surfactant flowing from the alveolus. The morphological data were consistent with this, for the osmiophilic film at the air–mucus interface was greatly thickened in the acid-exposed animals (15). The source of the additional lipids could have been from injured cell membranes or from lamellar bodies secreted by type II cells.

B. Cystic Fibrosis

The potential role of surfactant in the treatment of cystic fibrosis (CF) was recently reviewed (227). CF is due to an inherited mutation in the cystic fibrosis transmembrane conductance regulator (CFTR) gene on chromosome 7. The defect involves reduced chloride channel activity and ion transport abnormalities that, in turn, cause the increased viscosity and adhesivity of the mucus seen in patients with CF. Tam and Verdugo (228) have shown experimentally that the abnormally viscous mucus found in CF patients might result from defective hydration of the mucus by an altered composition of ions (i.e., Ca^{2+}; 229) in the extracellular fluid lining the mucosal surface. There is evidence that the lipid fraction in the tracheobronchial secretions is altered in CF (45) raising the possibility of an abnormality of airway surfactant in this condition (88,89). The properties of surfactant in stimulating clearance of particles and mucus, its role in maintaining airway hydration (223), its ability to fluidize mucus (121), and its antimicrobial properties, all would, in theory, appear to be of benefit in the treatment of CF.

C. Asthma

By definition, *asthma* is a recurrent reversible obstruction of the airways accompanied by bronchial hyperreactivity and inflammation. It may be triggered by exogenous or endogenous stimuli. Asthma has increased during the last decades, mainly in industrialized countries and, in epidemiological studies, is strongly associated with exposure to fine ($PM_{2.5}$) airborne particles (230–232) and specific allergens. Immune mechanisms as well as nonspecific stimuli can trigger an asthma attack. How inhaled allergens and irritant particulates are processed following deposition in the airways may have profound implications for the genesis of asthma and for the perpetuation of the asthmatic response.

There are many reasons to consider that surfactant may be important in the pathogenesis of asthma. Alveolar and airway surfactant, by lowering surface tension, are important for maintaining small airway patency. Alveolar surfactant, by lowering alveolar surface tension, maintains the tension on the bronchiolar walls and prevents their collapse. Alveolar surfactant may also be involved in the changes in parenchymal lung mechanics induced by hyperpnea in asthmatics (233). Airway surfactant, on the other hand, by preventing or delaying meniscus formation during expiration (51,91,92), maintains airway patency and prevents liquid accumulation in the lumen (82). These properties are inhibited by the presence of proteins (234) that are present during the acute asthmatic response (235).

Surfactant dysfunction has been demonstrated in a guinea pig model of allergic asthma (236), and in this model the airway narrowing can be alleviated by surfactant inhalation (237). Surfactant protein A is deficient in the bronchoalveolar fluid of some asthmatics (238). Recently, Kurashima et al. (239) have demonstrated that, during the early phase of an asthmatic attack, decreases in the surface activity of sputum from asthmatic patients were ameliorated during the late phase, possibly as a result of surfactant recruitment. Pilot studies have shown that surfactant inhalation may alleviate the symptoms of asthma (240).

Surfactant also enhances mucociliary clearance (117) and reduces particle toxicity (139). Mucociliary clearance is impaired in some asthmatics (241). Surfactant's role in promoting displacement and retention of particles in the airways may be important in determining the site and amount of antigen presentation. Enhanced oxygen free radical release by alveolar macrophages from asthmatic patients (242) might be influenced by the hydrophilic proteins in surfactant (185,186,221), or be suppressed by their lipid components (151,218,225). Recently, it has been proposed (67) that the hyperresponsiveness characteristic of asthma may result from the unmasking of surfactant-coated receptors in the airways. The immunosuppressive effects of the lipid component of surfactant (195,197), particularly its effects on IL-2 release and adhesion molecules (243), may also be important in dampening inflammatory reactions that occur at the surface of the airways. Finally, a surfactant layer may have important implications for airway responses to inhaled drugs (244,245).

IX. Summary

Retention of particles by surface and line tension forces exerted on inhaled particles by surfactant situated at the aqueous phase–air phase interface is the initial step of a complex cascade of defense mechanisms in the lungs. Surfactant coating of particles renders them more palatable to phagocytic cells, reduces their cytotoxicity, and enhances mucociliary clearance. Surfactant has important antimicrobial and antioxidant properties. Its role in particle-associated genotoxicity appears to be related to the surface properties of the particle. Given the complexity of the system and the multitude of interactions between inhaled particles and surfactant, it is necessary to examine the role of surfactant in diseases associated with particle exposures, such as some forms of acute alveolar injury, cystic fibrosis, and asthma. A knowledge of the mechanisms involved and, in particular, the role of surfactant will greatly enhance our ability to understand these diseases and to develop appropriate therapeutic strategies.

Acknowledgments

The authors thank Mr. W. Dong for technical assistance. This work was supported by the Swiss National Science Foundation (grant 32-32513.91), the Stanley Thomas Johnson Foundation (Switzerland), the MRC grant (MT-6435), the Alberta Heritage Foundation for Medical Research, Canada, and the Alberta and Canadian Lung Associations.

References

1. Gehr P, Green FHY, Geiser M, Im Hof V, Lee MM, Schürch S. Airway surfactant, a primary defense barrier: mechanical and immunological aspects. J Aerosol Med 1996; 9:63–181.
2. Gehr P, Geiser M, Im Hof V, Schürch S, Waber U, Baumann M. Surfactant and inhaled particles in the conducting airways: structural, stereological, and biophysical aspects. Microsc Res Technol 1993; 26:423–436.
3. Gehr P, Schürch S, Berthiaume Y, Im Hof V, Geiser M. Particle retention in airways by surfactant. J Aerosol Med 1990; 1:27–43.
4. Schürch S, Gehr P, Im Hof V, Geiser M, Green F. Surfactant displaces particles toward the epithelium in airways and alveoli. Respir Physiol 1990; 80:17–32.
5. Macklem PT, Proctor DF, Hogg JC. The stability of peripheral airways. Respir Physiol 1970; 8:191–203.
6. Gil J, Weibel ER. Extracellular lining of bronchioles after perfusion–fixation of rat lungs for electron microscopy. Anat Rec 1971; 169:185–200.
7. Im Hof V, Gehr P, Gerber V, Lee MM, Schürch S. In vivo determination of surface tension in the horse trachea and in vitro model studies. Respir Physiol 1997; 109: 81–93.
8. Im Hof V, Schürch S, Straub R, Gehr P. Surfactant in the trachea of the horse (abstr). Eur Respir J 1990; 3(suppl):257.
9. Holm BA. Surfactant inactivation in adult respiratory distress syndrome. In: Robert-

son B, van Golde LMG, Batenburg JJ, eds. Pulmonary Surfactant: From Molecular Biology to Clinical Practice. Amsterdam: Elsevier Science, 1992:665–684.

10. Neumann AW, Absolom DR, Francis DW, Omenyi SN, Spelt JK, Policova Z, Thomson C, Zingg W, van Oss CJ. Measurement of surface tensions of blood cells and proteins. Ann NY Acad Sci 1983; 416:276–298.
11. Gehr P, Im Hof V, Geiser M, Schürch S. The fate of particles deposited in the intrapulmonary conducting airways. J Aerosol Med 1991; 4:349–361.
12. Gehr P, Schürch S. Surface forces displace particles deposited in airways toward the epithelium. News in Physiological Sciences 1992; 7:1–5.
13. Mercer RR, Russel ML, Crapo JD. Mucous lining layers in human and rat airways (abstr). Am Rev Respir Dis 1992; 145:355.
14. Lee MM, Schürch S, Roth SH, Jiang X, Cheng S, Bjarnason S, Green FHY. Effects of acid aerosol exposure on the surface properties of airway mucus. Exp Lung Res 1995; 21:835–851.
15. Sims DE, Westfall JA, Kiorpes AL, Horne MM. Preservation of tracheal mucus by nonaqueous fixative. Biotech Histochem 1991; 66:173–180.
16. King RJ, Clements JA. Surface active materials from dog lung. II. Composition and physiological correlations. Am J Physiol 1972; 223:715–726.
17. Johansson J, Curstedt T. Molecular structures and interactions of pulmonary surfactant components. Eur J Biochem 1997; 244:675–693.
18. Clements JA. Functions of the alveolar lining. Am Rev Rev Respir Dis 1977; 115: 67–71.
19. Schürch S, Schürch D, Curstedt T, Robertson B. Surface activity of lipid extract surfactant in relation to film area compression and collapse. J Appl Physiol 1994; 77:974–986.
20. Schürch S, Bachofen H, Goerke J, Green F. Surface properties of rat pulmonary surfactant studied with the captive bubble method: adsorption, hysteresis, stability. Biochim Biophys Acta 1992; 1103:127–136.
21. Schürch S, Lee M, Gehr P. Pulmonary surfactant: Surface properties and function of alveolar and airway surfactant. Pure Appl Chem 1992; 64:1747–1750.
22. Keough KMW. Physical chemistry of pulmonary surfactant in the terminal air spaces. In: Robertson B, van Golde LMG, Batenburg JJ, eds. Pulmonary Surfactant: From Molecular Biology to Clinical Practice. Amsterdam: Elsevier Science, 1992: 109–164.
23. Schürch S, Possmayer F, Cheng S, Cockshutt AM. Pulmonary SP-A enhances adsorption and appears to induce surface sorting of lipid extract surfactant. Am J Physiol 1992; 263:L210–L218.
24. Suzuki Y, Fujita Y, Kogishi K. Reconstitution of tubular myelin from synthetic lipids and proteins associated with pig pulmonary surfactant. Am Rev Respir Dis 1989; 140:75–81.
25. Voorhout WF, Veenendaal T, Haagsman HP, Verkleij AJ, van Golde LM, Geuze HJ. Surfactant A is localized at the corners of the pulmonary tubular myelin lattice. J Histochem Cytochem 1991; 39:1331–1336.
26. Clark JC, Wert SE, Bachurski CJ, Stahlman MT, Stripp BR, Weaver TE, Whitsett JA. Targeted disruption of the surfactant protein B gene disrupts surfactant homeostatis, causing respiratory failure in newborn mice. Proc Natl Acad Sci USA 1995; 92:7794–7798.

27. Korfhagen TR, Glasser SW, Wert SE, Bruno MD, Daugherty CC, McNeish JD, Stock JL, Potter SS, Whitsett JA. *cis*-Acting sequences from human surfactant protein gene confer pulmonary-specific gene expression in transgenic mice. Proc Natl Acad Sci USA 1990; 87:6122–6126.
28. Cockshutt AM, Weitz J, Possmayer F. Pulmonary surfactant-associated protein A enhances the surface activity of lipid extract surfactant and reverses inhibition by blood proteins in vitro. Biochemistry 1990; 29:8424–8429.
29. Hallman M, Merritt TA, Akino T, Bry K. Surfactant protein A, phosphatidylcholine, and surfactant inhibitors in epithelial lining fluid. Am Rev Respir Dis 1991; 144:1376–1384.
30. Hallman M, Katsumi M, Wagner RM. Isolated lamellar bodies from rat lung: correlated ultrastructural and biochemical studies. Lab Invest 1976; 35:79–86.
31. Williams MC. Ultrastructure of tubular myelin and lamellar bodies in fast-frozen adult rat lung. Exp Lung Res 1982; 4:37–46.
32. Walker SR, Williams MC, Benson B. Immunocytochemical localization of the major surfactant apoproteins in type II cells, Clara cells and alveolar macrophages of rat lung. J Histochem Cytochem 1986; 34:1137–1148.
33. Voorhout WF, Veenendaal T, Kuroki Y, Ogasawara Y, van Golde LMG, Geuze HJ. Immunocytochemical localization of surfactant protein D (SP-D) in type II cells, Clara cells, and alveolar macrophages of rat lung. J Histochem Cytochem 1992; 40:1589–1597.
34. Eckenhoff RG, Somlyo AP. Rat lung type II cell and lamellar body: elemental composition in situ. Am J Physiol 1988; 254:C614–C620.
35. Hassett RJ, Engleman W, Kuhn C. Extramembranous particles in tubular myelin from rat lung. J Ultrastruct Res 1980; 71:60–67.
36. Haagsman HP, van Golde LMG. Lung surfactant and pulmonary toxicology. Lung 1985; 163:275–303.
37. Hawgood S, Benson BJ, Hamilton RL Jr. Effects of a surfactant-associated protein and calcium ions on the structure and surface activity of lung surfactant lipids. Biochemistry 1985; 24:184–190.
38. Williams MC, Hawgood W, Hamilton RL (1991). Changes in lipid structure produced by surfactant proteins SP-A, SP-B, and SP-C. Am J Respir Cell Mol Biol 1991; 5:41–50.
39. Yu SH, Possmayer F. Role of bovine pulmonary surfactant-associated proteins in the surface active property of phospholipid mixtures. Biochim Biophys Acta 1990; 1046:233–241.
40. Williams MC. Morphologic aspects of the surfactant system. In: Robertson B, van Golde LMG, Batenburg JJ, eds. Pulmonary Surfactant: From Molecular Biology to Clinical Practice. Amsterdam: Elsevier Science, 1992:87–107.
41. Wright JR, Clements JA. Metabolism and turnover of lung surfactant. Am Rev Respir Dis 1987; 135:426–444.
42. Bhaskar KR, O'Sullivan DD, Opaskar-Hincman H, Reid LM. Lipids in airway secretions. Eur J Respir Dis 1987; 71(suppl 153):215–221.
43. Bernhard W, von der Hardt H. Bronchial surfactant: phospholipid classes and phosphatidylcholine molecular species as indicators of its alveolar origin. Appl Cardiopulm Pathol 1995; 5(suppl 3):6–7.

44. Bernhard W, Haagsman HP, Tschernig T, Poets CF, Postle AD, van Eijk ME, von der Hardt H. Conductive airway surfactant: surface-tension function, biochemical composition, and possible alveolar origin. Am J Respir Cell Mol Biol 1997; 17: 41–50.
45. Slomiany A, Murty VLN, Aono M, Snyder CE, Herp A, Slomiany BL. Lipid composition of tracheobronchial secretions from normal individuals and patients with cystic fibrosis. Biochim Biophys Acta 1982; 710:106–111.
46. Hallman M. Lung surfactant phospholipids in the foetus, newborn, and in the adult; evidence of abnormality in respiratory failure. Ann Chir Gynaecol 1982; 196 (suppl):19–23.
47. Girod S, Fuchey C, Galabert C, Lebonvallet S, Bonnet N, Ploton D, Puchelle E. Identification of phospholipids on secretory granules of human submucosal gland respiratory cell. J Histochem Cytochem 1991; 39:193–198.
48. Widdicombe JG, Pack RJ. The Clara cell. Eur J Respir Dis 1982; 63:202–220.
49. Widdicombe JG. Role of lipids in airway function. Eur J Respir Dis 1987; 71(suppl)153:197–204.
50. Clements JA, Oyarzun MJ, Baritussion A. Secretion and clearance of lung surfactant: a brief review. Prog Respir Res 1981; 15:20–26.
51. Grotberg JB, Halpern D, Jensen OE. Interaction of exogenous and endogenous surfactant spreading rate effects. J Appl Physiol 1995; 78:750–756.
52. Adamson AW. Physical Chemistry of Surfaces. 5th ed. New York: John Wiley & Sons, 1990.
53. Weiss JM, Gebhardt KF, Ziegler H, Rensch H. Role of surfactant in peripheral transport mechanisms. Eur J Respir Dis 1987; 71:205–208.
54. Rensch H, von Seefeld H. Surfactant–mucus interaction. In: Robertson B, van Golde LMG, Batenburg JJ, eds. Pulmonary Surfactant: From Molecular Biology to Clinical Practice. Amsterdam: Elsevier Science, 1984:203–214.
55. Rensch H, Von Seefeld H, Gebhardt KF, Renzow D, Sell PJ. Stop and go particle transport in the peripheral airways? A model study. Respiration 1983; 44:346–350.
56. Massaro GD, Singh G, Mason R, Plopper CG, Malkinson AM, Gail DB. Biology of the Clara cell. Am J Physiol 1994; 266:L101–L106.
57. Yoneda K. Mucus blanket of the rat bronchus. Am Rev Respir Dis 1976; 114:837–842.
58. De Water R, Willems LNA, van Muijen GNP, Franken C, Fransen JAM, Dijkman JH, Kramps JA. Ultrastructural localization of bronchial antileukoprotease in central and peripheral human airways by a gold-labeling technique using monoclonal antibodies. Am Rev Respir Dis 1986; 133:882–890.
59. Ayers M, Jeffrey PK. Proliferation and differentiation in adult mammalian airway epithelium: a review. Eur Respir J 1988; 1:58–80.
60. Kim KC, Singh BN. Hydrophobicity of mucin-like glycoproteins secreted by cultured tracheal epithelial cells: association with lipids. Exp Lung Res 1990; 16:279–292.
61. Khoor A, Gray ME, Hull WM, Whitsett JA, Stahlman MT. Developmental expression of SP-A and SP-A mRNA in the proximal and distal respiratory epithelium in the human fetus and newborn. J Histochem Cytochem 1993; 41:1311–1319.

62. Auten R, Watkin RM, Shapiro DL, Horowitz S. Surfactant apoprotein A (SP-A) is synthesized in airway cells. Am J Respir Cell Mol Biol 1990; 3:491–496.
63. Khoor A, Stahlman MT, Gray ME, Whitsett JA. Temporal-spatial distribution of SP-B and SP-C proteins and mRNAs in developing respiratory epithelium of human lung. J Histochem Cytochem 1994; 42:1187–1199.
64. Schürch S, Goerke J, Clements JA. Direct determination of volume- and time-dependence of alveolar surface tension in excised lungs. Proc Natl Acad Sci USA 1978; 75:3417–3421.
65. Putz G, Goerke J, Clements JA. Surface activity of rabbit pulmonary surfactant subfractions at different concentrations in a captive bubble. J Appl Physiol 1994; 77:597–605.
66. Weibel ER, Gil J. Electron microscopic demonstration of an extracellular duplex lining layer of alveoli. Respir Physiol 1968; 4:42–57.
67. Hills BA. A mechanism for masking receptors with particular application to asthma. Med Hypotheses 1996; 46:33–41.
68. Hills BA. Oesophageal surfactant: evidence for a possible mucosal barrier on oesophageal epithelium. Aust NZ J Med 1994; 24:41–46.
69. Nakamura H, Tonosaki A, Washioka H, Takahashi K, Yasui S. Monomolecular surface film and tubular myelin figures of the pulmonary surfactant in hamster lung. Cell Tissue Res 1985; 241:523–528.
70. Ueda S, Kawamura K, Ishii N, et al. Ultrastructural studies on surface lining layer (SLL) of lungs: Part III. Jpn Med Soc Biol Interface 1984; 13:76–88.
71. Kalina M, Pease DC. The preservation of ultrastructure saturated in phosphatidylcholines by tannic acid in model systems and type II pneumocytes. J Cell Biol 1997; 74:726–741.
72. Roth J, Winkelmann H, Meyer HW. Electron microscopic studies in mammalian lungs by freeze-etching. IV. Formation of the superficial layer of the surfactant system by lamellar bodies. Exp Pathol 1973; 8:354–362.
73. Mazzone RW, Durand CM, West JB. Electron microscopy of lung rapidly frozen under controlled physiological conditions. J Appl Physiol Respir Environ Exerc Physiol 1978; 45:325–333.
74. Bastacky J, Lee CYC, Goerke J, Koushafar H, Yager D, Kenaga L, Speed TP, Chen YA. Alveolar lining layer is thin and continuous: low temperature scanning electron microscopy of rat lung. J Appl Physiol 1995; 79:1615–1628.
75. Sims DE, Horne MM. Heterogeneity of the composition and thickness of tracheal mucus in rats. Am J Physiol 1997; 273:L1036–L1041.
76. Thurston RJ, Hess RA, Kilburn KH, McKenzie WN. Ultrastructure of lungs fixed in inflation using a new osmium–fluorocarbon technique. J Ultrastruct Res 1976; 56:39–47.
77. Schürch S, Qanbar R, Bachofen H, Possmayer F. The surface-associated surfactant reservoir in the alveolar lining. Biol Neonate 1995; 67:61–76.
78. Groniowski J, Biczyskowa W. Structure of the alveolar lining film of the lungs. Nature 1964; 204:745–747.
79. Ries RE, Swift H. Twisted double-layer ribbons and the mechanism for monolayer collapse. Langmuir 1987; 3:853–855.

80. Kilburn KH. A hypothesis for pulmonary clearance and its implications. Am Rev Respir Dis 1968; 98:449–463.
81. Yager D, Kamm RD, Drazen JM. Airway wall liquid. Chest 1995; 107:105S–110S.
82. Yager D, Cloutier T, Feldman H, Bastacky J, Drazen JM, Kamm RD. Airway surface liquid thickness as a function of lung volume in small airways of the guinea pig. J Appl Physiol 1994; 77:2333–2340.
83. Sturgess JM. The mucous lining of major bronchi in the rabbit lung. Am Rev Respir Dis 1977; 115:819–827.
84. Van As A, Webster I. The morphology of mucus in mammalian airways. Environ Res 1974; 7:1–12.
85. Allegra L, Bossi R, Braga P. Influence of surfactant on mucociliary transport. Eur J Respir Dis 1985; 67(suppl 142):71–76.
86. Morgenroth K. Morphology of the bronchial lining layer and its alteration in IRDS, ARDS and COLD. Eur J Respir Dis 1985; 67(suppl 142):7–18.
87. Widdicombe JG. Introduction to endobronchial surface active phospholipids: morphology, biochemistry, function and therapeutic aspects. Eur J Respir Dis 1985; 67(suppl 142):1–5.
88. Girod S, Galabert C, Lecuire A, Zahm J-M, Puchelle E. Phospholipid composition and surface-active properties of tracheobronchial secretions from patients with cystic fibrosis and chronic obstructive pulmonary disease. Pedeatr Pulmonal 1992; 13: 22–27.
89. Girod S, Zahm J-M, Plotkowski C, Beck G, Puchelle E. Role of the physicochemical properties of mucus in the protection of the respiratory epithelium. Eur Respir J 1992; 5:477–487.
90. Hamm H, Fabel H, Bartsch W. The surfactant system of the adult lung: physiology and clinical perspective. Clin Invest 1992; 70:637–657.
91. Liu M, Wang L, Li E, Enhorning G. Pulmonary surfactant will secure free airflow through a narrow tube. J Appl Physiol 1991; 71:742–748.
92. Halpern D, Grotberg JB. Surfactant effects on fluid–elastic instabilities of liquid-lined flexible tubes: a model of airway closure. J Biomech Eng 1993; 115:271–277.
93. Evrensel CA, Khan MRU, Elli S, Krumpe PE. Viscous airflow through a rigid tube with a compliant lining: a simple model for the air–mucus interaction in pulmonary airways. J Biomech Eng 1993; 115:262–270.
94. Barnes GT, La Mer VK. The evaporation resistances of monolayers of long-chain acids and alcohols and their mixtures. In: La Mer VK, ed. Retardation of Evaporation by Monolayers: Transport Processes. New York: Academic Press, 1962:9–33.
95. Ikeda K, Sasaki T, Shimura S, Satoh M, Isihara H, Sasaki H, Takishima T, Saitoh Y, Nishiyama A. Effect of surfactant on bioelectric properties of canine tracheal epithelium. Respir Physiol 1990; 81:41–49.
96. Bissetti A. Pulmonary surfactant and respiratory infections. Respiration 1989; 55(suppl 1):45–48.
97. Pison U, Max M, Neuendank A, Weißach S, Pietschmann S. Host defence capacities of pulmonary surfactant: evidence for ''non-surfactant'' functions of the surfactant system. Eur J Clin Invest 1994; 24:586–599.

98. Roveri A, Bruni R, Baritussio A, Coassin M, Benevento M, Baiorino M, Ursini F. Antioxidant defences of rabbit alveolar lining fluid. Respiration 1989; 55(suppl 1): 68–73.
99. Kanner B, Glass JE. Surface viscosity and elasticity: significant parameters in industrial processes. In: Ross S, ed. Chemistry and Physics of Interfaces II. Washington, DC: American Chemical Society 1971:57.
100. Scriven LE, Sternling CV. The Marangoni effects. Nature 1960; 187:186–188.
101. Aveyard R, Clint JH. Particle wettability and line tension. J Chem Soc Faraday Trans 1996; 92:85–89.
102. Wallace JA, Schürch S. Line tension of a sessile drop on a fluid–fluid interface modified by a phospholipid monolayer. J Colloid Interface Sci 1988; 124:452–461.
103. Li D. Drop size dependence of contact angles and line tensions of solid–liquid systems. Colloids Surfaces 1996; 116:1–23.
104. Oliver JF, Huh C, Mason SG. Resistance to spreading of liquids by sharp edges. J Colloid Interface Sci 1977; 59:568–581.
105. Lay JC, Berry CR, Kim CS, Bennett WD. Retention of insoluble particles after local intrabronchial deposition in dogs. J Appl Physiol 1995; 79:1921–1929.
106. Lee MM. Structure and function of the extracellular layer of airspaces and its configuration following deposition of solid and liquid particles. PhD dissertation, The University of Calgary, May 1997:102–117.
107. Ilowite JS, Smaldone GC, Perry RJ, Bennett WD, Foster WM. Relationship between tracheobronchial particle clearance rates and sites of initial deposition in man. Arch Environ Health 1989; 44:267–273.
108. Geiser M, Cruz-Orive LM, Im Hof V, Gehr P. Assessment of particle retention and clearance in the intrapulmonary conducting airways of hamster lungs with the fractionator. J Microsc 1990; 169:75–88.
109. Ferin J. Pulmonary retention and clearance of particles. Toxicol Lett 1994; 72:121–125.
110. Scheuch G, Philipson K, Falk R, Anderson M, Svartengren M, Stahlhofen W, Camner P. Retention of particles inhaled in boli with and without induced bronchoconstriction. Exp Lung Res 1995; 21:901–916.
111. Stahlhofen W, Koebrich R, Rudolf G, Scheuch G. Short- and long-term clearance of particles from the upper human respiratory tract as a function of particle size. J Aerosol Sci 1990(suppl 1); 21:S407–S410.
112. Newhouse M, Sanchis J, Bienenstock J. Lung defense mechanisms [part 1]. N Engl J Med 1976; 295:990–996.
113. Green FHY, Lee MM, Roth SH, Karkhanis A, Schürch S, Schürch D, Bjarnason SG, Vincent R, Gehr P. Effects of solid and liquid acid particles on airway mucus (abstr). J Aerosol Med 1995; 8A:111.
114. Peatfield AC, Richardson PS. The action of dust in the airways on secretion into the trachea of the cat. J Physiol 1983; 342:327–334.
115. Persson CGA. Airway mucosal exudation of plasma. In: Takishima T, Shimura S, eds. Airway Secretion: Physiological Bases for the Control of Mucous Hypersecretion. New York: Marcel Dekker, 1994:451–467.

116. Eljamal M, Wong LB, Yeates DB. Capsaicin-activated bronchial- and alveolar-initiated pathways regulating tracheal ciliary beat frequency. J Appl Physiol 1994; 77:1239–1245.
117. Kakuta Y, Sasaki H, Takishima T. Effect of artificial surfactant on ciliary beat frequency in guinea pig trachea. Respir Physiol 1991; 83:313–322.
118. De Sanctis GT, Tomkiewicz RP, Rubin BK, Schürch S, King M. Exogenous surfactant enhances mucociliary clearance in the anaesthetized dog. Eur Respir J 1994; 7:1616–1621.
119. Gerber V, Gehr P, Straub R, King M, Im Hof V. Mucus quality on horse tracheal epithelium—microscopic grading based on transparency. Respir Physiol 1997; 107: 67–74.
120. Festa E, Saldiva PHN, King M. Effects of bovine surfactant (bLES) on rheological properties and mucociliary transport of respiratory secretions in cystic fibrosis (CF) patients (abstr). Am J Respir Crit Care Med 1995; 151:A314.
121. Motta C, Touillon AM, Simon G, Dastugue B. Active lipid: a potential fluididizer of cystic fibrosis mucus. In Lawson D, ed. Cystic Fibrosis: Horizons. Chichester: Wiley, 1984:337.
122. Davis JT, Rideal EK, eds. Interfacial Phenomena. 2d ed. New York: Academic Press, 1963:217–281.
123. Geiser M, Baumann M, Cruz-Orive LM, Im Hof V, Waber U, Gehr P. The effect of particle inhalation on macrophage number and phagocytic activity in the intrapulmonary conducting airways of hamsters. Am J Respir Cell Mol Biol 1994; 10:594–603.
124. Geiser M, Cruz-Orive LM, Waber U, Im Hof V, Gehr P. Particle retention in airways estimated by unbiased stereology and photometry. J Aerosol Med 1995; 8: 149–165.
125. Harmsen AG, Muggenburg BA, Burton-Snipes M, Bice DE. The role of macrophages in particle translocation from lungs to lymph nodes. Science 1985; 230: 1277–1280.
126. Oberdörster G, Ferin J, Lehnert BE. Correlation between particle size, in vivo particle persistence, and lung injury. Environ Health Perspect 1994; 102(suppl 5):173–179.
127. Lehnert BE. Correlation between particle size, in vivo particle persistence, and lung injury. Environ Health Perspect 1994; 102(suppl 5):173–179.
128. Brody AR, Roe MW, Evan JN, Davis GS. Deposition and translocation of inhaled silica in rat. Lab Invest 1982; 47:533–542.
129. Adamson IY. Radiation enhances silica translocation to the pulmonary interstitium and increases fibrosis in mice. Environ Health Perspect 1992; 97:233–238.
130. van Haarst JMW, de Wit HJ, Drexhage HA, Hoogsteden HC. Distribution and immunophenotype of mononuclear phagocytes and dendritic cells in the human lung. Am J Respir Cell Mol Biol 1994; 10:487–492.
131. Nelson DJ, McMenamin C, McWilliam AS, Brenan M, Holt PG. Development of the airway intraepithelial dendritic cell network in the rat from class II major histocompatibility (Ia)-negative precursors: differential regulation of Ia expression at different levels of the respiratory tract. J Exp Med 1994; 179:203–212.

132. McWilliam AS, Nelson D, Thomas JA, Holt PG. Rapid dendritic cell recruitment is a hallmark of the acute inflammatory response at mucosal surfaces. J Exp Med 1994; 179:1331–1336.
133. Wallace WE, Keane MJ, Mike PS, Hill CA, Vallyathan V. Mineral surface-specific differences in the adsorption and enzymatic removal of surfactant and their correlation with cytotoxicity. In: Mossman BT, Bégin RO, eds. Effects of Mineral Dusts of Cells. Berlin: Springer-Verlag, 1989:49–56.
134. Wallace WE Jr, Headley LC, Weber KC. Dipalmitoyl lecithin surfactant adsorption by kaolin dust in vitro. J Colloid Interface Sci 1975; 51:535–537.
135. Wallace WE Jr, Keane MJ, Vallyathan V, Hathaway P, Regad ED, Castranova V, Green FHY. Suppression of inhaled particle cytotoxicity by pulmonary surfactant and re-toxification by phospholipase: distinguishing properties of quartz and kaolin. Ann Occup Hyg 1988; 32:291–298.
136. Marks J. The neutralization of silica toxicity in vitro (abstr). Br J Ind Med 1957; 14:81.
137. Stringer B, Kobzik L. Alveolar macrophage uptake of the environmental particulate titanium dioxide: role of surfactant components. Am J Respir Cell Mol Biol 1996; 14:155–160.
138. Hill CA, Wallace WE, Keane MJ, Mike PS. The enzymatic removal of a surfactant coating from quartz and kaolin by P388D1 cells. Cell Biol Toxicol 1995; 11:119–128.
139. Wallace WE, Keane MJ, Mike PS, Hill CA, Vallyathan V, Regad ED. Contrasting respirable quartz and kaolin retention of lecithin surfactant and expression of membranolytic activity following phospholipase A_2 digestion. J Toxicol Environ Health 1992; 37:391–409.
140. Emerson RJ, Davis GS. Effect of alveolar lining material-coated silica on rat alveolar macrophages. Environ Health Perspect 1983; 51:81–84.
141. Vallyathan V, Shi X, Dalal NS, Irr W, Castranova V. Generation of free radicals from freshly fractured silica dust: potential role in acute silica-induced lung injury. Am Rev Respir Dis 1988; 138:1213–1219.
142. Cifuentes J, Ruiz-Oronoz J, Myles C, Nieves B, Carlo WA, Matalon S. Interaction of surfactant mixtures with reactive oxygen and nitrogen species. J Appl Physiol 1995; 78:1800–1805.
143. Gilliard N, Heldt GP, Gasser H, Redi H, Merritt TA, Spragg RG. Exposure of the hydrophobic components of porcine lung surfactant to oxidant stress alters surface tension properties. J Clin Invest 1994; 93:2608–2615.
144. Haddad IY, Ischiropoulos H, Holm BA, Beckman JS, Baker JR, Matalon S. Mechanisms of peroxynitrite-induced injury to pulmonary surfactants. Am J Physiol 1993; 265:L555–L564.
145. Haddad IY, Crow JP, Hu P, Yaozu Y, Beckman J, Matalon S. Concurrent generation of nitric oxide and superoxide damages surfactant protein A. Am J Physiol 1994; 267:L242–L249.
146. Krzanowski J. Oxidant-induced alterations of lung surfactant system. J Fla Med Assoc 1994; 81:49–51.
147. Matalon S, DeMarco V, Haddad IY, Myles C, Skimming JW, Schürch S, Cheng

S, Cassin S. Inhaled nitric oxide injures the pulmonary surfactant system of lambs in vivo. Am J Physiol 1996; 270:L272–L280.
148. Ryan SF, Ghassibi Y, Liau DF. Effects of activated polymorphonuclear leukocytes upon pulmonary surfactant in vitro. Am J Respir Cell Mol Biol 1991; 4:33–41.
149. Holm BA, Hudak BB, Keicher L, Cavanaugh C, Baker RR, Hu P, Matalon S. Mechanisms of H_2O_2-mediated injury to type II cell surfactant metabolism and protection with PEG-catalase. Am J Physiol 1991; 261(5 pt 1):C751–C757.
150. Jackson RM. Molecular, pharmacologic, and clinical aspects of oxygen-induced lung injury. Clin Chest Med 1990; 11:73–83.
151. Matalon S, Holm BA, Baker RR, Whitfield MK, Freeman BA. Characterization of antioxidant activities of pulmonary surfactant mixtures. Biochim Biophys Acta 1990; 1035:121–127.
152. Cantin AM, North SL, Hubbard RC, Crystal RG. Normal alveolar epithelial lining fluid contains high levels of glutathione. J Appl Physiol 1978; 63:152–157.
153. Salathe M, Guldimann P, Conner GE, Wanner A. Hydrogen peroxide-scavenging properties of sheep airway mucus. Am J Respir Crit Care Med 1995; 151:1542–1550.
154. Davis WB, Pacht ER. Extracellular antioxidant defenses. In: Crystal RG, West JB et al., eds. The Lung: Scientific Foundations. 2d ed. Philadelphia: Lippincott–Raven; 1997:2271–2278.
155. Cross C, Halliwell B, Allen A. Antioxidant protection: a function of tracheobronchial and gastrointestinal mucus. Lancet 1984; 1:1328–1329.
156. Craighead JE, Kleinerman J, Abraham JL, Gibbs AR, Green FHY, Harley RA, Ruttner JR, Vallyathan V, Juliano EB. Diseases associated with exposure to silica and non-fibrous silicate minerals. Arch Pathol Lab Med 1988; 112:673–720.
157. Dethloff LA, Gilmore LB, Brody AR, Hook GER. Induction of intra- and extracellular phospholipids in the lungs of rats exposed to silica. Biochem J 1986; 233: 111–118.
158. Heppleston AG, Wright NA, Stewart JA. Experimental alveolar lipo-proteinosis following the inhalation of silica. J Pathol 1970; 101:293–307.
159. Bégin R, Possmayer F, Ormseth MA, Martel M, Cantin A, Massé S. Effect of aluminum inhalation on alveolar phospholipid profiles in experimental silicosis. Lung 1989; 167:107–115.
160. Crouch E, Persson A, Chang D, Parghi D. Surfactant protein D. Increased accumulation in silica-induced pulmonary lipoproteinosis. Am J Pathol 1991; 139:765–766.
161. Vallyathan V, Green FHY, Schürch S, Leonard S, Wallace WE. Effect of oxygen radicals on surfactant activity [abstr]. FASEB J 1995; A973.
162. Ma JYC, Weber KC. Dipalmitoyl lecithin and lung surfactant adsorption at an air–liquid interface by respirable particles. Environ Res 1986; 41:120–129.
163. Schürch SF, Roach MR. Interference of bronchographic agents with lung surfactant. Respir Physiol 1976; 28:99–117.
164. Curti PC, Genghini M. Role of surfactant in alveolar defence against inhaled particles. Respiration 1989; 55(suppl 1):60–67.

165. Nieman GF, Clark WR Jr, Wax SD, Webb WR. The effect of smoke inhalation on pulmonary surfactant. Ann Surg 1980; 191:171–181.
166. Matulionis DH, Kimmel E, Diamond L. Morphologic and physiologic response of lungs to steroid and cigarette smoke: an animal model. Environ Res 1985; 36:298–313.
167. Mistretta A, Crimi N, Palermo F, Oliveri R, Vancheri C, Vigneri G, Gibellino F. Lung permeability in smokers after ambroxol treatment. Respiration 1989; 1:79–83.
168. Miller D, Bondurant S. Effects of cigarette smoke on the surface characteristics of lung extracts. Am Rev Respir Dis 85:692–696.
169. Schmekel B, Khan AR, Linden M, Wollmer P. Recoveries of phosphatidylcholine and alveolar macrophages in lung lavage from healthy light smokers. Clin Physiol 1991; 11:431–438.
170. Finley TN, Ladman AJ. Low yield of pulmonary surfactant in cigarette smokers. N Engl J Med 1972; 286:223–227.
171. Shirnamé-Moré L. Genotoxicity of diesel emissions. Part I: mutagenicity and other genetic effects. In: Diesel Exhaust: A Critical Analysis of Emissions, Exposure and Health Effects. Cambridge, MA: The Health Effects Institute, 1995:223–242.
172. King LC, Kohan MJ, Austin AC, Claxton LD, Huisingh JL. Evaluation of the release of mutagens from diesel particles in the presence of physiological fluids. Environ Mutagen 1981; 3:109–121.
173. Keane MJ, Xing S-G, Harrison JC, Ong T, Wallace WE. Genotoxicity of diesel-exhaust particles dispersed in simulated pulmonary surfactant. Mutat Res 1991; 260:233–238.
174. Wallace WE, Keane MJ, Hill CA, Xu J, Ong T-M. Mutagenicity of diesel exhaust particles and oil shale particles dispersed in lecithin surfactant. J Toxicol Environ Health 1987; 21:163–171.
175. Liu J, Keane MJ, Ong T, Wallace WE. In vitro genotoxicity studies of chrysotile asbestos fibers dispersed in simulated pulmonary surfactant. Mutat Res 1994; 320: 253–259.
176. Andersson B, Svanborg-Eden C. Attachment of *Streptococcus pneumoniae* to human pharyngeal epithelial cell. Respiration 1989; 55(suppl 1):49–52.
177. La Force FM, Kelley WJ, Huber GL. Inactivation of staphylococci by alveolar macrophages with preliminary observations on the importance of alveolar lining material. J Clin Invest 1973; 71:129–141.
178. O'Neill SJ, Lesperance E, Klass DJ. Human lung lavage surfactant enhances staphylococcal phagocytosis by alveolar macrophages. Am Rev Respir Dis 1984; 130: 1177–1179.
179. Brogden KA, De Lucca AJ, Bland J, Elliott S. Isolation of an ovine pulmonary surfactant-associated anionic peptide bactericidal for *Pasteurella haemolytica*. Proc Natl Acad Sci USA 1996; 93:412–416.
180. Coonrod JD. Role of surfactant free fatty acids in antimicrobial defences. Eur J Respir Dis 1987; 71(suppl 153):209–214.
181. Hoffman RM, Claypool WD, Katyal SL, Singh G, Rogers RM, Dauber JH. Augmentation of rat alveolar macrophage migration by surfactant protein. Am Rev Respir Dis 1987; 135:1358–1362.

182. Pison U, Wright J, Hawgood S. Specific binding of surfactant apoprotein SP-A to rat alveolar macrophages. Am J Physiol 1992; 262:L412–L417.
183. Malhotra R, Haurum J, Thiel S, Sim R. Interaction of C1q receptor with lung surfactant protein A. Eur J Immunol 1992; 22:1437–1445.
184. van Golde LMG. Potential role of surfactant proteins A and D in innate lung defense against pathogens. Biol Neonate 1995; 67(suppl 1):2–17.
185. van Iwaarden JF, Welmers B, Verhoef J, Haagsman HP, van Golde LMG. Pulmonary surfactant protein A enhances the host-defense mechanism of rat alveolar macrophages. Am J Respir Cell Mol Biol 1990; 2:91–98.
186. van Iwaarden JF, van Strijp JAG, Ebskamp MJM, Welmers B, Verhoef J, van Golde LMG. Surfactant protein A is an opsonin in the phagocytosis of herpes simplex virus type 1 by rat alveolar macrophages. Am J Physiol 1991; 61:L204–L209.
187. Wright JR, Youmans DC. Pulmonary surfactant protein A stimulates chemotaxis of alveolar macrophage. Am J Physiol 1993; 264:L338–L344.
188. Holmskov U, Malhotra R, Sim RB, Jensenius JC. Collectins: collagenous C-type lectins of the innate immune defense system. Immunol Today 1994; 15:67–74.
189. Hoppe H-J, Reid KBM. Collectins: soluble proteins containing collagenous regions and lectin domains, and their roles in innate immunity. Protein Sci 1994; 3:1143–1158.
190. Sastry K, Ezekowitz RA. Collectins: pattern recognition molecules involved in first line host defense. Curr Opin Immunol 1993; 5:59–66.
191. Kuan S-F, Rust K, Crouch E. Interactions of surfactant protein D with bacterial lipopolysaccharides. Surfactant protein D is an *Escherichia coli*-binding protein in bronchoalveolar lavage. J Clin Invest 1992; 90:97–106.
192. Zimmerman PE, Voelker DR, McCormack FX, Paulsrud JR, Martin WJ. 120-kD surface glycoprotein of *Pneumocystis carinii* is a ligand for surfactant protein A. J Clin Invest 1992; 89:143–149.
193. Downing JF, Pasula R, Wright JR, Twigg HL, Martin WJ. Surfactant protein A promotes attachment of *Mycobacterium tuberculosis* to alveolar macrophages during infection with human immunodeficiency virus. Proc Natl Acad Sci 1995; 92:4848–4852.
194. Blau H, Riklis S, Kravtsov V, Kalina M. Secretion of cytokines by rat alveolar epithelial cells: possible regulatory role for SP-A. Am J Physiol 1994; 266:L148–L155.
195. Thomassen MJ, Antal JM, Connors MJ, Meeker DP, Wiedemann HP. Characterization of Exosurf (surfactant)-mediated suppression of stimulated human alveolar macrophage cytokine responses. Am J Respir Cell Mol Biol 1994; 10:399–404.
196. Speer CP, Götze B, Curstedt T, Robertson B. Phagocytic functions and tumor necrosis factor secretion of human monocytes exposed to natural porcine surfactant (Curosurf). Pediatr Res 1991; 30:69–74.
197. Földes-Filep E, Sirois P, Filep JG. Pulmonary surfactant lipids inhibit prostanoid production of guinea pig alveolar macrophages. J Leukoc Biol 1994; 56:475–480.
198. Ansfield MJ, Kaltreider HB, Benson BJ, Caldwell JL. Immunosuppressive activity of canine pulmonary surface active material. J Immunol 1979; 122:1062–1066.
199. Sitrin BR, Ansfield MK, Kaltreider HB. The effect of pulmonary surface-active

material on the generation and expression of murine B- and T-lymphocyte effector functions in vitro. Exp Lung Res 1985; 9:85–97.
200. Lesur O, Mancini NM, Janot C, Chabot F, Boitout A, Polu JM, Gerard H. Loss of lymphocyte modulatory control by surfactant lipid extracts from acute hypersensitivity pneumonitis: comparison with sarcoidosis and idiopathic pulmonary fibrosis. Eur Resp J 1994; 7:1944–1949.
201. Woerndle S, Bartmann P. The effect of three surfactant preparations on in vitro lymphocyte functions. J Perinat Med 1994; 22:119–128.
202. Martling CR, Lundberg JM. Capsaicin sensitive afferents contribute to acute airway edema following tracheal instillation of hydrochloric acid or gastric juice in the rat. Anesthesiology 1988; 68:350–356.
203. Merritt TA, Amirkhanian JD, Helbock H, Halliwell B, Cross CE. Reduction of the surface–tension-lowering ability of surfactant after exposure to hypochlorous acid. Biochem J 1993; 295:19–22.
204. Green FHY, Schürch S, De Sanctis GT, Wallace JA, Cheng S, Prior M. Effects of hydrogen sulfide exposure on surface properties of lung surfactant. J Appl Physiol 1991; 70:1943–1949.
205. Muller B, Barth P, von Wichert P. Structural and functional impairment of surfactant protein A after exposure to nitrogen dioxide in rats. Am J Physiol 1992; 263: L177–L184.
206. Oosting RS, van Iwaarden JF, van Bree L, Verhoef J, van Golde LMG, Haagsman HP. Exposure of surfactant protein A to ozone in vitro and in vivo impairs its interactions with alveolar cells. Am J Physiol 1992; 262:L63–L68.
207. Curti PC, Genghini M. Role of surfactant in clearance of powders from the lung and possible preventive effect of ambroxol against pneumoconiosis including silicosis. Respiration 1985; 46:143–151.
208. Seeger W, Grube C, Günther A, Schmidt R. Surfactant inhibition by plasma proteins: differential sensitivity of various surfactant preparations. Eur Respir J 1993; 6:971–977.
209. Seeger W, Lepper H, Wolf HRD, Neuhof H. Alteration of alveolar surfactant function after exposure to oxidative stress and to oxygenated and native arachidonic acid in vitro. Biochim Biophys Acta 1985; 835:58–67.
210. Fuchimukai T, Fujiwara T, Takahashi A, Enhorning G. Artificial pulmonary surfactant inhibited by proteins. Am Physiol Soc 1987; 62:429–437.
211. Holm BA, Enhorning G, Notter RH. A biophysical-mechanism by which plasma proteins inhibit lung surfactant activity. Chem Phys Lipids 1988; 49:49–55.
212. Holm BA, Notter RH. Effects of hemoglobin and cell membrane lipids on pulmonary surfactant activity. J Appl Physiol 1987; 63:1434–1442.
213. Amirkhanian JD, Bruni R, Waring AJ, Taeusch HW. Inhibition of mixtures of surfactant lipids and synthetic sequences of surfactant proteins SP-B and SP-C. Biochim Biophys Acta 1991; 1096:355–360.
214. Hallman M, Spragg R, Harrell JH, Moser KM, Gluck L. Evidence of lung surfactant abnormality in respiratory failure. Study of bronchoalveolar lavage phospholipids, surface activity, phospholipase activity, and plasma myoinositol. J Clin Invest 1982; 70:673–683.

215. Keough KM, Parsons CS, Tweeddale MG. Interactions between plasma proteins and pulmonary surfactant: pulsating bubble studies. Can J Physiol Pharmacol 1989; 47:663–668.
216. Goodglick LA, Kane AB. Role of reactive oxygen metabolites in crocidolite asbestos toxicity to mouse macrophages. Cancer Res 1986; 46:5558–5566.
217. Vallyathan V, Mega JF, Shi X, Dalal NS. Enhanced generation of free radicals from phagocytes induced by mineral dusts. Am J Respir Cell Mol Biol 1992; 6: 404–413.
218. Ahuja A, Oh N, Chao W, Spragg RG, Smith RM. Inhibition of the human neutrophil respiratory burst by native and synthetic surfactant. Am J Respir Cell Mol Biol 1996; 14:496–503.
219. McElvancy NG, Crystal RG. Proteases and lung injury. In: Crystal RG, West JB, Weibel ER, Barnes PJ, eds. The Lung: Scientific Foundations. Philadelphia: Lippincott–Raven; 1997:2205–2218.
220. Pison U, Tam EK, Caughey GH, Hawgood S. Proteolytic inactivation of dog lung surfactant-associated proteins by neutrophil elastase. Biochim Biophys Acta 1989; 992:251–257.
221. Katsura H, Kawada H, Konno K. Rat surfactant apoprotein A (SP-A) exhibits antioxidant effects on alveolar macrophages. Am J Respir Cell Mol Biol 1993; 9:520–525.
222. Scarpelli EM, Mautone AJ. The surfactant system and pulmonary mechanics. In: Robertson B, van Golde LMG, Batenburg JJ, eds. Pulmonary Surfactant: From Molecular Biology to Clinical Practice. Amsterdam: Elsevier Science, 1984:119–170.
223. Guyton AC, Moffatt DS, Adair TH. Role of alveolar surface tension in transepithelial movement of fluid. In: Robertson B, van Golde LMG, Batenburg JJ, eds. Pulmonary Surfactant: From Molecular Biology to Clinical Practice. Amsterdam: Elsevier Science, 1984:71–186.
224. Berggren P, Lachmann B, Curstedt T, Grossmann G, Robertson B. Gas exchange and lung morphology after surfactant replacement in experimental adult respiratory distress syndrome induced by repeated lung lavage. Acta Anaesthesiol Scand 1986; 30:321–328.
225. Matalon S, Holm BA, Notter RH. Mitigation of pulmonary hyperoxic injury by administration of exogenous surfactant. J Appl Physiol 1987; 62:756–761.
226. Taeusch HW, Clements J, Benson S. Exogenous surfactant for human lung disease. Am Rev Respir Dis 1983; 128:791–794.
227. Puchelle E, De Bentzmann S, Zahm JM. Physical and functional properties of airway secretions in cystic fibrosis—therapeutic approaches. Respiration 1995; 462(suppl 1):2–12.
228. Tam PY, Verdugo P. Control of mucus hydration as a Donnan equilibrium process. Nature 1981; 292:340–342.
229. Potter JL, Matthews LW, Lemm J, Spector S. Studies on pulmonary secretions. II. Osmolality and the ionic environment of pulmonary secretions from patients with cystic fibrosis, bronchiectasis, and laryngectomy. Am Rev Respir Dis 1967; 96: 83–97.

230. Braun-Fahrlander C, Ackermann-Liebrich U, Schwartz J, Gnehm HP, Rutishauser M, Wanner HU. Air pollution and respiratory symptoms in preschool children. Am Rev Respir Dis 1992; 145:42–47.
231. Lipfert FW. Air Pollution and Community Health: A Critical Review and Data Sourcebook. New York: Van Nostrand Reinhold, 1994.
232. Pope CA III, Thun MJ, Namboodiri MM, Dockery DW, Evans JS, Speizer FE, Heath CW Jr. Particulate air pollution as a predictor of mortality in a prospective study of U.S. adults. Am J Respir Crit Care Med 1995; 151:669–674.
233. Kaminsky DA, Wenzel SE, Carcano C, Gurka D, Feldsien D, Irgin CG. Hyperpnea-induced changes in parenchymal lung mechanics in normal subjects and in asthmatics. Am J Respir Crit Care Med 1997; 155:1260–1266.
234. Enhorning G, Holm B. Disruption of pulmonary surfactant's ability to maintain openness of a narrow tube. J Appl Physiol 1993; 74:2922–2927.
235. Sanerkin NG, Evans DMD. The sputum in bronchial asthma: pathopneumonic patterns. J Pathol 1965; 89:66–73.
236. Liu M, Wang L, Enhorning G. Surfactant dysfunction develops when the immunized guinea pig is challenged with ovalbumin aerosol. Clin Exp Allergy 1995; 25: 1053–1060.
237. Kurashima K, Fujimura M, Tsujiura M, Matsuda T. Effect of surfactant inhalation on allergic bronchoconstriction in guinea pigs. Clin Exp Allergy 1997; 27:337–342.
238. Van de Graaf EA, Jansen HM, Lutter R, Alberts C, Kobesen J, De Vries IJ, Out TA. Surfactant protein A in bronchoalveolar lavage fluid. J Lab Clin Med 1992; 120:252–263.
239. Kurashima K, Fujimura M, Matsuda T, Kobayashi T. Surface activity of sputum from acute asthmatic patients. Am J Respir Crit Care Med 1997; 155:1254–1259.
240. Kurashima K, Ogawa H, Ohka T. A pilot study of surfactant inhalation for the treatment of asthmatic attack. Jpn J Allergol 1991; 40:160–163.
241. Pavia D, Lopez-Vidriero MT, Clarke SW. Mediators and mucociliary clearance in asthma. Bull Eur Physiopathol Respir 1987; 23(suppl 10):89S–94S.
242. Vachier I, Chanez P, Le Doucan C, Damon M, Descomps B, Godard P. Enhancement of reactive oxygen species formation in stable and unstable asthmatic patients. Eur Respir J 1994; 7:1585–1592.
243. Roth MD, Pinto M, Golub SH, Shau H. Pulmonary surfactant inhibits interleukin-2-induced proliferation and generation of lymphokine-activated killer cells. Am J Respir Cell Mol Biol 1993; 9:652–658.
244. Widdicombe JG. Airway liquid: a barrier to drug diffusion? Eur Respir J 1997; 10:2194–1297.
245. Hohlfeld J, Hoymann HG, Molthan J, Fabel H, Heinrich U. Aerosolized surfactant inhibits acetylcholine-induced airway obstruction in rats. Eur Respir J 1997; 10: 2198–2203.

15

Pathophysiological Mechanisms of Cardiopulmonary Effects

JOHN J. GODLESKI and ROBERT W. CLARKE

Harvard School of Public Health and
Brigham and Women's Hospital
Boston, Massachusetts

I. Introduction

Recent epidemiological studies show that exposures to particulate air pollution are associated with increased respiratory disease morbidity and mortality (1–8). Although mechanisms leading to these effects have not yet been delineated, these epidemiological studies offer important clues about potential mechanisms, such as that persons with chronic respiratory disease (asthma, chronic bronchitis) and cardiovascular disease are particularly susceptible (2,9–13). The theme of this chapter is that ambient air particles have intrinsic toxicity and are more harmful in the setting of preexisting pulmonary inflammation because they exacerbate both inflammatory and airway obstructive responses, as well as systemic effects manifested in the heart. Such processes can account for the increased morbidity and be related to the increased mortality seen in epidemiological studies, and they can specifically produce the cardiopulmonary events described in the epidemiological studies.

The approach of our laboratory to understand mechanisms of mortality and morbidity caused by ambient air particles uses animal models of human diseases associated with increased sensitivity in the epidemiological studies. Underlying concepts include (1) The effects of ambient particles are best defined using ''real-world'' ambient air particles unaltered by collection techniques; (2) the exposed populations should model human populations, and adverse effects should include measurable increased morbidity and mortality; (3) the use of concentrated airborne particles (CAPs) in animal exposures will permit the populations studied in the laboratory to be adequate to detect the modeled effect and to test mechanistic hypotheses. Based on these concepts, the cornerstones of our studies have been the utilization of (1) the Harvard Ambient Particulate Concentrator (HAPC), a newly developed device that can increase ambient particle concentrations by a factor of 30 times, without changing the physical or chemical characteristics of the particles (14,15); (2) a typical Northeastern United States urban aerosol with a usual fine particle concentration range of 5–15 $\mu g/m^3$, containing transported sulfur-containing acidic particles during the summer and local combustion product particulate in winter (16); (3) animal models of chronic bronchitis, asthma, pulmonary hypertension–inflammation, and coronary artery disease to model compromised human populations and to elucidate mechanistic effects (17–22); and (4) analytical capabilities to relate adverse effects to specific constituents in the exposure aerosol (23,24).

These cornerstones have allowed investigation into the biological responses induced by inhaled air pollution. Recent studies have shown the following: (1) Inhalation of CAPs results in as high as 37% mortality in animals with preexisting pulmonary inflammation, but at the concentrations studied there is no mortality in normal animals. (2) Inhalation of low concentrations (500 $\mu g/m^3$) of fuel oil fly ash particles (FAPs), as an example of a complex combustion-generated environmental particle, results in 42% mortality in animals with preexisting pulmonary inflammation and with this dose of FAPs; proinflammatory cytokines are found in the lungs and cardiac macrophages even in normal animals. (3) With exposure to environmental particles, significant cardiac electrophysiological alterations were found, even in normal animals, using highly sensitive techniques. (4) CAPs initiate production of oxidants and cytokines in inflammation-primed lung cells to levels comparable with highly toxic α-quartz; and reactive oxygen species directly induce proinflammatory cytokines, which may play pivotal roles in morbidity and mortality.

A central hypothesis derived from this data is as follows: Ambient air particles are complex mixtures with intrinsic toxicity. In concert with preexisting inflammation, particulate exposure results in stimulation of lung receptors and immune cells, release of reactive oxygen species (ROS), and induction of proinflammatory mediators that lead to local and systemic effects, which ultimately account for the epidemiological associations between adverse health effects and particulate air pollution. Hypothetical mechanistic pathways by which inhalation of ambient particles in urban air may lead to morbidity and mortality are outlined in Figure 1.

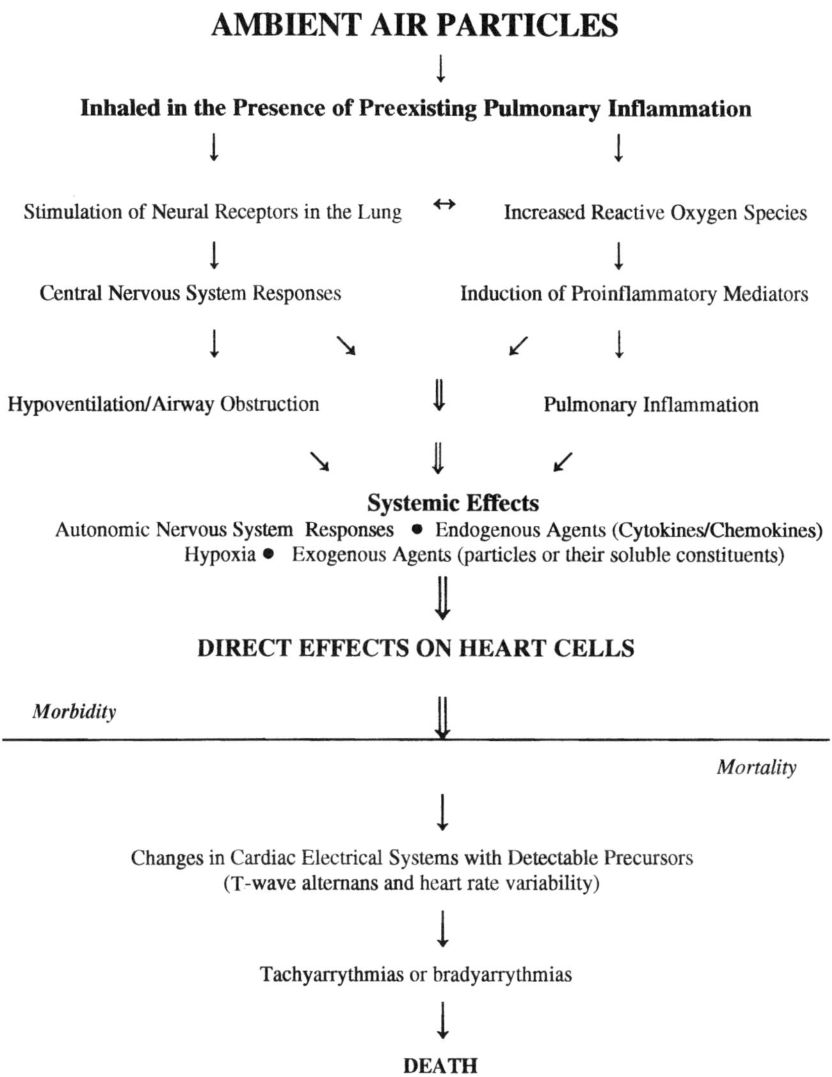

Figure 1 Hypothetical mechanistic pathways by which inhalation of concentrated ambient particles may lead to morbidity and mortality.

II. Rationale for Each Step in the Potential Mechanisms of Morbidity and Mortality

A. ROS as Intermediates of Particle-Induced Inflammation

Particle exposure has been specifically linked to induction of pulmonary inflammation. Amdur and Chen (25) reported increased neutrophil numbers and increased bronchoalveolar lavage (BAL) protein following exposure to acid-coated particles. Exposure to fly ash, a model of outdoor air pollution, induces severe pulmonary inflammation (26) marked by increased numbers of neutrophils (27) and increased lavageable protein (26). Interestingly, the observed pulmonary inflammation has been specifically related to the metal content of the fly ash particle, particularly iron, nickel, and vanadium (26). Other studies have pointed to the effectiveness of these transition metals in inducing reactive oxygen species (ROS) in lung cells (28,29).

Lung macrophages constitute the first line of defense in response to inhaled particles through phagocytosis and subsequently released ROS. These macrophages also produce a variety of proinflammatory and anti-inflammatory mediators on activation by external stimuli. These mediators include cytokines, growth factors, and products of arachidonic acid metabolism (30). Although the generation of ROS are necessary for host defense, they can also cause secondary damage to host tissue. Prolonged exposure to environmental particles and the recurring activation of macrophages could lead to unattenuated release of toxic ROS and proinflammatory mediators. The production of ROS has been implicated as a final common pathway of lung injury in exposure to numerous environmental agents, as well as during therapy with hyperoxia or quinoid drugs (31). Accumulating evidence of our studies (32,33) suggested that an oxidative stress alone is sufficient to trigger expression of neutrophil chemotactic cytokines (chemokines) and, thereby, contribute to acute and chronic pulmonary inflammation.

The induction of ROS synthesis in lung macrophages and epithelial cells by interaction with environmental particles (34,35) appears to be partially dependent on the metal content of the particle itself. Of the various transition metals found in urban air particles, we have recently demonstrated that vanadium and manganese, individually, are able to induce a rapid respiratory burst in lung macrophages (36–38). Both metals are able to activate the NADPH oxidase complex by separate intracellular signal transduction pathways, thereby generating ROS at the macrophage membrane (37). Intratracheal instillation of these metals induces a rapid neutrophil influx to the lung surface, with a concomitant expression in lung macrophages of mRNA for the neutrophil chemoattractant cytokines macrophage inflammatory protein (MIP)-2 and KC (38,39). Pretreatment of lung macrophages with the antioxidant *N*-acetylcysteine before vanadium or manganese exposure in vitro eliminates induction of the MIP-2 and KC genes in these cells (38). These observations, taken together, suggest ROS as an intermediate of particle-induced inflammation.

Arachidonic acid metabolism can be altered by oxidative stress (40–42) and changes in response to particles have also been observed. For example, exposure to coal dust resulted in an increase of macrophage numbers and an increase in thromboxane A_2 (TXA_2) and leukotriene B_4 (LTB_4) production, as well as a decrease of prostaglandin E_2 (PGE_2) production (43). Chen et al. (44) reported increased $PGF_{2\alpha}$ following exposure to acid sulfate-coated zinc oxide particles. Moreover, changes of arachidonic acid metabolites by coal dust can be attenuated by antioxidants (45). These modulations of arachidonic acid metabolism are important because the increase in TXA_2 and LTB_4 production could lead to broncho- and vasoconstriction and chemotaxis of polymorphonuclear neutrophils (PMN), whereas the increase in PGF_2 is associated with a decrease in vital capacity and diffusing capacity. Likewise, the decrease in PGE_2 production may also result in smooth-muscle constriction. Furthermore, oxidative stress alone induces airway constriction (46). The potential role of ROS and arachidonic acid metabolites as mediators of increased pulmonary inflammation, airway constriction, and changes in ventilation are potentially important mechanisms of response to inhaled ambient particles.

The interaction of inhaled particles, including CAPs, with macrophages leads to the production of ROS. ROS may further trigger the release of proinflammatory cytokines and arachidonic acid metabolites (47). These inflammatory mediators, inflammatory cytokines, and especially ROS may be responsible for adverse effects of CAPs, such as pulmonary inflammation, airway narrowing, and increased morbidity and mortality.

B. Role of Cytokines in Pulmonary Inflammation and Pulmonary Function

An important mechanistic clue related to the biological response to inhaled particles has been that many epidemiological studies associate preexisting inflammatory lung diseases with adverse effects of air particles. Recent investigations suggest a primary pathophysiological role for inflammation in exacerbations of pulmonary disease and focus on the presence of neutrophils in symptomatic chronic airway disease (48,49). The hypothesis, that airway function is modulated by inflammatory cells that are activated and sequestered within the lung, has become especially attractive in relation to both chronic bronchitis and asthma. Recent studies (50,51) show that neutrophil accumulation and increased airway responsiveness in asthma are correlated. The presence of pulmonary inflammation is a clear starting place to assess changes of morbidity and mortality.

Cytokines act as both proinflammatory mediators and effectors of pulmonary function, indicating their importance in the study of responses to inhaled particles. The focus on interleukin 8 (IL-8) and platelet factor-4 family cytokines as important mediators of inflammation is based on the biological properties of these peptides (52). IL-8 is primarily a neutrophil chemotactic and activating factor (53–55), and it appears to be relatively resistant to inactivation by plasma proteases (54). These features, plus that it is a product of many cell types, including lung macrophages (56), pulmonary epithelial cells, and fibroblasts, makes this cytokine a very likely candidate for a role in the exacerbation of chronic bronchitis and asthma associated with particle inhalation. Although IL-8 appears to be the primary chemokine responsible for the neutrophilia associated with pulmonary inflammation in humans (57), it is not expressed at the mRNA or protein level in rats. There is substantial evidence that two closely related members of the IL-8, platelet factor 4 family, KC and MIP-2 replace IL-8 in rats (18,58–62). Expression studies illustrate the role of these cytokines and the cytokines interleukin-1 (IL-1) and tumor necrosis factor (TNF) in response to environmental agents (63,64).

C. Death Is Often Ultimately Related to Cardiac Dysfunction

Although death may be attributable to many underlying conditions, the final common pathway remains the cessation of the heart electrical activity. With hospitalized patients, cardiac arrest is usually manifested by ventricular fibrillation, from which the patient may or may not be resuscitated. Sudden cardiac death, which claims over 350,000 lives annually in the United States, results from abrupt disruption of heart rhythm, also primarily in the form of ventricular fibrillation. Death in those instances is due not to extensive cardiac injury, but rather, to transient triggers that impinge on the electrically unstable heart (65–67). Identification of individuals at risk for sudden cardiac death remains a major objective in cardiology. Similarly, the specific mechanism linking ambient air particle exposure to death is unknown.

Quantification of T-wave alternans is a novel mechanistic approach to investigate cardiac changes because of the consistent occurrence of this phenomenon before fibrillation under diverse conditions, including coronary artery occlusion, hypothermia, Prinzmetal's vasospastic angina, and the long Q-T syndrome (68–70). Early studies (71) showed that psychological stress may have profound influences on ventricular arrhythmias during myocardial infarction in the conscious dog. Recent studies have solidified the importance of T-wave alternans as an index of cardiac vulnerability (72) and in ischemia (73). In studies, newly developed signal-processing techniques have been employed that permit simultaneous tracking of rapid changes in autonomic nervous system activity using heart rate variability and cardiac vulnerability by complex demodulation and T-wave alternans (73,74). These experiments have found that exposures to fly ash aerosols in the range of 1 mg/m^3 produce increasing amplitude of T-wave alternans, ST-segment elevation, and increasing frequency of apneic episodes. The alterations measured by these techniques suggest the importance of cardiac dysfunction in relation to inhalation of complex particles.

Few published reports have centered on inhaled particles resulting in cardiac abnormalities. One potential model for biological mechanistic studies of the association of inhaled ambient air particles and cardiac disease is environmental tobacco smoke (ETS). Epidemiological studies have shown an association between ETS exposure and both fatal and nonfatal heart disease (75,76). In experimental studies, ETS exposure has been associated with short-term cardiovascular effects, such as hypoxia (77,78), exercise ability (79,80), platelet and leukocyte activation, and with increased tissue damage following myocardial infarction (76). A recent study (81) reported acute cardiac mortality due to FAPs exposure in pulmonary hypertensive animals. In these studies, animals exhibited FAPs-associated arrthymias, including both bradycardia and tachycardia before death.

D. Role of Cytokines in Cardiac Dysfunction

In this chapter, the hypothesis is offered that cytokines may have both local and systemic effects. Levels of TNF (82–84) and IL-8 (85) increase in cardiac ischemia and myocardial infarction. Similarly, myocardial dysfunction in sepsis is related to TNF (86–87). These cytokines are also related to myocardial dysfunction in long-standing heart failure (88). These cytokines are produced by many cell types, including macrophages, and may be an amplification mechanism of inflammation. Whether amplification is by circulating cytokines or the possibility that particles or their soluble constituents reach the heart is unclear. Therefore, it is reasonable to assume that particles reaching the systemic circulation could be transported to cardiac macrophages whereby they may elicit a cytokine response (Fig. 2). In vitro effects of cytokines on isolated myocardial cells have been studied in various systems. Decreased contractility resulted from TNF (89–91), and IL-1 prolonged action potential duration (92). Both IL-1 and TNF induced arrhythmias in cardiac cells in vitro (93). Thus, relations of cytokines and myocardial abnormalities have been established, and it is suggested that the lung is a source of these cytokines as a result of particle inhalation. Moreover, in rodent studies with inhalation of environmental particles, the proinflammatory chemokine analogue MIP-2 can be found in cardiac macrophages, and this detection is markedly enhanced with preexisting pulmonary inflammation (22). In further study of cardiac macrophages in these FAP-exposed animals, particles with an analytical signature typical of fly ash may be found in their macrophages (see Fig. 2).

E. Hypoxia Resulting from Increasing Airway Obstruction or Hypoventilation in Concert with Pulmonary Inflammation Following Inhalation of Ambient Air Particles

In humans, elevated particulate air pollution has been associated with declines in lung function, increases in respiratory symptoms, and restricted activity

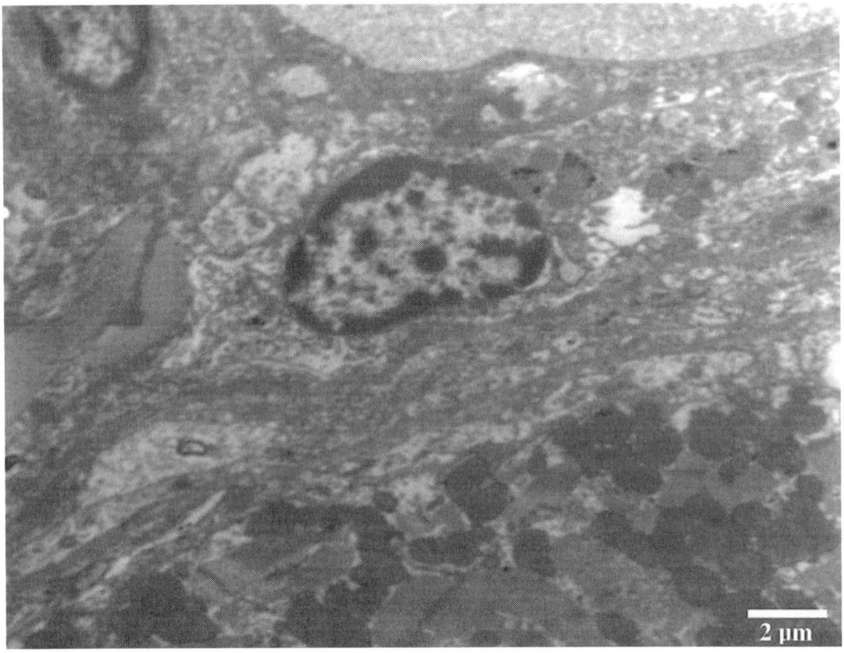

Figure 2 Electron micrograph of a resident macrophage from rat cardiac tissue that has phagocytosed environmental particles. Note the black opacities in the cytoplasm. Bar = 2 μm.

(7,8,10,94). There are also reports specifically linking air particle exposure with exacerbation of symptoms in patients with preexisting chronic bronchitis and declining pulmonary function (95,96). Studies of urban air pollution (97) using healthy rats have contained useful mechanistic clues, such as the demonstrated continued changes in all segments of the respiratory tract, as evidenced by increased airway resistance, secretory cell hyperplasia, ultrastructural ciliary alterations, and thick mucous accumulation. Our studies of the rat model of chronic bronchitis demonstrate mucous hypersecretion, airway obstruction, and increased airway responsiveness to inhaled aerosolized methacholine (17). Preliminary experiments from our laboratory, using rats with chronic bronchitis that are additionally exposed to CAPs, demonstrate significant bronchoconstriction and mortality (21,98). Significant bronchoconstriction and mortality are not detected in animals with SO_2-induced chronic bronchitis exposed to filtered air, rather than to CAPs, indicating the dangerously confounding role of CAPs with preexisting disease. Therefore, we have evidence that the airway obstruction present in rats with SO_2-induced chronic bronchitis is exaggerated following exposure to CAPs.

Mismatching of ventilation and blood flow is responsible for most of the defective gas exchange leading to hypoxia in pulmonary diseases (99). Studies with healthy mixed-breed dogs exposed to fly ash particles showed changes in breathing pattern and apnea. Substantial electrocardiogram changes, including ST segment elevation and T-wave alternans, have also been recorded. Both the pulmonary and cardiac findings make investigation of hypoxia as a mechanism leading to cardiac electrical instability an important component in this area of research. Similarly, airway obstruction caused by accumulation of mucus, inflammation, and bronchoconstriction detected in animals with chronic bronchitis and CAP exposure could result in nonuniform ventilation, and ultimately hypoxia.

F. Autonomic Mechanisms Resulting from Inhalation of CAPs and Affecting Cardiac Rhythm

In this hypothetical mechanistic scheme, it is postulated that electrocardiographic alterations produced by exposure to air pollutants will result partly from central nervous system (CNS)-mediated changes in cardiac autonomic tone. This supposition is based on the fact that the main cytokines that are released in response to air pollution can alter CNS activity. Also subjecting the lungs to noxious stimuli may elicit powerful cardiac reflexes that can alter sympathetic and parasympathetic activity. This is a critical consideration, because it is well established that both divisions of the autonomic nervous system exert a profound influence on the repolarization properties of the heart. These potential changes may play a vital role in the culminative response of inhaled particles on the cardiopulmonary system.

III. Studying Ambient Particles Using an Ambient Particle Concentrator

Acute health effects studies of several hundred children in Uniontown and State College, Pennsylvania, showed a linear relation between decrease in peak expiratory flow rates and particle acidity for a range up to the equivalent of 34 $\mu g/m^3$ of sulfuric acid, suggesting that the effect of exposure is greater under real-world conditions than under simulated chamber conditions (100). If we consider the strong associations shown by epidemiological studies of chronic and acute respiratory health effects of inhaled particles, it is unlikely that laboratory-produced aerosol exposures represent real-world particle exposures. Ambient aerosols are a complex amalgam of particles, gases, and vapors that comprise a variety of compounds the interactions of which may be the most critical feature. Although more complex exposures, such as diesel particles (101,102), combinations of simulated pollutant particle and gas combinations (25,103,104), mixtures of oxidant gases and sulfuric acid particles, or irradiated automobile exhaust (105) have sometimes been used, rarely, have inhalation studies attempted to reproduce the complex size distribution and particle composition characteristic of urban ambient particles (106). Most human and animal experiments have been carried out with relatively simple materials, such as sulfuric acid aerosols, silica, aluminum oxide, latex, iron oxide, or carbon.

The complex nature of particles has not been largely investigated in laboratory studies. Amdur (25) showed that the toxicity of acid sulfates was markedly increased when surface-adsorbed to zinc oxide particles. Anderson et al. (107) exposed subjects to carbon particles coated with sulfuric acid to simulate exposures of carbonaceous–acid aerosol particle mixtures. Hemenway et al. (104) and Clarke et al. (108) observed that sulfur dioxide transformed to sulfate species on a carbonaceous particle surface exacerbate suppression of alveolar macrophage phagocytosis and bactericidal activity, particularly in the presence of an environmental oxidant, ozone. Brain et al. (109) and Beck et al. (110) investigated the effects of soluble acid aerosols on the respiratory health of rats by instilling atmospheric particle filter extracts. Although these studies have made attempts to simulate ambient particle exposures, these approaches do not fully achieve a real-world situation.

An ambient particle concentrator has been developed that can increase the concentration of ambient air so that inhalation studies may be performed (Fig. 3; 14,15). The concentrator consists of a series of newly developed slit-nozzle virtual impactors, a series of honeycomb denuders, and a temperature–relative humidity control system. This system can concentrate ambient fine particles to more than 1000 $\mu g/m^3$ levels in a four-stage system and up to 300–1000 $\mu g/m^3$ levels in a three-stage system, without affecting their size or chemical composition. The concentrated aerosol has a particle size range from 0.1- to 2.5-μm–aerodynamic diameter, with a size fraction distribution identical with ambient air. Toxicological findings of severe lung injury and death with ultrafine Teflon combustion particles (111,112) as well as our own data identifying ultrafine particles in the lung macrophages of humans and animals (113) have been reported. The development of an ultrafine particle concentrator is an important goal of this area of research, particularly in light of their importance in toxicological responses to inhaled particles.

A. Harvard Ambient Particle Concentrator

Previous particle exposure studies have not used real ambient particles to investigate particle toxicity or develop dose–response relationships. Our laboratory has developed and evaluated a technique that can be used to separate and concentrate respirable particles from ambient air before their delivery to an inhalation exposure system (14,15). With this approach, particles are airborne throughout the

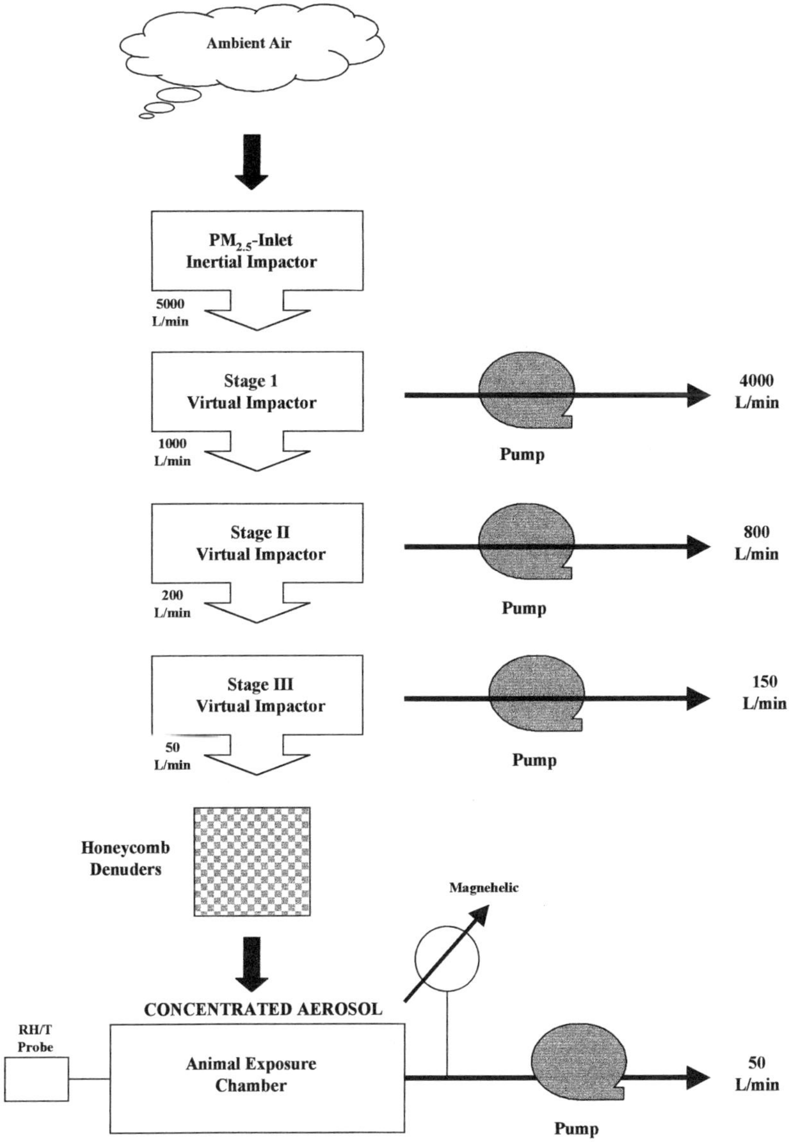

Figure 3 Schematic diagram of the ambient particle concentrating system used to conduct animal exposures. The RH/T probe measures relative humidity and temperature. Specific honeycomb denuders can be used to remove varying gaseous aerosol components (14,15). (From Ref. 14.)

concentration process by virtual impactors. Maximum concentrations are on the order of 30 times ambient levels. After the particles are concentrated, a series of honeycomb glass denuders can be added to remove specific acidic and oxidant gases. This preserves the particle and potential surface components, without interference of secondary agents. Finally, the inlet air is conditioned to constant temperature and relative humidity using an air-conditioning system, eliminating the effects of temperature and relative humidity.

B. Description of the Main Components of the HAPC Concentrating System

1. A high volume conventional impactor with a 2.5-µm cutoff size (separator)
2. Three virtual impactors in series, with a 0.1-µm cutoff size
3. A series of optional honeycomb denuders to remove oxidant and acidic gaseous pollutants from the concentrated aerosol supplied to the exposure chamber

The aerosol concentrator employs a series of virtual impactors, which are devices used for the classification of particles according to their aerodynamic size. A jet of particle-laden air is injected at a collection probe, which is slightly larger than the acceleration nozzle. Larger particles cross the airstreamlines and enter the collection probe, whereas smaller particles follow the deflected streamlines. To remove the larger particles from the collection probe, a fraction of the total flow is allowed to pass through the probe. This fraction of the airflow is referred to as the minor flow, which is typically 10–20% of the total flow. As a result, the concentration of the larger particles in the minor flow increases by a factor of Q_{tot}/Q_{min}, where Q_{tot} is the total flow entering the virtual impactor and Q_{min} is the minor flow. As the mass fraction of ambient particles smaller than approximately 0.1-µm–aerodynamic diameter is negligible (114–116), the minor flow of a virtual impactor with a 50% cutpoint on the order of 0.1 µm contains most of the fine ambient particulate mass.

C. Characterization of the Concentrating System

A three-stage HAPC was evaluated using room air as the test aerosol. The ambient levels of fine particulate mass ($PM_{2.5}$) and sulfate were determined using two Harvard-Marple impactors (HMI). The HMIs have been designed and characterized to have a 50% aerodynamic diameter cutpoint of 2.5 µm at a flow rate of 4 L/min with negligible interstage particle losses (< 0.2%) for particles smaller than 2.7-µm–aerodynamic diameter (117). Measurements were conducted by placing 47-mm Teflon filters downstream from the minor flow of stage III and the Harvard-Marple impactors (HMIs) and comparing the fine particulate mass and sulfate concentrations ($d_p < 2.5$ μm) determined by both samplers. The ratio of the concentration in the minor flow of stage III to the average concentration of the two HMIs gives an estimate of the enrichment of the concentration of fine ambient particle that was achieved. At the end of each run, the filters were weighed after equilibration in the constant humidity and temperature room. After their final weighing, the filters were extracted with 5 mL of ultrapure water and 0.100 mL ethanol, which wets the typically hydrophobic Teflon filters. Subsequently, the filters were sonicated for 15 min and analyzed for sulfate ions by ion chromatography (23). The fine mass concentration was increased by a factor of 26.9 (± 0.9), whereas the fine sulfate concentration was increased by a factor of 27.8 (± 1.0). Most importantly, the concentrator and ambient fine mass and sulfate concentrations were highly correlated ($R^2 = 0.93$ and 0.91, respectively).

Another important issue was to determine the particle size range distribution between ambient and concentrated aerosols (118). Specifically, microorifice uniform deposit impactors were placed downstream from the preselective $PM_{2.5}$ inlet and upstream from the stage III outlet. Particles were classified in four ranges: 0.15–0.25, 0.25–0.50, 0.50–1.0, and 1.0–2.5. The particle size fraction distributions in these ranges are clearly not affected by the concentrator (Fig. 4).

D. Exposure of Animals to CAPs

In our laboratory, dogs, rats, mice, and hamsters have been exposed to CAPs. We also have the capability to study various animal models of disease, including rats with monocrotaline-induced inflammation and chronic bronchitis, mice with asthma, and dogs with acute coronary occlusion to model an angina attack. These studies have provided the preliminary basis for investigations of the mechanisms of response described in the foregoing.

The first set of animal exposure studies was conducted by exposing Syrian hamsters to three different concentration levels for 6 hr: a control level (corresponding to typical indoor air; e.g., 5–15 μg/m^3), an intermediate level (fine mass concentration, 151.6 μg/m^3), and a high level (fine mass concentration, 386.7 μg/m^3). Pulmonary response was assessed at the end of exposure and at 24 hr afterward by performing BAL and measuring cells and other constituents in the lavage fluid. Parameters measured included lactate dehydrogenase, myeloperoxidase, hemoglobin, albumin, macrophage number, and cell differential. These experiments did not demonstrate any evidence of lung injury in these healthy animals. The observed exposure levels were as much as 30 times greater than normal ambient levels. This study demonstrated the feasibility of conducting animal exposures using the HAPC and supports the hypothesis that CAPs would usually have little effect on normal animals. In subsequent studies, described in the fol-

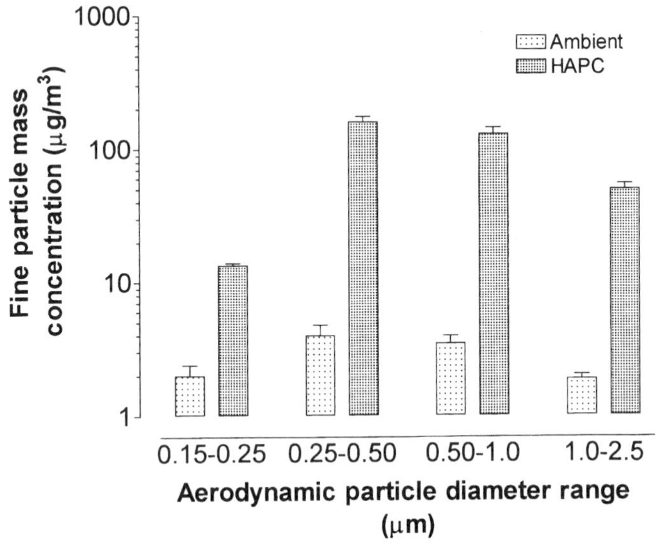

Figure 4 Mass comparison of size fractionation for ambient and concentrated particulate aerosols. Note the similar distribution patterns indicating that concentration does not alter the normal particle size distribution. (From Ref. 118.)

lowing, findings with normal rats as controls also showed no effects on mortality, but pulmonary morbidity parameters have demonstrated significant changes.

Investigation of chronic bronchitic rats exposed to CAPs provided necessary insight into the potential interactions of pulmonary inflammation and pulmonary function alteration that are hypothesized to be associated with downstream cardiac dysfunctions. Normal and chronic bronchitic rats were exposed to filtered air or ultrafine CAPs for 3 days ($\text{mean}_{\text{CAPs}} \approx 500\ \mu g/m^3$ for 6 hr/day). Twenty-four hours following the 3 days of exposure, pulmonary function was reassessed and BAL was performed. Pulmonary function changes were evident in both CAP-exposed groups, air controls, and chronic bronchitic diseased animals. Interestingly, the air controls exposed to CAPs exhibited changes in respiratory frequency and minute volume commonly associated with an irritant-type response (noxious stimuli). In contrast, the chronic bronchitis animals exposed to CAPs exhibited pulmonary function changes in respiratory function (RF), minute volume (MV), and peak expiratory flow, consistent with a bronchoconstrictive stress-type of response (119). Table 1 summarizes the inflammatory changes found, including neutrophil influx and elevated BAL protein owing to vascular permeability associated with CAPs exposure. The observed inflammation was

Table 1 Bronchoalveolar Lavage Parameter Measurements from Normal or Chronic Bronchitic 12-Week-Old Rats Exposed to Filtered Air or Concentrated Urban Air Particulates (CAPs)[a]

Parameter	Normal/air	CB/air	Normal/CAPs	CB/CAPs
Total cell counts ($\times 10^6$)	4.66	5.46	5.81	8.53*
BAL neutrophils ($\times 10^4$)	6.66	28.00	61.00*	142.03*
BAL lymphocytes ($\times 10^4$)	2.66	5.46	17.26*	49.10*
Lactate dehydrogenase (μg/mL)	56.95	112.00	97.64*	109.80
β-*N*-Acetylglucosaminidase (μg/mL)	52.58	36.72	71.26	35.46
Total BAL protein (μg/mL)	458.50	597.60	416.10	2475.00*

[a]Filtered air or CAPs exposures were 6 hr/day for 3 days. Bronchoalveolar lavage was performed 24 hr following exposures. Each value represents the mean of at least eight determinants. *, $p < 0.05$ as determined by *t*-test comparison of CAPs versus air groups.

relatively mild in air-exposed animals, whereas it was quite severe in chronic bronchitic animals, indicating a synergistic-type response (98).

Rat models of monocrotaline-induced pulmonary vascular injury–inflammation (120,121) and chronic bronchitis, with their appropriate controls have been used in exposures of groups of 16 animals to CAPs and groups of 16 normal or diseased animals exposed to filtered air at the same temperature, pressure, and flow, as a control. The concentration factor of outdoor air particles was approximately 30-fold. Exposures to CAPs resulted in significant mortality with monocrotaline-induced inflammation and significant mortality in animals with chronic bronchitis. Table 2 lists concentration, mortality, and pathological findings in these studies (21).

The greater mortality seen with chronic bronchitis compared with monocrotyline-induced inflammation is important. Monocrotyline animals had more PMNs and greater acute inflammation. Pathologically, inflammation was seen in all groups with these preexisting diseases, but animals with chronic bronchitis exposed to CAPs also exhibited evidence of significant bronchoconstriction. The presence of bronchoconstriction was enumerated in histological sections of all groups, comparing the number of constricted airways in animals that died during the exposure with those who survived exposure, but were killed afterward. Visible buckling of the epithelium was the main criteria and is illustrated in the photomicrographs of Figure 5.

Animals that died with chronic bronchitis had the most evidence of airway constriction by this measurement. Survivors with this disease had the second

Table 2 Mortality and Pathological Findings in Rats with No Preexisting Disease, Chronic Bronchitis, or Pulmonary Hypertension Following Exposure to CAPs for 6 hr/Day for 3 Days

Parameter\\group	Control	Monocrotaline	Chronic bronchitis
CAPs (μg/m^3 ± SD)	254 ± 45	228 ± 89	272 ± 40
% Mortality	0%	29%	37%*
Pathological findings on death or sacrifice	No inflammation Minimal bronchoconstriction	Acute inflammation in alveoli and interstitium Some bronchoconstriction	Airway inflammation, increased mucus Marked bronchoconstriction Interstitial edema Pulmonary vascular congestion

*$p < 0.05$.

highest level, followed by animals dying in the monocrotyline treatment group. Thus, the mechanism and role of inflammation and bronchoconstriction in mortality and morbidity is the major focus of this proposal using the chronic bronchitis model because of its significant mortality.

In BAL analysis of our surviving animals in the mortality studies just listed, the monocrotyline animals had about 80% neutrophils in both groups (CAPs and

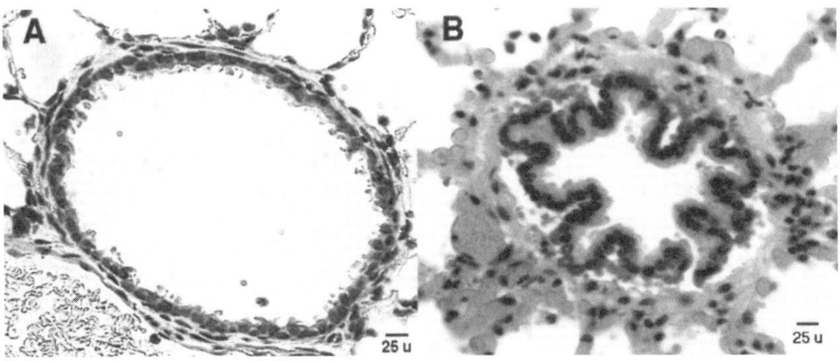

Figure 5 (A) Light micrograph of airways from a normal rat exposed to concentrated ambient particles (CAPs); (B) a chronic bronchitic rat exposed to CAPS that died following exposure for 6 hr/day for 3 days. Note the slight visible buckling of the epithelium in the normal rat exposed to CAPs. In contrast, note the severe bronchoconstriction in the airway of the chronic bronchitic, CAP-exposed rat and the cellular infiltrate in the airway lumen.

filtered air). There were no differences in total BAL neutrophils in these two groups. In rats with chronic bronchitis, CAPs exposure doubled the total number of BAL neutrophils. Another study using an asthma model, with exposure to CAPs, showed the number of macrophages, eosinophils, and neutrophils in BAL fluid doubled with exposure to CAPs, with no effect of CAPs exposure on normal controls. Thus, we have shown (1) significant mortality resulting from CAPs exposure, especially in animals with chronic bronchitis; (2) bronchoconstriction associated with death in both groups, but considerably more bronchoconstriction in the chronic bronchitis groups; and (3) potentiation of inflammation in the asthma and chronic bronchitis groups.

The greater bronchoconstrictive changes histologically and in measured pulmonary function in the chronic bronchitic animals combined with the more severe pulmonary inflammation solidified the hypothesized effect of inhaled particles. Extrapolating from these data, it is possible that the pulmonary inflammation causes changes in pulmonary function and the subsequent release of cytokines and other inflammatory mediators, which leads to cardiac alterations.

IV. Summary and Conclusions

An understanding of the mechanisms whereby inhaled particles cause acute morbidity and mortality has not yet been realized. Epidemiological evidence suggests that cardiopulmonary disease is a primary predecessor of these outcomes (8). Many of these studies have further suggested the importance of investigating fine and ultrafine particles as the primary particulate culprits.

Cardiopulmonary mortality as a result of particle inhalation may be the result of acute pulmonary injury that leads to subsequent cardiac electrical changes and, on occasion, death. It is hypothesized that inhaled ambient particles induce pulmonary inflammation and airway changes in individuals with cardiopulmonary disease. These airway changes most likely stem from an influx of inflammatory cells and changes in the airway lumen. The concomitant release of inflammatory mediators from lung cells, including macrophages, neutrophils, and epithelium, produce local and systemic alterations in cell responses and function. Organs undergoing systemic effects include the heart, in which the combination of cardiac inflammation, hypoxia, and pulmonary stress, lead to cardiac electrical changes, including T-wave alternans, that may eventually interrupt cardiac rhythm, resulting in sudden mortality.

Until now, toxicological studies have failed to adequately address the issue of inhaled particle toxicity relative to the foregoing mechanisms. Most studies have been limited by exposure protocols and the lack of clear-cut pathways for toxic effects. The best currently available studies have employed surrogate particles (26) or limited combinations of ambient pollutants to take into account atmospheric interactions (25,102). The development of ambient particle-concentrating systems is a significant advancement that will allow us to address these issues. At present, the HAPC provides an excellent technical solution for producing aerosols consisting of actual ambient particles. This system has allowed a new generation of particle studies that specifically address ambient atmospheres.

To date, increased pulmonary inflammation and decrements in pulmonary function have been clearly associated with CAPs exposure in animals with cardiopulmonary disease. Normal animals are also not immune to the effects of inhaled particulate matter; these animals have exhibited significant, albeit less severe, lung injury following particle exposure. The future of these studies lies in the investigation of the signaling pathways that are responsible for the sudden mortality observed. Given these data, it is clear that these pathways should be further delineated to develop potential measures to prevent sudden mortality and morbidity in exposed populations.

References

1. Schwartz J, Dockery DW. Particulate air pollution and daily mortality in Steubenville, Ohio. Am J Epidemiol 1992; 135:12–19.
2. Schwartz J, Dockery DW. Increased mortality in Philadelphia associated with daily air pollution concentrations. Am Rev Respir Dis 1992; 145:600–604.
3. Pope CA, Schwartz J, Ransom MR. Daily mortality and PM_{10} in Utah Valley. Arch Environ Health 1992; 47:211–217.
4. Ostro B. The association of air pollution and mortality: examining the case for interference. Arch Environ Health 1993; 48:336–342.
5. Spix C, Heinrich J, Dockery D, Schwartz G, Volksch G, Schwinkowski K, Collen C, Wichmann HE. Air pollution and daily mortality in Erfurt, East Germany, 1980–1989. Environ Health Perspect 1993; 101:518–526.
6. Dockery DW, Pope CA, Xu X, et al. An association between air pollution and mortality in six US cities. N Engl J Med 1993; 329:1753–1759.
7. Dockery DW, Pope CA. Acute effects of particulate air pollution. Annu Rev Publ Health 1994; 15:107–132.
8. Pope CA, Thun MJ, Namboodiri MM, et al. Particulate air pollution as a predictor of mortality in a prospective study of U.S. adults. Am J Respir Crit Care Med 1995; 151:669–674.
9. Bates DV, Sizto R. Hospital admissions and air pollutants in Southern Ontario: the acid summer haze effect. Environ Res 1987; 43:317–331.
10. Pope CA. Respiratory hospital admissions associated with PM_{10} pollution in Utah, Salt Lake, and Cache valleys. Arch Environ Health 1991; 46:9–97.
11. Sunyer J, Anto JM, Murillo C, et al. Effects of urban air pollution on emergency room admissions for chronic obstructive pulmonary disease. Am J Epidemiol 1991; 134:277–286.
12. Burnett RT, Dales R, Krewski D, Vincent R, Dann T, Brook JR. Associations be-

tween ambient particulate sulfate and admissions to Ontario hospitals for cardiac and respiratory diseases. Am J Epidemiol 1995; 142:15–22.
13. Sioutas C, Koutrakis P, Burton RM. A high-volume small cutpoint virtual impactor for separation of atmospheric particulate from gaseous pollutants. Particulate Sci Technol 1995; 12:207–221.
14. Sioutas C, Koutrakis P, Burton RM. A technique to expose animals to concentrated fine ambient aerosols. Environ Health Perspect 1995; 103:172–177.
15. Spengler JD, Thurston GD. Mass and elemental composition of fine and coarse particles in six U.S. cities. J Am Pollut Control Assoc 1983; 33:1162–1171.
16. Shore SA, Kobzik L, Long N, et al. Increased airway responsiveness to inhaled methacholine in a rat model of chronic bronchitis. Am J Respir Crit Care Med 1995; 151:1931.
17. Farone A, Huang S, Paulauskis JD, Kobzik L. Airway neutrophilia and chemokine mRNA expression in SO_2-induced bronchitis. Am J Respir Cell Mol Biol 1995; 152:345–350.
18. Sweeney TD, Skornik WA, Brain JD, Hatch V, Godleski JJ. Chronic bronchitis alters the pattern of aerosol deposition in the lung. Am J Respir Crit Care Med 1995; 151:482–488.
19. Nearing BD, Verrier RL. Simultaneous assessment of autonomic regulation and cardiac vulnerability during coronary occlusion and reperfusion by complex demodulation of heart rate variability and T-wave alternans. Circulation 1992; 86(suppl I):I639.
20. Godleski JJ, Sioutas C, Katler M, Koutrakis P. Death from inhalation of concentrated ambient air particles in animal models of pulmonary disease. Am J Respir Crit Care Med 1996; 153:A15.
21. Schwartz J, Morris R. Air pollution and hospital admissions for cardiovascular disease in Detroit, Michigan. Am J Epidemiol 1995; 142:123–125.
22. Killingsworth C, Alessandrini F, Krishna Murthy G, Catalano P, Paulauskis J, Godleski J. Inflammation, chemokine expression, and death in monocrotaline-treated rats following fuel oil fly ash inhalation. Inhal Toxicol 1997; 9:541–565.
23. Koutrakis P, Wolfson JM, Spengler JD. An improved method for measuring aerosol acidity: results from a nine-month study in St. Louis, MO and Kingston, TN. Atmos Environ 1988; 22:157–163.
24. Koutrakis P, Briggs SLK. Source apportionment of indoor aerosols in Suffolk and Onondaga counties, New York. Environ Sci Technol 1992; 26:521–527.
25. Amdur M, Chen L. Furnace-generated acid aerosols: speciation and pulmonary effects. Environ Health Perspect 1989; 79:147–150.
26. Dreher K, Jaskot R, Lehmann J, Richards J, McGee J, Ghio A, Costa D. Soluble transition metals mediate residual oil fly ash induced acute lung injury. J Toxciol Environ Health 1997; 50:285–305.
27. Killingsworth CR, Skornik WA, Gazula G, Katler M, Stearns RC, Paulauskis JD, Godleski JJ. Ultrafine copper oxide particles increase pulmonary inflammation and resistance in hamsters. Am J Respir Crit Care Med 1996; 153:A470.
28. Dye JA, Adler KB, Richards JH, Dreher KL. Epithelial injury induced by exposure to residual oil fly-ash particles: role of reactive oxygen species? Am J Respir Cell Mol Biol 1997; 17:625–633.
29. Kadiiska MB, Mason RP, Dreher KL, Costa DL, Ghio AJ. In vivo evidence of free

radical formation in the rat lung after exposure to an emission source air pollution particle. Chem Res Toxicol 1997; 10:1104–1108.
30. Sibille Y, Reynolds HY. State of the art: macrophages and polymorphonuclear neutrophils in lung defense and injury. Am Rev Respir Dis 1990; 141:471–501.
31. Halliwell B, Gutteridge JMC. Free Radicals in Biology and Medicine. Oxford: Clarendon Press, 1989.
32. Shi MM, Godleski JJ, Paulauskis JD. Effect of oxidative stress on inflammatory cytokine mRNA expression in rat alveolar macrophages. FASEB J 1995; 9:A346.
33. Shi MM, Godleski JJ, Paulauskis JD. Regulation of macrophage inflammatory protein-1α mRNA by oxidative stress. J Biol Chem 1996; 271:5878–5883.
34. Stringer B, Imrich A, Kobzik L. Lung epithelial cell (A549) interaction with unopsonized environmental particulates: quantitation of particle-specific binding and IL-8 production. Exp Lung Res 1996; 22:495–508.
35. Stringer B, Kobzik L. Priming of lung epithelial cell (A549) with TNF-a up-regulates IL-8 production in response to environmental particulates. Am J Respir Crit Care Med 1996; 153:A15.
36. Grabowski GM, Paulauskis JD, Godleski JJ. Vanadium-induced active oxygen radical production and phosphotyrosine phosphatase inhibition in rat lung macrophages. In: FASEB Summer Research Conference, Phosphatases, 1994.
37. Grabowski GM, Tsai CS, Paulauskis JD, Godleski JJ. Signal transduction in the metal-induced respiratory burst of lung macrophages. Am J Respir Crit Care Med 1996; 153:A240.
38. Tsai CS, Shi MM, Godleski JJ, Paulauskis JD. Manganese-induced pulmonary inflammation and increased expression of pro-inflammatory cytokines mRNA in rat lung cells. Am J Respir Crit Care Med 1996; 153:A614.
39. Pierce LM, Alessandrini F, Godleski JJ, Paulauskis JD. Vanadium-induced chemokine mRNA expression and pulmonary inflammation. Toxicol Appl Pharmacol 1996; 138:1–11.
40. Sedgewick JB, Berube ML, Zurier RB. Stimulus-dependent inhibition of superoxide generation by prostaglandins. Clin Immunopathol 1985; 34:205–215.
41. Forman HJ, Kim E. Inhibition by linoleic acid hydroperoxide of alveolar macrophage superoxide production: effect upon mitochondrial and plasma membrane potentials. Arch Biochem Biophys 1989; 274:443–452.
42. Robinson TW, Forman HJ. Dual effect of nitrogen dioxide on rat alveolar macrophage arachidonate metabolism. Lung Res 1993; 19:21–36.
43. Kuhn DC, Stanley CF, El-Ayouby N, Demers LM. Effect of in vivo coal dust exposure on arachidonic acid metabolism in the rat alveolar macrophage. J Toxicol Environ Health 1990; 29:157–168.
44. Chen L, Miller P, Amdur M. Effects of sulfur oxides on eicosanoids. J Toxicol Environ Health 1989; 28:99–109.
45. Demers LM, Kuhn D. Influence of mineral dusts on metabolism of arachidonic acid. Environ Health Perspect 1994; 102:97–100.
46. Misawa M, Nakano E. Airway constriction by xanthine/xanthine oxidase in guinea pigs in vivo. J Toxicol Environ Health 1993; 39:193–205.
47. Carter JD, Ghio AJ, Samet JM, Devlin RB. Cytokine production by human airway

epithelial cells after exposure to an air pollution particle is metal-dependent. Toxicol Appl Pharmicol 1997; 146:180–188.
48. Mullen J, Wright J, Wiggs B, et al. Reassessment of inflammation of airways in chronic bronchitis. Br Med J 1985; 291:1235–1239.
49. Thompson A, Daughton D, Robbins R, Ghafouri M, Oehlerking M, Rennard S. Intraluminal airway inflammation in chronic bronchitis. Am Rev Respir Dis 1989; 140:1527–1537.
50. Hutson P, Varley J, Sanjar S, et al. Evidence that neutrophils do not participate in the late phase airways response provoked by ovalbumin inhalation in conscious, sensitized guinea pigs. Am Rev Respir Dis 1990; 141:535–539.
51. Pauwels R, Kips J, Peleman R, Straeten MVD. The effect of endotoxin inhalation on airway responsiveness and cellular influx in rats. Am Rev Respir Dis 1990; 141: 540–545.
52. Baggiolini M, Walz A, Kunkel SL. Neutrophil-activating peptide-1/interleukin 8, a novel cytokine that activates neutrophils. J Clin Invest 1989; 84:1045–1049.
53. Detmers P, Lo S, Olsen-Egbert E, Walz A, Baggiolini M, Cohn Z. Neutrophil-activating protein-1/interleukin-8 stimulates the binding activity of the leukocyte adhesion receptor CD116/DC18 on human neutrophils. J Exp Med 1990; 171: 1155–1162.
54. Peveri P, Walz A, Dewald B, Baggiolini M. A novel neutrophil-activating factor produced by human mononuclear phagocytes. J Exp Med 1988; 167:1547–1599.
55. Thelen FM, Peveri P, Kernen P, Tscharner VV, Walz A. Mechanism of neutrophil activation by NAF, a novel monocyte derived peptide agonist. FASEB J 1988; 2: 2702–2706.
56. Strieter R, Chensue S, Basha M, Standiford T, Lynch J, Baggiolini M, Kunkel S. Human alveolar macrophage gene expression of interleukin-8 by tumor necrosis factor-alpha, lipopolysaccharide, and interleukin-1 beta. Am J Respir Cell Mol Biol 1990; 2:321–326.
57. Kunkel S, Standiford T, Kashara K, Streiter R. Interleukin-8 (IL-8): the major neutrophil chemotactic factor in the lung. Exp Lung Res 1991; 17:17–23.
58. Wolpe SD, Davatelis G, Sherry B, Beutler B, Hesse DG, Nguyen HT, Moldawer LL, Nathan CF, Lowry SF, Cerami A. Macrophages secrete a novel heparin-binding protein with inflammatory and neutrophil chemokinetic properties. J Exp Med 1988; 167:570–581.
59. Watanabe K, Kinoshita S, Nakagaw H. Purification and characterization of cytokine-induced neutrophil chemoattractant produced by epithelioid cell line of normal rat kidney. Biochem Biophys Res Commun 1989; 161:1093–1099.
60. Oquendo P, Alberto J, Wen D, Grayear JL, Deryuck R, Stiles CD. The platelet derived growth factor-inducible KC gene encodes a secretory protein related to platelet alpha-granule proteins. J Biol Chem 1989; 264:4133–4137.
61. Huang S, Paulauskis JD, Godleski JJ, Kobzik L. Expression of macrophage inflammatory protein-2 and KC mRNA in pulmonary inflammation. Am J Pathol 1992; 141:981–988.
62. Huang S, Paulauskis JD, Kobzik L. Rat KC cDNA cloning and mRNA expression in lung macrophages and fibroblasts. Biochem Biophys Res Commun 1992; 184: 922–929.

63. Frevert CW, Farone A, Danaee H, Paulauskis JD, Kobzik L. Functional characterization of the rat chemokine macrophage inflammatory protein-2. Inflammation 1995; 19:133–142.
64. Kobzik L, Huang S, Paulauskis JD, Godleski JJ. Particle opsonization and lung macrophage cytokine response: in vitro and in vivo analysis. J Immunol 1993; 151: 2753–2759.
65. Lown B, Verrier RL. Neural activity and ventricular fibrillation. N Engl J Med 1976; 294:1165–1170.
66. Zipes DP, Miyazaki T. The autonomic nervous system and the heart: basis for understanding interaction and effects on arrhythmia development. In: Zipes DP, Jalife J, eds. Cardiac Electrophysiology: From Cell to Bedside. Philadelphia: WB Saunders, 1990.
67. Corr PB, Yamada KA, Witkowski FX. Mechanisms controlling cardiac autonomic function and their relation to arrhythmogenesis. In: Fozzard HA, et al., eds. The Heart and Cardiovascular System. New York: Raven Press, 1986.
68. Smith JM, Clancy EA, Valeri CR, Ruskin JN, Cohen RJ. Electrical alternans and cardiac electrical instability. Circulation 1988; 77:110–121.
69. Schwarz PJ, Malliani A. Electrical alteration of the T-wave: clinical and experimental evidence of its relationship with the sympathetic nervous system and with the long Q-T syndrome. Am Heart J 1975; 89:45.
70. Rosenbaum DS, Jackson LE, Smith JM, et al. Electrical alternans and vulnerability to ventricular arrhythmias. N Engl J Med 1994; 330:235–241.
71. Corbalan R, Verrier RL, Lown B. Psychological stress and ventricular arrhythmias during myocardial infarction in the conscious dog. Am J Cardiol 1974; 34:692–696.
72. Verrier RL, Nearing BD. Electrophysiologic basis for T-wave alternans as an index of vulnerability to ventricular fibrillation. J Cardiovasc Electrophysiol 1994; 5:445–461.
73. Nearing BD, Verrier RL. Personal computer system for tracking cardiac vulnerability by complex demodulation of the T-wave. J Appl Physiol 1993; 74:2606–2612.
74. Nearing BD, Huang AH, Verrier RL. Dynamic tracking of cardiac vulnerability by complex demodulation of the T-wave. Science 1991; 252:437.
75. Wells A. Passive smoking as a cause of heart disease. J Am Coll Cardiol 1994; 24:546–554.
76. Zhu B, Sun Y, Sievers R, Glantz S, Parmley W, Wolfe C. Exposure to environmental tobacco smoke increased myocardial infarct size in rats. Circulation 1994; 89: 1282–1290.
77. Moskowitz W, Mosteller M, Schieken R, Hewitt J, Bodurtha J, Segrest J. Lipoprotein and oxygen transport alteration in passive smoking preadolescent children: the MCV Irwin study. Circulation 1990; 81:586–592.
78. Aronow W. Effect of passive smoking on angina pectoris. N Engl J Med 1978; 299:21–24.
79. Khalfen E, Klochkov V. Effect of passive smoking on the physical tolerance of ischemic heart disease patients. Terapevticheskii Arkhiv 1987; 59 (5):112–115.
80. McMurray R, Hicks L, Thompson D. The effects of passive inhalation of cigarette

smoke on exercise performance. Eur J Appl Physiol Occup Physiol 1985; 54:196–200.
81. Watkinson WP, Campen MJ, Costa DL. Cardiac arrhythmia induction after exposure to residual oil fly ash particles in a rodent model of pulmonary hypertension. Toxicol Sci 1998; 41:209–216.
82. Vaddi K, Nicolini FA, Mehta P, Mehta JL. Increased secretion of tumor necrosis factor-alpha and interferon-gamma by mononuclear leukocytes in patients with ischemic heart disease. Circulation 1994; 90:694–699.
83. Strieter RM, Kunkel SL, Bone RC. Role of tumor necrosis factor-alpha in disease states and inflammation. Crit Care Med 1993; 21:S447–S463.
84. Basaran Y, Basaran MM, Babacan KF, et al. Serum tumor necrosis factor levels in acute myocardial infarction and unstable angina pectoris. Angiology 1993; 44: 332–337.
85. Abe Y, Kawakami M, Kuroki M, et al. Transient rise in serum interleukin-8 concentration during acute myocardial infarction. Br Heart J 1993; 70:132–134.
86. Giroir BP, Horton JW, White DJ, et al. Inhibition of tumor necrosis factor prevents myocardial dysfunction during burn shock. Am J Physiol 1994; 267:H118–H124.
87. Tanaka N, Kita T, Kasai K, Nagano T. The immunocytochemical localization of tumour necrosis factor and leukotriene in the rat heart and lung during endotoxin shock. Virchows Arch 1994; 424:273–277.
88. Mann DL, Young JB. Basic mechanisms in congestive heart failure. Recognizing the role of proinflammatory cytokines. Chest 1994; 105:897–904.
89. DeMeules JD, Pigula FA, Mueller M, et al. Tumor necrosis factor and cardiac function. J Trauma 1992; 32:686–692.
90. Finkel MS, Oddis CV, Jacob TD, et al. Negative inotropic effects of cytokines on the heart mediated by nitric oxide. Science 1992; 257:387–389.
91. Yokoyama T, Vaca L, Rosen RD, et al. Cellular basis for the negative inotropic effects of tumor necrosis factor-alpha in the adult mammalian heart. J Clin Invest 1993; 92:2302–2312.
92. Li YH, Rozanski GJ. Effects of human recombinant interleukin-1 on electrical properties of guinea pig ventricular cells. Cardovasc Res 1993; 27:525–530.
93. Weisensee D, Bereiter-Hahn J, Schoeppe W, Low-Friedrich I. Effects of cytokines on the contractility of cultured cardiac monocytes. Int J Immunopharmacol 1993; 15:581–587.
94. Thurston G, Lippmann M, Bartoszek M, Fine J. Air pollution associations with asthma exacerbations, peak flow changes, and respiratory symptoms in children at a summer asthma camp. Am Rev Respir Dis 1993; 147:A632.
95. Williams MK. Sickness absence and ventilatory capacity of workers exposed to sulfuric acid mist. Br J Ind Med 1970; 27:61.
96. Gamble J, Jones W, Hancock J, Meckstroth RL. Epidemiological–environmental study of lead acid battery workers. III. Environ Res 1984; 35 (30).
97. Saldiva PHN, King M, et al. Respiratory alterations due to urban air pollution: an experimental study in rats. Environ Res 1992; 57:19.
98. Clarke R, Hatch V, Katler M, Koutrakis P, Love J, Krishna Murthy G, Stearns R, Sioutas C, Paulauskis J, Godleski J. Concentrated urban air particulate (CAPs)

inhalation induces pulmonary imflammation in normal and chronic bronchitic rats. Am Rev Respir Crit Care Med 1997; 155:A245.
99. West JB. Respiratory Physiology—the Essentials. Baltimore: Williams & Wilkins, 1990.
100. Neas L, Dockery D, Koutrakis P, Tollerud D, Speizer F. The association of ambient air pollution with twice daily peak expiratory flow rate measurements in children. Am J Epidemiol 1995; 141:111–122.
101. Eskelson CD, Chvapil M, Strom KA, et al. Pulmonary phospholipidosis in rats respiring air containing diesel particles. Environ Res 1987; 44:260–271.
102. Strom KA. Response of pulmonary cellular defenses to the inhalation of high concentrations of diesel exhaust. J Toxicol Environ Health 1984; 13:919–944.
103. Conner M, Lam H, Rogers A, Fitzgerald S, Amdur M. Lung injury in guinea pigs caused by multiple exposures to submicron zinc oxide mixed with sulfur dioxide in a humidified furnace. J Toxicol Environ Health 1985; 16:101–114.
104. Hemenway D, Clarke R, Frank R, Jakab G. Factors governing the mass-loading of aerosolized carbon black particles with acid sulfates, inhalation exposure, and alveolar macrophage phagocytosis. Inhal Toxicol 1996; 8:679–694.
105. Coffin DL, Blommer EJ. Acute toxicity of irradiated auto exhaust: its indication by enhancement of mortality from streptococcal pneumonia. Arch Environ Health 1967; 15:36–38.
106. Mauderly JL. Noncancer pulmonary effects of chronic inhalation exposure of animals to solid particles. In: Dungworth DL, Mauderly JL, Oberdorster G, eds. Toxic and Carcinogenic Effects of Solid Particles in the Respiratory Tract. Washington, DC: Academic Press, 1994:43–55.
107. Anderson KR, Avol EL, Edwards SA, et al. Controlled exposures of volunteers to respirable carbon and sulfuric acid aerosols. J Air Waste Manage Assoc 1992; 42: 770–776.
108. Clarke RW, Hemenway DR, Frank R, Jakab GJ. Impairment of lung defenses following simultaneous exposure to respirable particulate matter and sulfur dioxide occurs at high, but not low, relative humidity. The Proceedings of The Society of Experimental Biology and Medicine, 1995; 209:299.
109. Brain JD, Knudson DE, Sorokin SP, Davis MA. Pulmonary distribution of particles given by intratracheal instillation or by aerosol inhalation. Environ Res 1976; 11: 13–33.
110. Beck BD, Gerson B, Feldman HA, Brain JD. Lactate dehydrogenase isoenzymes in hamster lung lavage fluid after lung injury. Toxicol Appl Pharmacol 1983; 71: 59–71.
111. Oberdorster G, Gelein RM, Ferin J, Weiss B. Association of particulate air pollution and acute mortality: involvement of ultrafine particles? Inhal Toxicol 1995; 7:111–124.
112. Oberdorster G, Ferin J, Gelein R, Mercer P, Corson N, Godleski J. Low-level ambient air particulate levels and acute mortality/morbidity: studies with ultrafine Teflon particles. Am J Respir Crit Care Med 1995; 151:A66.
113. Godleski JJ, Hatch V, Hauser R, Christiani D, Gazula G, Sioutas C. Ultrafine particles in lung macrophages of healthy people. Am J Respir Crit Care Med 1995; 151:A264.

114. Whitby KT, Svendrup GM. California aerosols: their physical and chemical characteristics. Adv Environ Sci Technol 1980; 10:477.
115. McMurray P, Zhang X. Size distribution of ambient organic and elemental carbon. Aerosol Sci Technol 1990; 10:430–437.
116. Hitzenberger R, Puxbaum H. Comparisons of the measured and calculated specific absorption coefficients for urban aerosol samples in Vienna. Aerosol Sci Technol 1993; 18:323–345.
117. Marple V, Rubow KL, Turner W, Spengler JD. Low flow rate sharp cut impactors for indoor air sampling: design and calibration. J Air Pollut Control Assoc 1987; 37:1303–1307.
118. Sioutas C, Koutrakis P, Godleski JJ, Ferguson ST, Kim CS, Burton RM. Fine particle concentrators for inhalation exposures-effect of particle size and composition. J Aerosol Sci 1997; 28:1057–1071.
119. Clarke R, Catalano P, Krishna Murthy G, Sioutas C, Wolfson M, Koutrakis P, Godleski J. Inhalation of concentrated ambient particles (CAPs) induces pulmonary function alterations in normal and chronic bronchitic animals. Inhalation Tox 1999. In press.
120. Costa DL, Lehmann JR, Frazier LT, et al. Pulmonary hypertension: a possible risk factor in particulate toxicity. Am J Respir Crit Care Med 1994; 149:A840.
121. White SM, Roth RA. Progressive lung injury and pulmonary hypertension from monocrotaline. In: Cantor JO, ed. Handbook of Animal Models of Pulmonary Disease. vol 2. Boca Raton, FL: CRC Press, 1989.

16

Neurally Mediated Cardiopulmonary and Systemic Responses to Inhaled Irritants and Antigens

DONOVAN B. YEATES

University of Illinois at Chicago and
Veterans Affairs Chicago Health Care System
Chicago, Illinois

I. Introduction

The association between the presence of airborne irritants, including ozone, sulfur oxides, and particulates, and increased morbidity and mortality, is exacerbated in persons with compromised cardiopulmonary function, including congestive lung and heart diseases, as well as patients with asthma (see Chap. 5). This raises questions about the possible acute physiological sequellae that may be initiated or at least aggravated by inhaled irritants and antigens that precipitate these dire outcomes. In this chapter, I make intercomparisons between the neural reflexes activated by irritants and allergens and their efferent responses. These efferent responses include ventilation, bronchomotor tone, mucosal function, and cardiac performance. In addition, the invoked responses involve changes in pulmonary, visceral, and systemic vascular smooth-muscle tone that cause dramatic changes in pulmonary and systemic arterial pressures. In highlighting the similarities and differences in these responses, I hope to engender interest in research that will provide both insight into the potential pathophysiological mechanisms and targets for prophylactic and therapeutic intervention as well as provide a rationale for the reduction of exposure to inhaled irritants and antigens to persons at risk.

II. Irritant-Induced Cardiopulmonary Responses

The pulmonary chemoreflex, as its name suggests, is mediated by irritant activation of sensory nerves in the laryngeal, tracheobronchiolar [see Ref. 75], or alveolar regions of the lungs. It classically consists of apnea, followed by tachypnea together with bradycardia and systemic hypotension (1). An example of a pulmonary chemoreflex can be seen following spontaneous inhalation of one breath of ammonia vapor (Fig. 1). Following inhalation of the vapor above an 8 M solution,

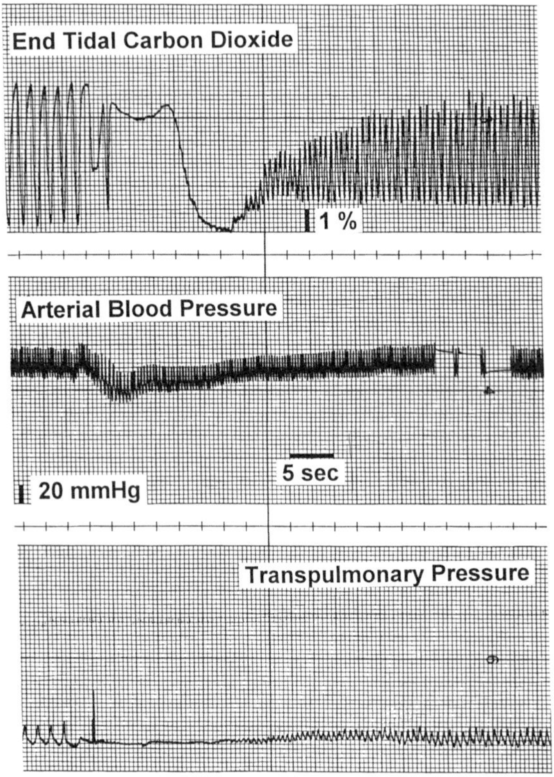

Figure 1 A beagle dog was anesthetized with propofol and etomidate and intubated. One 250-mL breath of ammonia vapor above an 8-M ammonia solution was administered to the dog. The end-tidal CO_2 shows an apnea followed by rapid, shallow breathing. The arterial pressure tracing demonstrates the short-lived decrease in heart rate and attendant hypotension. The transpulmonary pressure illustrates that the apnea and tachypnea was due to the absence of ventilatory drive, rather than airway occlusion.

there was an apnea followed by tachypnea, bradycardia, and a drop in femoral arterial pressure. This response was effectively over within 2 min. These responses were completely abrogated by cooling the vagosympathetic trunks to 0°C (Fig. 2). However, when a high concentration of ammonia vapor was delivered, this response was neither blocked by cooling the vagosympathetic trunks to 0°C (Fig. 3a) nor by bilateral vagotomy (see Fig. 3b). These data demonstrate that the neural responses low levels of irritants are transmitted by afferent nerves traversing the vagosympathetic trunks, and when high levels are encountered, the responses from ''sympathetic'' afferents play a larger role.

Pulmonary chemoreflexes can be initiated from sensory nerves in the laryngeal (2), bronchial, and alveolar regions of the lungs (3). Such pulmonary chemoreflexes, are activated by either nonspecific effects of sensory nerves (i.e., ammonia vapor), activation of J, or other receptors on unmylinated C-fibers, or by activating rapidly adapting receptors on myelinated nerves (1,3). At low irritant concentrations, neural transmission of these impulses centrally is by B and C fibers, primarily in the vagi (4,5). At higher concentrations there is evidence that sympathetic afferents are also involved. The neural impulses are centrally processed in the medulla, with the nucleus tractus solitarius (NTS) being a primary focal region (1,6), albeit higher cerebral centers are also involved (7). The resultant efferent neural pathways innervate multiple organs and tissues. Neural drive to the diaphragm and intercostal muscles control the ventilatory responses. There is an increase in breathing frequency at relatively low doses of irritants, and apnea, followed by rapid shallow breathing at higher doses. This can be interpreted in the following manner. The irritant-induced afferent neural impulses act on the central pattern generator to prematurely turn off inspiration, giving rise to rapid, shallow breathing. When the neural impulses become too frequent, the pattern generator is ''frozen,'' resulting in an apnea, the length of which is dose-dependent. When the intensity of these impulses decreases, there is the resultant rapid, shallow breathing. The role of this reflex in the genesis of dyspnea in humans is still speculative. In awake humans, conscious control of breathing will at least attempt to override this inhibition of respiratory drive. Neural drive to the heart causes a parasympathetically induced decrease in heart rate. The release of acetylcholine from efferent nerves in the systemic vasculature causes dilation of the vessels in the bronchi, skeletal muscle, and myocardium (1). This vasodilation, together with a decrease in heart rate, results in a marked decrease in systemic arterial pressure.

In addition to these ''classic'' responses, activation of sensory nerves can cause an increase in bronchial blood flow (8), bronchomotor tone (1), mucous secretion (9–12), and ciliary beat frequency (13), and possibly an increase of transepithelial fluid transport (14,15). In concert, these effects on the components of the mucociliary transport system are likely to cause an increase in mucociliary

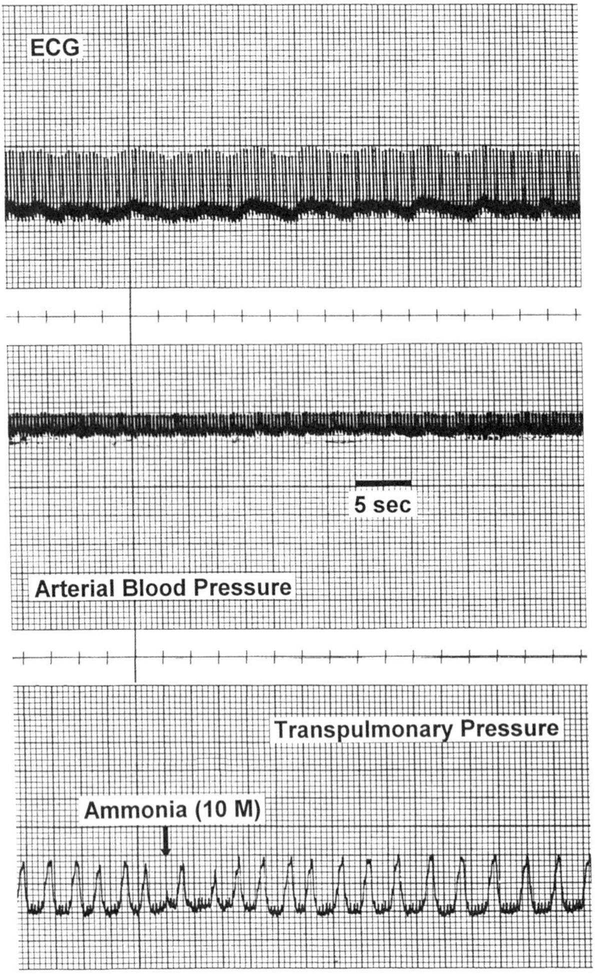

Figure 2 A beagle dog was anesthetized with thiamylal sodium (Surital) and intubated. The vagosympathetic trunks of this dog had previously been exteriorized and placed in skin tubes. This enabled the positioning of copper blocks, with templates of the skin tube milled out, to be placed on the skin tubes. These copper blocks were cooled to 0°C with thermoelectric elements with the excess heat conducted away by water flowing through the adjacent heat sink. A small jar containing 20 mL of 10-M ammonia solution was transiently placed in proximity to the endotracheal tube while the dog inhaled one breath. Following spontaneous inhalation of the ammonia vapor, there were no changes in ECG, arterial blood pressure, nor was there any tachypnea.

clearance. Teleologically, it can be argued that such a response from inhaled irritants (and allergens) is designed to remove the offending irritant from the airways. However, it has recently been proposed that the mucociliary transport system is under both excitatory and inhibitory neural control (15–17). This implies that stimulation of the mucociliary transport system can be affected by either the activation of excitatory neural pathways or, conversely, by the inhibition of inhibitory pathways. It also implies that either mucous secretion, ciliary activity, and possibly transepithelial ion and water transport can be reduced by activation of inhibitory pathways, or by inhibition of excitatory pathways. Protons and capsaicin activate overlapping subsets of sensory nerves by opening ion conductances of similar properties (18). It is possible that these proton-sensitive nerves constitute a set of sensory receptors for an inhibitory pathway. This inhibitory neural reflex could decrease mucociliary transport caused by SO_2 (16) and dry air (17). It may be that whether mucociliary clearance is fast or slow is of little consequence in terms of airway occlusion if airway secretions and ciliary activity are proportionately stimulated or inhibited. However, it is conceptually clear that if airway secretions are stimulated by an excitatory neural reflex and ciliary activity is slowed by an inhibitory reflex, mucus can accumulate in the airways, with a resultant loss of airway patency. This hypothesis has yet to be demonstrated. The predicted differential responses in these pathways could cause, or at least aggravate, obstructive airway diseases, such as bronchitis, cystic fibrosis, and asthma.

Organic irritants can cause a pulmonary chemoreflex. Such a response is shown in an anesthetized, spontaneously breathing dog in Figure 4. Here, the irritant was lauric acid and some heat-induced degradation products (possibly acrolein). On administration of the irritant there was an induced bradycardia and a marked and continued decrease in pulmonary artery pressure. On cessation of the challenge, there was an apneic period lasting for 63 sec, followed by rapid, shallow breathing, an increase in lung resistance, and a decrease in dynamic compliance. In this example, the response was prolonged, with the Po_2 decreasing from 94 mmHg (Pco_2 42 mmHg) before delivery of lauric acid to 60 mmHg (Pco_2 52 mmHg) 20 min after delivery of lauric acid. At 37 min, the Po_2 was 46 mmHg and Pco_2 76 mmHg. Considerable recovery was observed after 50 min, with Po_2 being 90 mmHg and Pco_2 being 39 mmHg.

Inhalation of irritants, such as ozone, can cause systemic effects. Inflammation causes a rise in heart rate and core temperature, whereas in rats, inhalation of the irritant gas, ozone (0.05 ppm), caused near maximal decreases in heart rate and core temperature within 10 min (20). It can be argued that the drop in heart rate and blood pressure (21,22), as well as the increase in breathing frequency (23), is due to parasympathetic responses resulting from the irritant-in-

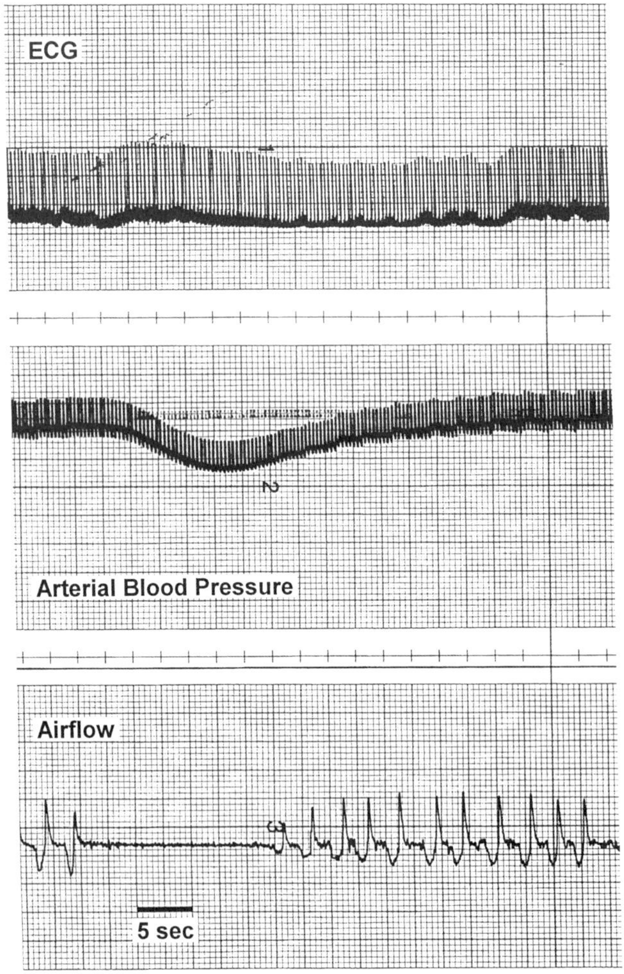

(a)

Figure 3 When the dog in Figure 2 inhaled a breath of ammonia vapor above a 14-M solution of ammonia, and the vagosympathetic trunks were cooled to 0°C, (a) the vapor still induced apnea and systemic arterial hypotension. (b) Neither the ammonia-induced apnea nor the hypotension were abolished by bilateral sectioning of the vagosympathetic trunks.

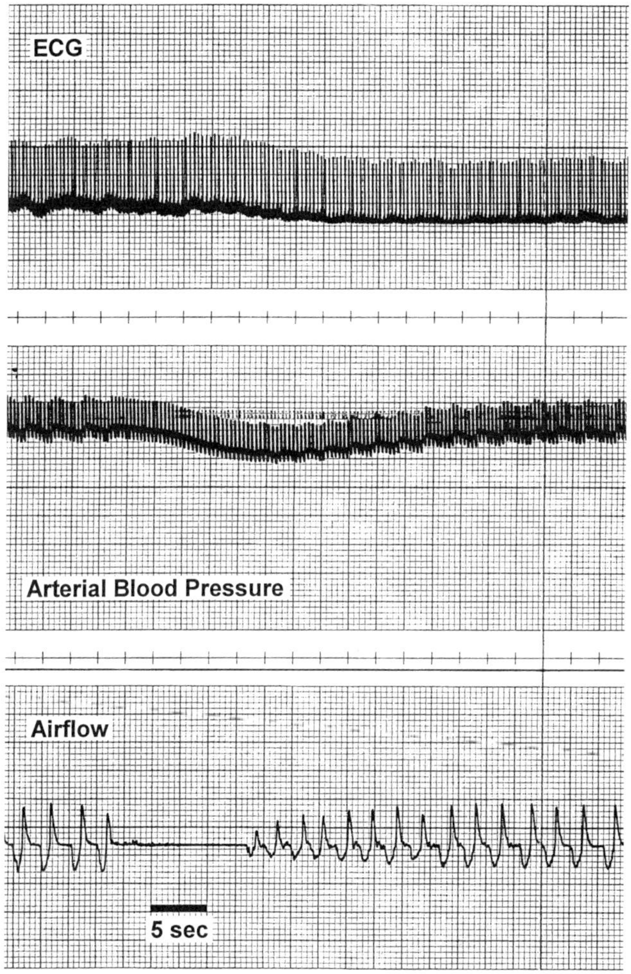

(b)

duced activation of mylinated and unmylinated sensory nerves, albeit the afferent role of pulmonary C-fibers has been questioned (24). In addition, activation of C-fibers and visceral nerves may have a general inhibitory effect on somatic components (1). The mechanisms responsible for these physiological responses have yet to be explicitly delineated. The decrease in core temperature and associated reduction in metabolism is a protective mechanism that is observable in

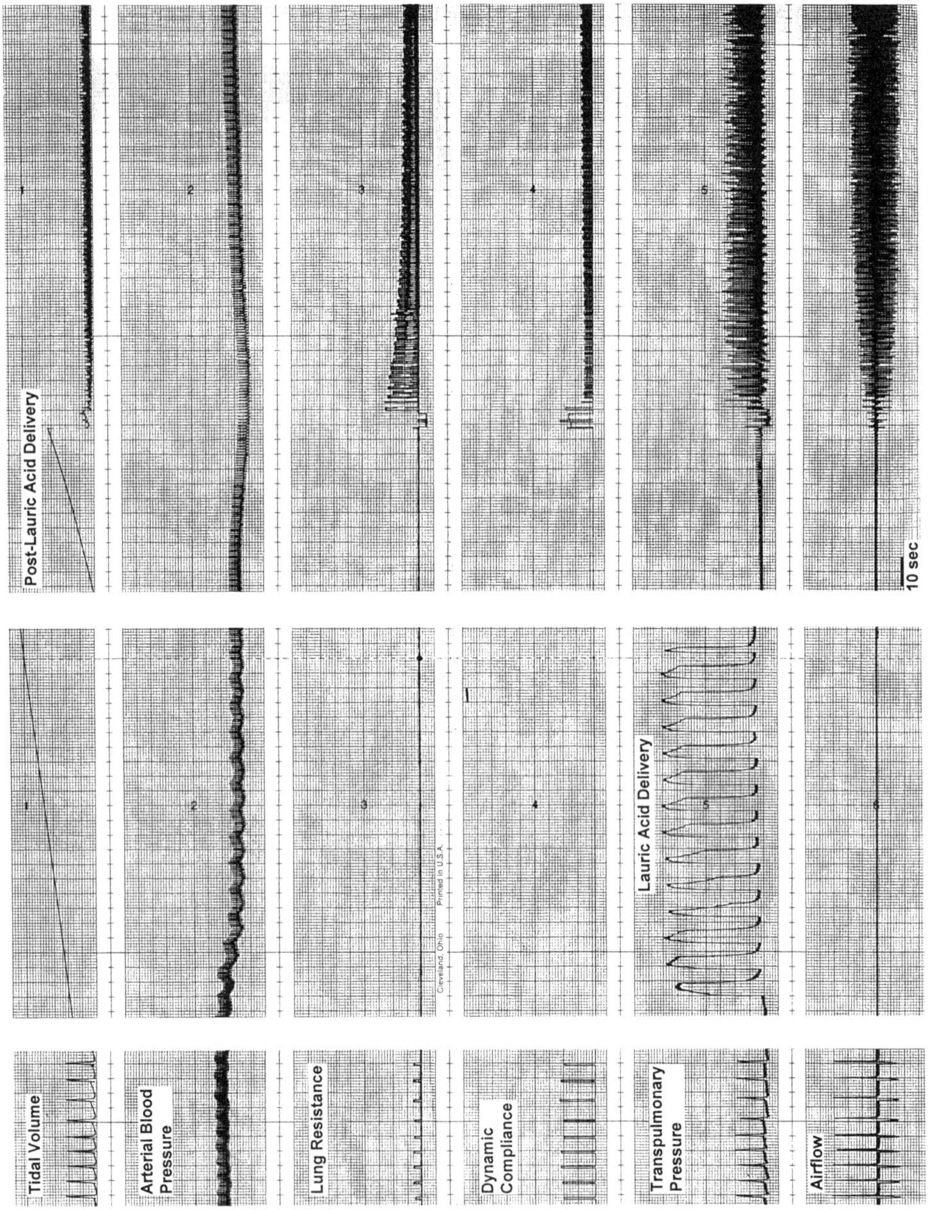
Tidal Volume
Arterial Blood Pressure
Lung Resistance
Dynamic Compliance
Transpulmonary Pressure
Airflow
Lauric Acid Delivery
Post-Lauric Acid Delivery
10 sec

rodents. Any role of this response in the morbidity and mortality in humans has yet to be demonstrated; however, the potential is apparent.

III. Effects of Pathology on the Pulmonary Chemoreflex

Lung congestion not only activates J receptors (25), it also augments the responses of rapidly adapting myelinated neurons to cigarette smoke (26). Experimental embolism causes an increase in lung resistance as well hyperreactively to acetylcholine that are both ablated by vagal blockade (27). Also, edema enhances the responses of J receptors to phenyl diguanide (28). These animal data are consistent with an increase in cholinergic tone in persons with chronic obstructive pulmonary disease (COPD; 29) and the beneficial role of anticholinergic therapy for the treatment of patients with obstructive lung disease (29,30). This congestion-induced neural hyperreactivity would indicate that this group of patients compose an ''at-risk'' population to inhaled irritants, consistent with epidemiological data. The increase in hypersensitivity seen in capsaicin-pretreated animals (24) could imply that at least a subset of these fibers is involved with inhibitory neural reflexes that oppose excitatory reflexes. This is also consistent with the airway hyperresponsiveness observed in persons with denervated lungs from lung transplantation. Thus, even in the absence of allergic hyperreactivity, persons with compromised lung function can, on physiological grounds, be predicted to be more susceptible to the acute effects of inhaled irritants.

IV. Antigen-Induced Cardiopulmonary and Systemic Responses

The striking similarities between the cardiovascular, ventilatory, and respiratory physiological responses to inhaled irritants and allergens implies that the irritant-induced pulmonary chemoreflex comprises a subset of the more profound allergen-induced anaphylactic cardiovascular and pulmonary collapse.

Figure 4 A beagle dog was anesthetized with thyamylal sodium (Surital) and intubated. The tidal volume, pulmonary artery pressure, lung resistance, dynamic compliance, transpulmonary pressure, and airflow are shown before and following administration of 14 breaths of an irritant. Lauric acid was heated, in a La Mer–type condensation generator (19), the vapor was condensed in a cold trap operated below 0°C. The response was due to the small particles and any vapors that were not deposited in this trap. This aerosol–vapor was administered for 14 breaths, using a time-controlled series of soleniod valves and thus only transpulmonary pressure and arterial pressure are displayed during the challenge.

All of the foregoing cardiovascular and ventilatory and respiratory responses—namely, apnea followed by tachypnea, bradycardia, and increased bronchial blood flow, as well as systemic hypotension—observed in the pulmonary chemoreflex are characteristic of an anaphylactic reaction (31). An example of the cardiopulmonary responses to an inhaled allergen in a spontaneously breathing dog is shown in Figure 5. There is an increase in transpulmonary pressure indicative of an increase in airways resistance and a decrease in dynamic compliance. There is a marked apnea followed by tachypnea, a marked bradycardia and hypotension. Albeit, there may be some compensatory increase in heart rate, the induced hypotension persists. This hypotension is probably, partly, mediated by the induction of nitric oxide (NO) through the parasympathetically induced activation of nitric oxide synthase (32,33).

In the dog, at least, cooling the vagosympathetic trunks to 0°C can afford immediate protection from the marked allergen-induced bradycardia and often cardiac arrythmias that result from an allergen challenge. The immediate neurogenic bradycardia and hypotension appear to be absent (Fig. 6). A later, but smaller, decrease in arterial pressure is still present. Moreover, both cooling the vagosympathetic trunks and anesthetization of the cervicothoracic ganglia with lidocaine appears to afford even greater protection. These data are consistent with the partial protective effect of vagotomy on death caused by anaphylaxis in the rat (34); airway obstruction (35,36) and tachypnea (37) in the dog; as well as the augmentation of pulmonary anaphylaxis by vagal stimulation in the guinea pig (38).

Neurogenic reflexes play a large role in all animal models of allergic hyperresponsiveness that are especially apparent in the immediate response to an acute antigen exposure. Concurrent with the anaphylactic responses, there is a marked increase in bronchomotor tone, which can be resistant to anticholinergic agents, indicating that, although there may be a cholinergic component, this component is not necessarly the major component in the presence of a direct mediator-induced increase in smooth-muscle tone. In the current treatment of asthma, anticholinergic agents are recommended to alleviate bronchoconstriction caused by increased parasympathetic activity (30,39,40). Thus, to study the role of mediator release from sensory nerves or other humoral mediators and cytokines released during anaphylaxis, the cholinergic and adrenergic components of these reflexes are often inhibited, or alternatively, isolated lung preparations are often used. Consequently, the importance of the central ''protective'' and pathogenic role of these central reflex responses is often overlooked. A question that remains is: Does inhibition of the neural pathways inhibit mediator release? There is evidence to support this contention.

In addition to the neural component of the immediate respiratory and cardiopulmonary responses, other humoral mediators play important, and often central, roles. In an allergen-induced anaphylaxis, the inhaled allergen cross-links

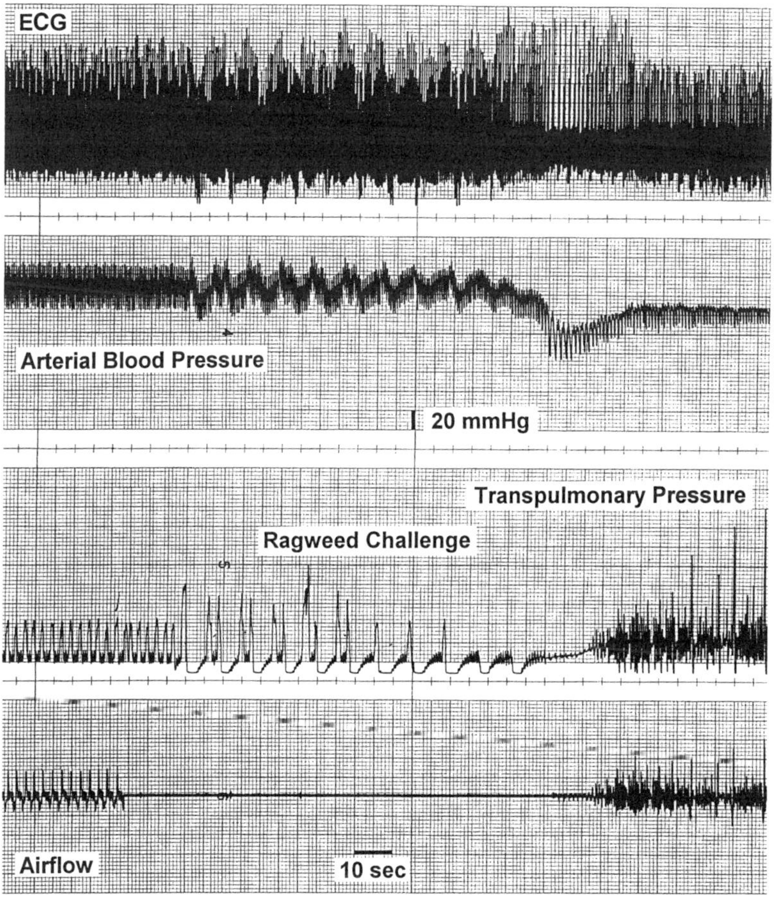

Figure 5 The cardiopulmonary responses to the inhalation of ragweed allergen using an inhalation pattern to preferentially deposit the allergen in the alveolar regions of the lungs of a ragweed-sensitized beagle dog is shown. The total dose of ragweed allergen deposited was 40 μg. Propofol was used as an anesthetic. The ECG, femoral arterial pressure, transpulmonary pressure, and airflow are shown before, during, and following the inhalation of 10 breaths of ragweed.

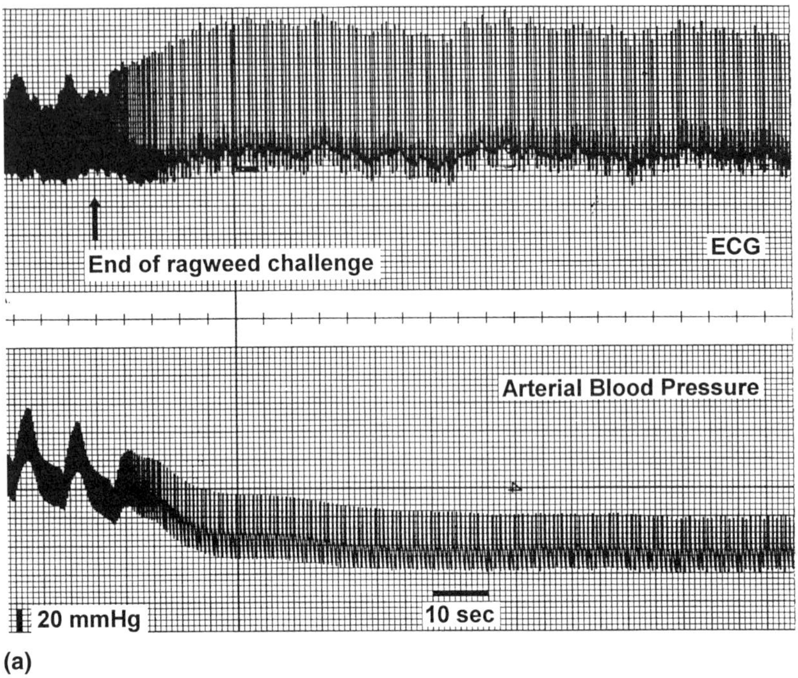

Figure 6 The ECG and blood pressure in a ragweed-sensitized dog that was challenged with 0.15 U/mL of ragweed allergen, (a) without neural blockade, (b) with cooling the vagosympathetic trunks to 0°C, and (c) cooling the vagosympathetic trunks to 0°C and anesthetizing the cervicothoracic ganglia with lidocaine. The slower heart rate under these conditions is indicative of the removal of sympathetic tone.

IgE bound to Fc regions of cellular receptors on mast cells, basophils, eosinophils, and monocytes, including macrophages (41). These cells, when activated, release preformed mediators such as histamine and tryptase, as well as activate the arachidonic acid metabolic pathways to liberate the eicosanoids, including the leukotrienes (i.e., LTD_4), and cyclooxygenase products (TXA_2, PGD_2) as well as the increasingly important roles of the cytokines. In addition, there is activation of complement factors C3a and C5a.

Immunologically sensitized cells are present both in the bronchial mucosa and in the alveolar regions of the lungs. The interstitial location (42) of many of these cells begs the question of how the inhaled allergen accesses these cells. Recently, data (43) have presented that indicate that the epithelium in persons with asthma, when compared with that of controls, lacks the ability to deactivate

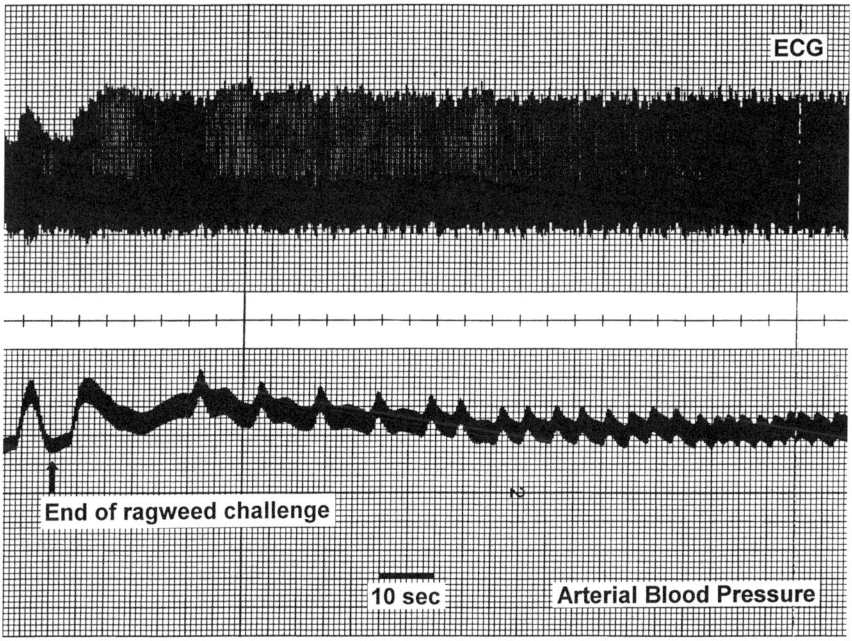
ECG
End of ragweed challenge
10 sec
Arterial Blood Pressure

(b)

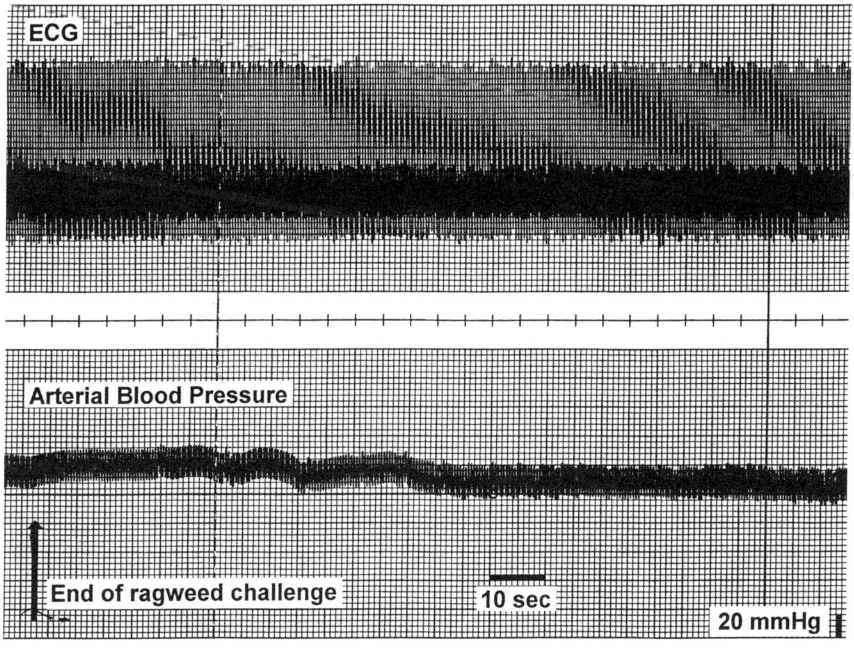
ECG
Arterial Blood Pressure
End of ragweed challenge
10 sec
20 mmHg

(c)

the allergen. These studies imply that the allergen may penetrate the epithelium in persons with asthma, but not that in healthy individuals.

The total number of immunologically primed cells is much greater in the alveolar regions of the lungs than in the bronchi. However, it can be predicted (44) that the surface concentration of particles is much larger in the bronchial airways than the alveolar regions. Thus, it is not surprising that we have demonstrated (31) that anaphylatic reactions are precipitated by deposition of the allergen either proximally or distally. Airborne allergens that deposit in the alveolar regions of the lungs can activate IgE-primed mast cells, macrophages, and basophils. Within 2 min of inhaling microgram masses of allergen, the mediators released activate receptors on sensory nerves as well as circulate within the blood, with the resultant classic anaphylactic reaction. This reaction can be so severe that there is (at least in the anesthetized dog), ventricular asystole, cardiac standstill, and arrhythmias, as well as cessation of breathing (up to 20 min; 31).

A characteristic of anaphylaxis, compared with the pulmonary chemoreflex, is a prolonged systemic circulatory collapse, analogous with, or leading to, circulatory shock (45). For inhaled ragweed allergen in ragweed-sensitized dogs, this hypotension is not compensated by a commensurate increase in heart rate. This indicates an allergen-induced impairment of the normal cardiovascular homeostatic regulatory mechanisms. The cardiovascular responses to inhaled allergens appears to differ from those caused by intravenous injection of antigens. In the later, there is sometimes a pronounced tachycardia (46); however, even in the presence of this tachycardia there is still a marked hypotension (46) indicative of circulatory collapse. Both increases and decreases of heart rate in humans have been observed in persons undergoing systemic anaphylaxis (47,48). Again, in humans, hypotension occurs despite any increase in heart rate (47,48). The major vasodilation causing this increased blood pool is in the splenic or visceral circulation. Administration of histamine can elicit many of the characteristics of anaphylaxis. However, antihistamines may attenuate, but they do not abrogate, the circulatory collapse caused by allergen-induced anaphylaxis (49). Also, unlike the systemic hypotension induced by histamine, this hypotension cannot be reversed by a balloon-induced increase in right atrial pressure (50). This decrease in systemic pressure is likely mediated by a combination of neural and humoral mechanisms. That blockade of vagosympathetic trunk abolishes, or at least markedly attenuates, the systemic circulatory collapse (see Fig. 6b), indicates that the reflex associated with anaphylaxis is also transmitted by the vagi to the visceral organs.

Compounding this profound systemic hypotension is a marked increase in pulmonary vascular resistance (49) caused by vasoconstriction of the pulmonary vasculature. This increase in pulmonary resistance, together with the increase in endothelial and epithelial permeability, give rise to interstitial and later flagrant airway and alveolar edema. This increase in tissue permeability appears to be mediated by the effector properties of sensory afferent nerves. These nerves, when stimulated, can release substance P (SP), calcitonin gene-related peptide (CGRP), and ATP. Of these, SP is associated with extravasation of plasma (51,52).

The airway mucosa also responds to an allergen challenge by an increase in transepithelial ion transport (53), an increase in mucous secretion (54–56), and a consequent marked stimulation of bronchial mucociliary clearance (31). The increase in mucous secretion in dogs is mediated by muscarinic and H_1 receptors (56), consistent with a histamine-induced vagal reflex. Thus, the airways of the lungs respond to an IgE-mediated challenge in a manner analogous with the gut, in which there is an increase in transepithelial ion and water transport and mucous secretion (57), with the removal of the offending antigen being effected by diurea and emesis, rather than ciliary activity and cough.

V. Cardiac Chemoreflex

The heart also responds to irritation by activation of a coronary chemoreflex, otherwise known as the classic Bezold–Jarish effect. This reflex also includes a fall in heart rate and blood pressure, and often, an alteration in the pattern of respiration (58). The heart and major vessels are innervated with sensory nerves, the reflex arcs of which traverse the vagi to synapse in the parasympathetic sensory ganglia. The afferents for this reflex, again run predominantly, but not exclusively, in the vagus nerves with a central medullary origin (59). Afferent nerves also traverse the middle thoracic ganglia to synapse in the dorsal root ganglia, from which information is processed centrally in the medulla (59). The postganglionic efferent nerves innervate the atria, ventricles, and nodal sites, suggesting central regulatory control in each of these sites (59). The heart (60), the gut (61), and most probably the lung, have intrinsic nervous systems. These facilitate intrinsic neural regulation within these large organs. These intrinsic nervous systems, in turn, are modulated by centrally mediated reflexes and events. The efferent traffic modulating the cardiac chronotropic and inotropic responses are transmitted by the vagi and sympathetic nervous system, with parasympathetic activity decreasing the heart rate and sympathetic activity increasing it. The role of this reflex in precipitating the changes in heart rate and arrhythmias caused by inhaled irritants is mostly speculative owing to the difficulty of determining the origin of the neural reflex. It can be predicted, however, that this reflex is more important when irritants cross the epithelial and endothelial barriers. This would include irritants of low molecular weight or high lipid solubility.

VI. Cardiac Anaphylaxis

Cardiac anaphylaxis is an acute ischemic dysfunction comprising coronary vasoconstriction and arrthythmias. The heart is repleat with interstitial mast cells

(62,63). In addition, interstitial basophils have also been reported. The heart itself can undergo anaphylactic responses in response to antigen challenge even when neurally decentralized (64). Ex vivo cardiac responses comprise an increase in coronary vascular resistance, heart rate, and PR interval; development of arrhythmias; and a transient increase followed by a decrease in contractile force. Concurrently, there is a release of histamine. Antigen challenge of the isolated sensitized mouse heart can elicit the outflow of histamine, leukotrienes, catecholamines, thromboxane, and prostacyclin, but not platelet-activating factor (PAF; 65). However, administration of PAF can mimic cardiac anaphylaxis and may play an important role. The roles of mast cells in the genesis of the profound anaphylactic systemic hypotension has been questioned (66). These data are consistent with the findings that antihistamines are relatively ineffective in attenuating this response. Anaphylaxis in mast cell-deficient mice still causes death (66). Bradykinin, a mediator released during anaphylaxis, is a specific bronchial C-fiber activator when administered to the bronchial circulation (67). When administered to the heart, it appears to specifically activate cardiac sympathetic afferents. Bradykinin is a coronary vasodilator, and its administration to the isolated heart can ablate the physiological responses, characteristic of cardiac anaphylaxis, through bradykinin, B_2 receptor activation (68).

The question of the genesis of the cardiac responses arises when the precipitating antigen is inhaled, rather than given intravenously; the latter is used in most experimental models of anaphylaxis. However, cardiovascular responses are elicited by the deposition of ragweed allergen, both proximally and distally (31), implying that cardiac anaphylactic reactions can be initiated either in the bronchial airways or the alveolar regions of the lungs.

There are several possible routes whereby such responses can be affected. First, there is a neural response, as evidenced by the analogous symptoms of the cardiac and pulmonary chemoreflexes. Second, mediators released from the inflammatory cells in the lungs are carried by the blood directly to the heart. Of note, C3a and C5a which are released during anaphylaxis activate cardiac, but not lung mast cells (62). Third, antigens may penetrate the airway and alveolar epithelium and enter into the vasculature and directly interact with cardiac mast cells and basophils. This latter pathway is likely important when small molecules, such as sodium diisocyanate, are inhaled, as these molecules form albumin–isocyanate conjugates that may be related to the induction of toluene diisocyanate hypersensitivity (69).

VII. Interaction Between Allergens and Irritants and Their Common Mechanisms

It is notable that extremely high concentration of irritants, such as ammonia vapor, are necessary to elicit a pulmonary chemoreflex, the physiological responses of which approach those elicited by microgram quantities of allergen. This implies that the activation of receptors on afferent nerves is extremely effective in precipitating a chemoreflex–anaphylactic response compared with that induced by inhalation of nonspecific irritants, such as ammonia. Organic particles, which presumably are not cleared as fast as ammonia, have a longer physiological response than ammonia, as already discussed.

It is quite clear that inhaled irritants and antigens deposited within the respiratory tract activate the sensory nerves. These afferent nerves appear to be primarily vagal, with sympathetic afferents having a larger role at higher levels of sensory excitation. The efferent impulses are transmitted by the vagi and sympathetic ganglia to multiple effector sites (organs). This includes, but probably is not limited to, the heart, the intercostal muscles, and diaphragm; the airway smooth muscle; the mucosal glands; and possibly, airway epithelial, as well as the bronchial, pulmonary, and systemic peripheral and visceral vasculatures. In addition, sensory nerves in both the lungs and heart have efferent functions. There are immunoneural interactions that activate sensory nerves and likely neuroimmune interactions at efferent nerve endings that amplify the responses to inhaled allergens. In sensitized animals or persons, it is possible that there are additional cellular processes that amplify the signals at the locations of both the sensory nerves and the postganglionic efferent motor responses. It is attractive to hypothesize that the cells that release mediators in response to allergen also become responsive to inhaled irritants when the Fc receptors are cross-linked with IgE, or that the nerves themselves are hypersensitive owing to increased densities of receptors or a lowering of the stimulus threshold. In addition, hypersensitivities of the central neural processing or ganglionic transmission are also possible.

Most studies on the cardiovascular and pulmonary responses to allergens have been conducted using very short challenges over several minutes, in contrast to investigations with inhaled irritants, for which both acute and chronic exposure have been more extensively studied. The responses to long-term low levels of allergens has received little attention. In a ragweed-sensitized dog exposed to 0.045 U/mL ragweed allergen over 21 min, a precipitous anaphylaxis was not observed, but rather a gradual decrease in arterial pressure from 160/90 to 140/90 mmHg (at 15 min), with the heart rate decreasing from 132 to 126 beats per minute. The Pao_2 decreased from 99 mmHg to 62 mmHg, despite an induced increase in ventilation. An increase in lung resistance and decrease in dynamic compliance was observed on cessation of the challenge. In addition, inhalation of low levels of allergens can cause hypersensitivity to acetylcholine (70) and enhance efferent neurotransmission (71). Thus, it is quite easy to envisage that the inhalation of low levels of environmental allergens and irritants could lead to a slow onset of severe respiratory distress in hyperresponsive persons and those with already compromised cardiopulmonary function.

The pulmonary chemoreflex is activated by laryngeal sensory nerves, and exposure of the oral cavity to allergens (presumably stimulating laryngeal afferents) markedly enhances the physiological responses to inhaled allergens (72–74). On this basis it can be argued that the protection from inhaled particles should include the ''nonrespirable'' particles larger than 10 μm, that will deposit within the mouth and larynx as well those that deposit in the bronchial and alveolar regions of the lungs.

It is also evident that inhaled particles and irritants, such as ozone and SO_2, can cause perturbations in both the lungs and the cardiovascular system that can potentially contribute to the increased morbidity and mortality observed with increasing levels of these pollutants. There is little doubt that these neural responses to inhaled irritants and antigen are increased in persons with hypersensitive airways, pulmonary congestion, and heart disease. Clearly, the roles of these irritants and allergens on these vital pulmonary and cardiovascular functions as well as the mechanisms whereby they defend the body or compromise its function need further delineation. This will help provide the needed mechanistic links between inhaled irritants and increased morbidity and mortality. In addition, it will lead to the identification of target sites for prophylactic and therapeutic intervention.

VIII. Summary and Conclusions

Irritants and allergens activate sensory nerves directly or by the release of mediators from inflammatory cells. Although mast cells and basophils appear to have some capacity to release mediators on exposure to irritants, direct evidence of the physiological responses from irritant-induced mediator release is sparse. It is a very attractive hypothesis that this type of nonimmune activation of inflammatory cells releases mediators of the anaphylactic responses to constitute an amplification mechanism contributing to the increase in morbidity and mortality in persons with compromised cardiopulmonary function or hyperresponsiveness to irritants and allergens.

The affector or target sites of inhaled irritants and allergens include, but are unlikely limited to, the larynx, tracheobronchiolar airways, alveoli, and heart, as well as the major blood vessels leading to and from the heart. The effector sites from activation of these tissues and organs include not only these organs or tissues and the interactions between them, but also remote organs and tissues including, but likely not limited to, the systemic, central, and visceral vasculatures.

It is quite clear that these multiple cardiopulmonary and systemic sequellae resulting from the release of mediators and the activation of sensory nerves in the lung and heart could contribute to impaired cardiovascular and pulmonary performance from inhaled environmental and occupational irritants and antigens.

Whereas considerable effort has gone into the investigation of the effects of environmental irritants and allergens on changes in bronchial smooth-muscle tone, as indicated by FEV_1, there is a dearth of information in the area of environmental toxicants' effects on cardiac or cardiovascular performance. The potential profound effects of inhaled irritants and antigens on cardiovascular performance has been documented over several decades; however, direct information relevant to the roles of these responses to the increase in morbidity and mortality in humans from inhaled particles and irritants is still awaiting causal verification.

Although, it has been documented that persons with airways diseases and asthma die of mucous-occluded airways, the pathogenic mechanisms leading to this occlusion are unknown. The hypothesis that this is due to an imbalance of irritant-activated excitatory and inhibitory neural pathways acting on mucous secretion and ciliary activity, respectively, requires investigation. Certainly, there is evidence that the excitatory cholinergic pathways are upregulated in animal models of allergic hyperresponsiveness and in persons with asthma and COPD. Any downregulation of the inhibitory pathways requires the further delineation of these pathways, followed by an evaluation of their roles in the maintenance of the homeostatic balance of the mucociliary transport system, as well as its responses to inhaled irritants and allergens.

If we are to understand the influence of inhaled irritants and allergens on humans and their contribution to morbidity and mortality, the potential systemic effects of irritants in humans and animal models of allergic hyperresponsiveness and compromised cardiopulmonary function must be evaluated and the mechanisms of these responses dclineated.

Acknowledgments

This work was funded in part by the National Institutes of Health, NIEHS R01 ES04317 and the Medical Service of the Department of Veterans Affairs. I am grateful for the technical help of Anthony V. Daza.

References

1. Coleridge HM, Coleridge JCG. Pulmonary reflexes: neural mechanisms of pulmonary defense. Annu Rev Physiol. 1994; 56:69–91.
2. Szeredaprzestaszewska M, Wypych B. Laryngeal constriction produced by capsaicin in the cat. J. Physiol Pharmacol 1996; 47:351–360.
3. Coleridge JCG, Coleridge HM. Afferent vagal C fibre innervation of the lungs and airways and its functional significance. Rev Physiol Biochem Pharmacol 1984; 99: 1–110.
4. Coleridge JCG, Coleridge HM, Schelegle ES, Green JF. Acute inhalation of O_3 stim-

ulates bronchial C-fibers and rapidly adapting receptors in dogs. J Appl Physiol 1993; 74:2345–2352.
5. Jones JF, Wang Y, Jordan D. Heart rate responses to selective stimulation of cardiac C-fibres in anaesthetized cats, rats and rabbits. J Physiol (Lond) 1995; 489:203–214.
6. Jansen ASP, Nguyen XV, Karpitsky V, Mettenleiter TC, Loewy AD. Central command neurons of the sympathetic nervous system: basis of the flight or flight response. Science 1995; 270:644–646.
7. Xu F, Frazed DT. Respiratory-related neurons of the fastigial nucleus in response to chemical and mechanical challenges. J Appl Physiol 1997; 82:1177–1184.
8. Pisarri TE, Coleridge JCG, Coleridge HM. Capsaicin induced bronchial vasodilation in dogs: central and peripheral neural mechanisms. J Appl Physiol 1993; 74:259–266.
9. Phipps RJ, Richardson RS. The effects of irritation at various levels of the airway upon tracheal mucus secretion in the cat. J Physiol 1976; 261:563–581.
10. Gallager JT, Kent PW, Passatore M, Phipps RJ, Richardson PS. The composition of tracheal mucus and the nervous control of its secretion in the cat. Proc R Soc Lond 1975; 192:49–76.
11. Kuo H, Rohde JAL, Barnes P, Rogers, DF. Cigarette smoke-induced airway goblet cell secretion: dose-dependent differential nerve activation. Am J Physiol 1992; 262: L161–L167.
12. Haxhiu MA, Haxhiu-Poskurica B, Moracic V, Carlo WA, Martin RJ. Reflex responses of tracheal submucosal glands in piglets. Respir Physiol 1990; 82:267–278.
13. Eljamal M, Wong LB, Yeates DB. Capsaicin activated bronchial and alveolar initiated pathways regulation tracheal ciliary beat frequency. J Appl Physiol 1994; 77: 1239–1245
14. Tamaoki J, Chiyotana A, Tagaya E, Takemura H, Konno K. Cholinergic control of rabbit transepithelial potential difference in vivo. Eur J Respir Dis 1966; 8:1632–1636.
15. Wong LB, Yeates DB. Dynamic of the regulation of ciliated epithelial function. Comm Theor Biol 1997; 4(2–3), 183–208.
16. Yeates DB. Inhibitory and excitatory neural regulation of the mucociliary transport system. In: Baum G, ed. Cilia, Mucus and Mucociliary Interactions. New York: Marcel Dekker, 1997:28–38.
17. Yeates DB, Katwala SP, Daugird J, Daza AV, Wong, LB. Excitatory and inhibitory neural regulation of tracheal ciliary beat frequency (CBF) activated by ammonia vapour and SO_2. Ann Occup Hyg 1997; 41(suppl 1):736–774.
18. Szallasi A, Blumberg PM, Lundberg JM. Proton inhibition of ^{3}H resiniferatoxin binding to vanilloid (capsaicin) receptors in rat spinal cord. Eur J Pharmacol 1995; 289:181–187.
19. Pillai RS, Yeates DB, Miller IF, Hickey AJ. Controlled release from condensation coated respirable aerosol particles. J Aerosol Sci 1994; 25:461–477.
20. Highfill JW, Watkinson WP. Ozone toxicity in the rat II. Modeling changes due to ambient temperatures and duration. J Appl Physiol 1996; 80:1811–1818.

21. Arito H, Uchiyama I, Yokoyama E. Acute effects of O_3 on EEG activity, sleep–wakefulness and heart rate in rats. Ind Health 1992; 30:23–24.
22. Uchiyama I, Simoura Y, Yokoyama E. Effects of acute exposure to ozone on heart rate and blood pressure of the conscious rat. Environ Res 1986; 41:529–537.
23. Watkinson WP, Aileru AA, Dowd SM, Doerfler DL, Tepper JS. Acute effects of ozone on heart rate and body temperature in the unanesthetized, unrestrained rat maintained at different temperatures. Inhal Toxicol 1993; 5:129–147.
24. Jimba M, Skornik WA, Killingsworth CR, Long NC, Brain JD, Shore SA. Role of C fibers in physiological responses to ozone in rats. J Appl Physiol 1995; 78:1757–1763.
25. Paintal AS. Mechanism of stimulation of type J pulmonary receptors. J Physiol 1969; 203:511–532.
26. Zang Z, Bonham AC. Lung congestion augments the responses of cells in the rapidly adapting receptor pathway to cigarette smoke in the rabbit. J Physiol (Lond) 1995; 484:189–200.
27. Islam MS, Zimmerman I, Ulmer WT. Relationship between pulmonary embolism, airway obstruction, and hypersensitivity of the airways in dogs. Respiration 1977; 34:105–112.
28. Anand A, Paintal AS, Whitteridge D. Mechanisms underlying enhanced responses of J receptors of cats to excitants in pulmonary edema. J Physiol 1993; 471:535–547.
29. Gross NJ, Skorodin CE. Cholinergic bronchomotor tone in COPD, estimation of its amount in comparison with that in normal subjects. Chest 1989; 96:856–870.
30. Barnes PJ. Current therapies for asthma, promise and limitations. Chest 1997; 111(suppl 2):17S–26S.
31. Yeates DB, Daza AV, Mussatto DM. Bronchial and alveolar allergen-induced anaphylaxis and the stimulation of bronchial mucociliary clearance in ragweed sensitized dogs. Proc Assoc Am Physicians 1997; 109:440–452.
32. Mitsuhata H, Takeuchi H, Sitoh J, Horiguchi Y, Shimizu R. An inhibitor of nitric oxide synthase, *N*-omega-nitro-L-arginine-methyl ester, attenuates hypotension but does not improve cardiac depression in anaphylaxis in dogs. Shock 1995; 6:447–453.
33. Modin A, Weitzberg E, Lundberg JM. Nitric oxide regulates peptide release from parasympathetic nerves and vascular reactivity to vasoactive intestinal polypeptide. Eur J Pharmacol 1994; 261:185–197.
34. Levy RM, Rose JE, Johnson JS. Effect of vagotomy on anaphylaxis in the rat. Clin Exp Immunol 1976; 24:96–101.
35. Gold WM, Kessler GF, Yu DYC. Role of the vagus nerve in experimental asthma in allergic dogs. J Appl Physiol 1972; 33:719–725.
36. Zimmerman I, Islam MS, Lanser K, Ulmer WT. Antigen-induced airway obstruction and the influence of vagus blockade. Respiration 1976; 33:95–103.
37. Cotton DJ, Bleeker-ER, Fisher SP, Graf PD, Gold WM, Nadel JA. Rapid shallow breathing after *Ascaris suum* antigen inhalation: role of the vagus nerves. J Appl Physiol Respir Environ Exerc Physiol 1977; 42:101–106.
38. Tocker JE, Gertner SB,Welton AF, Selig WM. Vagal stimulation augments pulmo-

nary anaphylaxis in the guinea pig lung. Am J Respir Crit Care Med 1995; 151: 461–469.

39. Chapman KR. An international perspective on anticholinergic therapy. Am J Med 1996; 100:2S–4S.
40. Fitzgerald JM, Grunfeld A, Pare PD, Levy RD, Newhouse MT, Hodder R, Chapman KR. The clinical efficacy of combination nebulized anticholinergic and adrenergic bronchodilators vs. nebulized adrenergic bronchodilator alone in acute asthma. Canadian Combivent Study Group. Chest 1997; 111:311–315.
41. Humbert M, Grant JA, Tabordabata L, Durham SR, Pfister R, Menz G, Barkans J, Ying S, Kay AB. High affinity IgE receptor (Fc-epsilon-RI)-bearing cells in bronchial biopsies from atopic and non atopic asthma. Am J Respir Crit Care Med 1996; 153:1931–1937.
42. Ammit AJ, Behir SS, Johnson PR, Armour CL, Black JL. Mast cell numbers are increased in smooth muscle of human sensitized isolated bronchi. Am J Respir Crit Care Med 1997; 155:1123–1129.
43. Mori L, Kleimberg J, Mancini C, Bellini A, Marini M, Mattoli S. Bronchial epithelial cells of atopic patients with asthma lack the ability to inactivate allergens. Biochem Biophys Res Commun 1995; 217:817–824.
44. Clarke SW, Yeates DB. Deposition and clearance. In: Murray JF, Nadel JA, eds. Textbook of Respiratory Medicine, vol 1. Philadelphia: WB Saunders, 1994:345–369.
45. Jacobsen J, Johnsen CR, Skov PS, Warberg J, Knigge U, Secher, NH. Cardiovasular and hormonal responses to anaphylactic shock in the pig. Clin Physiol 1995; 15: 81–90.
46. Martin TR, Ando A, Takeishi T, Katona IM, Drazen JM, Galli SJ. Mast cells contribute to the changes in heart rate, but not hypotension or death, associated with active anaphylaxis in mice. J Immunol 1993; 151:367–376.
47. Jacobsen J, Secher NH. Slowing of the heart during anaphylactic shock. Acta Anaesthesiol Scand 1988; 32:401–403.
48. Smith PL, Kagey-Sobotka A, Bleeker ER, Traystman R, Kaplan AP, Gralnick H, Valentine MD, Permutt S, Lichtenstein ER. Physiologic manifestations of human anaphylaxis. J Clin Invest 1980; 66:1072–1080.
49. Silverman HJ, Taylor WR, Smith PL, Kagey-Sobotka A, Permutt S, Lichtenstein LM, Bleecker ER. Effects of antihistamine on the cardiopulmonary changes due to canine anaphylaxis. J Appl Physiol 1988; 64:210–217.
50. Enjeti S, Bleecker ER, Smith PL, Rabson J, Permutt S, Traystman RJ. Hemodynamic mechanisms in anaphylaxis. Circ Shock 1983; 11:297–309.
51. Baluk P, Nadel JA, McDonald DM. Substance P-immunoreactive sensory axons in the rat respiratory tract: a quantitative study of their distribution and role of neurogenic inflammation. J Comp Neurol 1992; 319:586–598.
52. Persson CGA, Gustafsson B, Erjefalt B, Sundler F. Mucosal exudation of plasma is a noninjurious intestinal defense mechanism. Allergy 1993; 48:581–586.
53. Phipps RJ, Denas SM, Wanner A. Antigen stimulates glycoprotein secretion and ion fluxes in sheep trachea. J Appl Physiol Respir Environ Exerc Physiol 1983; 55:1593–1602.

54. King M, El-Azab J, Phillips DM, Angus GE. Antigen challenge and canine tracheal mucus. Int Arch Allergy Appl Immunol 1985; 77:337–342.
55. Shelhammer JH, Marom Z, Kaliner M. Immunologic and neuropharmacologic stimulation of mucous glycoprotein release from human airways in vitro. J Clin Invest 1980; 66:1400–1488.
56. Yamatake Y, Sagagawa S, Yanaura S, Kobayashi N. Involvement of histamine H_1 and H_2receptors in induced asthmas in dogs. Jpn J Pharmacol 1982; 27:791–797.
57. Cook HJ. Neuroimmune signaling in regulation of intestinal ion transport. Am J Physiol 1994; 266:G167–G178.
58. Evans RG, Ludbrook J, Michalicek J. Characteristics of cardiovascular reflexes originating from 5-HT receptors in the heart and lungs of unanesthetized rabbits. Clin Exp Pharmacol Physiol 1990; 17:665–679.
59. Standish A, Enquist LW, Schwaber JS. Innervation of the heart and its central medullary origin defined by viral tracing. Science 1994; 263:232–234.
60. Horackova M, Armour JA. Role of peripheral autonomic neurons in maintaining adequate cardiac function. Cardiovasc Res 1995; 30:326–335.
61. Costa M, Brooks SJ, Steele PA, Gibbins I, Burcher E, Kandiah CJ. Neurochemical classification of mysenteric neurons in the guinea-pig ileum. Neuroscience 1966; 75: 949–967.
62. Patella V, Marino I, Lamparter B, Arbustini E, Adt M, Marone G. Human heart mast cells: isolation, purification, ultrastructure, and immunologic characterization. J Immunol 1995; 154:2855–2865.
63. Genovese A, Stellato C, Marsella CV, Adt M, Marone G. Role of mast cells, basophils and their mediators in adverse reactions to general anesthetic and contrast media. Int Arch Allergy Immunol 1996; 110:13–22.
64. Regal JF and Heller LJ. Cardiac anaphylaxis in isolated guinea pig hearts perfused at constant flow or constant pressure. Proc Soc Exp Biol Med 1987; 185:193–200.
65. Mest HJ, Ponicke K, Heinroth I, Meissner N, Cheissler C. Relevance of mediators to cardiac parameters of isolated anaphylactic guinea-pig heart. Prostaglandins Leukot Essent Fatty Acids 1995; 53:21–29.
66. Martin TR, Akikazu A, Takeshi T, Katona IM, Drazen JM, Galli J. Mast cells contribute to the changes in heart rate but not hypotension or death, associated with anaphylaxis in mice. J Immunol 1993; 151:367–376.
67. Kaufman MP, Coleridge HM, Coleridge JCG, Baker DG. Bradykinin stimulates afferent vagal C-fibers in intrapulmonary airways in dogs. J Appl Physiol Respir Environ 1980; 48:511–517.
68. Rubin LE, Levi R. Protective role of bradykinin in cardiac anaphylaxis—coronary-vasodilating and antiarrythmic activities mediated by autocrine paracrine mechanisms. Circ Res 1995; 76:434–440.
69. Park HS, Nahm DH. Isocyanate-induced occupational asthma: challenge and immunologic studies. J Korean Med Sci 1996; 4:314–318.
70. Zimmerman I, Ulmer WT. Influence of low concentrations of allergens on the bronchial system. Respiration 1978; 35:87–95.
71. Kageyama N, Igarashi A, Ichinose M, Miura M, Yamauchi H, Tomaki M, Ishikawa

J, Sasaki Y, Shirato K. Chronic allergen exposure enhances cholinergic neurotransmission in sensitized guinea-pigs. Eur Respir J 1995; 8:752–754.
72. Zimmermann I, Kowalshi J, Curshmann P, Ulmer WT. Reaction following allergen inhalation via the mouth and via the tracheal tube in dogs. Lung 1976; 154:41–49.
73. Zimmermann I, Walkenhorst W, Ulmer WT. The role of the upper airways in antigen-induced bronchoconstriction. Respiration 179; 37:148–156.
74. Zimmermann I, Bugalho de Almeida AA, Ulmer WT. Partial sensory denervation of the upper respiratory tract on allergen- and histamine-induced bronchoconstriction. Respiration 1984; 45:394–405.
75. Smith H, ed. Human respiratory tract model for radiological protection. ICRP Publication 66. Ann ICRP 1994; 24.

Part Six

HEALTH CONSEQUENCES

17

Interaction of Inhaled Particles with the Immune System

M. IAN GILMOUR and HILLEL S. KOREN

U.S. Environmental Protection Agency
Research Triangle Park, North Carolina

I. Introduction

Several air pollution episodes documented over the last seven decades have been associated with significant increases in mortality in the exposed population. The most commonly cited events occurred in the Meuse Valley, Belgium, in 1930, Donora, Pennsylvania, in 1948, and in London, England, in 1952 (1). Daily death rates (primarily of respiratory and cardiovascular complications) during or immediately after these episodes increased up to ten times the normal level. More recent studies have reported that less extreme increases in airborne particulates, which occur regularly in urban and industrial areas of Europe and North America, are also associated with increased hospital admissions for pneumonia, asthma, and bronchitis (2,3). These acute effects are thought to occur most frequently in persons with preexisting cardiopulmonary disease (see Chaps. 15, 18, and 19), as a result of additional oxidative, neurogenic, and inflammatory stresses on an already weakened condition.

The extent to which air pollutant exposure also promotes the development of "new" disease has been demonstrated in experimental systems, but remains difficult to quantify by either epidemiological or clinical means. In animals, a broad range of airborne particulates ranging from vehicle exhaust and combustion products, to acid aerosols, metals, minerals, organic compounds, and cigarette smoke can interfere with the normal defense processes of the lung to enhance susceptibility to respiratory infections (4,5). Certain airborne particulates, such as diesel exhaust, can act as immunological adjuvants to increase the severity of pulmonary allergy and asthma (6). Although the carcinogenic and proinflammatory potential of airborne particulates are addressed elsewhere in this volume, this chapter will summarize the effects of inhaled particles on the immune system, and discuss the mechanisms by which ambient air particulate matter might promote the incidence, or exacerbate the severity of, infectious and allergic lung disease. Many of the findings described herein have also been established for gaseous air pollutants, such as O_3 and NO_2, and the reader is referred elsewhere (5–7) to reviews on oxidant air pollutants and the immune system.

A. The Challenge to the Respiratory Tract

During the course of a day the average healthy adult breathes between 10,000 and 20,000 L of air. If one assumes a conservatively low air particle burden of 10 $\mu g/m^3$, then the minimum mass of particles inhaled daily is at least 100 μg. This personal exposure is usually augmented according to the proximity of point and mobile source emissions, such as power plants and traffic; the dispersal of ground dust by mechanical agitation and wind; occupational exposure; and the level of indoor air contaminants, including house dust and environmental tobacco smoke. In addition to the myriad of nonreplicating entities, the lungs are also constantly challenged with a diverse range of organic materials and microbes.

Various specialized defense mechanisms have evolved in the mammalian respiratory tract to combat the daily assault of particles that, depending on their properties, may be inert, toxic, carcinogenic, allergenic, or infectious. These defenses include physical structures (e.g., nasal turbinates and hairs), to trap larger particles in the nose; mucociliary clearance and sneeze and cough reflexes, to expel particles from the upper airways; and phagocytic cells, to kill or detoxify, and clear inhaled materials from the alveolar region of the lung. The 40-some cells of the respiratory tract also interact to produce a complex mix of surfactant, enzymes, and mucus that maintains tissue homeostasis allowing gas exchange and protects the lung from toxic or infectious insult by an array of antioxidant and antimicrobial compounds.

If these ''first lines of defense'' are sufficiently stimulated or breached by an inhaled agent, the respiratory tract usually responds with the recruitment of additional phagocytic monocytes and neutrophils; an increased output of protective fluids, cytokines, and mediators; and for antigenic substances, the development of specific immunity. Most of these defense mechanisms are appropriate and protect the host from permanent injury, although the immune and inflammatory reactions may also cause tissue damage during allergic and autoimmune reactions, and other inflammatory conditions such as adult respiratory distress syndrome (ARDS).

Because of the complex exposures that individuals face every day, it is not surprising that the resulting host responses to inhaled agents take on different forms. Clinical studies and experiments in animals have contributed greatly to knowledge of the inflammatory and immune processes that occur after exposure to single agents, such as silica or pneumococcal bacteria. Research continues to unravel the mechanisms of fibrosis caused by silica inhalation, and for pneumococci, the pathogenetic mechanisms of bacterial pneumonia. An understanding of the interactions between the two agents, however, remains complicated, because biological responses in diseased tissue can be dramatically different from those observed during normal health. In addition, the timing and magnitude of exposures in relation to each other, the inherent susceptibility of the host, and the presence of biological redundancy in the immune system make for a potpourri of possible interactions that are only now beginning to be understood. The following sections will briefly describe the pulmonary immune system, and show evidence of how particle exposure can alter the immune system to enhance infectious and allergic lung disease.

B. Host Defenses

Despite the daily microbial assault that the respiratory tract experiences, even during normal breathing, the gas-exchange area of the lung is maintained in a remarkably sterile condition by the combined antimicrobial activity of the mucociliary, phagocytic, and immune systems (8,9). Nonspecific (innate) mechanical defenses include the cough reflex, physical barriers, such as nasal hair and turbinates, and the mucociliary apparatus of the airways that continuously sweeps particles and laden phagocytes to the pharynx for swallowing (10,11). Alveolar macrophages scavenge the airspaces and lower airways, engulfing foreign particles and cellular debris by phagocytosis (12). Polymorphonuclear leukocytes (PMNs) may also be recruited from the circulation to the lung in response to various proinflammatory chemoattractants to augment the usual phagocytic and bactericidal capacity of the macrophage (13). The magnitude and speed of the PMN influx varies with the nature of the stimulus, and endotoxin-coated (gram-negative) bacteria elicit a greater neutrophil response than gram-positive organisms (8). PMNs can also be responsible for several forms of acute lung injury caused by the release of toxic metabolites, inflammatory mediators, reactive oxygen species, and potent enzymes, such as elastase, collagenase, and cathepsin B (14,15).

Microrganisms are killed in phagocytes by an array of digestive enzymes, toxic oxygen species, and other antimicrobial agents. In addition to internalization and inactivation of microbes, macrophages, PMNs, and some epithelial cells secrete a variety of polypeptides that have antimicrobial activity. These include enzymes, such as lysozyme and complement components (16); cytokines, such as the interferons and tissue necrosis factor (TNF)-α (12); and small antimicrobial peptides, such as the defensin family (17). The importance of phagocytes in host defense is best illustrated in heritable chronic granulomatous disease (CGD). This usually fatal disease is characterized by a deficient ability of phagocytes to generate a respiratory burst by the production of reactive oxygen species (ROS), and results in recurrent bacterial and fungal infections (18). Natural killer (NK) cells make up another arm of the innate immune system and are important in recognizing and killing cells bearing viral and tumor antigens (19).

In addition to these innate pulmonary defense mechanisms, the respiratory epithelium and pulmonary lymph nodes are also populated with a contiguous network of dendritic cells that process inhaled proteins and present antigenic fragments (epitopes) to circulating and mucosal T lymphocytes (20,21). Soluble antigens can be processed either on the airway surface or in the peripheral lymph nodes after translocation by the bloodstream or lymphatics. Epithelial cells also express a variety of receptors important in cell signaling and adhesion, and can synthesize several mediators that regulate inflammatory and immune processes in the lung (Fig. 1). Other cell types, such as mast cells and goblet cells, are interspersed throughout the respiratory epithelium, and are available for cell–cell interaction by direct contact or by signaling through soluble mediators.

During the course of a primary infection, or after vaccination, foreign epitopes bound to accessory molecules on the surface of dendritic cells are presented to antigen-specific T- and B-lymphocyte populations. These cells are then activated to proliferate and expand into effector and memory subpopulations that circulate throughout the body and can home to particular mucosal sites, such as the respiratory and gastrointestinal tracts. The local specific immune response then eliminates the pathogen or neutralizes its toxic products with antibodies and through killing infected cells with cytotoxic $CD8^+$ T cells. Reinfection with the same agent is usually more limited because memory ($CD4^+$) T cells are available for rapid expansion into an effector population.

Once an individual has become immune through previous infection, vaccination, or by passive transmission of maternal antibody, these specific defenses effectively control most viral and bacterial pathogens. Depletion of the $CD4^+$ T-lymphocyte population, as occurs in acquired immunedeficiency syndrome (AIDS) leads to a general reduction in immune competence and an increased susceptibility to infectious and neoplastic disease (22). Similarly, IgA deficiency can result in increased risk of respiratory tract infection (23).

In contrast with reduced immune function, heightened (hypersensitive) responses to allergens or to self-antigens occurs in a significant percentage of the population and produces allergic and autoimmune disease (24). A brief descrip-

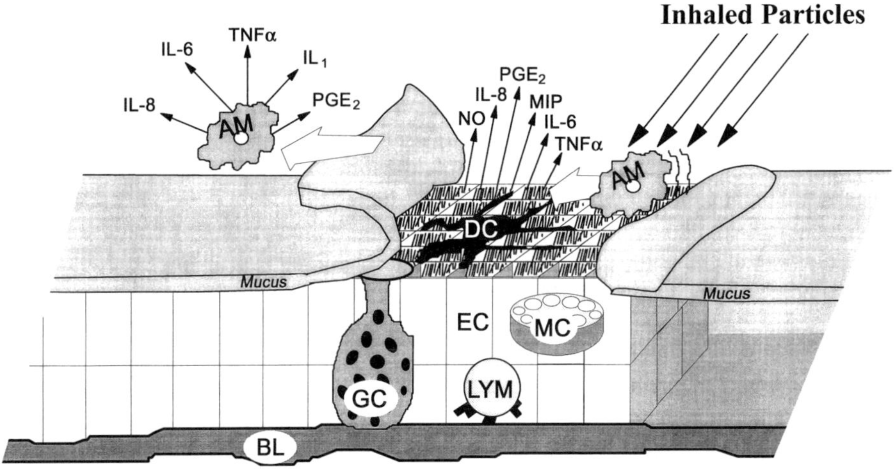

Figure 1 Schematic representation of the respiratory epithelium showing ciliated type II cells (EC), dendritic cells (DC), goblet cells (GC), submucosal lymphocytes (LYM), mast cells (MC), alveolar macrophages (AM), and basal lamina (BL). Exposure to particles causes epithelial cells and macrophages to release a variety of immunoreactive mediators.

tion of allergic immune responses and the consequences of particulate-enhanced immunity to allergens are discussed toward the end of this chapter.

A large database has been developed over the last four decades to describe how inhaled materials can perturb host defense mechanisms, resulting in enhanced susceptibility to infectious agents. These in vivo findings have, for the most part, been demonstrated in rodents, although extrapolation to humans is possible because of similarities in pulmonary defenses across mammalian species (25). More recent in vitro experiments have compared the antimicrobial capacity of human and rodent alveolar macrophages, thereby permitting prediction of immunotoxicity across different species (26,27). Although initial studies focused on fibrogenic materials, such as coal dust, silica, and cigarette smoke, recent experiments have also investigated diesel fumes, road dust, and ambient air particulate matter.

II. Particle-Enhanced Respiratory Infections

Respiratory tract infections constitute the most prevalent type of acute illness in the United States, and account for more days of debility than any other type of disease (28). Pneumonia and influenza are the fourth leading cause of death in Americans older than 65 years and the sixth in all age groups (29). Thirty percent (4.5 million) of all childhood deaths in the world each year are caused by respiratory infections, making these, along with diarrheal diseases, the most common form of preventable death (30). The lungs' array of defensive systems can normally protect against individual insults of microorganisms, particulates, and gases. The effectiveness of pulmonary clearance and immune mechanisms, however, may be reduced during elevated pollutant exposures. If an individual is then challenged with a virulent agent, the potential for infection is increased, because the host must now defend itself against the pathogen while experiencing reduced phagocytic ability, tissue inflammation, depression of specific immunity, and impaired mucociliary clearance (4). Despite the strong experimental evidence from animal studies supporting this concept, these effects have been difficult to demonstrate in humans because of (1) the complex pollutant exposure scenarios and recurrent natural epidemics of infection that occur at the population level, and (2) the risk of causing disease in clinical subjects. Nevertheless, studies of smokers and other individuals occupationally exposed to high levels of airborne particulates suggest an increased risk of pulmonary infection.

Smoking is the most significant risk factor for the development of bronchitis and emphysema, and it is associated with increased incidence and severity of respiratory infection (31). Children of smokers also have higher hospital admission rates for pneumonia and bronchitis, and experience a higher frequency and severity of viral lung infections than children in nonsmoking families (32). Exposure to other forms of smoke (e.g., wood smoke) also increases risk of respiratory infection in children (33). Occupational exposure to high levels of particulates in coal miners, for example, causes fibrosis and obstructive lung disease, as well as varying degrees of bronchitis that is often associated with increased incidence of infection (34). In the past, the prevalence of tuberculosis infection was 30 times higher among copper miners suffering from silicosis, compared with healthy miners (35), although this problem has subsided with the advent of BCG vaccination, effective chemotherapy, and reduced occupational exposure to silica.

Most of the definitive evidence for particles affecting the incidence of respiratory infection comes from animal studies. The first report of this phenomenon dates to a century ago when Durck (36) injected rabbits through the trachea with "dust" and exposed the animals to bacteria isolated from patients with pneumonia. The dust-exposed animals developed respiratory infections, whereas the controls remained healthy. In later studies guinea pigs exposed to a variety of dusts, including talc and cement, were more susceptible to tubercle bacilli than nonexposed controls (37). Similarly, rabbits injected in the trachea with tubercle bacilli and silica dust had more bacteria in lung sections and higher mortality of infection, compared with animals injected with either agent alone (38).

The interaction of particles and microbial pathogens in the lung has been most extensively studied with the streptococcal infectivity model. Mice exposed to irradiated automobile exhaust were more susceptible to a subsequent pulmonary infection following inhalation challenge with *Streptococcus zooepidemicus* (39). Out of 40 different types of particles instilled into the lungs of mice in this experimental system, 100-μg doses of bentonite, oil fly ash, salts (CdO, ZnO, $NaAsO_2$, $SnCl_2$, and $CoNO_3$), and ambient air particles (collected from Dusseldorf and Bochum in Germany) enhanced mortality to infection by more than 50% (40). Other dusts characterized as having intermediate potency (< 50% excess mortality) included an ambient air particle sample from Washington, D.C., three coal fly ash samples, powdered latex, BeO, and Fe_2O_3. Low-potency particles that did not enhance mortality significantly at the 100-μg dose level included samples of diesel and coal fly ash, an ambient air sample from St. Louis, Mount St. Helens volcanic ash, crystalline silica, CuO, Mn_3O_4, TiO_2, and PbO. Three of the dusts (Mt. St. Helens, Bochum, and residual oil fly ash) were retested in the streptococcal model (41), and the extent of particle-enhanced mortality was shown to be related to the amount of leachable iron on the particles (Fig. 2).

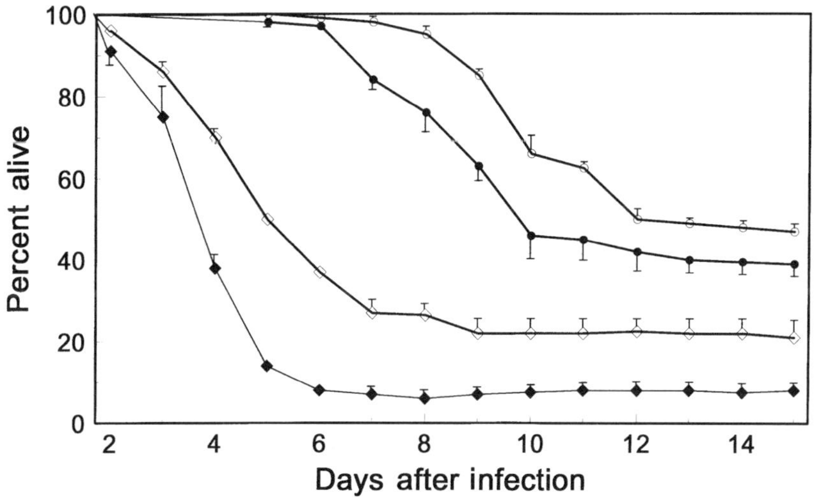

Figure 2 Mortality to streptococcal infection after intratracheal instillation of dusts increases with chelatable and total iron concentrations. Differences in mortality at 15 days were demonstrated for baghouse dust collected over Bochum, Germany (solid diamond), and a residual oil fly ash (open diamond) compared with those for saline (open circle) and Mount St. Helens dust (solid circle). (From Ref. 41.)

A. Impaired Pulmonary Clearance Mechanisms by Inhaled Particulates

Given that the successful eradication of pulmonary infection is based on the ability of the host to clear pathogens from the respiratory tract, knowledge of pulmonary defense mechanisms has been obtained largely through studies of the deposition and clearance of bacteria and viruses in the lungs of experimental animals. Much of the work has centered around the functional characteristics of alveolar macrophages (AM). These cells can be studied in terms of their ability to clear microbes or radiolabeled particles from the lung, or by testing their function after retrieval by bronchoalveolar lavage (BAL). Another approach is to assess the effect of in vitro particle exposure on AM cell functions, such as phagocytosis and microbicidal activity, enzyme release, and cytokine production. This latter technique has become a useful way to determine the relative potencies of different particles on human and animal AMs and, occasionally, to provide data for extrapolating animal toxicology data to potential human health effects in risk assessment paradigms (5).

During experimental infection in mice, 80–90% of an inhaled bolus containing 10^6 *Staphylococcus aureus* organisms are inactivated in vivo by murine AMs over a 4-hr period (42). By using a dual exposure system to demonstrate that particles can transport toxic substances to deeper areas of the lung, Jakab (43,44) showed that a 4-hr exposure to carbon black (10 mg/m^3), in conjunction with the cigarette smoke component acrolein (2.5 ppm) or formaldehyde (5 ppm), resulted in reduced intrapulmonary inactivation of *S. aureus*, compared with that found in animals exposed to any of the individual components. In addition, AMs retrieved from the dual-exposed animals had decreased phagocytic function ex vivo. Similarly, exposure to either carbon or acrolein alone did not affect influenza virus titers or the level of lung disease in mice; however, the combination of both aerosols resulted in increased pulmonary fibrosis caused by the interaction of viral antigens, antibodies, and complement (44). Enhanced disease was also noted when *Listeria monocytogenes* (for which clearance mechanisms rely on the development of T-cell–mediated enhancement of macrophage intracellular killing) was employed as the infectious agent.

Others have shown that the rate of intrapulmonary inactivation of inhaled *Escherichia coli* in the lungs of guinea pigs exposed for more prolonged periods to coal dust at 15 mg/m^3 (6 hr/day for 3 weeks) or cigarette smoke (1–2 cigarettes per day for 15 days) was less than control animals (45), and that mice exposed to aerosols of TiO_2 dust (20 mg/m^3, 23 hr/day) for 2 weeks were unable to clear an inhaled bolus of *Pasteurella haemolytica* organisms over a 4-day period (46). This latter finding was interpreted as being a result of macrophage ''overload'' with an inert dust.

Some studies have paradoxically shown that, under some exposure conditions, the pulmonary defenses can be temporarily stimulated, and are more proficient at handling inhaled microbes. Mice exposed to carbon black and acrolein enhanced clearance of *Proteus mirabilis* (44). These studies were attributed to the toxic exposure having induced a PMN influx that was then immediately available to ingest inhaled bacteria. In general, however, inhalation of particulates, ranging from coal dust, silica, and cigarette smoke, to inert particulates, such as talc dust and TiO_2 leads to reduced macrophage phagocytosis and impaired clearance of inhaled bacteria. This reduced phagocytic activity in the lung may arise from direct toxicity and damage to the cell (47), cellular overloading with particulate matter in the absence of toxicity (48), or by functional inhibition with mediators such as prostaglandin E_2 (49). Examples of impaired clearance of microorganisms after particle inhalation are presented in Table 1.

B. Particles Affecting Innate Immune Function

Although bacterial clearance studies and models of infection are useful for showing how particle inhalation can alter host resistance to infection, analysis of cell type and function after in vivo or in vitro particle exposure can produce more detailed information about the molecular and cellular processes affected by the toxicant. Overall interpretation of these experiments is difficult because some studies show suppression of phagocytosis and downregulation of immune cytokines, whereas others indicate an increase in these functions, suggesting a state of activation. These contradictory results can often be explained by differences in experimental protocols and culture techniques, the endpoints under study, species from which the cells are derived, and the type of particle used. It is well to keep the old toxicology adage in mind, however, that the dose makes the poison, and that subtoxic concentrations of substances can often be beneficial or at least stimulatory.

Lungs of cigarette smokers typically have elevated numbers of AMs that are laden with tar and other particulate components of the smoke. PMNs and lymphocytes are also present in greater numbers than in nonsmokers. Cultured AMs from smokers released more superoxide and have increased oxygen consumption compared with cells from nonsmokers (50), indicating a state of activation. In that study, the bactericidal activity was similar to cells lavaged from nonsmokers, whereas in another (51), AMs obtained from smokers had no differences in their ability to ingest the intracellular bacterium *Listeria monocytogenes*, but were less able to inactivate the organism. AMs retrieved from mice exposed to cigarette smoke showed no differences in chemotaxis or adherence properties, but had reduced capacity to bind and ingest *Candida albicans* particles (52). Thus, it would seem that cigarette smoking can result in brief activation of some

Table 1 Examples of Impaired Bacterial Clearance After Inhalation of Particulates

Particle type	Species/strain	Exposure conditions	Particle concentration (mg/m^3); size (μm)	Infectious agent	Ref.
Carbon black +5 ppm formaldehyde or 2.5 ppm acrolein	CD-1 mice	Nose and mouth only exposure, 4 hr	10,000; 2.45 MMAD	*Staphylococcus aureus*, *Listeria monocytogenes*	43,44
Coal dust	Guinea pigs	Whole-body exposure, 6 hr/day, 3 wk	15,000; 2.0 MMAD	*Escherichia coli*	45
Titanium dioxide	CBA mice	Whole-body exposure, 23 hr/day, 4 wk	20,000; 2.0 MMAD	*Pasteurella haemolytica*	46

biochemical defense mechanisms, such as oxidative burst, while decreasing other cell functions, such as phagocytosis and bactericidal activity. AMs lavaged from nonsmoking workers exposed to asbestos, silica, or coal dust over prolonged periods are generally in an activated state, as evidenced by their ability to release more superoxide anion and hydrogen peroxide which, although useful in microbial inactivation, may ultimately damage the epithelium (53). The long-term consequences of periodic or prolonged activation of these defense mechanisms are unknown.

Several studies have demonstrated that exposure to acid aerosols decreases the in vitro mobility and adherent properties of lavaged AMs from a variety of different species (10,11,54). Enhanced macrophage function has also been reported in rabbits 24 hr after inhalation of fine (0.3 mM) sulfuric acid particles (55), indicating that the effects may differ, depending on the time of assay or on the aerodynamic size of the aerosol. In dual particle-adsorbed vapor inhalation exposure experiments (56), in vivo exposure to carbon black and acrolein reduced ex vivo murine macrophage phagocytosis of opsonized red blood cells. Inhalation of smoke (57), lead oxide (58), and road dust (59) either decreases macrophage phagocytosis or reduces the expression of Fc receptors on the cells.

Recently, studies using both animal and human cells have reported the effect of in vitro particulate exposure on AM phagocytosis. Rat AMs exposed in vitro to acrolein or benzofuran adsorbed onto carbon black (60) ingested less opsonized sheep red blood cells than control cells (Fig. 3). Human peripheral blood monocytes exposed in vitro to particulate air samples collected from an industrial area in Germany had decreased phagocytic activity (61). Phagocytosis of particles, with and without opsonizing antibody, was also decreased by in vitro acid exposure and this effect was stronger in the guinea pig than in rats and rabbits, with human cells being the least sensitive of the species tested (26).

In addition to AM phagocytosis, several investigators have studied the release of mediators that are important in the generation of innate and specific immune responses, as well as in cellular activation. Again, caution is required when comparing different particles and experimental protocols, as well as the possible presence of bioactive agents such as LPS. AMs retrieved from rabbits exposed to 50–500 mg/m^3 H_2SO_4 showed a decreased ability to produce TNF-α, IL-1α and superoxide radical (62). In contrast, particulate air samples from Washington, D.C., and St. Louis caused increased release of TNF-α and IL-6 when incubated with either human or rat AMs (27; Fig. 4). Similarly, another group (63) reported increased gene expression for TNF-α, IL-1, IL-6, CINC, and MIP-2 in cultured rat AMs after in vitro incubation with urban air particles. In both these studies, the effects were attributed partly to endotoxin, because LPS could be detected in the samples by the limulus assay, and coincubation with polymyxin B reduced the cytokine responses. Although the consequences of cellular activation and proinflammatory cytokine release on the host defense network

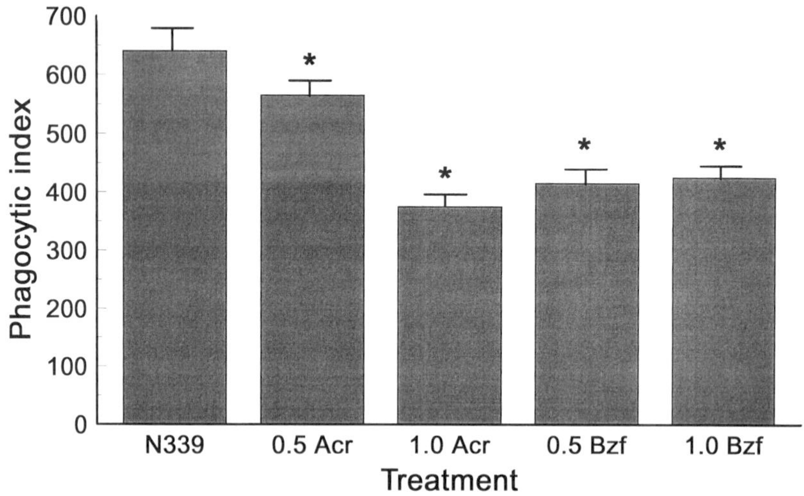

Figure 3 Phagocytosis of opsonized sheep red blood cells by rat alveolar macrophages preincubated with carbon black (N339) coated with 0.5 and 1.0 monolayer coverages of adsorbates (Acr, acrolein; Bzf, benzofuran). * indicates differences ($p < 0.05$) from carbon black N339 alone; $n = 8$. (From Ref 60.)

in toto are unclear, the involvement of cytokines in the development of fibrosis and other types of lung injury have received intensive investigation (see Chap. 10).

C. Particles Affecting Acquired Immune Function

The resolution of serious pulmonary infections, such as those caused by *M. tuberculosis* and *Streptococcus pneumoniae*, partly relies on the development of specific immunity. Cell-mediated immune responses consist of T-cell recognition and activation, which ultimately (through cytokines) direct AMs to kill obligate intracellular microbes, such as tubercle bacilli and *L. monocytogenes*. Humoral antibody production by T-cell–directed B lymphocytes results in opsonization and toxin neutralization, as occurs with *S. pneumoniae* and *Bordetella pertussis*. Viruses and obligate intracellular organisms are typically inactivated by the dual mechanisms of cytotoxic T cells and neutralizing antibody.

Several immune function assays measuring lymphocyte proliferation and antibody production to experimental antigens have been developed as surrogates for measuring protective immune responses. Mice exposed to carbon dust inhalation (2–4 mg/m^3) had a decreased number of antibody-forming cells in the spleen that was proportional to exposure time (64). In local mediastinal lymph nodes

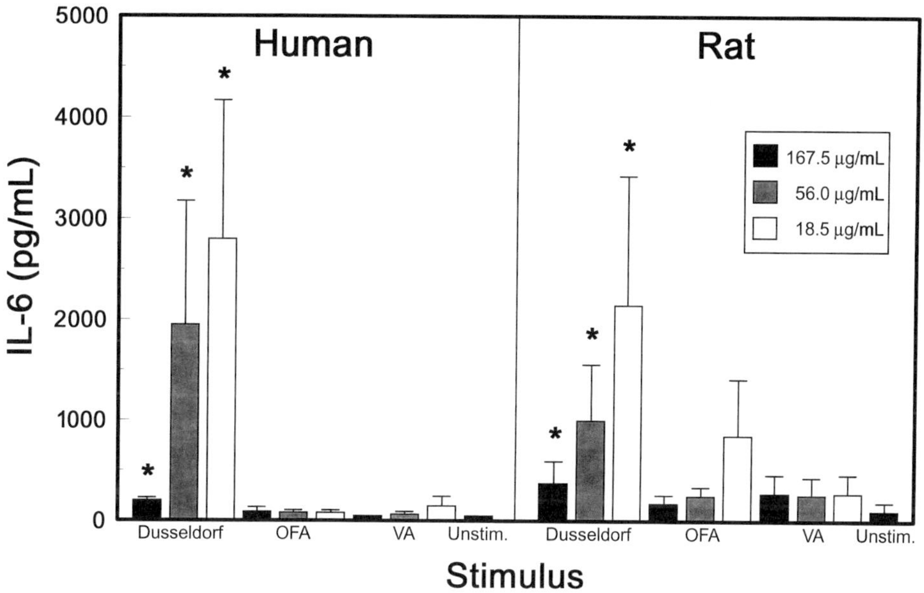

Figure 4 Interleukin-6 production by rat and human alveolar macrophages exposed to environmental particulates (Dusseldorf, oil fly ash [OFA]; volcanic ash [VA]). AMs were incubated overnight with varying amounts of particulate and supernates were assayed for IL-6 with a bioassay. * indicates significant differences ($p < 0.05$) from unstimulated controls; $n - 5$. (From Ref. 27.)

(MLN), antigen-specific cell proliferation was initially enhanced, but then decreased after 15 days exposure. In similar experiments, splenic T-cell responses to phytohemagglutinin mitogen (PHA) were depressed after 7 days exposure to carbon dust, but were enhanced thereafter (65). The same authors subsequently showed that silica inhalation suppressed the cellular and humoral responses to subsequent LPS challenge (66). Other laboratories have reported that long-term exposure to fly ash (67) or TiO_2 (68) suppresses both systemic and local antibody production and antigen-specific lymphocyte responses to inhaled antigen or bacteria. Inhalation of quartz or fly ash also suppressed primary IgM antibody responses in rats (69); however, no effects were seen on secondary immune response to recall antigen. The general pattern is that brief exposure to particulates may initially enhance or suppress cellular immune responses, depending on the nature of the particle, the host, and the anatomical location from which lymphocytes are sampled (local versus systemic). Long-term exposure, however, usually leads to suppression of most indicators of immune function. This pattern is best illustrated with cigarette smoke, for which transient exposure can temporarily elevate immune responsiveness, but prolonged exposure in mice, primates, and humans results in suppression of T-cell mitogen responses, antibody formation, NK-mediated cytotoxicity, and resistance to tumors (70).

Much of the particulate matter found in urban air is derived from combustion of fossil fuels and industrial discharges, and it contains varying amounts of metals, solvents, aromatic hydrocarbons, and other chemicals that modulate immune function. Of the metals, cadmium, vanadium, chromium, lead, and nickel have been most extensively studied and shown to decrease antibody formation, antigen processing, and lymphocyte proliferation in experimental animals, and, on occasion (e.g., lead), exposed populations (reviewed in 71–73). Organic compounds that show immunotoxic properties, such as benzene, trichloroethylene, dioxins, phenols, organotonins, and diester phorbol compounds are also found in the atmosphere at varying concentrations (see Chaps. 2 and 3) and have been shown experimentally to alter immune function (74). Although these studies offer evidence that organic chemicals and metal compounds can be immunotoxic, their role as cofactors in air pollutant-enhanced lung disease has not been fully explored.

When taken together, these studies show that prolonged exposure to a wide range of airborne particulates, and especially those containing toxic chemicals, can produce decreases in immune function. It is not yet clear at which point development of protective immunity is most affected. The generation of specific antibody, for example, arises only after antigen processing and presentation to T lymphocytes by accessory cells, notably macrophages and dendritic cells. Because air pollutant exposure suppresses AM phagocytosis, this could result in decreased antigen processing. Furthermore, dendritic cells, which exist in a contiguous network throughout the airway epithelium (75), may be directly affected by toxic exposure or, indirectly, by immunomodulatory mediators produced by proximal epithelial cells. Analysis of these primary signals and their effect on the subsequent generation of immunity will provide valuable mechanistic information on how air pollutant exposure can increase susceptibility to infectious agents.

III. Particle-Enhanced Allergic Lung Disease

Approximately 17% of the U.S. population suffers from some sort of allergic disease (76). Most of those individuals are hypersensitive to pollens or have atopic eczema. Six percent of the population has physician-diagnosed asthma, the prevalence of which has increased by approximately 30% over the last 15 years. Air pollution exposure has long been considered a risk factor for the exacerbation of asthma attacks in asthmatic individuals. Health care statistics in Canada and the United States show that hospital admissions for asthma increase during episodes of high ozone or airborne particulate levels and that bronchodilator use increases according to the level of particulate air pollution (77–80). In one report, a steel mill in Utah (which was the main contributor of particulate air pollution to the area), closed during the winter of 1986–1987. Peak concentrations of PM_{10} fell from 365 $\mu g/m^3$ to 113 $\mu g/m^3$, and this was associated with a 50% reduction in hospital admissions for respiratory disease, compared with adjacent years when the mill was operating (81). When the data were analyzed specifically for asthma and bronchitis, the investigators estimated that hospital admissions for these disorders were reduced by 4.2% for each 10-$\mu g/m^3$ drop in PM_{10} recorded over the 2-month period. Significantly, no differences in hospital admissions were observed in neighboring counties, which experienced no change in PM_{10} levels (82). A Japanese study showed that individuals living close to a major highway (hence, exposed to higher levels of automobile exhaust, latex from tires, and road dust) suffered more frequent and severe allergic reactions than cohorts living 5 miles (8 Km) from the highway, but with comparable levels of airborne pollen (83). Before describing experimental data supporting the epidemiological evidence, a brief description of pulmonary allergic disease is warranted.

A. Pulmonary Allergy

Allergic (hypersensitivity) lung disease is dependent on various host susceptibility factors, and interactions between antigens, accessory (antigen-presenting) cells, immune cells, and mediators. A central feature of pulmonary allergy is that it is immune-mediated and acquired following natural exposure to antigen. Several types of hypersensitivity reactions can occur (following reexposure to antigen), which have been broadly defined according to their time of onset, whether the effects are mediated by cells or antibody, and if the responses are directed against extrinsic or ''self''-antigens (24). Under this scheme, immediate (type I) hypersensitivity is caused by allergen-specific IgE antibodies, which bind to high-affinity Fcε receptors on the surface of mast cells in the airways. On reexposure to allergen, antigenic molecules cross-link immunoglobulin receptor sites, causing mast cell degranulation and release of vasoactive amines and other mediators responsible for acute inflammation and bronchoconstriction. Allergic alveolitis (type III) and delayed type hypersensitivity reactions (type IV) are caused by IgG–antigen complexes and cell-mediated reactions, respectively, and result in pulmonary inflammation, granuloma formation, and fibrosis. These reactions occur between 4 and 48 hr after allergen exposure and have a more chronic nature.

Ten years ago two types of CD4-positive T-helper lymphocytes termed Th1 and Th2 cells were identified in mice according to their contrasting cytokine production profiles and opposing functions in the generation of specific immune responses (84). Th1 cells produce interleukin-2 (IL-2), and interferon gamma

(IFN-γ), which are thought to evoke cell-mediated immune responses associated with protection against bacterial and viral pathogens. In contrast, Th2 cells produce IL-4, which stimulates IgE antibody production, and IL-5, which is a chemotactic and maturation factor for eosinophils. Th2 responses are associated with immediate-type hypersensitivity reactions to allergens and exposure or infection with protozoan parasites. Allergic (extrinsic) asthmatics usually display immediate (IgE-mediated) hypersensitivity reactions as well as later inflammatory (late-phase) responses that are thought to be controlled by T lymphocytes of the Th2 subphenotype. In addition, lung tissue and peripheral blood lymphocytes from persons with asthma have been shown to produce higher levels of IL-4 and IL-5, compared with normal persons (85).

B. Human Clinical Studies

Although the epidemiological data strongly suggest an interaction between inhaled particulate matter and the severity of asthma attacks, few controlled clinical studies have addressed this issue. In one report, a group of patients with allergic rhinitis and mild asthma were exposed to diesel exhaust particles (DEP) by nasal inhalation, and antibody-forming cells and free antibody were assessed in nasal washes at various times after challenge (86). Exposure to 0.3 mg DEP significantly enhanced IgE and IgG_4 antibody, but had no effect on other IgG subclasses, IgA, or IgM antibody. IgE-, but not IgA-forming cells were also increased in the nasal wash after DEP challenge and mRNA coding for a variety of epsilon heavy-chain variants was increased. The same group (87) later stimulated peripheral blood mononuclear cells or purified B cells from healthy human donors with IL-4 and anti-CD40 antibody along with organic extracts from diesel exhaust particles, and found that IgE production was increased by both types of cells compared with stimulated controls incubated with the organic extract vehicle. The results from these studies suggest that diesel particles may act as immunological adjuvants to enhance the induction of allergic (Th2) immune responses.

C. Animal Studies

Initial studies in animals have also shown that diesel exhaust particles have an adjuvant effect on IgE production. Mice immunized intraperitoneally with ovalbumin mixed with DEP had increased antigen-specific IgE antibody compared with mice that received ovalbumin alone (88). When antigen and DEP were administered into the nostrils of mice, antigen-specific IgE in the serum was dramatically enhanced compared with levels in control mice receiving ovalbumin alone (89). In a similar fashion, intratracheal instillation of DEP and ovalbumin enhanced lymphocyte proliferation and IL-4 production in the mediastinal lymph nodes 4–17 times control levels, and this effect was associated with increased serum IgE antibody (90). In a study from our laboratory, Brown Norway rats,

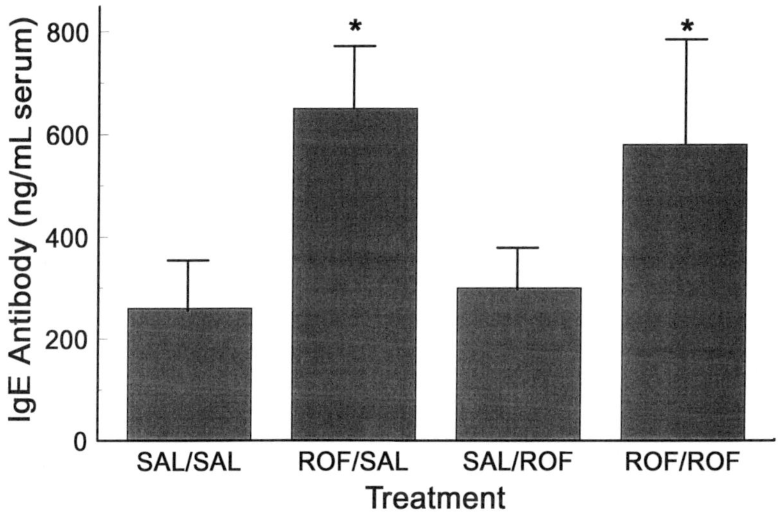

Figure 5 Total IgE in the serum of rats exposed to residual oil fly ash 3 days before sensitization with dust mite (ROF/SAL), 3 days before challenge (SAL/ROF), and 3 days before each immunization procedure (ROF/ROF). * indicates significant differences ($p < 0.05$) from controls (SAL/SAL). IgE was quantified by ELISA; $n = 5$.

instilled through the trachea with 1-mg residual oil fly ash (ROFA) 3 days before sensitization with house dust mite allergen, had increased levels of IgE antibody in the serum compared with controls (Fig. 5).

Each of these studies suggest that certain particles derived from emission sources have the ability to act as immunological adjuvants to promote both T-cell function and allergic IgE antibody production. In addition, it is becoming clear that, because these particles are also proinflammatory, they may exacerbate preexisting lung disease with additive or possibly even synergistic insult to the respiratory tract.

IV. Future Research Needs

Many epidemiological studies have shown that increases in particulate air pollution are associated with acute increases in morbidity and mortality (1). Mortality is thought to occur mainly in the elderly with preexisting pulmonary and cardiac disease, whereas morbidity is seen in younger, susceptible populations, such as those with asthma. Additional information identifying which individuals are at risk and their histories of exposure and health could contribute to the design of studies aimed at elucidating the mechanisms of the associations observed between ambient air PM_{10} levels, and enhanced morbidity and mortality. Further effort is also required to determine which particular chemical and biological components or physical properties (e.g., size) of airborne particulates can have effects on the immune system.

Most of the experimental evidence examining the effects of particles on the immune system has come from healthy young adult animals briefly exposed to high concentrations of particulates, such as silica, fly ash, cigarette smoke, and coal dust. These studies have so far demonstrated that inhaled particles can impair the ability of the pulmonary defenses to eliminate pathogens by several mechanisms, including slowing of the mucociliary escalator, reduced AM phagocytosis and microbial killing, alterations in lung lining fluid, and suppression of specific immune responses. As well as direct toxicity, these changes have been attributed to differences in lymphocyte trafficking, and the production of stress hormones, cytokines, and other mediators that can influence immune regulation and function. The effects are often reported in the absence of pathogenic insult, however, and the relative contributions of these functional defenses to overall host resistance in both healthy and diseased animals of different ages needs further study.

In an attempt to address this issue, Luster and colleagues (91) examined the concordance between a variety of immune function tests and changes in host resistance brought about by exposure to several chemicals known to produce immunotoxic effects. They found that decreases in antibody production and changes in lymphocyte phenotypic markers correlated best with enhanced susceptibility to infection by chemical exposure, but submitted that more complete algorithms of host defense, using different pathogens, need to be established. To this end, ''knockout mice,'' which are deficient in genes coding for (e.g., proinflammatory cytokines and other molecules important in resistance to infection) are being used to produce a more integrated view of the host defense network.

The epidemiological and experimental data also offer compelling evidence that airborne particulates can exacerbate asthma. One key question is whether particle inhalation can actually increase the incidence of asthma, as opposed to provoking exacerbation of existing disease. Most persons with asthma display ''nonspecific'' bronchial hyperresponsiveness to a wide range of inhaled substances, including cigarette smoke, hypertonic saline, and cold air. These challenges are not antigenic, but rather, behave as irritants in provoking bronchoconstriction. Although many of the early studies showed that air pollutants decreased immune responses, recent experiments have shown that airborne particulates can act as adjuvants to sway the immune response to a more allergic (Th2) phenotype. It is now becoming clear that a suppression of Th1 immune responses may coincide with an upswing in Th2 cell function, with subsequent increased IgE responses and enhanced immediate hypersensitivity reactions. This paradigm provides a rationale by which air pollutants can simultaneously enhance both allergic and infectious disease, despite the apparent contradiction of immunosuppression and immunoenhancement. Similar results have been obtained with other xenobiotic agents, such as metals, ultraviolet radiation (UVB), and oxidant gases (92). In UVB radiation, exposed keratinocytes release IL-10, which directs the immune response to a predominantly Th2 (IgE-producing) phenotype (93). Whether particles can act in a similar fashion on cells of the respiratory tract is unclear, although some urban air particulates cause epithelial cells and AMs to release proinflammatory cytokines. Particles ingested by AMs might further modulate immune function by affecting antigen trafficking and subsequent processing and presentation of antigen by dendritic cells in the airways.

There is a clear need to study the effect of brief and prolonged urban air particulate inhalation on healthy and diseased animals to investigate mechanisms of particulate-enhanced infectious and allergic lung disease. These experiments will require better animal models of human disease, as well as improved engineering techniques to either harness or create realistic pollution episodes. Finally, in vitro comparisons of human and animal cells will provide a rational basis for extrapolating from animal toxicology data to potential health effects in humans.

Acknowledgments

MIG is funded by Cooperative Agreement 817643 with the U.S. Environmental Protection Agency. The authors are grateful to Drs. L. Birnbaum, P. Bromberg, and R. Smialowicz for critical review of the manuscript.

Disclaimer

The research described in this chapter has been reviewed by the National Health and Environmental Effects Research Laboratory, U.S. Environmental Protection Agency, and approved for publication. Approval does not signify that the contents necessarily reflect the views and policies of the agency.

References

1. Pope CA, Dockery DW, Schwartz J. Review of epidemiological evidence of health effects of particulate air pollution. Inhal Toxicol 1995; 7:1–18.
2. Ostro BD. The association of air pollution and mortality: examining the case for inference. Arch Environ Health 1993; 48:336–342.
3. Dockery DW, Pope AC. Acute respiratory effects of particulate air pollution. Annu Rev Public Health 1994; 15:107–132.
4. Gardner DE. Effects of airborne gases and airborne particles on lung infections. In: McGrath JJ, Barnes CD, eds. Air Pollution: Physiological Effects. New York: Academic Press, 1982:48–79.

5. Selgrade MJK, Gilmour MI. Effects of gaseous air pollutants on immune responses and susceptibility to infections and allergic disease. In: Dean JH, Luster MI, Munson AE, Kimber I, eds. Immunotoxicology and Immunopharmacology. New York: Raven Press, 1994:395–411.
6. Gilmour MI. Interaction of air pollutants and pulmonary allergic responses in experimental animals. Toxicology 1995; 105:335–342.
7. Jakab GJ, Spannhake EW, Kleeberger SR, Canning BJ, Gilmour MI. The effects of ozone on immune function. Environ Health Perspect 1995; 103:77–89.
8. Green GM, Jakab GJ, Low RB, Davis GS. Defense mechanisms of the respiratory membrane. Am Rev Respir Dis 1977; 115:479–514.
9. Reynolds HB. Integrated host defense against infections. In: Crystal RG, West JB, eds. The Lung: Scientific Foundations. New York: Raven Press, 1991:1899–1911.
10. Schlesinger RB. The interaction of inhaled toxicants with respiratory tract clearance mechanisms. Crit Rev Toxicol 1990; 20:257–285.
11. Schlesinger RB. Interaction of gaseous and particulate pollutants in the respiratory tract: mechanisms and modulators. Toxicology 1995; 105:315–325.
12. Koren HS, Becker S. Antimicrobial defense mechanisms. In: Crystal RG, West JB, eds. The Lung: Scientific Foundations. New York: Raven Press, 1991:747–769.
13. Sibille Y, Reynolds HY. Macrophages and polymorphonuclear neutrophils in lung defense and injury. Am Rev Respir Dis 1990; 141:471–501.
14. Henson PM, Johnston RB. Tissue injury in inflammation: oxidants, proteinases and cationic proteins. J Clin Invest 1987; 79:669–674.
15. Weiss SJ. Tissue destruction by neutrophils. N Engl J Med 1989; 320:365–376.
16. Brown EJ. Complement receptors, adhesion and phagocytosis. Infect Agents Dis 1992; 1:63–70.
17. Lehr RI, Lichtenstein AK, Ganz T. Defensins: antimicrobial and cytotoxic peptides of mammalian cells. Annu Rev Immunol 1993; 11:105–128.
18. Liebow AA. Pulmonary angiitis and granulomatosis. Am Rev Respir Dis 1973; 108: 1–18.
19. Herberman R, Djeu J, Kay D, et al. Natural killer cells: characteristics and regulation of activity. Immunol Rev 1989; 44:43–70.
20. Haley PJ. Immunological responses within the lung after inhalation of airborne chemicals. In: Gardner D, Crapo JD, McClellan RO, eds. Toxicology of the Lung. 2nd ed. New York: Raven Press, 1993:389–416.
21. Murray MJ, Driscoll KE. Immunology of the respiratory tract. In: Parent RE, ed. Comparative Biology of the Normal Lung. Boca Raton, FL: CRC Press, 1991:725–746.
22. Edelman AS, Zolla-Pazner S. AIDS: a syndrome of immune dysregulation, dysfunction, and deficiency. FASEB J 1989; 3:22–30.
23. Plebani A, Ugazio AG, Monafo V. Selective IgA deficiency; an update. Curr Prob Dermatol 1989; 18:66–78.
24. Daniele RP. Immunology and Immunologic Diseases of the Lung. Boston: Blackwell Scientific, 1988.
25. Selgrade MJK, Cooper K, Devlin RB, Van Loveren H, Biagini RE, Luster MI. Im-

munotoxicity: bridging the gap between animal research and human health effects. Fundam Appl Toxicol 1995; 24:13–21.
26. Schlesinger RB, Fine JM, Chen LC. Interspecies differences in the phagocytic activity of pulmonary macrophages subjected to acidic challenge. Fundam Appl Toxicol 1992; 19:584–589.
27. Becker S, Soukup JM, Gilmour MI, Devlin RB. Stimulation of human and rat alveolar macrophages by urban air particulates: effects on oxidant radical generation and cytokine production. Toxicol Appl Pharmacol 1996; 141:637–648.
28. Dixon RE. Economic costs of respiratory tract infections in the United States. Am J Med 1985; 78(6B):45–51.
29. Chretien J, Holland W, Macklem P, Woolcock A. Acute respiratory infections in children: a global public health problem. N Engl J Med 1984; 310:982–984.
30. Berman S. Epidemiology of acute respiratory infections in children of developing countries. Rev Infect Dis 1991; 13:454–462.
31. Marcy TW, Merril WW. Cigarette smoking and respiratory tract infection. Clin Chest Med 1987; 8:381–391.
32. Department of Health and Human Services. The health consequences of smoking; chronic obstructive lung disease. A report of the Surgeon General. Rockville, MD: DHHS 1984.
33. Honicky RE, Osborne JS, Apcom CA. Symptoms of respiratory illness in young children and the use of wood burning stoves for indoor heating. Pediatrics 1985; 75:587–593.
34. Calder MA, Lutz W, Schonell ME. A 5 year study of bacteriology and prophylactic chemotherapy in patients with chronic bronchitis. Br J Dis Chest 1968; 62:93–108.
35. Paul R. Silicosis in northern Rhodesia copper mines. Arch Environ Health 1961; 2: 96–102.
36. Durck H. Studien uber Aetiologie und Histologie der Pneumonie im Kindesalter und der Pneumonie im Allgemeinen. Dtch Arch Klin Med 1896; 58:368–444.
37. Cesa Bianchi D. Staubinhalation und Lungentuberkulose. Z Hyg Infektionskrankh 1913; 73:166–181.
38. Kettle EH. The relation of dust to infection. Proc R Soc Med 1930; 24:79–94.
39. Coffin DL, Blommer EJ. Acute toxicity of irradiated auto exhaust. Arch Environ Health 1967; 15:36–38.
40. Hatch GE, Boykin E, Graham JA, Lewtas J, Pott F, Loud K, Mumford JL. Inhalable particles and pulmonary host defense: in vivo and in vitro effects of ambient air and combustion particles. Environ Res 1985; 36:67–80.
41. Pritchard RJ, Ghio AJ, Lehmann, JR, et al. Oxidant generation amd lung injury after particulate air pollutant exposure increases with the concentration of associated metals. Inhal Toxicol 1996; 8:457–478.
42. Green GM, Kass EH. The role of the alveolar macrophage in the clearance of bacteria from the lung. J Exp Med 1964; 119:167–176.
43. Jakab GJ. Relationship between carbon black particulate-bound formaldehyde, pulmonary antibacterial defenses, and alveolar macrophage phagocytosis. Inhal Toxicol 1992; 4:325–342.

44. Jakab GJ. The toxicologic interactions resulting from inhalation of carbon black and acrolein on pulmonary antibacterial and antiviral defenses. Toxicol Appl Pharmacol 1993; 121:165–175.
45. Rylander R. Pulmonary defense mechanisms to airborne bacteria. Acta Physiol Scand 1968; 306(supp):8–89.
46. Gilmour MI, Baskerville A, Taylor FGR, Wathes CM. The effect of titanium dioxide inhalation on the pulmonary clearance of *Pasteurella haemolytica* in the mouse. Environ Res 1989; 50:157–172.
47. Menzel DB. Ozone: an overview of its toxicity in man and animals. J Toxicol Environ Health 1984; 13:183–204.
48. Morrow PE. Dust overloading of the lungs: update and appraisal. Toxicol Appl Pharmacol 1992; 113:1–12.
49. Canning BJ, Hmieleski RR, Spannhake EW, Jakab GJ. Ozone reduces murine alveolar and peritoneal macrophage phagocytosis: the role of prostaglandins. Am J Physiol 1991; 261:L277–L282.
50. Hoidal JR, Niewoehner DE. Lung phagocytic recruitment and metabolic alterations induced by cigarette smoke in humans and in hamsters. Am Rev Respir Dis 1982; 126:548–552.
51. King TE, Savici D, Campbell PA. Phagocytosis and killing of *Listeria monocytogenes* by alveolar macrophages: smokers versus nonsmokers. J Infect Dis 1988; 158: 1309–1316.
52. Ortega E, Barriga C, Rodriguez AB. Decline in the phagocytic function of alveolar macrophages from mice exposed to cigarette smoke. Comp Immunol Microbiol Infect Dis 1994; 17:77–84.
53. Rom WN, Bitterman PB, Rennard SI, Cantin A, Crystal RG. Characterization of the lower respiratory tract inflammation of nonsmoking individuals with interstitial lung disease associated with chronic inhalation of organic dusts. Am Rev Respir Dis 1987; 136:1429–1434.
54. U.S. Environmental Protection Agency. An acid aerosols issue paper: health effects and aerometrics: Research Triangle Park, NC: Office of Health and Environmental Assessment, EPA report no. EPA-600/8-88-005F. Available from NTIS, Springfield, VA; PB91–125864, 1989.
55. Chen LC, Fine JM, Qu QS, Amdur MO, Gordon T. Effects of fine and ultrafine sulfuric acid aerosols in guinea pigs: alterations in alveolar macrophage function and intracellular pH. Toxicol Appl Pharmacol 1992; 113:109–117.
56. Jakab GJ, Hemenway DR. Inhalation co-exposure to carbon black and acrolein suppresses alveolar macrophage phagocytosis and TNF-a release and modulates peritoneal macrophage phagocytosis. Inhal Toxicol 1993; 5:275–289.
57. Moores HK, Janigan DT, Hajela RP. Lung injury after experimental smoke inhalation: particle associate changes in alveolar macrophages. Toxicol Pathol 1993; 21: 521–527.
58. Zelikoff JT, Parsons E, Schlesinger RB. Inhalation of particulate lead disrupts pulmonary macrophage-mediated functions important for host defense and tumor surveillance in the lung. Environ Res 1993; 62:207–222.
59. Zeigler B, Bhalla DK, Rasmussen RE, Kleinman MT, Menzel DB. Inhalation of resuspended road dust, but not ammonium nitrate decreases the expression of the pulmonary macrophage Fc receptor. Toxicol Lett 1994; 71:197–208.

60. Jakab GJ, Risby TH, Sehnert SS, Hmieleski RB, Gilmour MI. Suppression of alveolar macrophage membrane receptor-mediated phagocytosis by model particle adsorbate complexes: physico-chemical moderators of uptake. Environ Health Perspect 1991; 89:169–174.
61. Hadnagy W, Seemayer NH. Inhibition of phagocytosis of human macrophages induced by airborne particulates. Toxicol Lett 1994; 72:23–31.
62. Zelikoff JT, Schlesinger RB. Modulation of pulmonary immune defense mechanisms by sulfuric acid: effects on macrophage-derived tumor necrosis factor and superoxide. Toxicology 1992; 76:271–281.
63. Dong W, Lewtas J, Luster MI. Role of endotoxin in tumor necrosis factor alpha expression from alveolar macrophages treated with urban air particles. Exp Lung Res 1996; 22:577–592.
64. Zarkower A, Morges W. Alteration in antibody response induced by carbon inhalation: a model system. 1972; Infect Immun 5:915–920.
65. Miller SD, Zarkower A. Effects of carbon dust inhalation on the cell mediated immune response in mice. Infect Immun 1974; 9:534–539.
66. Miller SD, Zarkower A. Silica-induced alterations of murine lymphocyte immunocompetence and suppression of B lymphocyte immunocompetence. A possible mechanism. J Reticuloendothel Soc 1976; 19:46–61.
67. Eskew ML, Zarkower A, Scheuchenzuber WJ, Graham JA. Effects of fly ash inhalation on murine immune function: effect on systemic responses. Environ Res 1982; 28:375–385.
68. Gilmour MI, Wathes CM, Taylor FGR. Pulmonary clearance of *Pasteurella haemolytica* and immune responses in mice following exposure to titanium dioxide. Environ Res 1989; 50:184–194.
69. Bice DDE, Hahn FF, Benson J, Carpenter RL, Hobbs CH. Comparitive lung immunotoxicity of inhaled quartz and coal combustion fly ash. Environ Res 1987; 43: 374–389.
70. Johnson JD, Houchens DP, Kluwe WM, Craig DK, Fisher GL. Effects of mainstream and environmental tobacco smoke on the immune system in animals and humans: a review. Crit Rev Toxicol 1990; 20:369–395.
71. U.S. Environmental Protection Agency. Air quality criteria for lead. Research Triangle Park, NC: Office of Health and Environmental Assessment, EPA report no. EPA-600/8-83-028aF-dF.4v. Available from NTIS, Springfield, VA; PB87–142378, 1986.
72. Newcombe DS, Esa AH. Immunotoxicity of organophosphorus compounds. In: Newcombe DS, Rose NR, Bloom JC, eds. Clinical Immunotoxicology. New York: Raven Press, 1992:349–363.
73. Kowoleko M, McCabe MJ, Lawrence DA. Metal induced alterations of immunity. In: Newcombe DS, Rose NR, Bloom JC, eds. Clinical Immunotoxicology. New York: Raven Press, 1992:401–419.
74. Saboori AM, Newcombe DS. Environmental chemicals with immunotoxic properties. In: Newcombe DS, Rose NR, Bloom JC, eds. Clinical Immunotoxicology. New York: Raven Press, 1992:365–400.
75. Holt PG, Schon-Hegrad MA, Oliver J, Holt BJ, McMenamin PG. A contiguous network of dendritic antigen presenting cells within the respiratory epithelium. Int Arch Allergy Appl Immunol 1990; 91:155–159.

76. U.S. Department of Health and Human Services. Guidelines for the diagnosis and management of asthma. Publication 91-3042. Bethesda, MD: National Institutes of Health, 1991.
77. Bates DV, Sizto R. Hospital admissions and air pollutants in Southern Ontario: the acid summer haze effect. Environ Res 1987; 43:317–331.
78. Pierson WE, Koenig JQ. Respiratory effects of air pollution on allergic disease. J Allergy Clin Immunol 1992; 90:557–565.
79. Cody RP, Weisel CP, Birnbaum G, Lioy PJ. The effect of ozone associated with summertime photochemical smog and the frequency of asthma visits to hospital emergency departments. Environ Res 1992; 58:184–194.
80. Roemer W, Hoek G, Brunekreef B. Effect of ambient winter air pollution on respiratory health of children with chronic respiratory symptoms. Am Rev Respir Dis 1993; 147:118–124.
81. Pope CA. Respiratory disease associated with community air pollution and a steel mill, Utah Valley. Am J Public Health 1989; 79:623–628.
82. Pope CA. Respiratory hospital admissions associated with PM-10 pollution in Utah, Salt Lake, and Cache Valleys. Arch Environ Health 1991; 46:90–97.
83. Ishizaki T, Koizumi K, Ikemori R, et al. Studies of prevalence of Japanese cedar pollinosis among the residents in a densely cultivated area. Ann Allergy 1987; 58: 265–270.
84. Mosmann TR, Coffman RL. Two types of mouse T helper clone: implication for immune regulation. Immunol Today 1987; 8:233–236.
85. Robinson DS, Hamid Q, Ying S, et al. Predominant Th2-like bronchoalveolar T lymphocyte population in atopic asthma. N Engl J Med 1992; 326:298–304.
86. Diaz-Sanchez D, Dotson AR, Takeaka H, Saxon A. Diesel exhaust particles induce local IgE production in vivo and alter the pattern of messenger RNA isoforms. J Clin Invest 1994; 94:1417–1425.
87. Takenaka H, Zhang K, Diaz-Sanchez D, Tsien A, Saxon A. Enhanced human IgE production results from exposure to the aromatic hydrocarbons from diesel exhaust: direct effects on B cell IgE production. J Allergy Clin Immunol 1995; 95:103–115.
88. Muranaka M, Suzuki S, et al. Adjuvant activity of diesel exhaust particulates for the production of IgE antibody in mice. J Allergy Clin Immunol 1986; 77:616–623.
89. Takafuji S, Suzuki S, Koizumi K, et al. Diesel exhaust particulates inoculated by the intranasal route have an adjuvant activity for IgE production in mice. J Allergy Clin Immunol 1987; 79:639–645.
90. Fujimaki H, Nohara O, Ichinose T, Watanabe N, Saito S. IL4 production in mediastinal lymph node cells in mice intratracheally instilled with diesel exhaust particles and antigen. Toxicology 1994; 92:261–268.
91. Luster MI, Portier C, Pait DG, et al. Risk assessment in immunotoxicology II. Relationships between immune and host resistance tests. Fundam Appl Toxicol 1993; 21:71–82.
92. Selgrade MJ, Lawrence DA, Ullrich SE, Gilmour MI, Schuyler MR, Kimber I. Modulation of T-helper populations; potential mechanisms of respiratory hypersensitivity and immune suppression. Toxicol Appl Pharmacol 1997; 145:219–229.
93. Ulrich SE. Mechanism involved in the systemic suppression of antigen presenting cell function by UV irradiation. J Immunol 1994; 152:3410–3416.

18

Cardiopulmonary Consequences of Particle Inhalation

MARK W. FRAMPTON and MARK J. UTELL

University of Rochester Medical Center
University of Rochester School of Medicine and Dentistry
Rochester, New York

JONATHAN M. SAMET

Johns Hopkins University
Baltimore, Maryland

I. Introduction

Increases in the concentration of fine particles in the air are associated with increases in mortality. The excess deaths are predominantly from respiratory causes, but deaths from cardiovascular causes are affected as well. This association has been observed in many cities worldwide; and perhaps most remarkably, remains strong at low particle concentrations previously thought to be without adverse health effects. The mechanisms by which particulate pollution induces health effects at such low mass concentrations remain unclear. Determining the biological mechanisms involved has been identified as a high-priority research need in the United States (1) and other countries. As suggested by the word cardiopulmonary this chapter will explore hypotheses and evidence linking particle exposure with both respiratory and cardiac dysfunction and disease.

We will begin by considering the epidemiological database and its implications for mechanisms of health effects. The following sections explore the respiratory and cardiac diseases that may confer increased susceptibility to the effects of particle exposure, and discuss the experimental approaches being taken to move from speculation to understanding of the mechanisms involved.

II. Implications of Epidemiological Data

A. Overview

During the last decade there has been a remarkable expansion of the epidemiological literature on the health effects of air pollution in general and of particulate air pollution in particular.

The studies, conducted not only in the United States, but in other developed countries and in developing countries, have addressed effects of particles on measures of both mortality and morbidity (Table 1). The studies have included ecological (group-level) studies of the time–series design and also analytical (individual-level) studies of the cross-sectional or cohort design. The expansion of the epidemiological evidence reflects the completion of several large epidemiological studies and the development of new statistical methods for time–series analysis that can be readily applied to public use databases. During this decade, final results of several major epidemiological studies have been reported, including the Six-Cities Study in the United States (2) and the 24-Cities Study (3) in the United States and Canada.

Many time–series studies have addressed the associations between daily mortality counts and pollutant levels, after taking into account weather and temporal trends in mortality. These studies have considered total mortality, exclusive of external causes, and also cause-specific mortality, with focus on cardiac and respiratory causes of death. Total mortality counts are a relatively nonspecific outcome category, because a priori considerations of pathogenesis indicate that effects of particulate air pollution would be anticipated primarily on deaths from chronic cardiac and respiratory conditions and from respiratory infections, including pneumonia and influenza. To date, two studies have linked air pollution exposure with mortality on a longer time frame (4,5). These studies are viewed as pivotal because they indicate possible longer-term effects from particulate pollu-

Table 1 Mortality and Morbidity Measures Considered in Epidemiological Studies of Particulate Air Pollution

Mortality
Long-term mortality: total and cause-specific
Short-term mortality: total and cause-specific
Morbidity
Long-term hospitalization rates
Daily hospitalization rates
Rates of emergency room visits for respiratory diseases
Respiratory symptom occurrence
Physiological indicators

tion and suggest that the day-to-day associations between air pollution and mortality may have consequences for shortening life. The studies of morbidity have also been conducted throughout the world. Coherence is anticipated between the findings of investigations on mortality and morbidity (6).

Associations of particulate pollution with mortality should be paralleled by associations with appropriate morbidity measures, whether investigated using an ecological or an analytical design. For example, an association between particulate air pollution and mortality should be mirrored in associations of particulate pollution with hospitalization rate or with individual-level measures of outcome, such as occurrence of cardiac ischemia or need for medication for angina pectoris. To date, studies of hospitalization rates in the United States have primarily addressed elderly persons because of the availability of data from the Health Care Financing Administration for Medicare participants. Emergency room visit rates have been considered as an outcome as well, but coverage extends to all ages.

Analytic or individual-level studies have been directed either at the effect of air pollution exposure on respiratory health generally, or on the status of persons with conditions (e.g., asthma) that make them more susceptible to air pollution than the population in general. The Six-Cities Study, a prospective cohort study, and the 24-Cities Study, a cross-sectional study, were of the general design. The ''panel'' study, a short-term cohort study involving relatively intensive assessment of outcome, has been used to assess the effects of air pollution on susceptible persons. Typically, a panel of participants is enrolled and asked to maintain a diary of symptom status and medication use, and physiological measurements, such as peak expiratory flow rate (PEFR) may be made. New methods for data analysis have also made this design more informative than previously (7,8).

B. Summary of Findings

The recent epidemiological data have been extensively reviewed (see, e.g., 9–14). Table 2, drawing from these reviews, provides a summary of the findings. The table is intended to focus our consideration of pathophysiological mechanisms and should not be considered an interpretative summary of this lengthy and controversial literature.

The general pattern of findings for daily mortality counts indicates effects of particulate pollution on older persons, particularly those with chronic heart and lung diseases. Effects of particulate pollution have tended to be greater for heart and lung disease than for other causes (15), and increased risk has also been found for elderly persons (16). The general pattern of findings has been interpreted as reflective of the effects of air pollution on a pool of individuals made susceptible by age and the presence of underlying heart and lung disease (17,18). Individuals in this susceptible pool are postulated to have either chronic

Table 2 Summary of Findings of Epidemiological Studies of Particulate Air Pollution and Morbidity and Mortality Measures

Mortality	
	Measures of particulate air pollution are associated with daily mortality counts, both for total deaths and for cardiac and respiratory causes.
	Measures of particulate air pollution are associated with total mortality and with cardiopulmonary mortality over periods of years.
Morbidity	
	Measures of particulate air pollution are associated with daily rates of hospitalization for cardiac and respiratory causes.
	Measures of particulate air pollution are associated with adverse effects on persons with asthma, including emergency room and other outpatient visits, and symptom occurrence and lung function level.
	Measures of particulate air pollution are associated with indicators of respiratory health in children.

obstructive pulmonary disease (COPD) or chronic ischemic heart diseases; these same individuals would be at increased risk for more severe respiratory infections because of the underlying chronic condition (19,20). Hospitalization data for the elderly are consistent with the mortality pattern, showing positive associations between particulate indicators and hospitalization rates for heart disease, chronic obstructive pulmonary disease, and pneumonia (13). Morbidity findings indicate that persons with asthma are also adversely affected; deaths from asthma are rare and, consequently, the association of air pollution with daily mortality rates from asthma cannot be evaluated.

The studies of children indicate a variety of nonspecific effects, including increased chronic symptoms, such as cough and bronchitis, and reduced lung function, presumed to represent a reduced rate of lung growth. Associations have also been shown with day-to-day symptom reports (9,14).

C. Populations at Risk

Thus, several lines of evidence suggest that persons in the population at risk from inhaled particles are those with severe heart and lung diseases. The newer findings mirror the historical record from times of much higher exposures. In the London fog of 1952, the proportion of deaths attributed to heart and lung diseases increased during the dates of the fog (21). Additionally, because heart disease is the leading cause of death in the United States, any effect of particulate air pollution on total mortality would be expected to reflect at least an adverse effect on persons with heart disease.

The principal diagnostic labels assigned to this potentially susceptible group in the population by virtue of having chronic heart or lung disease would include coronary artery disease or ischemic heart disease, inclusive of persons with a history of myocardial infarction or coronary artery bypass surgery, COPD, and asthma. Persons with coronary artery disease have atherosclerotic narrowing of the coronary arteries, which deliver blood to the heart. Persons with COPD have physiologically significant impairment of lung function, most often from underlying emphysema and airways narrowing caused by smoking. *Asthma* has been defined as an inflammatory disorder of the airways with accompanying airways hyperresponsiveness and the clinical manifestation of variable airflow obstruction (22). Other groups considered to be potentially susceptible include persons affected by pneumonia or other severe respiratory infections, and infants and the elderly in general.

The conditions associated with susceptibility, ischemic heart disease, asthma, and COPD, are common, and the total pool of potentially susceptible individuals is large. Estimates have been made on the sizes of these potentially susceptible groups. The American Lung Association (23) has published estimates of their numbers in its publication, *Breath in Danger II*. For particulate matter, the groups assumed to be at risk in the report include preadolescent children ($\leq$ 13 years old), the elderly ($\geq$ 65 years old), and persons with preexisting respiratory disease, including COPD and asthma. Population data from the 1990 Census were used at the county level. Estimates of the population having COPD and asthma were based on the National Health Interview Survey; these national data were applied at the county level. Nonattainment was based on 1991 data from the U.S. Environmental Protection Agency (EPA).

In 1991, 74 cities and countries, with a total population of 40,208,738, were in nonattainment for PM_{10}. These cities and counties included 8,468,492 preadolescent children, 4,581,242 elderly persons, 610,874 children younger than 18 years of age with asthma, 1,068,385 adult asthmatics, and 2,227,190 persons with COPD. These categories are not exclusive and cannot be totaled. If persons with coronary heart disease were also considered at risk from PM_{10} then an additional 1,600,000 persons, or about 4% of the total population, would be added. Although these estimates should be considered as only approximate, they signal a basis for public health concern. On the other hand, the numbers of persons in these susceptibility groups who are truly fragile and vulnerable to premature death are likely to be substantially smaller than the American Lung Association's estimates. Furthermore, the purported susceptibility of preadolescents has been based on anticipated increased lung doses of pollutants because of outdoor activity, and not on intrinsically greater susceptibility, in comparison with older persons.

D. Synthesis

Evidence from mortality and morbidity studies suggest that particulate air pollution affects a sizeable pool of frail and older persons, with underlying chronic heart and lung diseases. Short-term associations have been found that link daily counts of events to air pollution on the same or recent days. This temporal pattern of association implies that underlying mechanisms of injury respond rapidly to inhalation of particles, with consequences that adversely affect the functioning of the lungs and of the heart. Elsewhere in this chapter we consider the potential mechanisms, which include increased susceptibility to respiratory infection, or greater severity of respiratory infections; airways inflammation, leading to impaired ventilation–perfusion relations and less efficient gas exchange; alveolar inflammation, possibly with release of mediators that have systemic effects; and precipitation of pulmonary edema from increased lung permeability.

The prolonged effects of particulate air pollution measures on mortality imply that higher exposures could accelerate the occurrence of the disease and contribute to a more severe clinical picture. Enhanced inflammation in the airways and alveoli is a potential mechanism underlying these associations.

III. Cardiopulmonary Diseases of Concern

What respiratory diseases confer increased susceptibility to adverse effects of inhaled particles, and why? Epidemiological studies suggest that the observed increases in mortality occur among persons with underlying respiratory and cardiac disease, particularly the following: COPD, pneumonia, and ischemic heart disease. Morbidity studies indicate that persons with asthma are also adversely affected by exposure to particulate pollution, with ambient particle concentrations associated with increased symptoms, medication use, and visits to hospital emergency rooms. Increases in deaths on high-particle days are the greatest among the elderly, suggesting that aging, independently of underlying respiratory or cardiac disease, may be associated with increased susceptibility.

A. Chronic Obstructive Pulmonary Disease

The term *COPD* encompasses various pathophysiological states associated with obstruction to airflow. The obstruction is relatively fixed, differentiating this condition from asthma, in which reversibility or variability in airflow obstruction is a cardinal feature. There are three main pathophysiological elements seen in patients with COPD (Table 3): chronic bronchitis, emphysema or acinar enlargement, and narrowing of small, distal airways (24). For a given patient, the relative involvement with these three types of pathology determines in part the symptoms, signs, and course of COPD. The pathophysiology of these disease types may confer different susceptibilities to the effects of air pollutant exposure. However, the information available for analysis in epidemiological studies, generally death or discharge diagnoses, does not permit distinction between the types of disease;

Table 3 Pathophysiological Elements in COPD

Chronic bronchitis	
	Mucus hypersecretion
	Mucous gland enlargement
	Smooth muscle hyperplasia
	Bronchial wall thickening
	Inflammation
Emphysema	
	Acinar enlargement
	Alveolar capillary destruction
	Increased lung compliance
Small airways disease	
	Inflammation
	Fibrosis

the relative susceptibilities of persons with these disease subsets to the effects of particle exposure have not been assessed.

Both airway inflammation and narrowing, as well as the loss of lung parenchyma and elastic tissue, contribute to the collapse of small airways during the expiratory phase of breathing. Destruction of lung tissue leads to a reduction in the number of functioning lung units or alveoli, so that remaining lung units must accomplish a larger portion of the net gas exchange. In COPD patients, the proportion of dead space ventilation is increased, compared with normal individuals. To maintain gas exchange, total ventilation must be increased, thereby increasing the exposure to particles and other pollutants. Each remaining functional lung unit, therefore, is exposed to increased concentrations of inhaled particulate matter compared with the normal lung (6,24). Exposure to ozone, a gaseous pollutant that is often part of the atmospheric pollutant mix, appears to alter particle distribution in the lung (25), which may further increase the dose of particles to susceptible lung units. Mismatching of ventilation and perfusion, as well as a shortened capillary transit time, contribute to exertional hypoxemia, which may precipitate myocardial ischemia in the presence of coronary artery disease.

Smoking is, by far, the most important etiological risk factor for COPD; occupational exposures also contribute. Genetic deficiency of the α_1-protease inhibitor enzyme is another proved, but rare, cause. Other postulated risk factors include increased airways responsiveness to nonspecific stimuli, asthma, childhood respiratory infections, and air pollution (24). The potential role of particulate air pollution in the causation of COPD or other respiratory diseases remains unclear.

The mechanisms by which particle exposure may cause adverse effects in patients with COPD have not been determined. However, several potential factors are summarized in Table 4. Insights may be gained by examining the factors that contribute to the frequent occurrence of exacerbation in COPD. One of the most important of these is infection. The airways of patients with chronic bronchitis are often colonized with microorganisms, such as *Haemophilus influenzae* and *Moraxella catarrhalis*. These organisms rarely cause respiratory infections in healthy adults, but frequently participate in the worsening of COPD and chronic bronchitis (24), evidence that host defense mechanisms are impaired. Mucociliary clearance is slowed, leading to retention of secretions and bacteria. Exposure to particles could increase susceptibility to infectious complications of COPD by further impairing mucociliary clearance, by increasing adhesion of bacteria to epithelial cells, by altering natural host resistance factors in epithelial cells or mucus as a consequence of epithelial injury, by impairing alveolar macrophage function, or by impairing specific or nonspecific functions of the immune system (see Chap. 17). Such effects could also increase susceptibility to respiratory viral infections, important contributors to declining lung function and death in patients with COPD.

Inflammation is almost universally present in the airway of patients dying of obstructive lung disease. Particle exposure may contribute to progression of disease by enhancing inflammation. Airway edema often accompanies influx of inflammatory cells, with resultant airway narrowing, worsening obstruction, and increased airway responsiveness. Reducing airway inflammation is an important goal of modern therapy of COPD as well as asthma.

B. Asthma

In contrast with COPD, asthma is often a disease of the young and otherwise healthy; the incidence is highest in the first 10 years of life. It is a very common

Table 4 Potential Mechanisms by Which Particle Exposure May Worsen COPD

Altered mucociliary clearance
Epithelial injury
Increased bacterial adherence
Altered alveolar macrophage function
Reflex bronchoconstriction
Increased airway inflammation
Increased particle deposition
Increased susceptibility to viral infection

condition, affecting from 3 to 6% of the U.S. population. The hallmark features of asthma are reversible airway obstruction, hyperresponsiveness, and inflammation (22). A growing body of evidence implicates allergic sensitization in the etiology of asthma. Even in persons with mild asthma, endobronchial biopsies reveal evidence for airway epithelial injury and infiltration with eosinophils and polymorphonuclear leukocytes. Products released from activated eosinophils, such as eosinophil cationic protein (ECA) and major basic protein (MBP), contribute to airway injury and continued inflammation. The Th2 lymphocyte, which preferentially expresses interleukins (IL)-4 and IL-5, may drive airway responses toward the recruitment and retention of eosinophils (26) in patients with asthma.

Table 5 shows the mechanisms by which particle exposure may contribute to asthma exacerbations. Note that asthma and COPD share several potential pathogenetic mechanisms, particularly epithelial injury, airway inflammation, and bronchoconstriction. Viral infections often precipitate asthma exacerbations, perhaps by interfering with the elaboration of bronchodilator substances by epithelial cells, or by worsening the underlying airway inflammation. Viral respiratory infections, such as influenza, increase nonspecific airway responsiveness, which can persist for weeks (27). Airway responsiveness to nitrate particles increases during influenza infection in otherwise healthy individuals (28); impairment of antiviral host defense by particle exposure, therefore, would be expected to increase the frequency and severity of asthma exacerbations.

The prevalence of asthma has increased dramatically in developed countries over the past 20 years, and air pollution has been proposed as a contributing factor. However, ambient pollutant concentrations have been decreasing during the period in which asthma mortality has been increasing, suggesting other causes may be more important. A recent study comparing the incidence of asthma in eastern versus western Europe found a higher incidence of asthma in western Europe, where pollution levels were lower (29). Mortality caused by asthma is

Table 5 Potential Mechanisms by Which Particle Exposure May Worsen Asthma

Increased susceptibility to viral infection
Increased airway inflammation
Reflex bronchoconstriction
Increased responsiveness to allergen challenge
Increased allergen sensitization
Increased responsiveness to other pollutants
Increased nonspecific airway responsiveness
Epithelial injury

relatively rare, accounting for about 3–5% of respiratory deaths (30); therefore, the association of particle exposure with mortality cannot be explained by increases in asthma deaths alone.

Nevertheless, considerable evidence suggests that particulate pollution contributes to exacerbations of asthma. Atmospheric particle levels have been linked with worsening of symptoms, decrements in lung function, increased hospital admissions for asthma, and increased medication use (31–33). Recent clinical studies demonstrate that exposure to ozone increases airway inflammation in patients with mild asthma (34,35). Whether exposure to ambient particles also exacerbates airway inflammation in asthma has not been demonstrated. However, two recent studies suggest that exposure to acid aerosols either followed by (36), or in combination with (37), ozone exposure may increase airway responsiveness to ozone in subjects with asthma, at concentrations of acid aerosol well below those known to cause changes in lung function or airway inflammation in the absence of ozone (38).

Given the central role of inflammation in the cause and persistence of asthma, it is plausible that enhancement of airway inflammation is a mechanism by which particle exposure may worsen asthma. More specifically, it will be important to determine whether atmospheric pollutant exposure further shifts the cellular inflammatory response in the airways to favor a Th2 lymphocyte response, with an increase in susceptibility to allergic sensitization or responsiveness. Recent studies in humans (39) and in animal models of allergy (40) suggest that exposure to relatively low concentrations of nitrogen dioxide increases responsiveness to allergen exposure. Other possible mechanisms include direct injury to epithelial cells, increases in reflex bronchoconstriction, or increased nonspecific airway responsiveness.

C. Pneumonia

Atmospheric particle concentrations have been linked with hospital admissions for pneumonia among the elderly (41). Pneumonia is a common complication of COPD, and it is often the precipitating terminal event. An increase in the incidence of pneumonia would thus be consistent with adverse effects on patients with COPD or other chronic respiratory diseases. All of the host defense factors listed in the foregoing for COPD could be important in particle effects on the risk of developing pneumonia: interference with host defense mechanisms would be expected to increase this common cause of respiratory morbidity and mortality. Data are lacking that would allow assessment of particle effects on defense against specific pathogens important in humans, such as *Streptococcus pneumoniae*.

D. Cardiovascular Disease

An increase in deaths caused by ischemic heart disease has been repeatedly linked with particulate air pollution (6,42). Among the possible explanations are the following: (1) respiratory deaths can be misclassified as cardiac deaths; (2) respiratory and cardiac disease often coexist, and respiratory exacerbations may precipitate cardiac events; and (3) pollutant exposure may initiate events with direct cardiac consequences. Recent preliminary studies in healthy and compromised animals from the laboratories of the U.S. Environmental Protection Agency (43) and from Harvard (44) have suggested that inhalation of particulate pollutants may induce changes in cardiac rhythm or repolarization. Cigarette smoking is associated with a reversible decrease in heart rate variability in otherwise healthy subjects (45). Depressed heart rate variability seems to represent a subclinical form of cardiac involvement in respiratory disease, and may prove to be a sensitive indicator of cardiac–pulmonary interactions following pollutant exposure.

Sudden, unexpected death is usually classified as cardiac in etiology, assumed to be due to ischemic heart disease or an arrhythmia. Death from asphyxia caused by acute bronchospasm could be erroneously classified as a cardiac cause of death. In addition, exacerbations of COPD can precipitate cardiac arrhythmias or myocardial infarction in patients with significant underlying heart disease (6,42). Severe COPD is often complicated by cor pulmonale, or chronic failure of the right ventricle caused by pulmonary hypertension and hypoxemia. Deaths caused by cor pulmonale may be misclassified as primary cardiac deaths, although the precipitating event may be a pulmonary insult.

There is little evidence to suggest that exposure to particulate air pollution has direct cardiac effects, either in healthy or compromised individuals. However, there is growing evidence indicating that inflammatory processes are important contributors in the development of atherosclerosis and coronary artery occlusion (46). A recent study found plasma concentrations of C-reactive protein to be a risk factor for the subsequent development of myocardial infarction (47). C-reactive protein is one of the ''acute-phase reactants'' recognized as a systemic marker of the response to inflammation. Moreover, these same blood samples showed that levels of soluble intercellular adhesion molecule-1 (ICAM-1) were predictive of cardiac events (48), providing evidence that endothelial activation is associated with cardiovascular risk. Acute inflammatory responses can be accompanied by increases in plasma viscosity and blood coagulation factors, such as fibrinogen, factor VII, and plasminogen activator inhibitor (49). If exposure to particulate air pollution contributes to a systemic acute-phase response, with accompanying increases in blood coagulability or viscosity, the risk of coronary artery occlusion may be increased in individuals with critical coronary lesions.

Particle exposure may affect cardiovascular health by other indirect mechanisms. For example, the obstructive sleep apnea syndrome (OSAS) is a very common condition, with well-known adverse cardiovascular effects. It occurs in persons whose body habitus is characterized by a narrow posterior pharyngeal airway; the relaxation of upper airway musculature during the rapid eye movement phase of sleep leads to upper airway obstruction, apnea, hypoxemia, and subsequent arousal. The hypoxemic episodes are often associated with changes in cardiac rate and rhythm, and sufferers are at increased risk for adverse cardiac events, and for the development of pulmonary hypertension and cor pulmonale. The disease worsens with upper respiratory infections, periods of nasal obstruction, and during the postoperative period. Exposure to particulate air pollution could either worsen upper airway obstruction through nasal or pharyngeal irritation, or enhance the severity of hypoxemic episodes by increasing ventilation–perfusion mismatching (42). Obstructive sleep apnea is extremely common, with prevalence estimates ranging between 1% in Israeli industrial workers and 42% in an elderly nursing home population (50), and it often goes unrecognized. Many deaths from this disorder may be misclassified as cardiac deaths, and a small pollutant-related effect could potentially affect large numbers of susceptible individuals.

E. Aging

The increases in mortality associated with particulate air pollution are greatest among the elderly. The prevalence of COPD and other chronic respiratory diseases increases with age. However, many physiological changes associated with aging may increase susceptibility to particle effects. Virtually all components of the respiratory system are affected by aging (51), including spirometry, diffusing capacity for oxygen, lung elastic recoil, chest wall compliance, and inspiratory muscle strength. In addition, maximal oxygen uptake and maximal cardiac output decline with age. The elderly are more susceptible to respiratory infections, partly because of age-related declines in specific immune responsiveness.

The elderly may be more susceptible to particle exposure because of a lifetime of exposure to environmental agents, including particulate air pollution, as well as previous respiratory infections. In one study, healthy elderly (65–78 years), nonsmoking volunteers had increased neutrophils, immunoglobulin content, and IL-6 levels in bronchoalveolar lavage fluid when compared with 20- to 36-year-old subjects (51). Thus even in the healthy elderly, years of exposure to external challenges may induce airway inflammation and, thereby, increase susceptibility to a subsequent challenge.

F. Synthesis

Figure 1 presents a mechanistic schema linking particle exposure with both respiratory and cardiovascular effects. It must be recognized that there is currently

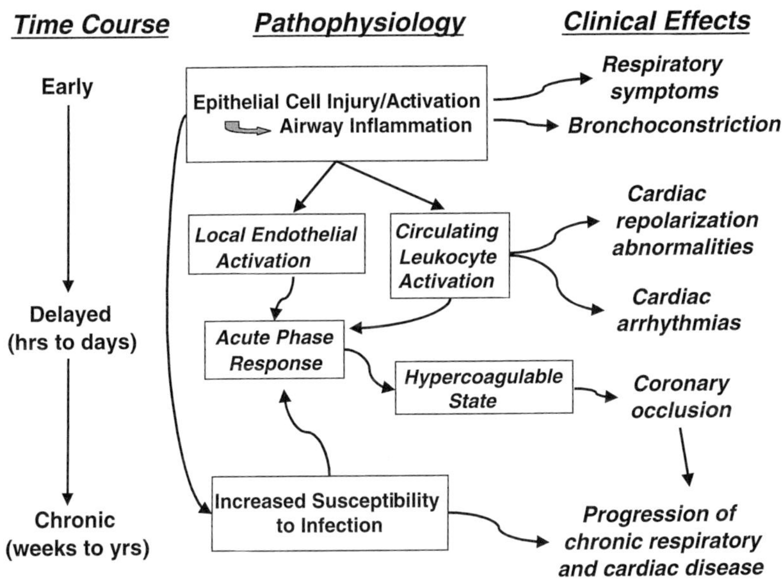

Figure 1 Conceptual model linking exposure to ambient air pollution particles with respiratory and cardiovascular health effects.

very little direct evidence in support of this conceptual model. However, the interaction between epithelium, endothelium, and marginating leukocytes during the inflammatory response has been elucidated in some detail (52), and it is now recognized that vascular inflammatory processes play a role in the progression of coronary artery disease (53). Recent epidemiological studies have suggested that variations in ambient air pollution levels are associated with subtle changes in heart rate (54) and blood viscosity (55). Experimental studies are needed to test this and other hypotheses explaining the association between low-level particle exposure and health effects.

IV. Lessons from Experimental Exposure Studies

In remarkable contrast to the observed association between ambient level particle exposure and mortality, animal exposure studies have often shown minimal or no effects at exposure levels manyfold higher than ambient. Human exposure studies, although few, have also not shown evidence of adverse effects from particle exposure. For example, healthy human volunteers have been exposed to sulfuric acid aerosols at concentrations of 1000 $\mu g/m^3$ or higher for several hours, with no clinical respiratory effects (38,56). Anderson et al. (57) exposed healthy and asthmatic volunteers to 0.5-μm–carbon particles, with and without a coating of sulfuric acid, at a relatively high concentration of 250 μg/m^3 for 1 hr, and found no significant effects on symptoms, pulmonary function, or airways responsiveness. Although several studies have demonstrated that persons with asthma are more sensitive than healthy subjects for bronchoconstriction following exposure to acid aerosols, concentrations an order of magnitude higher than ambient have generally been required to demonstrate effects, even in this sensitive population (56).

This apparent discrepancy between experimental exposures and epidemiological findings has been attributed variously to the following: (1) epidemiological findings may reflect an association, but not a cause–effect relation; (2) the wrong particles may have been studied; (3) studies have not included the appropriate animal model of human disease, or the most susceptible human population; (4) studies have primarily focused on respiratory endpoints and may have overlooked systemic or cardiac effects; and (5) effects represent an interaction among the ''mix'' of particles, gases, organic materials, and chemical species in ambient air.

Recent and ongoing experimental approaches are attempting to address these possibilities. A single experimental approach is unlikely to answer the important questions, and a multidisciplinary approach is necessary, including in vitro and in vivo studies. In both animal and human exposure studies, model particles designed to reproduce important characteristics of size and chemical composition of the ambient aerosol are being employed. For example, particles in the ultrafine-size range (smaller than about 50 nm) appear to have the capability to avoid alveolar macrophage clearance mechanisms, and to penetrate the respiratory epithelium more readily than larger particles (58). These extremely small particles, therefore, may have a greater propensity to induce endothelial or systemic effects following exposure. The technology has been developed to concentrate the fine-particle fraction of outdoor air for use in experimental exposures of both humans and animals (59), providing a novel way to assess the potential toxicity of an ambient particle mixture. Detailed assessment of systemic and cardiovascular endpoints, including a variety of markers of cardiovascular disease, are being incorporated in clinical exposure studies. Finally, animal models of human disease, genetically engineered mouse models, and human populations with increased susceptibility are being incorporated to determine the nature and mechanisms of increased susceptibility.

V. Summary

Exposure to particles in the air is associated with increased mortality in the elderly with chronic lung or heart disease. The mortality data are coherent with data on hospitalization for COPD, pneumonia, asthma, and heart disease, and suggest that a sizable pool of chronically ill individuals are susceptible to the acute effects of exposure to particles in the air. In addition, the course of their chronic illness may be accelerated by prolonged exposure to particles, although data supporting this hypothesis are limited.

The experimental database has yet to provide insights into the mechanisms by which exposure to very low levels of particles exacerbate both respiratory and cardiac disease. We and others have speculated on the mechanisms and relations that could be involved, and tools are being developed to test these hypotheses in field studies, animal exposure studies, and human clinical studies.

References

1. Environmental Protection Agency. Executive Summary. In: Particulate Matter Research Needs for Human Health Risk Assessment to Support Future Reviews of the National Ambient Air Quality Standards for Particulate Matter. Research Triangle Park, NC: National Center for Environmental Assessment, 1998.
2. Speizer FE, Fay ME, Dockery DW, Ferris BG Jr. Chronic obstructive pulmonary disease mortality in six U.S. cities. Am Rev Respir Dis 1989; 140:S49–S55.
3. Dockery DW, Cunningham J, Damokosh AI, Neas LM, Spengler JD, Koutrakis P, Ware JH, Raizenne M, Speizer FE. Health effects of acid aerosols on North American children: respiratory symptoms. Environ Health Perspect 1996; 104:500–505.
4. Dockery DW, Pope CA III, Xu X, Spengler JD, Ware JH, Fay ME, Ferris BG Jr, Speizer FE. An association between air pollution and mortality in six U.S. cities. N Engl J Med 1993; 329:1753–1759.
5. Pope CA III, Thun MJ, Namboodiri MM, Dockery DW, Evans JS, Speizer FE, Health CW Jr. Particulate air pollution as a predictor of mortality in a prospective study of U.S. adults. Am J Respir Crit Care Med 1995; 151:669–674.
6. Bates DV. Health indices of the adverse effects of air pollution: the question of coherence. Environ Res 1992; 59:336–349.
7. Zeger SL, Liang KY. Longitudinal data analysis for discrete and continuous outcomes. Biometrics 1986; 42:121–130.
8. Schwartz J, Wypij D, Dockery DW, Ware J, Zeger S, Spengler JD, Ferris BG Jr. Daily diaries of respiratory symptoms and air pollution: methodological issues and results. Environ Health Perspect 1991; 90:181–187.
9. Dockery DW, Pope CA III. Acute respiratory effects of particulate air pollution. Annu Rev Public Health 1994; 15:107–132.
10. Bascom R, Bromberg PA, Costa DA, Devlin R, Dockery DW, Frampton MW, Lambert W, Samet JM, Speizer FE, Utell MJ. State of the art review: health effects of outdoor air pollution. Part 1. Am J Respir Crit Care Med 1996; 153:3–50.
11. Bascom R, Bromberg PA, Costa DL, Devlin R, Dockery DW, Frampton MW, Lambert W, Samet JM, Speizer FE, Utell M. Health effects of outdoor air pollution. Part 2. Am J Respir Crit Care Med 1996; 153:477–498.
12. U.S. Environmental Protection Agency (EPA), Office of Air Quality Planning and

Standards. Review of the National Ambient Air Quality Standards for particulate matter: policy assessment of scientific and technical information. OAQPS Staff paper. Research Triangle Park, NC: U.S. Government Printing Office, 1996:EPA-452\R-96-013.
13. Dockery D, Pope A. Epidemiology of acute health effects: summary of time-series studies. In: Wilson R, Spengler J, eds. Particles in Our Air: Concentrations and Health Effects. Cambridge: Harvard School of Public Health, 1996:123–147.
14. Pope A, Dockery D. Epidemiology of chronic health effects: cross-sectional studies. In: Wilson R, Spengler J, eds. Particles in Our Air: Concentrations and Health Effects. Cambridge: Harvard School of Public Health, 1996:149–168.
15. Spengler JD, Dockery DW, Turner WA, Wolfson JM, Ferris BG Jr. Long-term measurements of respirable sulfates and particles inside and outside homes. Atmos Environ 1981; 15:23–30.
16. Samet JM, Zeger SL, Kelsall JE, Xu J, Kalkstein LS. Air pollution, weather, and mortality in Philadelphia 1973–1988. In: Particulate Air Pollution and Daily Mortality: Analyses of the Effects of Weather and Multiple Pollutants. Cambridge, MA: Health Effects Institute Research Report, 1997.
17. Schwartz J. Air pollution and daily mortality: a review and meta-analysis. Environ Res 1994; 64:36–52.
18. Spix C, Heinrich J, Dockery D, Schwartz J, Volksch G, Schwinkowski K, Collen C, Wichmann HE. Air pollution and daily mortality in Erfurt, East Germany, 1980–1989. Environ Health Perspect 1993; 101:518–526.
19. Monto AS, Ross HW. The Tecumseh study of respiratory illness. X. Relation of acute infections to smoking, lung function and chronic symptoms. Am J Epidemiol 1978; 107:57–64.
20. Glezen WP, Decker M, Perrotta DM. Survey of underlying conditions of persons hospitalized with acute respiratory disease during influenza epidemics in Houston, 1978–1981. Am Rev Respir Dis 1987; 136:550–555.
21. Brimblecombe P. The Big Smoke: A History of Air Pollution in London Since Medieval Times. London: Methuen, 1987.
22. U.S. Department of Health and Human Services (USDHHS). Guidelines for the diagnosis and management of asthma. National Asthma Education Program Expert Panel Report. Bethesda, MD: U.S. Government Printing Office, 1991: Publ. No.-91-3042.
23. American Lung Association. ''Breath in Danger II.'' Estimation of Populations-at-Risk of Adverse Health Consequences in Areas Not in Attainment with National Ambient Air Quality Standards of the Clean Air Act. Washington, DC: American Lung Association, 1993.
24. Weinberger SE. Medical progress: recent advances in pulmonary medicine. N Engl J Med 1993; 328:1389–1397.
25. Foster WM, Silver JA, Groth ML. Exposure to ozone alters regional function and particle dosimetry in the human lung. J Appl Physiol 1993; 75:1938–1945.
26. Frampton MW. Asthma, lymphocytes, and dendritic cells. Chest 1993; 103:986–987.
27. Hall WJ, Douglas RG, Hyde RW, Roth FK, Cross AS, Speers DM. Pulmonary mechanics after uncomplicated influenza A infection. Am Rev Respir Dis 1976; 113:141–147.

28. Utell MJ, Aquilina AT, Hall WJ, Speers DM, Douglas RG, Gibb FR, Morrow PE, Hyde RW. Development of airway reactivity to nitrates in subjects with influenza. Am Rev Respir Dis 1980; 121:233–241.
29. von Mutius E, Fritzsch C, Weiland SK, Roll G, Magnussen H. Prevalence of asthma and allergic disorders among children in united Germany: a descriptive comparison. Br Med J 1992; 305:1395–1399.
30. U.S. Bureau of the Census. Statistical Abstract of the United States: 1992. 112th ed. Washington, DC: Author, 1992.
31. Thurston GD, Lippmann M, Scott MB, Fine JB. Summertime haze air pollution and children with asthma. Am J Respir Crit Care Med 1997; 155:654–660.
32. Pope CA 3d, Dockery DW, Spengler JD, Raizenne ME. Respiratory health and PM_{10} pollution. Am Rev Respir Dis 1991; 144:668–674.
33. Dusseldorp A, Kruize H, Brunekreef B, Hofshreuder P, de Meer G, van Oudvorst AB. Associations of PM_{10} and airborne iron with respiratory health of adults living near a steel factory. Am J Respir Crit Care Med 1995; 152:1932–1939.
34. Basha MA, Gross KB, Gwizdala CJ, Haidar AH, Popovich J Jr. Bronchoalveolar lavage neutrophilia in asthmatic and healthy volunteers after controlled exposure to ozone and filtered purified air. Chest 1994; 106:1757–1765.
35. Scannell C, Chen L, Aris RM, Tager I, Christian D, Ferrando R, Welch B, Kelly T, Balmes JR. Greater ozone-induced inflammatory responses in subjects with asthma. Am J Respir Cell Mol Biol 1996; 154:24–29.
36. Frampton MW, Morrow PE, Cox C, Levy PC, Condemi JJ, Speers D, Gibb FR, Utell MJ. Sulfuric acid aerosol followed by ozone exposure in healthy and asthmatic subjects. Environ Res 1995; 69:1–14.
37. Linn WS, Anderson KR, Shamoo DA, Edwards SA, Webb TL, Hackney JD, Gong H Jr. Controlled exposures of young asthmatics to mixed oxidant gases and acid aerosol. Am J Respir Crit Care Med 1995; 152:885–891.
38. Frampton MW, Voter KZ, Morrow PE, Roberts NJ Jr, Culp DJ, Cox C, Utell MJ. Effects of H_2SO_4 aerosol exposure in humans assessed by bronchoalveolar lavage. Am Rev Respir Dis 1992; 146:626–632.
39. Devalia JL, Rusznak C, Wang J, Khair OA, Abdelaziz MM, Calderon MA, Davies RJ. Air pollutants and respiratory hypersensitivity. Toxicol Lett 1996; 86:169–176.
40. Gilmour MI. Interaction of air pollutants and pulmonary allergic responses in experimental animals. Toxicology 1995; 105:335–342.
41. Schwartz J. Air pollution and hospital admissions for the elderly in Detroit, Michigan. Am J Respir Crit Care Med 1994; 150:648–655.
42. Utell MJ, Frampton MW. Particles and mortality: a clinical perspective. Inhal Toxicol 1995; 7:645–655.
43. Watkinson WP, Campen MJ, Costa DL. Cardiac arrhythmia induction after exposure to residual oil fly ash particles in a rodent model of pulmonary hypertension. Toxicol Sci 1998; 41:209–216.
44. Godleski JJ, Sioutas C, Verrier RL, Killingsworth CR, Lovett E, Murthy GGK, Hatch V, Wolfson JM, Ferguson ST, Koutrakis P. Inhalation exposure of canines to concentrated ambient air particles [abstr]. Am J Respir Crit Care Med 1997; 155:A246.
45. Stein PK, Rottman JN, Kleiger R. Effect of 21 mg transdermal nicotine patches and smoking cessation on heart rate variability. Am J Cardiol 1996; 77:701–705.

46. McLaughlin MA, Fuster V. The three mechanisms for coronary artery disease progression: insights into future management. Mt Sinai J Med 1995; 62:265–274.
47. Ridker PM, Cushman M, Stampfer MJ, Tracy RP, Hennekens CH. Inflammation, aspirin, and the risk of cardiovascular disease in apparently healthy men. N Engl J Med 1997; 336:973–979.
48. Ridker PM, Hennekens CH, Roitman-Johnson B, Stampfer MJ, Allen J. Plasma concentration of soluble intercellular adhesion molecule 1 and risks of future myocardial infarction in apparently healthy men. Lancet 1998; 351:88–92.
49. Seaton A, MacNee W, Donaldson K, Godden D. Particulate air pollution and acute health effects. Lancet 1995; 345:176–178.
50. Redline S, Young T. Epidemiology and natural history of obstructive sleep apnea. Ear Nose Throat J 1993; 72:20-1–24-26.
51. Meyer KC, Ershler W, Rosenthal NS, Lu X-G, Peterson K. Immune dysregulation in the aging human lung. Am J Respir Crit Care Med 1996; 153:1072–1079.
52. Lukacs NW, Strieter RM, Kunkel SL. Leukocyte infiltration in allergic airway inflammation. Am J Respir Cell Mol Biol 1995; 13:1–6.
53. Maseri A. Inflammation, atheroscerosis, and ischemic events—exploring the hidden side of the moon. N Engl J Med 1997; 336:1014–1016.
54. Peters A, Perz S, Doring A, Stieber J, Wichmann HE. Increased heart rate during an air pollution episode. Am J Respir Crit Care Med 1998; 157:A880.
55. Peters A, Doring A, Wichmann HE, Koenig W. Increased plasma viscosity during an air pollution episode: a link to mortality? Lancet 1997; 349:1582–1587.
56. Utell MJ, Frampton MW. Sulfur dioxide and sulfuric acid aerosols. In: Rom WM, ed. Environmental and Occupational Medicine. 3rd ed. Philadelphia: Lippincott–Raven, 1998:627–635.
57. Anderson KR, Avol EL, Edwards SA, Shamoo DA, Peng R-C, Linn WS, Hackney JD. Controlled exposures of volunteers to respirable carbon and sulfuric acid aerosols. J Air Waste Manage Assoc 1992; 42:770–776.
58. Stearns RC, Murthy GGK, Skornik W, Hatch V, Katler M, Godleski JJ. Detection of ultrafine copper oxide particles in the lungs of hamsters by electron spectroscopic imaging. ICEM 13-Paris 1994; July 17–22:763–764.
59. Sioutas C, Koutrakis P, Burton RM. A technique to expose animals to concentrated fine ambient aerosols. Environ Health Perspect 1995; 103:172–177.

19

Effects of Particulate Air Pollution Exposures

DOUGLAS W. DOCKERY

Harvard School of Public Health
Boston, Massachusetts

C. ARDEN POPE III

Brigham Young University
Provo, Utah

FRANK E. SPEIZER

Harvard Medical School and
Brigham and Women's Hospital
Boston, Massachusetts

I. Introduction

In the past decade, an abundance of epidemiological studies have reported adverse health effects associated with environmental exposure to airborne particulate matter at the relatively low concentrations found currently in the United States and other developed countries. Toxicological and clinical studies have not reported adverse health effects from controlled exposures to models of particulate matter except at extremely high concentrations (see Chap. 18). The estimated risks associated with particulate matter at concentrations observed in most developed countries are small; that is, excess relative risks of 20% or less. The ability of epidemiology to detect relative risks of this magnitude has been questioned (1). Moreover, the lack of supporting toxicological and clinical evidence has raised questions about the validity and generalizability of these epidemiological findings (2). Nevertheless, these findings have been robust and consistent across many settings, and have stimulated a revision of the ambient air quality standards for particulate matter in the United States (3).

II. Characteristics of Particulate Air Pollution

Particulate air pollution is a mixture of solid, liquid, or solid and liquid particles suspended in the air (see Chap. 2). These suspended particles vary in size, composition, and origin. The largest particles, called the *coarse fraction* (or *mode*), are mechanically produced by breaking up larger solid particles (4). The amount of energy required to break these particles into smaller sizes increases as the size decreases, which effectively establishes a lower limit for the production of these coarse particles of approximately 1 μm.

Smaller particles, called the *fine fraction* or *mode*, are largely formed from gases. The smallest particles, less than 0.1 μm, are formed by nucleation; that is, condensation of low-vapor–pressure substances formed by high-temperature vaporization or by chemical reactions in the atmosphere to form new particles (nuclei). Particles in this *nucleation range* or *mode* grow by coagulation—that is, the combination of two or more particles to form a larger particle; or by condensation—that is, condensation of gas or vapor molecules onto the surface of existing particles. Some gases produced in combustion are subsequently converted in atmospheric reactions to low-vapor–pressure substances. For example, sulfur dioxide (SO_2) is oxidized in the atmosphere to form sulfuric acid (H_2SO_4). Nitrogen dioxide (NO_2) is oxidized to nitric acid (HNO_3) which, in turn, reacts with ammonia (NH_3) to form ammonium nitrate (NH_4NO_3). The particles produced by intermediate reactions of gases in the atmosphere are called *secondary particles*. Secondary sulfate and nitrate particles are the dominant component of fine particles in the United States.

Aerodynamic particle size is the most important characteristic influencing deposition in the respiratory system (see Chap. 5). Particles larger than 10-μm–aerodynamic diameter are largely deposited in the nose and mouth and do not penetrate into the lungs. Particles smaller than 1-μm–aerodynamic diameter are more likely to penetrate deeply into the lungs and deposit in the smaller conducting airways and the gas-exchange regions of the lung. Thus, the submicron particles produced by combustion processes are also those particles most likely to be deposited in the lower airways and alveoli of the lungs.

In 1987, the U.S. Environmental Protection Agency (EPA) redefined the National Ambient Air Quality Standard (NAAQS) for particles based on the mass concentration of particles smaller than 10-μm–aerodynamic diameter (PM_{10}; 5). This 10-μm cutoff focused monitoring and regulatory efforts on particles of a size that would be deposited in, and damaging to the conducting airways and the gas-exchange areas of the respiratory system during mouth breathing (6). Thoracic particles, the basis for occupational particle standards, have a 50% cutpoint at 10 μm, although they have a less sharp size cut (7).

Largely because of health concerns associated with fine particles, the EPA has defined a new standard for particles less than 2.5-μm–aerodynamic diameter ($PM_{2.5}$; 3). This will result in control strategies being focused on combustion-related particles. The occupational definition of respirable particle specifies a 50% cut at 4 μm (6).

III. Epidemiological Evidence of Health Effects

The hazard of episodes of high air pollution was recognized in the first half of this century, when episodes of extreme air pollution were associated with increased deaths and morbidity in the Meuse Valley, Belgium, in 1934 (8) and in Donora, Pennsylvania, in 1947 (9). However, it was the air pollution episodes of December 1952 in London that provided the first quantitative air pollution exposure data and the most convincing evidence of the hazard.

On Thursday, December 4, 1952, a slow-moving anticyclone came to a halt over the city of London (10). Fog developed over the city, and particulate and sulfur pollution began accumulating in the stagnating air mass. Smoke and sulfur dioxide concentrations built up over the following 3 days. On Monday, the polluted fog began to ease, and by Tuesday conditions were back to normal. Mortality records showed that deaths increased in a pattern very similar to that of the pollution measurements (Fig. 1). It was estimated that 4000 extra deaths were attributable to this pollution episode (11).

Although the London 1952 episode identified the hazard of extreme air pollution episodes, it did not identify the specific agent within the mix of pollutants that was responsible for the observed health effects, nor did it establish whether similar effects could be seen at lower concentrations.

By the 1970s, a link had been well established between respiratory disease and particulate or sulfur oxide air pollution, but there remained disagreement on the level of pollution that would significantly affect human health. In reviewing research published between 1968 and 1977, Holland and several other prominent British scientists (12) concluded that particulate and related air pollution at high levels posed a hazard to human health, but that health effects of particulate pollution at lower concentrations could not be "disentangled" from health effects of other factors. Other reviewers (13–16) concluded that the epidemiological evidence showed that human health may be adversely affected by particulate pollution even at relatively low concentrations.

Recent epidemiological studies have convincingly shown adverse health effects with particulate pollution at levels common in urban areas of the developed world. More specific and precise measures of both pollution exposures and health endpoints, plus advances in analytical techniques have permitted the evaluation of pollution associations that would not have been possible in the 1970s.

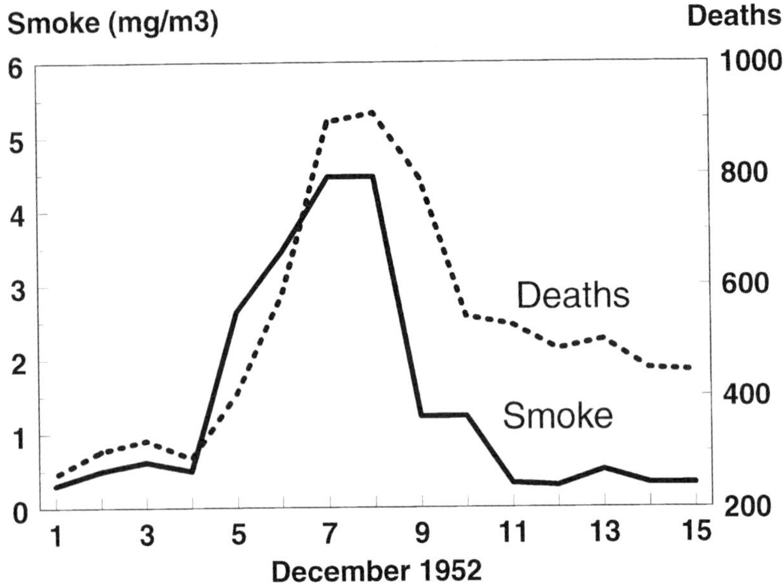

Figure 1 Daily mean pollution concentrations and daily number of deaths during the London fog episode of 1952.

A. Mortality Associated with Short-Term Exposures

Recent epidemiological studies have highlighted the association of particulate air pollution with increased daily mortality in a score of communities around the world. In 1990, Schwartz and Marcus (17) published a reanalysis of daily mortality counts and daily British Smoke (an estimate of particle mass determined from blackness of sample) and SO_2 measurements for the winters of 1959–1972 in London. This time series was originally compiled by MacFarlane (18) and had been analyzed by several investigators (19,20). After sorting the data by particle concentrations, as estimated by British Smoke, and averaging each 20 consecutive observations, Schwartz and Marcus showed a striking nonlinear association between daily mortality and particulate air pollution (Fig. 2). These analyses indicate that mortality increased with increasing smoke concentrations down to the lowest measured concentrations. Positive, statistically significant associations remained after adjustment for possible confounding by temperature and season in multiple regression. In addition, multiple regression analyses showed that the estimated association with particulates was stable after adjustment for SO_2, whereas the estimated association with SO_2 was substantially reduced after adjustment for the smoke measurements. This suggests that the deserved association

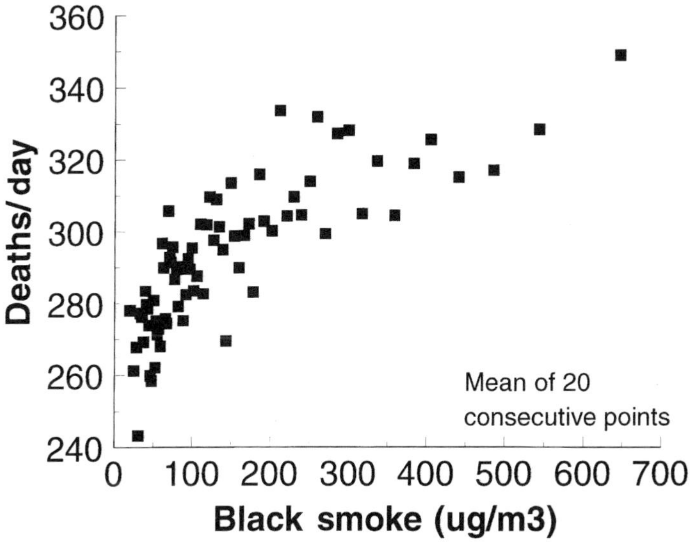

Figure 2 Average daily mortality in Greater London for period April 1, 1965 through December 31, 1972 versus British Smoke ($\mu g/m^3$). Each point represents average of 20 days sorted by smoke. (From Ref. 17.)

with SO_2 was due to particulate air pollution, rather than SO_2 itself. That is, the observed SO_2 association was due to confounding by particulate air pollution.

Analyses of the association of daily mortality in two cities in the United States—Steubenville, Ohio (21), and Philadelphia, Pennsylvania (22), confirmed the London findings based on daily measurements of particles (measured as total suspended particulates; TSP) and of SO_2. Both of these analyses suggested that daily mortality was associated with the much lower particle concentrations observed currently in the United States and other developed countries, even after adjustment for SO_2 exposures.

In addition to the analyses of Philadelphia and Steubenville, increased daily mortality has been reported to be associated with total suspended particulate air pollution concentrations in Detroit, Michigan (23), Cincinnati, Ohio (24), Erfurt, Germany (25), and Beijing, China (26). Positive associations with British Smoke measures of particles have been reported in Athens, Greece (27) and Amsterdam, the Netherlands (28). However, the lack of specific upper size cut for these particulate exposure measures and the site-specific character of the particle size distribution makes it difficult to compare associations across studies. Eight studies (Fig. 3) have reported associations between daily mortality and PM_{10} in Birmingham, Alabama (29); Chicago, Illinois (30); Los Angeles, California (31);

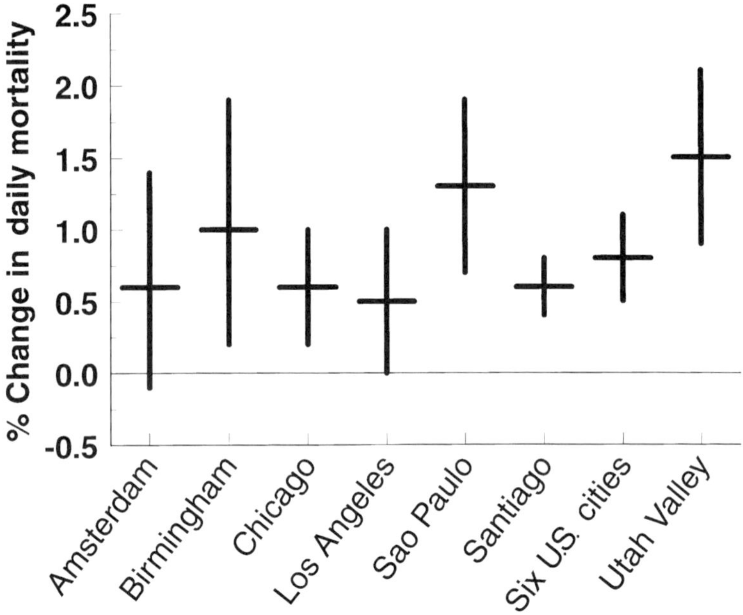

Figure 3 Estimated percentage increase in daily mortality (95% confidence interval) associated with each 10-µg/m^3 increase in PM_{10} concentration in studies specifically assessing effects of PM_{10}.

Utah Valley, Utah (32); six other U.S. cities (33); Amsterdam, the Netherlands (28); Sao Paulo, Brazil (34); and Santiago, Chile (35).

There is good consistency in the estimated effect of PM_{10} across these studies. Effect estimates range between 0.5 and 1.6% increase in daily mortality for each 10-µg/m^3 increase in PM_{10} concentration. A weighted mean of the study-specific effect estimates, with inverse variance weights (36) gives a combined effect estimate for these studies of 0.7% (95% CI; 0.6–0.9%) increase in daily mortality for each 10-µg/m^3 increase in PM_{10}.

Confounding by Time-Varying Covariates

Epidemiological studies suffer from the weakness that observed associations with a specific exposure may result from an unmeasured association with an unknown or uncontrolled factor correlated with *both* exposure and disease; that is, from a confounder. Time–series studies have the advantage that many major causes of increased mortality (such as smoking, hypertension, or even age) cannot confound the observed associations with particulate air pollution because these factors do not vary with daily pollution exposures. This is not to say that response may not differ by these factors. Indeed, the mortality effects of particulate air pollution are most strongly seen in the elderly (21,22,37,38), which indicates that age is an effect modifier. Unfortunately, data on smoking or preexisting chronic diseases are not available in the data sets of daily deaths used in these analyses, so the potential for stronger (or weaker) effect estimates among smoking or chronically debilitated subjects has not been evaluated.

Other time-varying factors, such as season and weather conditions and changes in base population, are potential confounders in these analyses. Indeed weather and seasonal factors are consistently strong predictors of daily mortality. Thus, it is important to control for these time-varying factors in the analysis.

How sensitive are the observed associations to confounding by season and weather? Although confounding is a potentially important issue in these studies, comparisons of effect estimates with and without control of weather have not shown these factors to be important confounders of the particulate air pollution associations once season effects are controlled. This is not to suggest that weather is not an important predictor of mortality, but rather, that it does not confound the particulate air pollution associations. The reason for this apparent inconsistency may be that the weather characteristics that are most strongly associated with mortality, such as temperature, are only weakly associated with particulate air pollution exposures. On the other hand, those weather factors most strongly associated with particulate air pollution, such as wind speed, are only weakly associated with daily mortality. Thus, although both air pollution and daily mortality are strongly associated with weather factors, the specific weather factors associated with each are different and largely independent.

Confounding by Other Pollutants

A more serious issue is control of confounding by copollutants. If the hypothesis is that particulate air pollution is associated with daily mortality, then correlated copollutants would act as confounders if they were themselves causally associated with mortality. Possible confounding by various copollutants has been considered in many of the previously cited studies. Other pollutants are included in the regression models to produce estimates of the effect of particulate matter adjusted for these copollutants. Ostro et al. (35) reported a lack of confounding of the particle–mortality association by SO_2, O_3, and CO in a study in Santiago, Chile, although quantitative comparisons of the effect estimates were not reported. Dockery and Schwartz (39) summarized the results from studies in which the particle–mortality association was evaluated quantitatively in regression analyses for confounding by SO_2, O_3, and CO. In seven published studies that assessed the effects of particles and SO_2 simultaneously, the estimated univariate effect of a 10-$\mu g/m^3$ increase in PM_{10} across all studies was a 0.9% (95% CI;

0.7–1.0%) increase in daily mortality. After adjustment for SO_2, the combined effect estimate for PM_{10} was 0.7% (95% CI; 0.5–0.9%). Similar results were found in four studies that assessed confounding by CO, and three that assessed confounding by O_3. Thus, although there was some reduction in the effect estimates for particles, a positive association was found even after adjustment for each of the copollutants. On the other hand, it is generally found that the estimated effect of the posited confounder (e.g., SO_2, O_3, or CO) is substantially reduced after adjustment for particulate air pollution.

An alternative method for control of confounding by other pollutants is through restriction. If the proposed confounding pollutant is not present or has little variation, it cannot confound the association. Although in most communities particulate air pollution is highly correlated with sulfur oxides and other pollutants, a few communities have provided settings with exposure to particles in the presence of low exposures to other pollutants.

Fairley (40) reported an analysis of daily mortality in Santa Clara Country, California, for the winters of 1980–1982 and 1984–1986. Daily mortality was positively associated with levels of particles measured as Coefficient of Haze, a measure of light transmission through a sample collected on a filter. When expressed in terms of equivalent PM_{10}, the estimated effect was 0.9% (95% CI; 0.2–1.5%) increase in total daily mortality per 10-$\mu g/m^3$ PM_{10} (39). Santa Clara has very limited emissions of SO_2 and, because this analysis was limited to winter, very low O_3 concentrations. Thus, it is unlikely that the observed particle associations were confounded by these pollutants.

A similar case of control of confounding by copollutants was reported in a study in Utah Valley, Utah (32). Utah Valley is approximately 1400 m above sea level and is bordered on the east by the Wasatch Mountains and on the west by the Lake Mountains. Shallow winter temperature inversions trap locally generated particulate air pollution near the valley floor. SO_2, O_3, and NO_2 concentrations are low during these winter inversions, but PM_{10} concentrations are often above the U.S. ambient air quality standard of 150 $\mu g/m^3$ (41). Total mortality increased 1.5% with each 10-$\mu g/m^3$ increase in 5-day mean PM_{10} concentration.

On the other hand, in communities with very high concentrations of O_3, such as Los Angeles (31), or very high SO_2, such as eastern Europe (25), associations with particulate air pollution are still found that are comparable in magnitude with the estimates from other communities. Thus, even though these copollutants may be causally associated with mortality, they do not substantially confound the observed particulate air pollution associations with mortality.

Lagged Associations

Increased mortality is consistently reported to be associated with particle concentrations 1–5 days before death. It would violate a basic assumption of causality if exposures were not concurrent with or preceding the observed effect. The pattern of daily mortality during the 1952 London fog episode showed that mortality peaked after the maximum air pollution exposures and remained high in the weeks after the episode compared with the week before (see Fig. 1). In the analysis of Utah Valley deaths, Pope et al. (32) considered lag structures up to 7 days and found the strongest associations with the 5-day moving average—that is, with the mean PM_{10} of the current day and the 4 previous days.

It is not unreasonable to expect that a brief exposure may lead to death (or other adverse event) of some individuals on 1 day, but that others may linger on before dying the next or even the following day. Thus, the response to a brief exposure could be distributed over several following days. Methods for estimating distributed lag functions have been developed in econometrics, and their application to epidemiological time–series data has been described by Pope and Schwartz (42).

Harvesting

A weakness of time–series studies is that those individuals who die as a result of pollution exposure cannot be identified. The associations of mortality with particle air pollution are stronger in the elderly (21,22,37,38), and deaths are associated with chronic respiratory or cardiovascular problems (43). But it is not clear who is dying. Are they people who would have died within the next couple of days anyway? Is air pollution "harvesting" those who were on the verge of mortality? If so, the few days' loss of life expectancy may not have major public health significance.

If harvesting is occurring, then there should be fewer deaths than expected following an air pollution or other episode that produces excess deaths. Following the London 1952 episode, there was no indication of lower-than-expected mortality following the episode (see Fig. 1). In fact, the observed number of deaths per day in the week following the episode was substantially higher than the number of deaths per day before the episode. Spix et al. (25) looked for a negative correlation between the number of deaths in the preceding period (up to 2 weeks) and deaths associated with air pollution episodes. There was an indication of weak harvesting, but the effect was small compared with the estimated air pollution effect.

If harvesting were operating in the mortality time–series, then each increase in mortality should be balanced by a subsequent decrease in mortality. Thus, the change in the annual mortality rate should be less than expected on the basis of the change in mean particle concentrations. Between August 1, 1986, and September 1, 1987, the major source of particulate air pollution in Utah Valley, a steel mill, was closed by a labor dispute. During the 13 months that the mill was not operating, average particulate air pollution concentrations dropped from 50- to 35-$\mu g/m^3$ PM_{10} (32). Based on the 1.5% increase in mortality for each 10-$\mu g/$

m^3 PM_{10} observed in the valley, a 2.3% reduction in mortality would be expected. There was actually a 3.2% reduction in overall mortality during this period. Moreover, associations between city-specific mortality rates and mean particulate pollution rates have been observed in cross-sectional studies. For example, Pope et al. (44) show that age-, sex-, and race-adjusted mortality rates increased with particle concentrations in 151 communities with sulfate measures in 1980 (Fig. 4). These observed differences in mortality rates suggest that the increased deaths associated with short-term particulate air pollution exposures are not balanced by decreased mortality in the following days.

Particle Characteristics

Schwartz et al. (33) assessed the specific associations of fine ($PM_{2.5}$) versus coarse (between 2.5- and 10-μm) particles with daily mortality in six U.S. cities. Fine particles were consistently associated with total daily mortality in all six

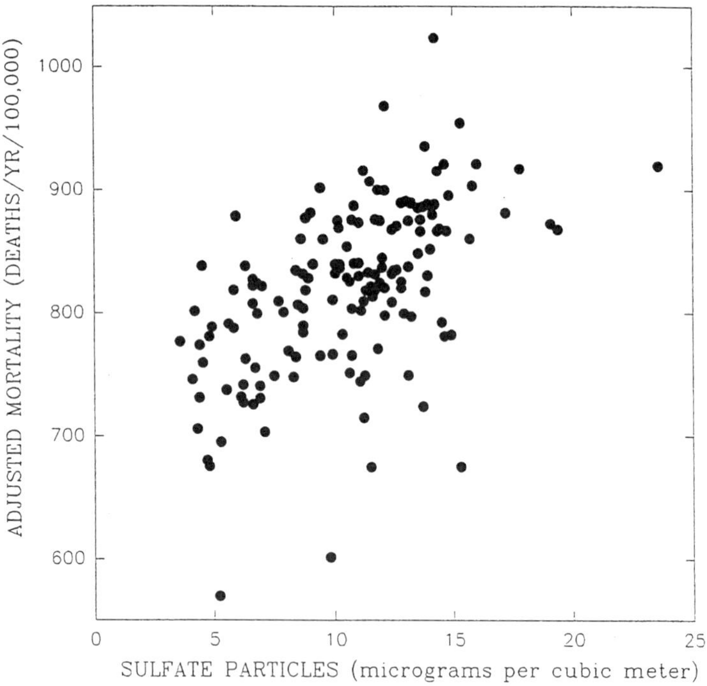

Figure 4 Age-, sex-, and race-adjusted city-specific mortality rates for 1980 plotted against mean concentrations of total sulfate air pollution levels for 1980 for 151 metropolitan areas in the United States. (From Ref. 54.)

cities. Coarse particles were associated with mortality only in the single city, Steubenville, Ohio, where there was a high correlation between fine and coarse particles.

Lippman (45) has suggested that the observed associations may be specifically associated with the acidity of the particulates. Indeed, several analyses have suggested that increased mortality in London in the 1960s was more strongly associated with the acidity of the particles than with the blackness measured as British Smoke (46,47). However, Schwartz et al. (33) failed to find any association between aerosol acidity and mortality in contemporary U.S. data.

B. Cause-Specific Mortality

If total daily mortality is associated with particulate air pollution, then there should be marked differences in the magnitude of this effect by cause of death. Seven mortality studies (21,22,24,29,32,40,48) have provided a breakdown by broad cause-of-death categories (Fig. 5). Cardiovascular deaths accounted for about 45% of all deaths in these studies. Effect estimates for cardiovascular deaths ranged between 0.7 and 1.8% (weighted mean 1.4%; 95% CI; 1.0–1.8%) increase for each 10-μg/m^3 PM_{10}. Respiratory deaths, which were 2–8% of the

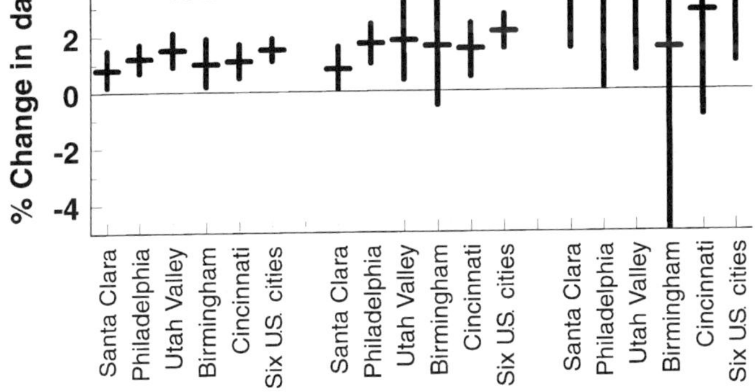

Figure 5 Estimated percentage increase (95% CI) in total, cardiovascular, and respiratory mortality associated with each 10-μg/m^3 increase in estimated PM_{10} concentration in studies specifically assessing cause-specific mortality.

total, had effect estimates between 1.5 and 3.7% (weighted mean 3.5%; 95% CI, 2.0–4.7%) increase for each 10-μg/m^3 PM_{10}. No associations with cancer or with other causes of death were reported in any of these studies. Thus, the strongest associations consistently are observed with respiratory and cardiovascular mortality, although confidence intervals are much wider for these specific causes.

C. Hospital Usage

If daily particulate pollution levels are associated with daily mortality, then associations should also be expected with increased hospital admissions and emergency department visits. In a unique natural experiment, Pope (41,49) observed that hospital admissions of children for respiratory disease in Utah Valley dropped by over 50% during the winter of 1986–1987 compared with adjacent years. During this winter, the strike by workers at the local steel mill led to much lower PM_{10} concentrations—a mean of 51 μg/m^3 and maximum of 113 μg/m^3, compared with a mean of 90 μg/m^3 and a maximum of 365 μg/m^3 in the previous year. Regression analyses estimated a 4.2% decrease in asthma and bronchitis admissions and a 7.1% decrease in all respiratory admissions of children associated with a 10-μg/m^3 decrease in the 2-month mean PM_{10} concentration. No associations were found with all other, (i.e. nonrespiratory) hospital admissions.

Burnett and colleagues (50) reported increased respiratory hospital admissions in southern Ontario for the summers of 1983–1988, associated with increased sulfate concentrations. Sulfate particles make up more than half of the fine particle mass ($PM_{2.5}$) in southern Ontario. These sulfate particle associations were independent of associations with ozone exposures. Thurston and colleagues have reported associations of respiratory hospital admissions with $PM_{2.5}$ concentrations in Toronto, Ontario (51), and sulfate particles in New York City and Buffalo, New York (52).

Hospital admissions for asthma were reported to increase in association with particles in both the Ontario and both New York studies. Schwartz (38) has reported associations between daily PM_{10} concentrations and daily hospital admissions for asthma among the elderly (65+ years) in Detroit, Michigan. These studies indicate that asthma hospital admissions increase by about 1.0% (95% CI, 0.4–1.6%) for each 10-μg/m^3 increase in PM_{10} (Fig. 6). An analysis of asthma emergency department visits in Seattle, Washington (53), found an increase of 3.4% (95% CI, 0.9–6%) associated with each 10-μ/m^3 increase in PM_{10}.

Schwartz estimated the association between daily PM_{10} exposures and hospital admissions for pneumonia among the elderly in Birmingham, Alabama (54), Detroit, Michigan (38), and Minneapolis–St. Paul, Minnesota (55) (see Fig. 6). These studies give a combined estimated increase of 1.4% (95% CI; 0.7–7.0%) in pneumonia admissions for each 10-μg/m^3 increase in PM_{10}. These associations do not imply that particulate air pollution is producing new cases of pneumonia,

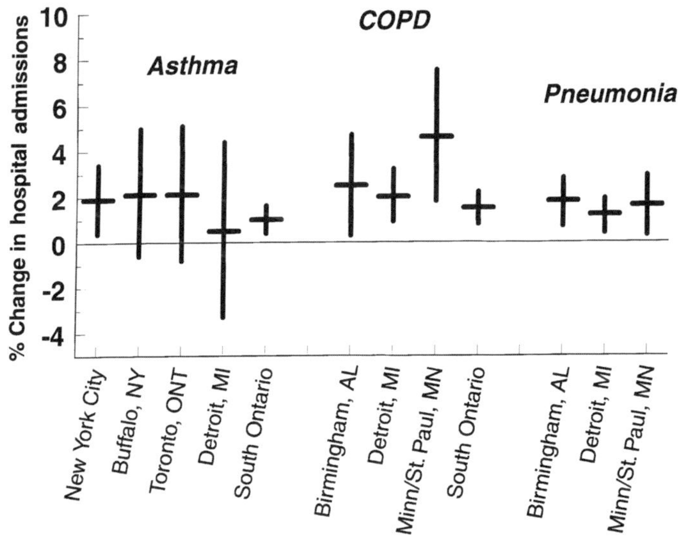

Figure 6 Estimated percentage increase (95% CI) in hospital admissions for asthma, chronic obstructive pulmonary disease (COPD), and pneumonia associated with each 10-$\mu g/m^3$ increase in estimated PM_{10} concentration.

but rather, that particulate pollution is aggravating existing pneumonia cases sufficiently to send patients to the hospital.

Schwartz also reported increased admissions for aggravation of chronic obstructive pulmonary disease (COPD) in these same cities (38,54,55). Burnett et al. (53) found increased hospital admissions for COPD associated with sulfate particles in southern Ontario. These studies suggest an increase of 2.4% (95% CI; 1.5–3.4%) in hospital admissions for COPD associated with each 10-$\mu g/m^3$ increase in PM_{10}. Emergency department visits for COPD were associated with Black Smoke concentrations in Barcelona (56,57). The estimated effect corresponded to a 2.3% (95% CI; 1.4–3.2%) increase in emergency visits for COPD associated with a 10-$\mu g/m^3$ increase in PM_{10} (36).

The evidence of increased cardiovascular mortality suggests that associations should also be observed for cardiovascular hospital admissions. Indeed, Schwartz (58) and Burnett et al. (50) have reported increased cardiovascular admissions associated with increased particle concentrations in Detroit and southern Ontario (Fig. 7). These two analyses suggest a 1.0% (95% CI; 0.5–1.4%) increase in congestive heart failure (ischemia), a 0.6% (95% CI; 0.3–0.9%) increase in coronary artery disease, and a 0.5% (95% CI; −0.1 to +1.1%) increase in dysrythmias, for each 10-$\mu g/m^3$ increase in PM_{10}.

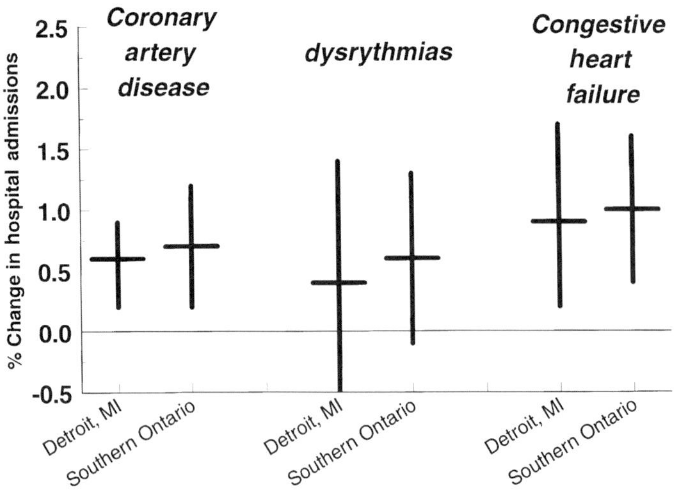

Figure 7 Estimated percentage increase (95% CI) for hospital admissions for cardiovascular disease associated with each 10-μg/m³ increase in estimated PM_{10} concentration.

D. Asthma Attacks

Hospital admission and emergency department visit data suggest that short-term particle exposures may be associated with asthma attacks. To assess the association of air pollution and other time-varying factors with exacerbation of asthma, daily reports have been collected in defined cohorts; that is, panels, of asthmatics.

Winter studies of asthmatic children with chronic respiratory symptoms in the Netherlands (59) and of asthmatic adults in Denver, Colorado (60) both found substantial increases in reported asthmatic attacks associated with particle exposures. Ostro et al. (48) found that children in an asthma summer camp in Los Angeles had increased attacks of shortness of breath associated with increased PM_{10} concentrations. These studies give a combined effect estimate of 8.8% (95% CI; 6.9–11.4%) increase in asthma attacks associated with 10-μg/m³ PM_{10}.

The use of bronchodilators has been evaluated as a measure of exacerbation in a panel of asthmatics in the Netherlands (59) and panels of symptomatic children and asthmatic patients in the Utah Valley (61). The weighted mean of these studies gives an estimated effect of a 2.3% (95% CI; 1.5–4.5%; 36) increase in bronchodilator use associated with each 10-μg/m³ increase in PM_{10}.

E. Respiratory Symptoms

Daily diaries of respiratory symptoms are a commonly used method of evaluating acute changes in respiratory health status associated with air pollution. In a commonly applied study design, panels of subjects (e.g., school children) record the presence of specific respiratory symptoms daily on weekly or monthly calendars. These symptom reports are often aggregated into upper respiratory symptoms (runny or stuffy nose, sinusitis, sore throat, wet cough, head cold, hayfever, and burning or red eyes) and lower respiratory symptoms (wheezing, dry cough, phlegm, shortness of breath, and chest discomfort or pain). In addition, cough, the most frequently reported symptom, is often analyzed separately.

Studies of lower respiratory symptoms have been conducted during winter periods in panels of children in Utah Valley (61,62), the Netherlands (63,64), and during summer periods in panels of children in six U.S. cities (53) and Pennsylvania (65). The combined weighted average from these studies gives an estimated effect of 3.0% (95% CI; 1.5–4.5%; 36) increase in lower respiratory symptoms with each 10-$\mu g/m^3$ increase in daily mean PM_{10} concentrations. For upper respiratory symptom reports, the weighted average effect estimate was only a 0.7% (95% CI; −0.1 to 1.5%; 36) increase in upper respiratory symptoms with each 10-$\mu g/m^3$ increase in daily mean PM_{10}.

Cough reports were analyzed in three of these studies as well as in a winter diary study in the Netherlands (59), a study of two Swiss cities (66), and the summer diary study in Uniontown (65) and State College, Pennsylvania (67). The weighted mean effect estimate from these studies was a 1.3% (95% CI; 0.5–2.0%; 36) increase in cough associated with each 10-$\mu g/m^3$ increase in daily mean PM_{10}.

F. Lung Function

Lung function is a sensitive indicator of acute response to ozone in controlled exposure and chamber studies (68). Repeated measures of lung function in panels of subjects also have been used to evaluate the effect of particulate air pollution episodes.

Panels of elementary school children in Steubenville, Ohio, had their lung function measured weekly before, during, and after particulate and sulfur dioxide episodes during four periods in 1978 through 1980 (69). Forced expired volume in three-quarters of a second ($FEV_{0.75}$) was reported to decline following these episodes, and remained depressed for up to 2 weeks following the episode. In a reanalysis of the Steubenville data, Brunekreef et al. (70) found the strongest association with increased mean total suspended particulates over the previous 5 days. A study of weekly lung function measurement of school children in the Netherlands (71) following a sulfur dioxide and particulate episode, in January 1985, reported decreases in forced expired volume in 1 sec (FEV_1) that were similar in magnitude and in lag structure to those observed in Steubenville. Subsequent studies of panels of school children with weekly lung function measurements (63,64) have also shown FEV_1 to be inversely associated with PM_{10} concentrations.

Pope and Kanner (72) analyzed repeated FEV_1 measurements in a panel of adult COPD patients participating in the Lung Health Study. Measurements were taken 10–90 days apart. An 0.2% decrease in FEV_1 for each 10-$\mu g/m^3$ increase in daily PM_{10} was reported.

Taken together, these studies found a decrease of between 0.05 and 0.35% or a weighted average of 0.15% (95% CI; 0.09–0.21%) decrease in FEV_1 associated with each 10-$\mu g/m^3$ increase in daily mean PM_{10}.

Peak flow measurements have been widely used as a simple, inexpensive indicator of lung function. Peak flow measurements were made in the weekly panel studies of school children in the Netherlands (63,64). In these two studies, peak flow declined approximately 0.16% for each 10-$\mu g/m^3$ increase in PM_{10}.

In two studies in the winters of 1989–1990 and 1990–1991 in Utah Valley, Utah (61,62), panels of school children measured their peak flow daily before going to bed. In both cases, small but significant reductions in peak flow were found associated with increased mean PM_{10} concentrations that day. In both studies there appeared to be associations between lower peak flow and higher PM_{10} concentrations for up to 5 preceding days, and stronger associations were found when these lag structures were included in the models. Similar winter panel studies of school children have been conducted in the Netherlands (59). Effects were observed between evening peak flow and daily mean PM_{10} concentrations, and 7-day mean PM_{10} concentration, which were similar to those observed in Utah.

A panel study of children was conducted in the summer of 1992 in Uniontown, Pennsylvania (65), and the summer of 1993 in State College, Pennsylvania (76), to evaluate peak flow changes in areas of high aerosol acidity. Although the strongest associations were found with aerosol acidity, there was also an association between evening peak flow and daily mean PM_{10} that was consistent with the estimates from other studies.

In summary, studies of repeated measure of lung function consistently show a small decrement in FEV_1 (weighted mean 0.15%; 95% CI; 0.09–0.25%) and peak flow (weighted mean 0.08%; 95% CI; 0.05–0.11%) associated with each 10 $\mu g/m^3$ in PM_{10} daily mean concentration. There is a strong suggestion in these data that changes in lung function may reflect the cumulative exposure of several (5–7) days preceding the measurement.

G. Summary of Short-Term Effects

Evidence from these selected epidemiological studies shows a *consistency* of effects across independent analytic studies with different investigators in different settings and suggests a *coherence* of effects across a range of related health outcomes. Table 1 presents the estimated effects for specific health indicators of each 10-$\mu g/m^3$ increase in 1- to 5-day–mean PM_{10}, averaged over the studies cited in this review following methods used previously (36). Although much

Table 1 Overall Estimates Across Cited Epidemiological Studies of Percentage Change in Health Indicators for Each 10-μg/m³ Increase in PM_{10} Concentration for Exposures of 1–5 Days

Parameter	% Change
Increase in daily mortality	
Total deaths	0.7
Respiratory deaths	3.5
Cardiovascular deaths	1.4
Increase in respiratory hospital admissions	
Asthma	1.0
COPD	2.4
Pneumonia	1.4
Increase in cardiovascular hospital admissions	
Congestive heart failure	1.0
Coronary artery disease	0.6
Dysrythmias	0.5
Exacerbation of asthma	
Asthma attacks	8.8
Bronchodilator use	2.3
Increases in respiratory symptoms	
Upper respiratory	0.7
Lower respiratory	3.0
Cough	1.3
Decreased lung function	
FEV_1 and $FEV_{0.75}$	0.15
Peak flow	0.08

attention has been given to the reports of increased daily mortality associated with acute effects of PM_{10} exposures, it is clear that these exposures are similarly associated with a wide range of indicators of respiratory and cardiovascular disease (morbidity).

IV. Effects of Long-Term Exposures

The effects of short-term (1- to 5-day) exposures to particulates may accumulate over longer periods to produce a chronic irreversible effect on health. Long-term effects may also include effects of low or moderate exposure that persist for a long time. These health effects may include chronic diseases with long-term latencies, such as cancer, chronic cardiovascular disease, or chronic pulmonary disease.

Prolonged exposure studies compare mortality and morbidity health outcomes among communities with different levels of air pollution. Exposure is based on summaries of air pollution of a year or more. These long-term studies are based on geographic, rather than temporal, differences in air pollution exposure. Thus, the samples of people in epidemiological studies of long-term effects are defined by the communities in which they live. Cross-sectional studies in which exposure and health status are determined at a single point in time suffer from several weaknesses, which we will describe. Cohort studies in which sample populations are followed for many years are very costly and time-consuming. Thus, the available database assessing long-term effects is much more limited than that for brief exposures.

A. Mortality Studies

Population-Based (Ecological) Mortality Studies

Many cross-sectional studies have found increased mortality of long-term exposure associated with air pollution. In 1964, Martin (11) reported that overall annual respiratory mortality (as opposed to episodic mortality) in the Greater London region was significantly related to smoke (particulate) levels. In 1970, Lave and Seskin (74) reported that city-specific mortality rates in the United States were positively correlated with sulfates and other measures of particulate air pollution.

The work of Lave and Seskin has been followed by several cross-sectional studies in the late 1970s and 1980s that attempted to define and refine air pollution–mortality associations based on population or ecological data (75–81). These studies consistently observed that city-specific mortality rates were positively associated with fine or sulfate particulate pollution levels. For example, the plot of age- and sex-adjusted mortality rates for 151 U.S. metropolitan areas for 1980 plotted against the mean sulfate concentrations in these communities is very suggestive of a positive association (see Fig. 4; 44). Regression-modeling techniques have been used to control for other risk factors by inclusion of population characteristics, such as average age, sex, and race distributions; indicators of smoking; education levels; income levels; poverty rates; housing density; and other demographic characteristics.

Although population-based cross-sectional studies suggest that air pollution contributes to human mortality, these studies have severe limitations and have been largely discounted for several reasons. First is the size of the estimated association. If taken literally, these studies suggest that as much as 3–9% of urban mortality in the United States is associated with particulate air pollution. Given that air pollution levels in the United States are relatively low, such a large mortality effect has been considered implausible.

A more explicit weakness of the cross-sectional population-based studies is the concern that the observed association was due to confounding. Because of their cross-sectional ecological design, these population studies could not directly control for differences in cigarette smoking and other risk factors on an individual level, but only based on population average characteristics. Thus, there is substantial potential for residual confounding in these regression models. Second, these studies were questioned because of the instability of the estimated associations. The magnitude and statistical significance of the estimated pollution effect was sensitive to model specification; the choice of social, demographic, and other variables included in the models; and the choice of study areas used in the analysis.

Prospective Cohort Mortality Studies

Recently, the results of three prospective cohort mortality studies have been reported (44,82,83). The design of these cohort studies has addressed weaknesses in the cross-sectional analyses of population statistics. Cohort studies analyze the incidence of health effects in a sample of individuals whose relevant personal characteristics are recorded along with the exposures in question. Measurement of smoking, sex, age, occupation, and other individual characteristics for each participant in the study allow for direct adjustment for hypothesized confounders.

However, such studies are costly and time-consuming. Large amounts of information are collected on large numbers of people who are followed for long periods. The Seventh-Day Adventists study (85) followed about 6000 white, nonsmoking, long-term California residents prospectively for 6–10 years. Cumulative exposure to total suspended particulates (TSP) and ozone was estimated for each individual in the study. Mortality was not consistently associated with TSP. Measures of inhalable particulate (PM_{10}) or fine particulate ($PM_{2.5}$) pollution were not considered in this analysis. Two other large prospective cohort studies specifically evaluate the mortality effects of fine particulate air pollution in urban populations in the United States.

Harvard Six-Cities Study

The Six-Cities Study (83) followed 8111 adults living in six U.S. cities: Watertown, Massachusetts; Harriman, Tennessee; St. Louis, Missouri; Steubenville, Ohio; Portage, Wisconsin; and Topeka, Kansas prospectively for 14–16 years. The six cities were selected to be representative of the range of particulate air pollution in the United States in the mid-1970s. TSP, PM_{10}, $PM_{2.5}$, SO_4, H^+, SO_2, NO_2 and O_3 levels were monitored in each community. Although TSP concentrations dropped over the study periods, fine particulate and sulfate pollution concentrations were relatively constant. Survival data were analyzed using multivariate Cox proportional hazards regression. Differences in the probability of survival among the cities were statistically significant ($p < 0.01$). Mortality risks were most strongly associated with cigarette smoking. After controlling for individual differences in age, sex, cigarette smoking, body mass index, education, and occupational exposure, differences in relative mortality risks across the six cities were strongly associated with differences in particulate pollution levels in those cities. Associations between mortality risk and air pollution were stronger for respirable particles and sulfates, as measured by PM_{10}, $PM_{2.5}$, and SO_4, than for TSP, SO_2, aerosol acidity (H^+), or ozone. The association between mortality risk (indicated as a mortality rate ratio) and fine particulate air pollution was consistent and nearly linear (Fig. 8), with no apparent ''no-effects'' threshold level above the ambient level in the least-polluted city (Portage). The adjusted total mortality-rate ratio for the most-polluted of the cities compared with the least polluted was 1.26 (95% CI; 1.08–1.47). Fine particulate pollution was associated with cardiopulmonary mortality and lung cancer mortality (not statistically significant), but not with the mortality from other causes analyzed as a group (Table 2).

American Cancer Society 151-City Study

Similar results were observed in a much larger prospective cohort study (44) of approximately 500,000 adults participating in the American Cancer Society (ACS) Cancer Prevention Study II (CPS-II). Individual risk-factor data were col-

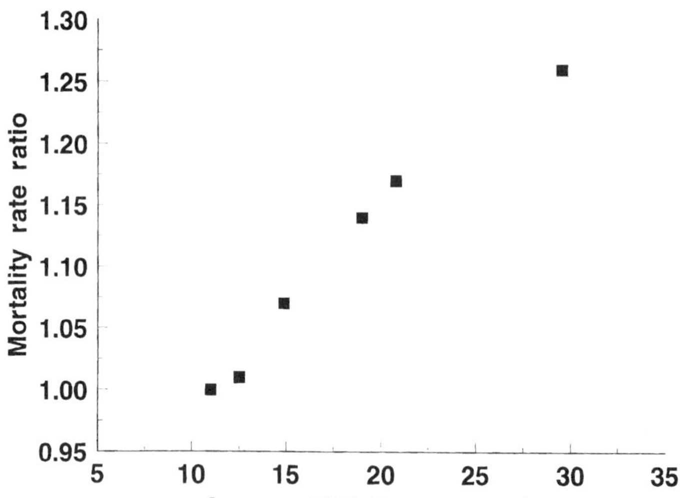

Figure 8 Estimated city-specific mortality rate ratios adjusted for age, sex, smoking, education, and body mass index, plotted against mean $PM_{2.5}$ concentrations in six U.S. cities. (From Ref. 73.)

Table 2 Estimated Increase in Lifetime Mortality Risk Associated with Each 6.5-$\mu g/m^3$ Increase in Fine Particles ($PM_{2.5}$)[a] in Prospective Cohort Studies

Parameter/study	% Increase in mortality
Total mortality	
All subjects	
Six-Cities Study	8.4% (2.7%, 14.4%)
American Cancer Society	4.3% (2.3%, 6.3%)
Never-smokers	
Six-Cities Study	6.3% (−3.6%, 17.1%)
American Cancer Society	5.4% (1.8%, 9.1%)
Cardiopulmonary mortality	
Six-Cities Study	8.4% (2.7%, 14.4%)
American Cancer Society	7.4% (4.3%, 10.6%)
Lung cancer	
Six-Cities Study	11.6% (−7.0%, 34.1%)
American Cancer Society[b]	5.7% (1.9%, 9.6%)
All other mortality[c]	
Six-Cities Study	0.3% (−8.0%, 9.5%)
American Cancer Society[c]	0.2% (−1.5%, 5.9%)

[a]Approximately equivalent to 10-$\mu g/m^3$ increase in PM_{10} (50).
[b]Based on 3.6-$\mu g/m^3$ increase in mean SO_4 concentration. Associations with $PM_{2.5}$ 0.8% (−5.8%, 7.8%) for lung cancer, 1.8% (−2.1%, 5.9%) for other.
[c]Not cardiovascular, respiratory, or lung cancer.

lected on enrollment in 1982 and vital status determined for 8 years through 1989. Exposure to particulate air pollution was based on fine particle ($PM_{2.5}$) measurements made in 50 metropolitan areas and sulfate measurements in 151 metropolitan areas by the EPA in 1980. Mortality relative risk ratios were estimated using multiple Cox proportional hazards regression, adjusting for age, sex, race, cigarette smoking, pipe and cigar smoking, exposure to passive cigarette smoke, occupational exposure, education, body mass index, and alcohol use. Additionally, weather variables that accounted for relatively hot or cold conditions were included. Adjusted rate ratios of total mortality for the most-polluted compared with the least-polluted communities were estimated to be 1.15 (95% CI; 1.09–1.22) and 1.17 (95% CI; 1.09–1.26) when using sulfate concentration (range 19.9 $\mu g/m^3$) and fine particulate concentration (range 24.9 $\mu g/m^3$), respectively. For total, cardiopulmonary, and lung cancer mortality, the associations with sulfate particles were highly statistically significant (see Table 2). For total and cardiopulmonary mortality, significant associations were also found using fine particulate matter as the index of air pollution levels. The association between air pollution and all-cause and cardiopulmonary mortality was observed for both men and women and for smokers and nonsmokers.

Implications of Prospective Cohort Mortality Results

These prospective cohort studies confirm that the associations between mortality and sulfate or fine particulate air pollution observed in the population-based cross-sectional studies persist even when individual differences in age, sex, race, smoking, body mass index, and other individual risk factors are controlled in regression analyses. Moolgavkar and Luebeck (84) have suggested that these associations may be attributable to residual confounding by smoking. Indeed cigarette smoking was an important predictor of increased mortality in both studies. However, careful control of smoking did not affect the observed air pollution associations. Furthermore, the association with particulate air pollution remained even when only never-smokers were included in the analyses (see Table 2).

If the results from these studies are interpreted literally, the annual number of deaths in the United States attributed to fine particulate air pollution levels over background levels can be estimated. The National Resources Defense Council estimated that approximately 64,000 deaths per year were attributable to fine particulate air pollution in 239 U.S. cities, with a range of estimates between approximately 28,000 and 124,000 deaths per year (85). Although these studies do not allow air pollution-related deaths to be estimated with much precision, they suggest long-term exposure to air pollution continues to be an important contributor to early mortality.

Ultimately, the question is not how many deaths are attributable to particulate air pollution, but whether these associations represent substantial loss of life expectancy. In the Six-Cities Study, the estimated effect of air pollution across the range of exposures for never-smokers was 1.19 (95% CI; 0.90–1.57). Applying this increased probability of death at each age between 25 and 85 years for the U.S. population (86) gives a decrease in life expectancy of 2.0 years (95% CI; 1.2–5.1 years). The American Cancer Society estimates for effect of fine particles on never-smokers [relative risk of 1.22 (95% CI; 1.07–1.39)] would similarly estimate decreased life expectancy of 2.3 years (95% CI; 0.8–3.7 years). For comparison, based on the Six-Cities Study results, smoking one pack of cigarettes per day starting at age 25 would lead to a decreased life expectancy of 8.5 years.

B. Chronic Respiratory Disease in Adults

Several recent studies have evaluated the associations between particulate air pollution and chronic respiratory disease in adults. Portney and Mullahy (87) merged health data from the 1979 National Health Interview Survey (NHIS) with routinely collected air pollution measurements. They reported that a combined index of emphysema, chronic bronchitis, or asthma was associated with total suspended particulate concentrations (Table 3). Schwartz (88) merged ambient measurements of total suspended particulates with health data collected in the first National Health and Nutrition Examination Survey (NHANES I). Increased reporting of chronic bronchitis and doctor-diagnosed respiratory illness was associated with higher particulate exposures (see Table 3). These associations persisted, and were stronger in magnitude, when the sample was restricted to never-smokers.

Abbey and colleagues (82,89,90) have been following a cohort of Seventh-Day Adventists living in California who were enrolled in 1977. These subjects were selected because of their very low smoking rates and the heterogeneity of their air pollution exposures. Those who had lived at least 11 years in areas of Southern California identified as having high or low pollution were compared on the basis of chronic respiratory status (91). Residents of the higher-pollution area had a 15% higher rate of COPD than residents in the lower-pollution area, after adjusting for age, sex, occupational exposure, race, and past smoking history. This included chronic bronchitis, asthma, and emphysema. Euler et al. (92) used the same population sample and found a statistically significant association between past TSP exposure and chronic respiratory disease. Past TSP exposure was based on residence zip-code history. As noted earlier, however, analysis of data from this cohort did not generally observe mortality effects with TSP. Abbey et al. (90) have recently reported associations between estimated respirable partic-

Table 3 Increase in Reporting of Chronic Respiratory Disease in Adults Associated with Increased Long-Term Mean Particulate Concentrations: 10-μg/m^3 PM_{10}; 6.5-μg/m^3 $PM_{2.5}$; 21.7-μg/m^3 TSP

Disease/Cohort	Particle-type	% Increase	Refs.
Doctor diagnosed respiratory illness			
NHANES I	TSP	13.5% (4.6%, 23.1%)	88
Chronic bronchitis			
NHANES I	TSP	7.6% (2.3%, 13.2%)	88
7th-Day Adventists	$PM_{2.5}$	4.4% (−0.0%, 9.0%)	90
Obstructive airway disease			
7th-Day Adventists	$PM_{2.5}$	2.8% (−3.1%, 9.0%)	90
Asthma			
7th-Day Adventists	$PM_{2.5}$	2.5% (−5.2%, 10.8%)	90
Emphysema, chronic bronchitis, or asthma			
1979 NHIS Survey	TSP	14.1% (−78%, 494%)	87

ulate ($PM_{2.5}$) exposures and increased chronic bronchitis, obstructive airway disease, and asthma (see Table 3).

C. Respiratory Symptoms and Illness in Children

Cross-sectional surveys of children have consistently found increased reporting of bronchitic symptoms and cough associated with particulate air pollution. As noted earlier, whereas epidemiological studies of chronic effects may adjust for individual characteristics, the air pollution exposures are determined by community. Results from multiple city studies, such as the Six-Cities (88) and the 24-Cities (93) studies, provide some of the most convincing epidemiological evidence for associations. Both of these studies attempted to assess the influence of particulates on the respiratory health of children living primarily in the eastern United States. Increased reporting of bronchitis was associated with particulate air pollution in both the Six- and 24-Cities Studies (Table 4). Increased chronic cough was also associated with particulates in the Six-Cities Study.

On the other hand, increased particulate air pollution was not associated with increased reporting of asthma or persistent wheeze in either of these studies (see Table 4). Thus, although short-term exposures to particulate air pollution clearly exacerbate existing asthma, there is no indication in these data that long-term exposures to particulate air pollution increases the prevalence of asthma in these children.

Table 4 Increase in Reported Respiratory Symptoms on Illness in Children Associated with Increased Long-Term Mean Particulate Exposures: 6.5-$\mu g/m^3$ $PM_{2.5}$ or $PM_{2.1}$

Disease/Cohort	Particle size	% Increase	Ref.
Bronchitis			
6 U.S. cities	$PM_{2.5}$	21.4% (−6.5%, 57.5%)	97
24 U.S. cities	$PM_{2.1}$	19.3% (−4.0%, 48.4%)	93
Chronic cough			
6 U.S. cities	$PM_{2.5}$	24.3% (−21.3%, 96.2%)	97
24 U.S. cities	$PM_{2.1}$	−8.3% (−23.4%, 9.7%)	93
Persistent wheeze			
6 U.S. cities	$PM_{2.5}$	0.0% (−17.6%, 21.3%)	97
24 U.S. cities	$PM_{2.1}$	−9.3% (−22.9%, 6.8%)	93
Asthma			
6 U.S. cities	$PM_{2.5}$	−12.5% (−28.4%, 7.0%)	97
24 U.S. cities	$PM_{2.1}$	−13.4% (−32.8%, 11.7%)	93

D. Long-Term Differences in Lung Function

Lung function declines irreversibly during adulthood. Smoking, occupational, and environmental exposures accelerate the loss of lung function with age. Reduced lung function is a very strong predictor of increased total mortality. Thus, deficits of lung function are taken as early indicators of disease. Holland and Reid (94) made a cross-sectional comparison of British male postal employees in London and in smaller country towns, where levels of SO_2 and particulate pollution were about half those in the metropolis. Accounting for cigarette-smoking levels, significant decrements of FEV_1 were reported in London employees, compared with those in the provinces.

There have been several recent studies that have evaluated associations between measures of lung function (forced vital capacity, FVC; FEV_1; the first three-quarters of a second, $FEV_{0.75}$; and peak expiratory flow, PEF) and particulate pollution levels in the United States (Table 5). These studies include analysis of data from both the first and second National Health and Nutrition Examination Surveys (NHANES I and NHANES II; 95,96), analysis of children's lung function data from the Harvard Six-Cities Study (97), and analysis of children's lung function from 24 U.S. cities (98). The effects of air pollution on lung function were estimated after adjusting for individual differences in age, race, sex, height,

Table 5 Percentage Change in Pulmonary Function Associated with Increased Long-Term Mean Particulate Concentrations: 10-$\mu g/m^3$ PM_{10}; 6.5-$\mu g/m^3$ $PM_{2.5}$; 21.7-$\mu g/m^3$ TSP

Function/Cohort	Particle type	% Change	Ref.
FVC			
NHANES I (49 cities)	TSP	−1.3% (−0.6%, −2.0%)	95
NHANES II	TSP	−1.3% (−0.3%, −2.2%)	96
24 U.S. cities	$PM_{2.1}$	−1.4% (−2.2%, −0.6%)	98
FEV_1			
NHANES I (49 cities)	TSP	−0.8% (−0.3%, −1.3%)	95
NHANES II	TSP	−1.1% (−0.1%, −2.0%)	96
24 U.S. cities	$PM_{2.1}$	−1.2% (−2.1%, −0.4%)	98
$FEV_{0.75}$			
24 U.S. cities	$PM_{2.1}$	−1.2% (−2.0%, −0.4%)	98
6 U.S. cities	TSP	−1.3% (−3.1%, 0.6%)	97
Peak flow			
NHANES I (49 cities)	TSP	−2.4% (−1.2%, −3.6%)	95
24 U.S. cities	$PM_{2.1}$	−1.7% (−2.2%, −1.1%)	98

and weight, and controlling for smoking or restricting the analysis to never-smokers.

All of these studies observed small negative associations between lung function and particulate air pollution. In the Six-Cities Study, which had the least statistical power, the association was weak and statistically insignificant. In each of the other studies, the association was small, but statistically significant. The results suggest that an increase in long-term particulate exposure, equivalent to approximately 10-$\mu g/m^3$ PM_{10} was typically associated with a 1–2% decline in lung function. Furthermore, as reported in the 24 Cities Study (98), the risk of relatively large deficits in lung function (15% or more) was much higher in the more-polluted cities, suggesting detrimental effects of respirable particulates or particulate acidity on normal lung growth and development.

E. Summary of Long-Term Effects

As with the effects of short-term exposures, long-term exposures are associated with a range of health indicators, including increased mortality, increased chronic respiratory disease, increased respiratory symptoms, and decreased lung function. These effects of prolonged exposure represent the cumulative effects of repeated exposure to short-term episodes, plus the net effects of the dose of particles accumulated over many years. In particular, the observed increases in lifetime mortality are substantially greater than the cumulative effects of the repeated short-term exposures alone. In addition, there is the suggestion of increased lung cancer mortality, a health endpoint generally not observed to be increased in the short-term studies.

For both adults and children, chronic cough and bronchitis are associated with increased particulate air pollution. However, wheeze and asthma were associated with chronic particulate exposures only among adults, but not in studies of children. This may reflect the very different characteristics of asthmatic symptoms and disease in children and the elderly.

Deficits of 1–2% in pulmonary function were associated with long-term exposures to particulate air pollution to each 10-$\mu g/m^3$ equivalent PM_{10}. For context, adult nonsmokers lose approximately 1% of their lung capacity each year. Thus, a 1% deficit in lung function is approximately equivalent to 1 year of aging.

V. Conclusions

Current epidemiological evidence suggests that respirable particulate air pollution, at levels common to many urban and industrial areas, contributes to human morbidity and mortality. Long-term, repeated exposure increases the risk of chronic respiratory disease and the risk of cardiorespiratory mortality. Short-term exposures can exacerbate existing cardiovascular and pulmonary disease and increase the number of persons in a population who become symptomatic, who require medical attention, or who die. The pattern of cardiopulmonary health effects associated with particulate air pollution that has been observed by epidemiological studies is the strongest evidence of the health effects of this pollution. Nevertheless, the epidemiological studies have important limitations that stem largely from the use of people who are living in uncontrolled environments, and who are exposed to complex mixtures of particulate air pollution.

In addition to providing limited information about biological mechanisms, current epidemiological studies provide relatively meager information on linkages between ambient and personal exposures, and are unable to fully explore the relative health effects of various constituents of air pollution. Furthermore, the relations between the relative importance of prolonged versus brief exposures remains unclear. Much of the recent epidemiological effort has focused on effects of short-term exposure, primarily because of the relative availability of relevant time–series data sets. However, the effects of long-term exposure may be more important in terms of overall public health relevance. Such research is also needed to provide a better understanding of susceptible populations. For example, individuals susceptible to serious effects of brief exposure may be only those with existing respiratory or cardiovascular disease; but, a much larger segment of the population may eventually be seriously effected by extended, long-term exposure.

Mass concentration of inhalable particles is only one measure of a complex mixture of gaseous and particulate air pollution to which people are exposed. PM_{10} includes a wide array of potentially toxic chemical species. Therefore, it is presumptuous to assign these observed health effects solely to the mass concentration of particulates. On the other hand, the consistency of these observed effects across so many communities suggests that, lacking an explicit hypothesis, these associations are assigned to a nonspecific definition of inhalable or fine particle concentrations common to urban areas.

The physical and chemical characteristics of ambient particles are generally unknown and so are impossible to duplicate in controlled animal- or human-exposure studies. Many of the health effects of particles are thought to reflect the combined action of the diverse components in the pollutant mix. Until controlled animal- and human-exposure studies identify the active component(s) of these complex mixtures and can characterize their underlying mechanisms of toxicity, it is prudent to ascribe health effects observed by epidemiologists to the undifferentiated particle mass, rather than to any specific component.

The results of epidemiological studies of transient effects of particulate air pollution, particularly those describing associations with cardiovascular mortality, have been called into question because of the lack of a biologically plausible mechanism (2,99). Although the specific biological mechanism for these brief increases in mortality is unclear, the internal consistency of the mortality studies and the external consistency with evidence of abrupt increases in morbidity measures suggest that these results are not artifacts.

Research into mechanisms of the adverse health effects of PM_{10} mass concentrations observed in recent epidemiological studies needs to be undertaken in controlled exposure studies of humans and animals. It is only through integration of the complementary evidence from laboratory animal and controlled human exposure studies with the results from epidemiological studies that the risk of particle exposures can be fully evaluated. Nevertheless, these recent epidemiological studies implicate particulate air pollution as contributing to respiratory morbidity and mortality, even at exposure levels below the current ambient air quality standards in the United States and in Europe.

Acknowledgments

This review was supported in part by National Institute of Environmental Health Sciences grant ES-00002.

References

1. Taubes G. Epidemiology faces its limits. Science 1995; 269:164–169.
2. Utell M, Samet JM. Particulate air pollution and health. New evidence on an old problem. Am Rev Respir Dis 1993; 147:1334–1335.
3. U.S. Environmental Protection Agency, Friday, July 18, 1997. 40 CFR Part 50. National Ambient Air Quality Standards for particulate matter, Final Rule. Federal Register 62(138):38651–38701.
4. Friedlander SK. Smoke, Dust and Haze: Fundamentals of Aerosol Behavior. New York: John Wiley & Sons, 1978. pp. 5–7.
5. U.S. Environmental Protection Agency. Wednesday, July 1, 1987. 40 CFR Part 50. Revisions to the National Ambient Air Quality Standards for Particulate Matter: Final Rules. Federal Register 52(126):24634–24669.
6. Miller FJ, Gardner DE, Graham JA, Lee RE Jr, Wilson WE, Bachmann JD. Size considerations for establishing a standard for inhalable particles. J Air Pollut Control Assoc 1979; 29:610–615.
7. 1993–1994 Threshold Limit Values and Biological Exposure Indices. Cincinnati, OH: ACGIH, 1993.
8. Firket J. Fog along the Meuse Valley. Trans Faraday Soc 1936; 32:1192–1197.
9. Shrenk HH, Heimann H, Clayton GD, Gafafer WM, Wexler H. Air pollution in Donora, PA: epidemiology of the unusual smog episode of October 1948, Preliminary Report. Public Health Bulletin No. 306 Washington, DC: Public Health Service, 1949.

10. Brimblecombe P. The Big Smoke: A History of Air Pollution in London Since Medieval Times. London: Methuen & Co., 1987.
11. Martin AE. Mortality and morbidity statistics and air pollution. Proc R Soc Med 1964; 57:969.
12. Holland WW, Bennett AE, Cameron IR, et al. Health effects of particulate pollution: reappraising the evidence. Am J Epidemiol 1979; 110:525–659.
13. Bates DV. The health effects of air pollution. J Respir Dis 1980; 1:29–37.
14. Ellison JM, Waller RE. A review of sulphur oxides and particulate matter as air pollutants with particular reference to effects on health in the United Kingdom. Environ Res 1978; 16:302–325.
15. Shy CM. Epidemiologic evidence and the United States air quality standards. Am J Epidemiol 1979; 110:661–671.
16. Ware JH, Thibodeau LA, Speizer FE, Colome S, Ferris BG Jr. Assessment of the health effects of atmospheric sulfur oxides and particulate matter: evidence from observational studies. Environ Health Perspect 1981; 41:255–276.
17. Schwartz J, Marcus A. Mortality and air pollution in London: a time series analysis. Am J Epidemiol 1990; 131:185–194.
18. MacFarlane A. Daily mortality and environment in English conurbations. 1: Air pollution, low temperature, and influenza in greater London. Br J Prev Med 1977; 31: 54–61.
19. Mazumdar S, Schimmel H, Higgins ITT. Relation of daily mortality to air pollution: an analysis of 14 London winters, 1958/59–1971/72. Arch Environ Health 1982; 37:213–220.
20. Ostro B. A search for a threshold in the relationship of air pollution to mortality: a reanalysis of data on London winters. Environ Health Perspect 1984; 58:397–399.
21. Schwartz J, Dockery DW. Particulate air pollution and daily mortality in Steubenville, Ohio. Am J Epidemiol 1992; 135:12–19.
22. Schwartz J, Dockery DW. Increased mortality in Philadelphia associated with daily air pollution concentrations. Am Rev Respir Dis 1992; 145:600–604.
23. Schwartz J. Particulate air pollution and daily mortality in Detroit. Environ Res 1991; 56:204–213.
24. Schwartz J. Particulate air pollution and daily mortality in Cincinnati, Ohio. Environ Health Perspect 1994; 102:186–189.
25. Spix C, Heinrich J, Dockery DW, Schwartz J, Volksch G, Schwinkowski K, Collen C, Wichmann, HE. Air pollution and daily mortality in Erfurt, East Germany, 1980–1989. Environ Health Perspect 1993; 101:518–525.
26. Xu X, Gao J, Dockery DW, Chen Y. Air pollution and daily mortality in residential areas of Beijing, China. Arch Environ Health 1994; 49:216–222.
27. Touloumi G, Pocock SJ, Katsouyanni K, Trichopoulos D. Short term effect of air pollution on daily mortality in Athens: a time series analysis. Int J Epidemiol 1994; 23:957–967.
28. Verhoeff AP, Hoek G, Schwartz J, van Wijuen JH. Air pollution and daily mortality in Amsterdam, the Netherlands. Epidemiology 1996; 7:225–230.
29. Schwartz J. Air pollution and daily mortality in Birmingham AL. Am J Epidemiol 1993; 137:1136–1147.
30. Ito K, Kinney PL, Thurston GD. Variations in PM-10 concentrations within two

metropolitan areas and their implications for health effects analyses. Inhal Toxicol 1995; 7:735–745.
31. Kinney PL, Ito K, Thurston GD. A sensitivity analysis of mortality/PM10 associations in Los Angeles. Inhal Toxicol 1995; 7:59–69.
32. Pope CA III, Schwartz J, Ransom MR. Daily mortality and PM_{10} pollution in Utah Valley. Arch Environ Health 1992; 47:211–217.
33. Schwartz J, Dockery DW, Neas LM. Is daily mortality associated specifically with fine particles? J Air Waste Manage Assoc 1996; 46:2–14.
34. Saldiva PHN, Pope CA III, Schwartz J, Dockery DW, Lichtenfels AJ, Salge JM, Barone I, Bohm GM. Air pollution and mortality in elderly people: a time series study in Sao Paulo, Brazil. Arch Environ Health 1995; 50:159–163.
35. Ostro B, Sanchez JM, Aranda C, Eskeland GS. Air pollution and mortality: results of a study of Santiago, Chile. J Exp Anal Environ Epidemiol 1996; 6:97–114.
36. Dockery DW, Pope CA III. Acute respiratory effects of particulate air pollution. Annu Rev Public Health 1994; 15:107–132.
37. Samet JM, Zeger SL, Berhane K. The association of mortality and particulate air pollution. In: HEI Report, 1995.
38. Schwartz J. Air pollution and hospital admissions for the elderly in Detroit, Michigan. Am J Respir Crit Care Med 1994; 150:648–655.
39. Dockery DW, Schwartz J. Particulate air pollution and mortality. Epidemiology 1996; 7:213–214.
40. Fairley D. The relationship of daily mortality to suspended particulates in Santa Clara County, 1980–1986. Environ Health Perspect 1990; 89:159–168.
41. Pope CA III. Respiratory disease associated with community air pollution and a steel mill, Utah Valley. Am J Public Health 1989; 79:623–628.
42. Pope CA III, Schwartz J. Time series for the analysis of pulmonary health data. Presented at the joint ATS/ERS Workshop on the Analysis of Longitudinal Respiratory Data, Barcelona, September 21–22, 1995.
43. Schwartz J. What are people dying of on high air pollution days? Environ Res 1994; 64:26–35.
44. Pope CA III, Thun MJ, Namboodiri MN, Dockery DW, Evans JS, Speizer FE, Health CW Jr. Particulate air pollution as a predictor of mortality in a prospective cohort study of U.S. adults. Am J Respir Crit Care Med 1995; 151:669–674.
45. Lippmann M. Airborne acidity: estimates of exposure and human health effects. Environ Health Perspect 1985; 63:63–70.
46. Lippmann M, Ito K. Separating the effects of temperature and season on daily mortality from those of air pollution in London: 1965–1972. Inhal Toxicol 1995; 7:85–97.
47. Ito K, Thurston GD, Hayes C, Lippmann M. Associations of London, England daily mortality with particulate matter, sulfur dioxide, and acidic air pollution. Arch Environ Health 1993; 48:213–220.
48. Ostro BD, Lipsett MJ, Mann JK, Braxton-Owens H, White MC. Air pollution and asthma exacerbations among African-American children in Los Angeles. Inhal Toxicol 1995; 7:711–722.
49. Pope CA III. Respiratory hospital admissions associated with PM_{10} pollution in Utah, Salt Lake, and Cache Valleys. Arch Environ Health 1991; 46:90–97.

50. Burnett RT, Dales RE, Krewski D, Vincent R, Dann T, Brook JR. Associations between ambient particulate sulfate and admissions to Ontario hospitals for cardiac and respiratory diseases. Am J Epidemiol 1995; 142:15–22.
51. Thurston GD, Ito K, Hayes CG, Bates DV, Lippman M. Respiratory hospital admissions and summertime haze air pollution in Toronto, Ontario: consideration of the role of acid aerosols. Environ Res 1994; 65:271–290.
52. Thurston GD, Ito K, Kinney PL, Lippmann M. A multi-year study of air pollution and respiratory hospital admissions in three New York State metropolitan areas: results for 1988 and 1989 summers. J Expos Anal Environ Epidemiol 1992; 2:429–450.
53. Schwartz J, Slater D, Larson TV, Pierson WE, Koenig JQ. Particulate air pollution and hospital emergency room visits for asthma in Seattle. Am Rev Respir Dis 1993; 147:826–831.
54. Schwartz, J. Air pollution and hospital admissions for the elderly in Birmingham, AL. Am J Epidemiol 1994; 139:589–598.
55. Schwartz J. PM_{10}, ozone, and hospital admissions for the elderly in Minneapolis-St. Paul, Minnesota. Arch Environ Health 1994; 49:366–374.
56. Sunyer J, Anto JM, Murillo C, Saez M. Effects of urban air pollution on emergency room admissions for chronic obstructive pulmonary disease. Am J Epidemiol 1991; 134:277–286.
57. Sunyer J, Saez M, Murillo C, Castellsague J, Martinez F, Anto JM. Air pollution and emergency room admissions for chronic obstructive pulmonary disease: a 5-year study. Am J Epidemiol 1993; 137:701–705.
58. Schwartz J, Morris R. Air pollution and hospital admissions for cardiovascular disease in Detroit, Michigan. Am J Epidemiol 1995; 142:23–35.
59. Roemer W, Hock G, Brunekreef B. Effect of ambient winter air pollution on respiratory health of children with chronic respiratory symptoms. Am Rev Respir Dis 1993; 147:118–124.
60. Ostro BD, Lipsett MJ, Wiener MB, Selner JC. Asthmatic response to airborne acid aerosols. Am J Public Health 1991; 81:694–702.
61. Pope CA III, Dockery DW, Spengler JD, Raizenne ME. Respiratory health and PM_{10} pollution: a daily time series analysis. Am Rev Respir Dis 1991; 144:668–674.
62. Pope CA III, Dockery DW. Acute health effects of PM_{10} pollution on symptomatic and asymptomatic children. Am Rev Respir Dis 1992; 145:1123–1128.
63. Hoek G, Brunekreef B. Acute effects of a winter air pollution episode on pulmonary function and respiratory symptoms of children. Arch Environ Health 1993; 48:328–335.
64. Hoek G, Brunekreef B. Effects of low level winter air pollution concentrations on respiratory health of Dutch children. Environ Res 1994; 64:136–150.
65. Neas LM, Dockery DW, Koutrakis P, Tollerud DJ, Speizer FE. The association of ambient air pollution with twice daily peak expiratory flow rate measurements in children. Am J Epidemiol 1995; 141:111–122.
66. Braun-Fahrlander C, Ackermann-Liebrich U, Schwartz J, Gnehm HP, Rutishauser M, Wanner HU. Air pollution and respiratory symptoms in preschool children. Am Rev Respir Dis 1992; 145:42–47.
67. Neas LM, Dockery DW, Burge H, Koutrakis P, Speizer FE. Fungus spores, air pol-

lutants and other determinants of peak expiratory flow rate in children. Am J Epidemiol 1996; 143:797–807.
68. Lippmann M. Health effects of ozone—a critical review. J Air Pollut Control Assoc 1989; 39:672–695.
69. Dockery DW, Ware JH, Ferris BG Jr, Speizer FE, Cook NR, Herman SM. Change in pulmonary function in children associated with air pollution episodes. APCA J 1982; 32:937–942.
70. Brunekreef B, Kinney PL, Ware JH, Dockery DW, Speizer FE, Spengler JD, Ferris BG Jr. Sensitive subgroups and normal variation in pulmonary function response to air pollution episodes. Environ Health Perspect 1991; 90:189–193.
71. Dassen W, Brunekreef B, Hoek G, Hofschreuder P, Staatsen B, de Groot H, Schouten E, Biersteker K. Decline in children's pulmonary function during an air pollution episode. J Air Pollut Control Assoc 1986; 36:1223–1227.
72. Pope CA III, Kanner RE. Acute effects of PM_{10} pollution on pulmonary function of smokers with mild to moderate chronic obstructive pulmonary disease. Am Rev Respir Dis 1993; 147:1336–1340.
73. Neas LM, Dockery DW, Burge H, Koutrakis P, Speizer FE. Fungus spores, air pollutants, and other determinants of peak expiratory flow rate in children. Am J Epidemiol 1996; 143:797–807.
74. Lave LB, Seskin EP. Air pollution and human health. Science 1970; 169:723–733.
75. Lave LB, Seskin EP. Air Pollution and Human Health. Baltimore: The Johns Hopkins University Press, 1977.
76. Mendelsohn R, Orcutt G. An empirical analysis of air pollution dose–response curves. J Environm Econ Manage 1979; 6:85–106.
77. Chappie M, Lave L. The health effects of air pollution: a reanalysis. J Urban Econ 1982; 12:346–376.
78. Lipfert FW. Air pollution and mortality: specification searches using SMSA-based data. J Environ Econ Manage 1984; 11:208–243.
79. Evans JS, Tosteson T, Kinney PL. Cross-sectional mortality studies and air pollution risk assessment. Environ Int 1984; 10:55–83.
80. Ozkaynak H, Thurston GD. Associations between 1980 U.S. mortality rates and alternative measures of airborne particle concentration. Risk Anal 1987; 7:49–61.
81. Lipfert FW, Malone RG, Daum ML, Mendell NR, Yang CC. A Statistical Study of the Macroepidemiology of Air Pollution and Total Mortality. Prepared for the Office of Environmental Analysis United States Department of Energy, 1988.
82. Abbey DE, Mills PK, Petersen FF, Beeson WL. Long-term ambient concentrations of total suspended particulates and oxidants as related to incidence of chronic disease in California Seventh-Day Adventists. Environ Health Perspect 1991; 94:43–50.
83. Dockery DW, Pope CA III, Xu X, Spengler JD, Ware JH, Fay ME, Ferris BG Jr, Speizer FE. An association between air pollution and mortality in six U.S. cities. N Engl J Med 1993; 329:1753–1759.
84. Moolgavkar SH, Luebeck EG. A critical review of the evidence on particulate air pollution and mortality. Epidemiology 1996; 7:420–428.
85. Shprentz DS, Bryner GC, Shprentz JS. Breath-Taking: Premature Mortality Due to Particulate Air Pollution in 239 American Cities. New York: Natural Resources Defense Council, 1996.

86. National Center for Health Statistics. Vital Statistics of the United States, 1980. Life Tables. Vol II, Section G. Department of Health and Human Services Publication No. (PHS) 84–1104.
87. Portney PR, Mullahy J. Urban air quality and chronic respiratory disease. Reg Sci Urban Econ 1990; 20:407–418.
88. Schwartz J. Particulate air pollution and chronic respiratory disease. Environ Res 1993; 62:7–13.
89. Abbey DE, Petersen F, Mills PK, Beeson WL. Long-term ambient concentrations of total suspended particulates, ozone, and sulfur dioxide and respiratory symptoms in a nonsmoking population. Arch Environ Health 1993; 48:33–46.
90. Abbey DE, Hwang BL, Burchette RJ, VanCuren T, Mills PK. Estimated long-term ambient concentrations of PM_{10} and development of respiratory symptoms in a nonsmoking population. Arch Environ Health 1995; 50:139–152.
91. Hodgkin JE, Abbey DE, Euler GL, Magie AR. COPD prevalence in nonsmokers in high and low photochemical air pollution areas. Chest 1984; 86:830–838.
92. Euler GL, Abbey DE, Magie AR, Hodgkin JE. Chronic obstructive pulmonary disease symptom effects of long-term cumulative exposure to ambient levels of total suspended particulates and sulfur dioxide in California Seventh-Day Adventist residents. Arch Environ Health 1987; 42:213–222.
93. Dockery DW, Damokosh AI, Neas LM, Raizenne M, Spengler JD, Koutrakis P, Ware JH, Speizer FE. Health effects of acid aerosols on North American children: respiratory symptoms and illness. Environ Health Perspect 1996; 104:500–505.
94. Holland WW, Reid DD. The urban factor in chronic bronchitis. Lancet 1965; 1:445.
95. Chestnut LG, Schwartz J, Savitz DA, Burchfiel CM. Pulmonary function and ambient particulate matter: epidemiological evidence from NHANES I. Arch Environ Health 1991; 46:135–144.
96. Schwartz J. Lung function and chronic exposure to air pollution: a cross-sectional analysis of NHANES II. Environ Res 1989; 50:309–321.
97. Dockery DW, Speizer FE, Stram DO, Ware JH, Spengler JD, Ferris BG Jr. Effects of inhalable particles on respiratory health of children. Am Rev Respir Dis 1989; 139:587–594.
98. Raizenne M, Neas LM, Damokosh AI, Dockery DW, Spengler JD, Koutrakis P, Ware JH, Speizer FE. Health effects of acid aerosols on North American children: pulmonary function. Environ Health Perspect 1996; 104:506–514.
99. Waller RE, Swan AV. Invited commentary: particulate air pollution and daily mortality. Am J Epidemiol 1992; 135:20–22.

AUTHOR INDEX

Italic numbers give the page on which the complete reference is listed.

A

B

D

E

F

G

H

K

L

N

P

Q

R

S

T

U

V

W

Z

SUBJECT INDEX

A

D

M

O

P

Q

R

S

T